PEDIATRIC CRITICAL

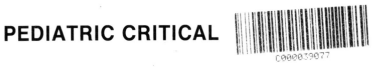

C000039077

PEDIATRIC CRITICAL CARE

Edited by

Janis Bloedel Smith, R.N., M.S.N.

Instructor
College of Nursing
University of Delaware
Newark, Delaware

DELMAR PUBLISHERS INC.®

NOTICE TO THE READER

Publisher and author do not warrant or guarantee any of the products described herein or perform any independent analysis in connection with any of the product information contained herein. Publisher and author do not assume, and expressly disclaim, any obligation to obtain and include information other than that provided to them by the manufacturer.

The reader is expressly warned to consider and adopt all safety precautions that might be indicated by the activities described herein and to avoid all potential hazards. By following the instructions contained herein, the reader willingly assumes all risks in connection with such instructions.

The publisher and author make no representations or warranties of any kind, including but not limited to, the warranties of fitness for particular purpose or merchantability, nor are any such representations implied with respect to the material set forth herein, and the publisher and author take no responsibility with respect to such material. The publisher and author shall not be liable for any special, consequential or exemplary damages resulting, in whole or in part, from the readers' use of, or reliance upon, this material.

The authors and publisher have made a conscientious effort to ensure that the drug information and recommended dosages in this book are accurate and in accord with accepted standards at the time of publication. However, pharmacology is a rapidly changing science, so readers are advised, before administering any drug, to check the package insert provided by the manufacturer for the recommended dose, for contraindications for administration, and for added warnings and precautions. This recommendation is especially important for new, infrequently used, or highly toxic drugs.

For information, address Delmar Publishers Inc.,
2 Computer Drive West, Box 15-015
Albany, New York 12212

Printed in the United States of America
Published simultaneously in Canada
By Nelson Canada
A Division of The Thomson Corporation

10 9 8 7 6 5 4 3 2 1

ISBN 0-8273-4374-4

To my family:

Mom and Dad
Becki, Michael, Lynn, and Carolyn

Jerry and Scott

CONTRIBUTORS

Sherry Waples Benica, R.N., B.S.N.
Former Head Nurse
Pediatric Intensive Care (Acute)
The Children's Hospital of Philadelphia
Philadelphia, Pennsylvania

Kathleen M. Corse, R.N., B.S.N.
Nursing Supervisor
The Children's Hospital of Philadelphia
Philadelphia, Pennsylvania

Susan B. De Jong, R.N., B.S.N.
Head Nurse
Pediatric Intensive Care (Isolation)
The Children's Hospital of Philadelphia
Philadelphia, Pennsylvania

Mary Howell Giblin, R.N., B.S.N.
Staff Nurse
Pediatric Intensive Care (Acute)
The Children's Hospital of Philadelphia
Philadelphia, Pennsylvania

Donna H. Groh, R.N., M.S.N.
Assistant Director of Nursing
Children's Hospital of Los Angeles
Los Angeles, California

Diane S. Jakobowski, R.N., B.S.N.
Graduate Student
Pediatric Nurse Specialist Program
Gwynedd-Mercy College
Gwynedd Valley, Pennsylvania
Former Nursing Coordinator
Nutrition Support Service
The Children's Hospital of Philadelphia
Philadelphia, Pennsylvania

Janet A. Koehler, R.N., B.S.N.
Staff Education Instructor
Pediatric Intensive Care Units
The Children's Hospital of Philadelphia
Philadelphia, Pennsylvania

Linda E. Lambert, R.N., M.S.
Nurse Supervisor
Intensive Care Nursery
University of Maryland Hospital
Baltimore, Maryland

Susan Carmody McCandless, R.N., B.S.N.
Former Staff Education Instructor
Pediatric Intensive Care Units
The Children's Hospital of Philadelphia
Philadelphia, Pennsylvania

Margaret D. Rielly, R.N., M.S.N.
Nursing Coordinator
Adolescent Unit
University of Massachusetts Medical Center
Worcester, Massachusetts

PREFACE

Nurses who provide pediatric critical care use an expanding body of knowledge in their care of seriously ill or injured children and their families. As the body of knowledge has grown, so has the need for expert clinical nursing skills and judgment. This book has been written from the perspective that nursing expertise is crucial in the successful critical care management of seriously ill children. The pediatric intensive care nurse is an essential partner in the provision of health care—a partner with other health care professionals who are committed to the well-being of children and families.

Pediatric Critical Care has taken a straightforward approach to the knowledge that critical care nurses need to practice. Chapter 1 details the effects of serious illness and hospitalization on children and parents and identifies nursing interventions that assist families in coping positively with the stress that such experiences evoke. Chapters 2 through 7 each begin with a review of selected aspects of physiology related to a body system that provides the foundation for principles of nursing care of children with respiratory, cardiac, neurological, neuromuscular, or renal disorders and shock or traumatic injury. Nursing assessment is detailed next in each chapter. Then follows a thorough explanation of the pathophysiology and critical care management of a variety of the disorders which necessitate pediatric intensive care. Chapter 8 examines nutritional support of critically ill children. Chapter 9 is devoted to the provider of critical care nursing and presents an analysis of the sources of stress in intensive care settings and strategies to deal with them successfully.

It is hoped that this book will become a valuable reference for nurses who practice in pediatric critical care. The contributors are a group of authors who have considerable experience and expertise in the provision of intensive nursing care. Most of all, it is hoped that this book will contribute to the care of children and parents who require pediatric critical care. It is for them that we continue to study and learn.

Janis Bloedel Smith

ACKNOWLEDGMENTS

As a group, the editor and contributors of *Pediatric Critical Care* have received the assistance of a large number of individuals who have provided special service during the preparation of the manuscript. Colleagues have provided criticism and suggestions, mothers and secretaries have spent long hours at the typewriter. We jointly express our sincere thanks to:

Hud Allender, M.D.

Betty Armstrong

Sandra Autman, R.N., M.S.N.

Muriel N. Babbitt

Millie Boettcher, R.N.

Violet Breckbill, R.N., Ph.D.

Kathleen Brodeur

Derek Bruce, M.D.

Arthur Cooper, M.D.

Loretta Forlaw, R.N., M.S.N.

Craig Langman, M.D.

Pat Meyers, R.N.

Nancy Miller, R.N., M.S.N.

Michael Norman, M.D.

William Primack, M.D.

David Swedlow, M.D.

Rita Talley, R.N., B.S.

Jane Waples

Moritz Ziegler, M.D.

In addition, the encouragement and support of Andy Fleschner and Craig Percy warrant special note and appreciation. We also thank Craig and his colleague Peter D'Epiro for the painstaking editorial preparation of this text.

Janis Bloedel Smith

CONTENTS

PEDIATRIC CRITICAL CARE

CHAPTER 1

NURSING PROCESS IN PEDIATRIC CRITICAL CARE

Janis Bloedel Smith

The provision of lifesaving intensive care to infants and children has made remarkable progress in recent years. This progress, however, does not extend to the emotional care of children who require critical care, nor to that of their families or the individuals who provide the intensive care. Technical advances have far outstripped advances in the *human* care of critically ill children and their families. The critical care nurse has been described as a vital "monitor" in the intensive care unit, responsible for minute-by-minute, sophisticated, and accurate assessment of patients, as well as for their often complex physical care. But the nurse is also the "human-to-human monitor," responsible for the constant assessment of the ill child's and family's reactions to critical care.[1] In this role, too, the ICU nurse must provide high-quality care.

The purpose of this chapter is twofold: first, it reviews the effects of hospitalization on children and their parents by examining the stressors these individuals face, their coping abilities, and the impact of critical illness on each group; second, it applies the nursing process in the critical care milieu by examining its application to the nurse's role as a human-to-human monitor.

EFFECTS OF HOSPITALIZATION ON CHILDREN

It is generally accepted that illness and hospitalization during childhood constitute a substantial threat to the child and represent a situational crisis of significant magnitude. Behavioral disturbances following even brief hospitalization for relatively minor treatments or illnesses include sleep disturbances, alterations in feeding patterns, regression in toilet training, increases in clinging behaviors, etc.[2,3] How the individual child responds to hospitalization is determined in large part by the ability of the child to cope in a positive manner with the stresses that result from hospitalization.

Stressors

The most stressful aspects of hospitalization during childhood are related to three distinct characteristics of the hospital experience: separation from parents and/or significant others, loss of self-control, and subjection to painful and/or intrusive procedures. Each of these characteristics has a different meaning for children of different ages and must be considered in light of the child's developmental status.

Infants. The greatest stress of illness and hospitalization for infants is separation from parents. Once the child has formed a firm bond to the parents and experienced the onset of "stranger anxiety," no other caretaker can be substituted for the parents without evoking protest from the infant. At the age of 3 months, infants already demonstrate a selective preference for their parents. During serious illness, protest behavior may not be obvious because the infant may not be physically capable of expressing it. It nevertheless seems likely that the infant still has a strong desire for closeness to the parents. Hospitalized infants rest and feed better when assured of the continuing presence of one or both parents.

The infant who requires hospitalization is also stressed by pain and intrusion. Despite the inability to verbalize, the infant's reaction to painful or intrusive procedures with generalized body movement leaves little doubt that pain is indeed felt and experienced. Before approximately 6 months of age, infants do not appear to remember painful experiences and, therefore, are not apprehensive about potentially painful procedures. After this age, infants are able to anticipate pain and react intensely with physical struggling and resistance.

Infants are engaged in active learning about their environment. Their primary mode of exploration is through motor activity, which is also an important coping mechanism for this age group. Immobilization represents an additional stress on the infant who is restricted from releasing tension and seeking comfort when motor activity is restrained.

Toddlers. Separation from parents remains a crucial factor in hospitalization of the toddler. A child of this age may react to impending separation with vigorous physical protest and clinging to parents if physically capable of doing so. The sicker child may be unable to protest physically, but will often cry out for the parents and, when left without them, cry inconsolably. Even when critical illness prohibits behavioral response to separation from parents, the toddler requires the close and consistent presence of parents.

Struggling with the developmental crisis of establishing autonomy, the toddler delights in new physical skills and abilities. Self-control is maintained through the use of ritualistic behavior, which permits the child to view the ever-expanding world as reliable and subject to control. Serious illness and hospitalization restrict the child's ability to exercise these newly gained physical abilities and disrupt the usual rituals through which the toddler maintains control of self as separate from parents. Little, if anything, in the typical intensive care environment is familiar or comforting to the child. The world is no longer safe, reliable, or available for exploration, and the child's ability to maintain self-control is severely threatened.

The toddler has poorly defined body image and boundaries and, therefore, responds in a similar way to either painful or intrusive procedures. Examination of the ears or measurement of rectal temperature evokes the same response as venous cannulation or intramuscular medication administration because pain and intrusion are equally threatening and offensive.

Preschoolers. Preschoolers possess remarkable physical and verbal activities that often make them appear more mature than they actually are. Although language skills are often highly developed in preschoolers, their thought processes are characterized by egocentricity, precausal and preconceptual logic, and magical thinking.

Egocentric thinking in these young children is demonstrated by their inability to accept a point of view different from their own and, in fact, by their failure to realize that different points of view actually exist. Preschoolers are thus restricted by a totally subjective view of the world.

Precausal thinking is characterized by the predominance of psychological and/ or moral explanations of events. Naturally occurring events are considered either to be caused by people or ordered by some supernatural being, rather than to be the result of physical or mechanical forces. For example, a preschooler who is asked why boats float may respond that boats float to carry people. These children may believe that illness is either ordered by some supernatural power or that it results from some personal wrongdoing. Therefore, hospitalization may be conceived as punishment for real or imagined misdeeds.

Preconceptual thinking prevents the young child from forming concepts based on the multiple characteristics of an object or individual. All vehicles with wheels may be characterized as cars, and all nurses may be viewed as administrators of pain, based on a single experience with a nurse from whom an injection was received. Words have very personal, subjective meanings for preschool children; yet, because they use language so well, others may assume that they understand the true meaning of all the terms they use.

Magical thinking and **fantasy** characterize the preschooler's view of the world. These children are unable to separate fantasy from reality and, therefore, the fear of ghosts, monsters, supernatural forces, robbers, and kidnappers is common. Hospital sights and sounds can evoke imaginings far more frightening than reality.

Preschoolers have often had experience with separation from their parents, and they cope with this successfully when healthy and well. During illness and hospitalization, however, these children need the safety and reliability of having their parents consistently close to them. A predominant fear of this age group is being alone. Illness and hospitalization, frightening in many ways, can only intensify this fear.

Because of the tremendous cognitive development that takes place during the preschool years, children of this age group feel extremely powerful. These feelings are instrumental in the preschooler's ability to maintain self-control. In the totally unfamiliar hospital environment, feelings of omnipotence and, consequently, of self-control, are lost. This loss is inextricably linked to the unknown and uncertain.

Preschool children are especially vulnerable to the threats of pain and intrusion because of the psychosexual conflicts of this age group. Mutilation and castration anxieties are paramount, and, therefore, preschoolers often need to reassess their own body integrity and receive reassurance of it from others.

School-age children. School-age children are increasingly capable of objective thought and of understanding that reality is not always as they perceive it. In fact, they have learned to question their own perceptions, as well as those of others. They may thus be reluctant to accept the expertise or explanations of others.

In addition, these children understand the concept of causation. Imaginary fears are less common, as are illogical explanations of events. However, when unknown or highly personal events are involved, these children may revert to precausal thinking. As a result, it cannot be assumed that children of this age understand the mechanisms of illness or the reasons for hospitalization. For example, the school-age diabetic child may believe that diabetes is related to the consumption of excessive amounts of candy.

School-age children have usually established a social sphere and support system outside their immediate family. However, since this age group spans the years between 6 and 12, a variety of behaviors related to separation from parents may be observed in these children. Once again, stress related to illness and hospitalization is likely to make these children more vulnerable to separation from their parents and to increase their need for the close and reliable presence of parents. School-age children also suffer as the result of separation from their peer group and larger family group, which involves the concomitant loss of their productive role in the family and at school. They are likely to worry about falling behind or failing at school, and they may also fear losing their friends during the absence that hospitalization necessitates. They may feel threatened, rejected, isolated, and depressed.

Loss of self-control is especially disturbing to school-age children. Hospitalization results in forced dependence and deprives these children of their ability to make choices about their own lives and activities. Loss of privacy is also a threat to self-control, as is the loss of a productive role in school and within the family. These industrious children may feel very unimportant, or even worthless, because their families and schools continue despite their absence. Fear of the unknown also contributes to feelings of having lost self-control. In contrast to the vague, generalized fears of preschoolers, school-age children usually have very specific fears related to things they do not understand. The school-age child is accustomed to mastering the environment through learning and is especially threatened by whatever is unknown or not understood.

School-age children generally maintain a great deal of composure when confronted with painful or intrusive procedures. Although verbal protest is not uncommon, they demonstrate little fear, overt resistance, or physical protest. Despite their outward composure, these children are very fearful of physical injury, illness, and death. Painful procedures necessitated by serious illness and hospitalization may intensify this fear. Intrusive procedures are often perceived as an invasion of personal privacy and, therefore, are also often threatening to these children.

Adolescent. Adolescents often have a wide and varied support system and also evince the intellectual development and ability to think abstractly and to conceptualize. In addition, their communication skills are well developed. While maturation in all these areas aids in coping with stress, adolescents may actually have their positive coping obstructed by aspects of their own development. For example, the adolescent's cognitive abilities in abstraction and conceptualization may facilitate the clouding of relevant issues with less important data. Their communication skills can serve to camouflage their true feelings.

The adolescent's anxiety about separation during illness and hospitalization is primarily the fear of separation from peers and the concomitant loss of group status and acceptance. Because of the adolescent's massive need for comformity, deviations from the group norm are poorly tolerated and concerns about illness may be exaggerated.

Being hospitalized fosters feelings of depersonalization and dependency, which are very threatening to the adolescent engaged in the psychic struggle for independence and individual identity. The adolescent may be reluctant to depend on others, especially parents, because dependence prevents the achievement of a new level of self-control. Serious illness also threatens the adolescent's self-control in that it calls into question the individual's potential for adult fulfillment.

Painful and/or intrusive procedures are met with rigid self-control. Physical resistance and aggression are unusual in the adolescent, although verbal aggression is quite common. Permanent disability and death are predominant fears of the adolescent patient and are intensified by pain. As with the school-age child, invasive procedures are perceived as an invasion of personal privacy. Provision of the greatest possible degree of privacy is crucial for this age group.

Coping

A child's capacity for coping positively with a stressful situation is determined by a variety of factors.[4,6] Most of all, coping is influenced by the child's developmental stage. Developmental status not only affects how a child perceives a given situation, but it is also related to the range of responses available to the child. Although all aspects of coping are dependent to some degree on the child's developmental status, there are a number of other factors that influence coping during childhood and that affect the child's ability to adapt to and master the stresses of illness and hospitalization.

Defense mechanisms.   Defense mechanisms are unconscious ways of thinking or behaving that serve to meet the needs of the personality. Because defense mechanisms require a certain level of cognitive development, the range of defense mechanisms available to the young child is not as broad as that available to the older child or adolescent. Table 1-1 lists the defense mechanisms available to children at various levels of maturation.

Young children, who have a smaller repertoire of available defense mechanisms, employ mechanisms that are often considered undesirable or even pathological in older children, adolescents, or adults. For all individuals, however, regardless of age, whichever defense mechanism assists in coping with a stressful situation is helpful rather than harmful, at least for limited periods of time.

**TABLE 1-1   Defense Mechanisms Available
by Developmental Stage**

Stage	Defense mechanism
Infants	Discrete defense mechanisms not identifiable
Toddlers and preschoolers	Regression
	Denial
	Repression
	Projection
School-age child	Regression
	Denial
	Repression
	Projection/displacement
	Sublimation
	Reaction formation
Adolescent	Regression
	Denial
	Repression
	Projection/displacement
	Sublimation
	Reaction formation
	Rationalization
	Intellectualization

Regression is an example of a defense mechanism that is difficult for both parents and nurses to accept, but that is nevertheless frequently used by hospitalized children. Regression may be defined as temporary retreat or reversion "to an earlier stage of behavior in order to retain or regain mastery of a stressful, anxiety-producing, or frustrating situation, thus achieving self-gratification and protection."[7] Regression allows the child to minimize energy output and conserve strength for recuperation from illness. It also permits the child to accept the caring provided by others. These behaviors are possible because regressed children make fewer demands on themselves.

The child who regresses during periods of acute illness and hospitalization usually loses the most recently acquired skill. Toilet training may be "forgotten," or the child may suddenly call for the bottle that was recently given up. Lost skills will be rapidly relearned, however, as the child regains trust in the environment and as recuperation restores available energy. The regressed child may also cry a great deal, particularly when parents are present. Rather than constituting a negative behavior, crying with parents permits the child to release tension and demonstrates a feeling of safety in relating strong emotion to the parents. Regression is an unhealthy response to stress only if the child is unable to remaster previously learned skills and becomes fixated at a previously abandoned developmental phase.

Denial is another example of a defense mechanism often regarded as pathological. Denial is necessary, however, at least for short time periods, whenever stress is acute. It represents the ability to ward off aspects of the environment that are excessively threatening in order to maintain hope. Like regression, denial is an unhealthy response only if it persists unreasonably and interferes with acceptance of a permanent aspect of reality.

Level of parental coping. Because of the very close relationship between parents and children, as well as the dependence that children normally experience in relating with their parents, the level of parental coping during the stress of a child's illness and hospitalization also affects how the child copes. Children tend to accept what their parents accept. In addition, parental anxiety, transmitted to children despite attempts to disguise it, makes the child more anxious. It has been shown that the negative reactions to hospitalization frequently demonstrated by children can be significantly diminished and even avoided by providing parents with information about what will occur and how they can assist their child and by supporting their positive coping responses.[8]

The environment and its support systems. Factors such as family life-style and cultural background determine a child's reaction to new and challenging situations. Children who have had previous opportunities to master new situations are likely to have greater self-esteem than those who have not had similar experiences. The hospital setting can provide an environment for mastery if the child receives moderate amounts of appropriate stimulation and is offered opportunities for autonomy and independent exploration, which also serve to enhance self-esteem.

Because parents are the most important component of the child's support system, features of the parent-child relationship are also correlated with the child's coping abilities. When there is a high "degree of fit" between parents and their child, the parents tend to provide their youngster with a great deal of emotional support when a new situation is encountered. In addition, they are more likely to respect and foster their child's abilities. There is probably no adequate substitute for parental love, encouragement, and support.

Previous coping experiences.   Maturation of cognitive skills permits the child to recall previous experiences with stressful or challenging situations. If the child has coped successfully with stressful experiences in the past, there is a sense of gratification as the child recalls the experience with pride. Such a child is likely to use similar coping strategies in a new stressful situation. On the other hand, the child who has been unsuccessful in attempts to master new situations is likely to remember the experiences as frustrating ones and to lack confidence about the abilities needed to succeed when challenged. This child is likely to react negatively to new situations and to view them and his or her personal abilities with doubt.

Temperament.   Children, like adults, are distinct individuals with innate qualities that determine their particular temperament. The qualities that characterize the individual child's temperament include the level and extent of motor activity, regularity of the daily schedule, response to new objects or persons, adaptability to change, sensitivity to stimuli, intensity of response, general mood (e.g., friendly, unfriendly, pleasant, etc.), degree of distractibility, and attention span or persistence in a given activity.[9] Characteristics such as regularity of bodily functions and daily schedule, confident response to new stimuli, pleasant mood, and persistence in challenging activities are likely to be found in the child who copes well with new situations. A child with the opposite temperament characteristics is likely to respond negatively to new situations and to have more difficulty with coping.

Range of positive coping resources.   Murphy has identified four resources which, if present in the environment or if part of the child's individual temperament, are likely to promote successful coping.[10] The first is a varied range of sources of gratification. Not only must the environment offer a variety of possible sources of gratification, but the child must be able to accept alternative sources of gratification or alternative solutions to problems when frustrated. Second, the child who has a positive, outgoing attitude toward life is likely to have a broader range of positive coping resources and to possess the pride, courage, and resilience necessary to mobilize resources after frustration or disappointment. The third characteristic of positive coping is flexibility of coping mechanisms, which permits the child to select from whatever defense mechanisms are available and to use a variety of coping mechanisms in a constructive manner. Finally, both environment and child must be tolerant of retreat and regression. This requires that the child feel secure about self and certain of acceptance by those in the environment, despite regressed behavior.

Intervening variables.   In addition to the above variables, coping ability is also determined by two intervening variables. First, the nature and severity of the illness have an influence on how hospitalized children view their environment and their place within it. Serious illness also limits the amount of energy available to the child for coping with stress. A second intervening variable that influences the child's coping ability is the nature and timing of the information the child receives in preparation for hospitalization. The opportunity to prepare in advance for the events of hospitalization permits the child to mobilize coping strategies and "try on" the role of patient before the actual event. Emergency admission to the hospital as the result of illness or injury deprives the child of the opportunity to practice for the role of patient and to receive anticipatory support and encouragement from parents.

Reaction to Critical Care

The behavioral response of adult critical care patients to life-threatening illness and intensive care has been described as the "intensive care syndrome."[11,12] This syndrome refers to a transient period of delirium or psychotic behavior characterized by confusion, disorientation, and delusions or hallucinations of a paranoid nature. Similar behavior has not been reported in children who require critical care. Little attention, however, has been given to the systematic study of children's behavioral responses to serious illness and life-threatening situations or to the critical care necessitated by such illness.

Children in critical care units have been described as withdrawn, solemn, passive, and preoccupied with their physical condition.[13,14] It is reasonable to suppose that the amount of energy required for physical recuperation from serious illness or major surgery is enormous and may preclude other behaviors. On the other hand, children in critical care units often react intensely to painful and intrusive procedures. Even the removal of ECG electrodes can elicit vigorous protest and physical resistance from the young child. It is likely that the extent and duration of procedures that are painful and/or intrusive leave the child with little reserve to withstand even comparatively minor episodes of discomfort. Perceived passivity and withdrawal may also be related to the nearly total loss of self-control that these seriously ill children experience. In addition, withdrawal may assist the child in denying aspects of the environment that are intolerable.

Although children in the critical unit may appear withdrawn, it has been demonstrated that they are acutely aware of their environment and can recall it in detail.[15,16] School-age children are reported to be aware of infants and other children in the ICU and to be concerned for their welfare.[16] It is also clear that children do understand the nature of serious illness and impending death. Children in the hospital ask the same questions that adults do: "Why am I in the hospital? What is wrong with me?"[17]

EFFECTS OF HOSPITALIZATION ON PARENTS

Children hospitalized as the result of critical illness cannot be adequately cared for if the needs of their families are not met. All individuals—patients, nurses, physicians, etc.—are products of a family unit and derive a part of their individual identity from their identity within a family. Children identify closely with their parents, whereas parents see themselves reflected in the lives of their children. The role of nurses caring for critically ill children must be expanded to include assisting parents and other family members to cope with the sick child's illness while maintaining family functioning. The stress resulting from a child's illness and hospitalization affects the parents in a number of ways, requiring them to use a variety of coping skills in order to care for the sick child and maintain family life.

Stressors

Hospitalization of a child evokes a great deal of stress within the child's family. Parents are called on to accomplish a variety of new tasks in order to understand and manage their child's illness, assist their sick child to understand and cope with the illness, and meet the ongoing needs of all other family members.[18] To master these tasks, parents must confront and deal with the very personal stress elicited by the hospitalization of their child. Aspects of this stress involve loss of their role as parents, guilt, and anxiety.

Loss of the parental role.   When a child requires hospitalization, it becomes necessary for parents to release to virtual strangers a portion of their responsibility as their child's primary caretakers. Parents in today's fast-paced, urban society are unaccustomed to accepting assistance or support from others in meeting the needs of their family, and their self-esteem and self-control may be threatened by their need to do so. In addition, parents may not be permitted (or may not be able) to participate in their child's care. They may thus experience increased feelings of helplessness and worthlessness because they feel that there is nothing that they can do to help their child.

Guilt.   Parents typically respond with some degree of guilt to illness or injury that requires the hospitalization of their child. This feeling is actually a common reaction of parents whenever their children become ill, but is magnified many times when the nature of the child's illness and hospitalization is critical. Guilt feelings most often have no basis in the real events that necessitated the child's hospitalization, because parents are only rarely directly responsible for causing their child's illness or injury. This fact does not appear to significantly lessen parents' guilt feelings, which are often present even when the hospitalization has been planned or scheduled. It is as if parents incriminate themselves for somehow having failed to protect the child from pain and suffering, and they thus accept responsibility for causing the illness, failing to prevent it, or not noticing its onset. Parents may evince their feeling of guilt in expressions such as "if only I hadn't sent him to the store on his bike," "I should have kept him inside after school," or "we should have taken him to the doctor earlier," or "he seems so little to be hurting so badly." It is understandable that parents have such feelings of guilt and failure: parents in our society are held responsible for their children's health, appearance, behavior, performance, achievements, and mistakes.[17]

Anxiety.   A child's illness or hospitalization causes great anxiety in the parents. In part, this reaction results from the guilt and loss of role that parents of hospitalized children experience. In addition, parents may be faced with grave uncertainty about their child's prognosis and with intense, disorienting emotions. They may be unable to grasp the complex, unfamiliar information with which they are provided, make practical arrangements for themselves or their family, or support their ill child. This paralysis of parents' abilities to function maturely and independently is characteristic of an anxiety reaction. Parents may even verbalize their inability to act with expressions such as "I just don't know what to do." This reaction is generally short-lived, however, and, within a period of hours to days, most parents begin to cope with the stresses related to the child's illness and hospitalization and to accomplish the tasks demanded of them.

Coping

How parents cope with the stress resulting from the serious illness and hospitalization of their child depends on a variety of factors. Human development is a lifelong process, and parents, as well as children, continue to develop. Therefore, whenever a family attempts to master a stressful situation, their responses depend on the personal resources and vulnerabilities that they bring to the situation. Coping is not a static process, but a dynamic one that requires continuous effort to maintain. Successful parental coping is dependent on the healthy use of a variety of defense mechanisms, the level of the partner's coping, the environment and its support systems, previous coping experiences, individual temperament, and a number of intervening variables.

Defense mechanisms. Mature individuals have a broad repertoire of defense mechanisms available to meet the needs of the personality (*see* Table 1-1). Healthy use of defense mechanisms permits the individual to maintain daily functioning despite intense stress. This is true regardless of the defense mechanism selected. Therefore, it is inaccurate and misleading to label some personality defenses as positive and others as negative. For example, parents of a seriously ill child often use denial as a mechanism that relieves them of a portion of the psychological burden of their child's illness. Life-threatening illness or a terminal prognosis cannot be accepted and dealt with either immediately or with ease. As with the grieving process, small pieces of the experience are accepted one after another. Use of denial permits parents to maintain hope, which is an *essential* component of coping. Without hope, parents may withdraw from their child and from each other.

When parents of a critically ill child are asked how they manage to cope with their child's illness, typical responses are "we just take one day at a time" or "we don't let ourselves think that the treatment might not work." These parents are not indicating lack of acceptance of the gravity of their child's illness; they are merely not permitting themselves to think of all the negative aspects of the situation at one time. This defense is necessary if parents are to assist their sick child and simultaneously maintain family functioning. Denial prevents emotional overload, acute anxiety, panic, and the inability to function.[17]

Parents of critically ill children are likely to use a variety of other defense mechanisms as they cope with the stress produced by this frightening situation. Because the defense mechanisms that any one parent selects for use depend on intensely personal characteristics of that individual, it is crucial that the particular mechanisms selected be supported by the health care team. In addition, coping with serious illness and critical care is a complicated process for the child, who is dependent, in large part, on the level of parental coping. Support of the parents' coping strategies permits them to assist their child's attempts at coping.

Level of partner's coping. Ideally, parents share a close relationship in which each assists the other in coping with stressful situations. As evidenced, however, by the soaring divorce rate, relationships between parents are not always loving or supportive. Criticial illness in a child can threaten the best parental partnerships and puts a serious strain on the less secure relationships. The quality of the parents' relationship and the level of each partner's coping influence the response of the other parent to the stress of illness and hospitalization of a child. Parents must be able to trust each other before trust can be extended to others. This trust is illustrated by either parent's ability to accept and support the other's coping strategies. Ideally, parents cope in ways that complement each other. Successful coping permits both parents to maintain their own needs and the integrity of their relationship.

The environment and its support systems. Cultural background and family life-style influence how individuals respond to any stressful situation. These factors also influence the quantity and quality of support that families receive from individuals in their environment. In general today's nuclear family exists in far greater isolation than was characteristic of previous eras. Extended families no longer live or work together. Upward mobility has separated the generations, often by thousands of miles. In addition, people often do not know their own neighbors. As a result, parents today have less direct access to a supportive network of family members and friends.

The relative isolation of the nuclear family has also resulted in decreased expectations for help and assistance from others. Adults do not expect to receive help from others (or, for that matter, to need it), but are determined to succeed unassisted. As a consequence, parents may not be comfortable about asking others for help even when it is necessary. They may fear rejection or reproach, or feel threatened by their need for assistance. It is fortunate, however, that the experience of a crisis situation, such as the hospitalization of a child, appears to make individuals more open to assistance from others. Successful coping depends at least partly on parental acceptance of assistance from the environment.

Previous coping experiences. Parents are likely to face the experience of hospitalization of a child with some previous experience of adversity. In general, previous experiences that resulted in mastery enhance an individual's self-esteem, whereas frustrating experiences lead to lack of confidence. However, because there is no relationship like that between parent and child, it is unreasonable to expect the parent who is successful in other aspects of life to cope well and the less successful parent to have more difficulty with coping. Previous positive coping experiences are helpful, but do not necessarily predict the parent's ability to cope with the child's illness and hospitalization.

Temperament. Parents are distinct individuals whose particular temperament is determined by innate personal qualities. No two individuals can be expected to react to the serious illness of a child in exactly the same way. Perhaps the only generalization possible is that all parents of sick children are anxious. As a result, the parent's actual temperament may be temporarily obscured. A feature of temperament that assists parents' efforts at coping is the range of positive coping resources available to them.

Intervening variables. Parents' coping ability, like that of their children, is also determined by two intervening variables (*see* p. 7). First, the nature and severity of the child's illness influence how parents view their situation. Serious or life-threatening illness disrupts previous life-style and menaces parental self-esteem. Second, parents' ability to cope with the stress of hospitalization of their child is influenced by the nature and timing of the information that parents receive in preparation for the hospitalization and throughout its course. This information is crucial to the parents' understanding and management of their child's illness—the first steps in coping positively with the stress of the hospitalization of a child.

Reaction to Critical Care

Because of the unique relationship between parents and their children, it seems plausible that parents would react to the serious illness or injury and subsequent critical care of their child in a manner unlike any other situation. This appears to be true of at least the intensity of the parents' reaction; however, there are certain similarities between parents' reactions to critical care and other stress-induced human responses, such as grief. A universal reaction in the first moments and even days following a crisis in one of shock and disbelief. Familiar reality is disrupted, giving way to intensified responses, loss of control, and the inability to regain one's bearings. The perceived world of the critical care unit undoubtedly intensifies these feelings of being out of touch with reality. The environment is one of unfamiliar sensory stimuli and general urgency.[19]

The next feeling to develop in parents of the critically ill child is a keen sense of deprivation, similar to that experienced with the death of a loved one.[20] This sense of loss is related both to the real loss of the child's spontaneous affection and to the perceived loss of the parental role. With the dawning of this painful awareness, parents generally begin to move from the isolation that characterizes the shock and disbelief phase to stages where the situation can be dealt with more directly. Parents often spend much time and energy attempting to collect information and understand every aspect of their child's illness. They may seek out, talk with, and compare details with other parents. They may question all members of the intensive care staff closely. The purpose of this activity is to transform the stressful situation into a problem that can be dealt with on a cognitive level. The attempt to achieve cognitive mastery of a situation is characteristic of the defense mechanism of intellectualization, but it also serves to assist parents in understanding and managing their child's illness.

Parents may experience feelings of anger as they develop an increased cognitive awareness of their child's illness or injury. This anger may be directed against themselves or each other as the result of guilty feelings related to their perception of themselves as parents who have somehow failed. They may even feel anger toward children who are well and toward their parents.[21] This anger may be expressed in bickering with each other or it may be directed at the critical care staff.

Some parents will find solace in prayer and religious practices. Prayer may involve bargaining with God: parents may try to "make a deal" with God, promising to be perfect parents in return for the recovery of their child.

The outcome of the child's illness greatly influences the parents' continuing reaction to the critical care their child is receiving. If the child recovers and grows well, the parents' efforts at coping are reinforced in an immediate and positive way. When the outcome remains uncertain for an extended period of time, parents are called on to cope with increased stress. These individuals report an intense need to believe that there is hope. When a child dies despite efforts at critical care, parents are faced with a new and even more demanding situation. These parents reenter the cycle of experiences characteristic of grief.

NURSING PROCESS IN CRITICAL CARE

Nurses who provide critical care to children and their families have a unique opportunity to affect these individuals. The seriousness of a child's illness when intensive care is required, and the child's and family's reaction to the serious illness and intensive care, encourage closeness between the professional staff and the family. When people are in crisis they are more open to assistance from others. Because critical care nurses meet these families at the point of crisis, they are often able to influence them in ways that assist their adaptation to the illness and promote family functioning. Parents have described the impact of their first meeting with the intensive care nurse and how that individual remained an especially important person to them and to their child throughout hospitalization.[22] In addition, critical care nurses spend a great deal of time with the child and parents and thus have a continuing opportunity to interact with these families and provide emotional support.

The critical care nurse applies the nursing process to the emotional care of hospitalized children and their families. As the human-to-human monitor, the nurse first *assesses* the child's and family's response to the illness and ICU environment and continues ongoing assessment of their coping strategies and their need for information and support. Next, based on the assessment data, the nurse designs specific *interventions* aimed at minimizing the stresses experienced by child and family and at promoting their coping abilities. Continued assessment of the status of child and family permits the nurse to *evaluate* the extent of their success in managing the child's illness based on the nursing interventions provided.

The goal of intensive emotional care of critically ill children and their families is to reunite the family at a level of functioning at least as effective as that at which the family unit operated before the crisis of critical illness and hospitalization. Crisis can lead to growth in the family relationship. Nurses have an important role in promoting such a positive outcome through the application of the nursing process.

Assessing

Assessment of the response of children and their parents to hospitalization and intensive care provides the foundation for the planning and implementing of nursing interventions. It is necessary to assess each individual—child, mother and father—as well as the family as a unit. Accurate assessment requires skilled observation and creative listening. Just as critical care nurses must know what to look for in an electrocardiogram, so must their observation of the critically ill child's and the family's emotional responses be guided by a knowledge of the aspects of hospitalization that particularly distress children of different ages and their parents, as well as the knowledge of typical coping responses. This prevents nurses from misunderstanding or misinterpreting the child's or family's responses. For example, despite the fact that children are observed to be quiet and withdrawn in the ICU environment, it cannot be assumed that they are unaware of events around them or unconcerned about what is occurring. When parents express hope for a positive outcome for their child with an extremely grave prognosis their denial is not unrealistic, but rather an expression of an essential component of coping. It is imperative that critical care nurses assess and interpret the responses of child and family accurately.

Intervening

Specific nursing interventions designed to minimize the stress associated with a child's hospitalization and promote the family's coping abilities are based on the assessment of the child's and parents' emotional responses and a knowledge of the needs these individuals typically experience. In general, children and parents need to trust themselves, each other, and the professionals caring for them; to be informed about what is and will be happening; to be guided and supported as they attempt to cope with the crisis in which they are engulfed; and to receive adequate human and physical resources to maintain coping.[18]

These needs are best met when parents are encouraged to participate in all aspects of their child's hospitalization. The parents' place is at their child's bedside: the parents' comforting presence minimizes the child's fear and stress related to separation and maintains the parents in their role. When a child experiences a life-threatening illness or undergoes major surgery, however, it is difficult, if not impossible, for the parents to relate to the child as the same individual they knew and loved before the catastrophe. Instead, parents undergo a process by which they reclaim their child.[23] This process has three phases: physical contact, care-giving, and identity.[23,24]

During the first phase, parents reestablish their relationship with their child through physical contact by touching, stroking, and holding while they talk to their child. This behavior is quite similar to that observed during the parent-newborn acquaintance process, which provides the basis for parent-infant bonding. Parents appear to be reestablishing the child's intactness as a prerequisite for a continuing relationship. The child is undoubtedly comforted by the familiar touch and voice of the parents.

In the second phase of reclaiming their child, parents begin to resume their role as physical caretakers. They may assist with bathing, grooming, dressing, and feeding their child. If the child's normal developmental status has been compromised, as by a severe neurological injury or illness, parents may perform these tasks even for an adolescent. In addition, any seriously ill child needs to regress in order to maintain ego integrity; comforting physical care from parents, however, can assist the child in regaining development skills. As the parents become more comfortable with providing the routine physical care with which they are familiar, they may begin to participate in caring for their child's special physical needs, such as range-of-motion exercises or stoma care. It seems essential to the reclaiming process and the healthy reintegration of the family that parents *first* provide typical parental care to their child and only *secondly* undertake care of the child's special needs.

The final phase of the reclaiming process is identification. Parents in this third phase identify and reincorporate the child as their own, a member of their family. They often bring photographs of the child and family from home and characterize the child by means of personal observations. They talk of experiences they shared with their child to the health care personnel and to the child. This behavior serves a dual purpose. First, it reorients the child to familiar events that define the past and the future. Second, it serves to acquaint the nurses and physicians with the child as a healthy person. This is the beginning of the parents' ability to act as their child's advocate. They have come to realize that they know their child better than anyone else, and they feel sufficiently secure in this realization to tell others how they or their child would like things to be. At this point, parents may question, or even demand changes in, their child's medical or nursing care.

Parents generally do not move spontaneously through these phases of reclaiming their child; they need assistance and support. The following is a list of specific nursing practices that encourage parents of a critically ill child to reassume their parental role:

1. Encouraging and strengthening parents in their role and never interfering with parenting, because health care professionals cannot take the place of parents.
2. Giving parents access to their child on a continuous, 24-hour basis.
3. Preparing parents for the sights and sounds of the ICU (including how their child will look) before their initial visit with their child.

4. Introducing the parents to the nurses and physicians responsible for their child's care.

5. Identifying for parents the individual with final authority for their child's care, since many individuals may be involved in meeting the child's physical needs.

6. Providing accurate, concise, and complete information to parents about their child's illness, condition, and the plan of care.

7. Repeating explanations to parents as often as necessary.

8. Providing the parents with holistic information about their child.

9. Informing parents of the rules and regulations of the ICU.

10. Assuring parents that their child needs them and that they are irreplaceable in meeting their child's needs.

11. Providing verbal and nonverbal encouragement to parents as they begin to touch, talk to, or care for their sick child.

12. Encouraging parents to bring the child reminders of life at home and to tell nurses and physicians about their child's personality and behavior while well and healthy.

13. Listening carefully, attentively, and respectfully to parents as they express their concerns for their child.

14. Assisting parents to become aware of their unexpressed needs by verbally labeling them.[25]

15. Accepting the legitimacy of the parents' feelings whether or not they are congruent with those of the health care professionals.[25]

While assisting parents with supporting their child, nurses in critical care settings should promote the parents' healthy use of defense mechanisms. Because denial is so frequently used by parents, but so often troubling to health care providers, nurses must be especially perceptive about the use of this defense mechanism. The parents' *defense* does not require the nurse's or physician's *offense*.[26] Instead, parents need to be supported in the expression of their hopes for their child, as well as of their fears and concerns.

Besides the presence of parents, there are specific nursing interventions that minimize stress for the critically ill child and promote coping. The interventions vary widely depending on the developmental stage of the child and the limitations imposed by the nature and severity of the child's illness. Table 1-2 presents specific nursing practices that minimize stress and promote coping in hospitalized children. Modification may be necessary, but these interventions are nevertheless easily incorporated into nursing care.

Evaluating

The emotional status of the seriously ill child and the family can rarely be fully or accurately evaluated during critical care. The defense mechanisms used by both may obscure their true level of functioning. That families remain intact during the acute crisis of critical illness is testimony to the remarkable resilience of the human spirit and to the profound capacity that parents have for coping. Positive signs of parents' coping include their ability to seek information about their child's care and treatment, form trusting relationships with health care professionals, maintain hope, and support their ill child. Evidence that the seriously ill child is

TABLE 1-2 Nursing Interventions to Minimize Stress and Promote Coping

Age group	Stressor	Interventions to promote coping
Infant	Separation	1. Encourage parents to stay with their infant as much as possible. 2. Provide consistent caretakers.
	Pain/intrusion	1. Investigate the reason for an infant's crying. 2. Initiate self-comforting behaviors, such as sucking, by bringing the infant's fingers toward the mouth. 3. Decrease stimulation by holding the infant's arms close to the body or by swaddling. 4. Talk quietly to the infant. 5. Use touch to soothe the infant by stroking, patting, holding, or cuddling.
	Immobilization	1. Provide changes in position by using an infant seat or by holding, rocking, or turning the infant. 2. Remove restraints periodically to permit free movement under close supervision. 3. Provide whatever exploration of the environment is possible in the crib or playpen or on the floor. 4. Provide stimulation and opportunities for visual exploration with colorful mobiles, pictures, mirrors, and soft toys.
Toddler	Separation	1. Encourage parents to stay with their toddler as much as possible. 2. Provide consistent caretakers. 3. Preserve ties to home by obtaining transitional objects, family photos, tape recordings of the family, objects from home, and by talking about home and family. 4. Teach parents that withdrawal is a response to stress and helps the child to conserve energy.
	Pain/intrusion	1. Accept that the toddler cannot differentiate pain from intrusion. 2. Expect vigorous protest behavior and carry out painful procedures as quickly as safety permits. 3. Teach parents that protest behavior is a healthy response. 4. Comfort the child with holding and cuddling after painful procedures and assist parents to do the same. 5. Provide "safe" times and places in which painful or intrusive procedures are prohibited. 6. Provide rest periods between stressful procedures.
	Loss of self-control	1. Continue rituals observed at home. 2. Provide opportunities for autonomy by permitting choices.

TABLE 1-2 (Continued)

Age group	Stressor	Interventions to promote coping
		3. Provide as much physical activity as safety permits.
		4. Provide for exploration of the environment to whatever extent possible.
		5. Accept regression and teach parents that this is a healthy response and that their toddler will remaster "lost" skills quickly after recovery.
Preschooler	Separation	1. (See corresponding section under *Toddlers.*)
		2. Teach parents that their young child still needs the reassurance of their continuing presence, especially when ill, and that fear of being alone is common in this age group.
	Pain/intrusion	1. Assist the child to cooperate with procedures by providing information about them and about what is expected of the child.
		2. Set realistic limits on undesirable behavior.
		3. Provide the child with opportunities to practice for potentially stressful procedures.
		4. Reassure the child that procedures are necessary and are not punishment.
		5. Use touch to convey comforting, warmth, and caring.
		6. Reassure the child about body intactness.
	Loss of self-control	1. Provide opportunities for self-expression.
		2. Encourage autonomy by permitting choices and participation in self-care.
		3. Make reality-oriented statements to the child.
		4. Use play as a vehicle for teaching the child and encouraging expression of feelings. Utilize the child's ability to fantasize constructively.
School-age child	Separation	1. Encourage parents to visit regularly and reliably.
		2. Provide consistent caretakers.
		3. Respond to withdrawn behavior or verbalization of loneliness with increased attention and closeness.
		4. Encourage communication with siblings and schoolmates.
		5. Keep the child informed about events at home and school.
	Pain/intrusion	1. Provide privacy during procedures.
		2. Encourage the child's ability to learn through repetition by teaching about upcoming events well in advance.
		3. Accept aggressive verbal protests while setting realistic limits on undesirable behavior.
		4. Provide activities for the release of aggression.
	Loss of self-control	1. Encourage the child to explain what he knows about his situation.

TABLE 1-2 (Continued)

Age group	Stressor	Interventions to promote coping
		2. Teach by means of honest explanations, diagrams, models, and actual equipment.
		3. Encourage the child to participate in self-care.
		4. Permit the child to make decisions and direct care whenever possible.
		5. Provide the child with meaningful tasks to perform. Use positive reinforcement for helpful behaviors.
Adolescent	Separation	1. Encourage parents to visit regularly and reliably.
		2. Provide consistent caretakers.
		3. Assist parents in understanding their adolescent's need to be in control while recovering.
		4. Support communication with peers by providing flexible visiting for peers whenever feasible.
		5. Respect the adolescent's need to conform to peer expectations.
		6. Encourage verbalization of feelings with regard to peers, peer pressure, etc.
	Pain/intrusion	1. Provide secure privacy during procedures.
		2. Assist the adolescent to prepare for stressful procedures.
		3. Accept aggressive verbal behavior without retaliating.
		4. Encourage verbalization of fears related to death or disability.
	Loss of self-control	1. Encourage the adolescent's active participation in care.
		2. Consult the adolescent about the plan of care.
		3. Be flexible about hospital routines whenever possible.
		4. Promote cognitive mastery by asking the adolescent to explain what he or she knows.
		5. Be aware of intellectualization. Clarify misconceptions.
		6. Accept temporary withdrawal.
		7. Encourage expression of emotion by reflecting the adolescent's feelings.
		8. Respect the adolescent's need for independence.

coping may be seen during recovery as the child responds to the parents and staff and begins to resume developmentally appropriate behavior.

The long-term effects of critical illness during childhood on parents, their child, and family functioning have not yet been studied. Despite the absence of conclusive data, critical care nurses must continue to care intensely for those children and parents for whom they represent the vital human-to-human monitor in the ICU. Only by such caring can the stress of critical illness be minimized and the coping abilities of all the individuals involved be promoted.

REFERENCES

1. Roberts. 3.
2. Fagin.
3. Pitrello and Sanger. 5.
4. Vipperman and Rager.
5. Murphy and Moriarty. 7.
6. Murphy. (1962) 77.
7. Audette.
8. Visintainer and Wolfer.
9. Thomas et al.
10. Murpy. (1961)
11. Kornfeld.
12. Katz.
13. Berlin.
14. May.
15. Barnes. (1974)
16. Barnes. (1975)
17. Ross.
18. Hymovich.
19. Gowan.
20. Parks. 6–7.
21. Surveyer.
22. Bell.
23. Schraeder.
24. Jay.
25. Strauss.
26. Green.

BIBLIOGRAPHY

Audette, M. S. 1974. The significance of regressive behavior for the hospitalized child. *Maternal-Child Nursing Journal*. **3:**31–40.

Barnes, C. 1974. School-age children's recall of the intensive care unit. *ANA Clinical Sessions*. Appleton-Century-Crofts, Norwalk, Conn. 73–79.

Barnes, C. 1975. Levels of consciousness indicated by responses of children to phenomena in the intensive care unit. *Maternal-Child Nursing Journal*. **4:**215–290.

Bell, G. 1976. Moths and butterflies. *Pediatric Nursing*. **2:**36–41 (May/June).

Berlin, C. 1970. The pediatric intensive care unit. *Medical Annals of the District of Columbia*. **9:**483–486,493.

Fagin, C. 1966. Pediatric rooming-in: its meaning for the nurse. *Nursing Clinics of North America*. **1:**83–93.

Gowan, N. J. 1979. The perceptual world of the intensive care unit: an overview of some environmental considerations in the helping relationship. *Heart & Lung*. **8:**340–344.

Green, M. 1979. Parent care in the intensive care unit. *American Journal of Diseases of Children*. **113:**1119–1120.

Hymovich, D. P. 1976. Parents of sick children: their needs and tasks. *Pediatric Nursing*. **2:**9–13.

Jay, S. 1977. Pediatric intensive care: involving parents in the care of their child. *Maternal-Child Nursing Journal*. **6:**195–204.

Katz, N. M. 1972. Delirium in surgical patients under intensive care. *Archives of Surgery*. **104:**310–313.

Kornfeld, D. S. 1969. Psychiatric view of the intensive care unit. *British Medical Journal*. **1:**108–110.

May, J. A. 1972. Psychiatric study of a pediatric intensive therapy unit. *Clinical Pediatrics*. **11:**76–82.

Murphy, L. B. 1961. Preventive implications of development in the preschool years. *In* Caplan, G., editor 1961. Prevention of Mental Disorders in Children. Basic Books, Inc., New York. 234–235.

Murphy, L. B. 1962. The Widening World of Childhood. Basic Books, Inc. New York.

Murphy, L. B., and A. E. Moriarity. 1976. Vulnerability, Coping, and Growth. Yale University Press, New Haven.

Parks, C. M. 1973. Bereavement: Studies of Grief in Adult Life. International Universities Press, Inc., New York.

Pitrello, M., and S. Sanger. 1980. Emotional Care of Hospitalized Children. J. B. Lippincott Co., Philadelphia. Second edition.

Roberts, J. L. 1976. Behavioral Concepts and the Critically Ill Patient. Prentice-Hall, Inc., Englewood Cliffs, N. J.

Ross, J. W. 1980. Childhood cancer: the parents, the patients, the professionals. *Issues in Comprehensive Pediatric Nursing*. **4:**7–16.

Schraeder, B. D. 1980. Attachment and parenting despite lengthy intensive care. *Maternal-Child Nursing.* **5:**37–41.

Strauss, S. J. 1981. Abuse and neglect of parents by professionals. *Maternal-Child Nursing.* **6:**157–160.

Surveyer, J. A. 1976. Coma in children: how it affects parents. *Maternal-Child Nursing.* **1:**17–21.

Thomas, A., S. Chess, and H. Birch. 1970. The origin of personality. *Scientific American.* **223:**102–109.

Vipperman, J. F., and P. M. Rager. 1980. Childhood coping: how nurses can help. *Pediatric Nursing.* **6:**12–18.

Visintainer, M. A., and J. A. Wolfer. 1975. Psychological preparation for surgical pediatric patients: effect on children's and parents' stress responses and adjustment. *Pediatrics.* **56:**187–201.

CHAPTER **2**

THE RESPIRATORY SYSTEM

Susan B. De Jong
Susan Carmody McCandless

The respiratory system of children is unique because it is changing and developing with growth. At birth, the respiratory system is relatively small but, with the onset of breathing, the lungs begin to grow rapidly. Primary growth results from an increase in the number and size of alveoli and a change in alveolar shape. This process, which continues until 12 years of age, serves to increase the area utilized for gas exchange. Growth also occurs with the branching of the peripheral bronchioles.

Growth of the respiratory tree proceeds much more rapidly than that of the vertebral column. This causes changes in the angle of access to the trachea as the respiratory system develops—an important fact to remember when positioning the child for emergency respiratory procedures (*see* p. 76–77).

Secondary growth occurs when the respiratory tree lengthens and enlarges. This change is relative to body growth, particularly height: the taller the child, the greater the surface area of the lungs.[1]

The growth of smooth muscle in the airway also occurs rapidly. At birth, there is a minimal amount, but by the fifth month there is sufficient muscle to respond to various irritants by contraction and bronchospasm. The development of smooth muscle is complete at the age of 1 year, when it is comparable to that of the adult.

The character of respirations also changes as a child grows. Until age 6 or 7, the child's breathing is primarily abdominal because of the more horizontal position of the rib cage. After age 6 or 7, the child begins to breathe using the thoracic muscles. This change is due to the maturation of the thoracic muscles and the increasing rigidity of the child's thorax.

These factors are significant because they can contribute to the respiratory problems of the child at various ages (e.g., younger children are more prone to airway obstruction and more vulnerable to atelectasis). On the other hand, children may recover faster and suffer fewer long-term effects of respiratory disease than adults because the respiratory tract is still developing and growing.

SELECTED ASPECTS OF RESPIRATORY PHYSIOLOGY

Control of Respiration

Control and regulation of respiration are maintained by a central respiratory control and a complex system of receptors.

The central respiratory control is composed of groups of neurons located in the medulla oblongata and the pons. When stimulated, these neurons initiate impulses (sent to various receptors throughout the body) that correct problems in respiration. In the medulla there are two groups of neurons, one group responsible for inspiration and the other for both inspiration and expiration.

Within the pons there are two centers, an apneustic and a pneumotaxic center. The apneustic center is responsible for ending normal inspiration. The pneumotaxic center is responsible for patterning respiration, regulating the apneustic center for correct timing, and responding to stimuli received from peripheral receptors.

Normal respiration is achieved when central respiratory control is mediated by stimuli from mechanical and chemical receptors in the body. These receptors include (1) intrapulmonary receptors, (2) peripheral chemoreceptors, (3) peripheral arterial chemoreceptors, and (4) central medullary chemoreceptors.

Intrapulmonary receptors (Table 2-1) are mechanical receptors within the chest that are frequently responsible for dyspnea and tachypnea. They directly alter tidal volume and regulate the timing of inspiration and expiration.

Peripheral chemoreceptors are chemical receptors that sense changes in pH within the tissues and evoke hyperpnea. This explains why during exercise the respiratory control center is stimulated to increase tidal volume by means of hyperventilation. This reflex compensates for the increased production of lactic acid during exercise by causing the excretion of greater amounts of carbon dioxide.

Peripheral arterial chemoreceptors (Table 2-2) are chemical receptors that are responsive to hypoxia and acidosis. They are important in maintaining ventilatory control and normal carbon dioxide tension.

The central medullary chemoreceptors (Table 2-2) are responsive to changes in the cerebrospinal hydrogen-ion concentration that occur when carbon dioxide crosses the blood-brain barrier. This carbon dioxide readily binds with water to

TABLE 2-1 Intrapulmonary Receptors

Type	Location	Stimulated by	Response to stimulation
Stretch receptors	Smooth muscle of small airways	Stretching or increase in lung volume	Sympathetic stimulation: bronchodilation, increased heart rate, impulses to central control inhibiting inspiration
Irritant receptors	Between airway epithelial cells.	Chemical irritants, smoke, dust, ammonia, histamine	Reflex hyperpnea, bronchoconstriction
"J" receptors	Wall of pulmonary capillaries	Disruption of the alveolar wall from pulmonary edema or pneumonia	Hyperpnea, hyperventilation

"J" receptors; juxtacapillary receptors

TABLE 2-2 Arterial and Central Chemoreceptors

Type	Location	Stimulated by	Response to stimulation
Peripheral Carotid bodies	At bifurcation of carotid arteries	Hypoxia, acidosis, increase in hy-drogen-ion con-centration, and hypercapnia	Hyperventilation
Aortic bodies	Distributed around aortic arch		Hyperventilation
Central	Ventral surface of brainstem	Increase in hydro-gen ions from dissociation of carbonic acid	Hyperventilation

form carbonic acid. Because carbonic acid dissociates easily, it causes the cerebrospinal hydrogen-ion concentration to rise, thereby stimulating respiration. Thus, the effect of carbon dioxide on respiration is related to its dissociation and the consequent movement of hydrogen ions into the cerebrospinal fluid.

The blood-brain barrier is readily permeable to gases such as oxygen and carbon dioxide, whereas it is less permeable to hydrogen and bicarbonate ions. This explains why respiratory acidosis is a more powerful ventilatory stimulus than metabolic acidosis, given the same change in serum pH or hydrogen ion concentration.

Mechanics of Respiration

For gas exchange to occur, air must move from the atmosphere into the lungs. When the lungs are at rest, intrapulmonic pressure is equal to atmospheric pressure. In order for gas to enter the lungs, atmospheric pressure must become greater than intrapulmonic pressure. A pressure gradient is established between the atmosphere and the alveoli by the active contraction of the chest muscles. With contraction, the diaphragm moves downward and the intercostal muscles pull the ribs upward and forward. This muscular movement increases the size of the lungs and decreases intrapulmonic pressure. Gas then flows into the lungs until a pressure equilibrium is reached. This is the process of inspiration. Expiration occurs as the contracted muscles relax and the elastic recoil of lung tissue forces gas out of the lungs. Expiration is normally a passive occurrence.

Stages of Respiration

The primary function of the respiratory system is to deliver oxygen to body tissues and remove carbon dioxide from them after cellular metabolism has taken place. Respiration is an ongoing process that is accomplished in four stages: ventilation, distribution, diffusion, and transportation. Disruptions in any of the four stages can result in respiratory failure. (Table 2-3 defines the stages of respiration and lists the causes of their disruption, the diseases associated with these disruptions, and appropriate nursing assessments of a child with any of these disorders.)

TABLE 2-3 Problems Associated with the Stages of Respiration

Stage of respiration	Definition	Causes of disruption	Diseases associated with disruptions	Nursing assessments
Ventilation	The movement of gas into and out of the lungs	Inadequate gas volume Narrowed/obstructed airways Impaired respiratory stimulation	Hypoventilation Hyperventilation Croup Epiglottitis Asthma Tracheal stenosis Brain injury Depression of the respiratory center	Observe respiratory rate, depth, pattern, and quality Assess color; note any cyanosis Listen to breathing; note any noise associated with respiration Observe chest excursion with respiration; note any use of accessory muscles Evaluate breath sounds Inspect secretions; be aware of any culture growth in sputum or blood Investigate any abnormal drug levels found in serum blood samples
Distribution	The movement of gas to the alveoli once inside the lungs	Neuromuscular diseases Impaired lung compliance Skeletal deformities	Werdnig-Hoffmann paralysis Guillain-Barré syndrome Infant botulism Myasthenia gravis Pneumothorax Postoperative splinting Asthma Bronchopulmonary dysplasia Pneumonia Scoliosis Kyphosis Pectus excavatum Flail chest Penetrating chest wounds Bronchopulmonary dysplasia	

Process	Definition	Factors	Conditions	Nursing interventions
Diffusion	The movement of gas across the alveolar-capillary membrane	Increased tissue thickness Decreased tissue area Altered pressure gradient	Asthma Cystic fibrosis Pulmonary edema Pneumonia Atelectasis Acidosis Alkalosis *Pneumocystis carinii* pneumonia	Follow arterial blood gas results and end-tidal CO_2 and $TcPO_2$ values Observe chest x-ray Evaluate vital signs, cardiac output, hemoglobin, hematocrit, and capillary refill Monitor electrocardiogram and filling pressures
Transportation	The movement of gas in the blood to and from the tissues	Decreased blood flow Impeded blood flow Decreased hemoglobin Ventilation-perfusion inequalities	Anemia Shock Pulmonary edema Acidosis Alkalosis Abnormal red blood cells (sickle cell anemia, thalassemia) Decreased cardiac output (hemorrhage, congestive heart failure)	

CO_2, carbon dioxide; $TcPO_2$, transcutaneous partial pressure of oxygen.

Ventilation. Ventilation is the movement of air into and out of the lungs. This process is regulated by the brain and involves the muscles of the chest. Effective ventilation provides an adequate gas volume for maintaining homeostasis in the body. The volume of gas available to the lungs from a single breath is known as the tidal volume. Normal tidal volume in children is generally estimated to be 7 to 10 ml/kg of body weight. Not all of the gas that enters the lungs reaches the alveoli for gas exchange. Less than 3 ml/kg remains in the airways and is referred to as wasted ventilation. The remainder of the gas is distributed throughout the alveoli to take part in alveolar ventilation and represents the volume of gas truly available for gas exchange.

Effective ventilation requires an adequate gas volume, an intact respiratory center to stimulate respiration, and patent airways for the gas to travel to the lungs.

Distribution. The distribution stage of respiration provides for adequate movement of gas to the alveoli once it has arrived in the lungs. Normally, the distribution of gas in the lungs is uneven and position-dependent. In the upright position, gas is distributed in increasing amounts from the upper to the lower lobes, with the lower lobes ventilating more thoroughly than the upper. In the supine position, the distribution is more evenly regulated from base to apex, but the posterior lung receives more gas than the anterior. In the lateral position, the dependent lung is more thoroughly ventilated.

Effective distribution of gas in the alveoli is dependent on patent alveoli, lung compliance, an intact neuromuscular system, and adequate chest-wall structure. (Lung compliance, a measurement of the elasticity of the lungs depends on normal pressures in the intrathoracic cavity, intact pleurae, and adequate surfactant.)

Diffusion. The diffusion stage of respiration involves the movement of gas across the alveolar-capillary membrane. This movement is determined by three factors: tissue area, tissue thickness, and the pressure gradient between alveolar and capillary blood. Diffusion across the membrane is described by Fick's law, which states that the rate of transfer of a gas through a sheet of tissue is proportional to the tissue area and inversely proportional to the tissue thickness.[2] Infants and young children have less alveolar surface area for gas exchange than older children or adults because respiratory system growth is not complete until 12 years of age. Normally, in the adult, the alveolar-capillary membrane is very thin (less than 0.5 micron), with an area of approximately 50 to 100 square meters. These dimensions enhance gas transfer. In addition, gas transfer is regulated by the partial pressure of oxygen (PO_2) and the partial pressure of carbon dioxide (PCO_2) in the blood and alveoli. On the average, the normal partial pressure of oxygen in the alveoli (PAO_2) is 95-100 mmHg; in the pulmonary artery (PaO_2) it is 40 mmHg. The normal partial pressure of carbon dioxide in the alveoli ($PACO_2$) is 40 mmHg; in the pulmonary artery ($PaCO_2$) it is 46 mmHg. The difference between the partial pressure of each gas creates a pressure gradient. This gradient promotes gas exchange: it causes gas to flow from the higher pressure region to the lower until equilibrium is achieved. It is because of this pressure gradient that oxygen moves from the alveoli to the pulmonary capillaries and carbon dioxide moves from the bloodstream to the alveoli. Diffusion of carbon dioxide across the membrane occurs as rapidly as the diffusion of oxygen even though the pressure gradient is much smaller. This is because the rate at which gas diffuses also depends on the solubility of the gas. Since carbon dioxide has a much higher solubility than oxygen, it diffuses about 20 times more rapidly. Therefore, carbon dioxide transfer can occur as fast as oxygen diffusion, despite a much smaller gradient.

Disruptions in diffusion occur when the tissue area is decreased, tissue thickness is increased, or the pressure gradients of oxygen and carbon dioxide are altered by pathology.

Transportation. The final stage of respiration is transportation. During this stage, oxygen, now dissolved in plasma or carried by hemoglobin, travels to the tissues where it is exchanged for carbon dioxide. The effectiveness of the transportation stage is dependent on adequate circulation, particularly on pulmonary blood flow. Hemoglobin must be available, as well as a sufficient cardiac output to supply blood to the pulmonary circulation. Normally, the distribution of blood flow in the lungs is uneven and (as with the distribution of gas) position-dependent. Blood flow to the lungs decreases from bottom to top in the upright position, and is more evenly distributed in the supine position and during exercise. Because of the uneven distribution of gas and blood flow, some areas of the lungs are not always ventilated, and some areas of the pulmonary circulation do not always have blood circulated through them. As a result a small percentage of pulmonary venous blood returns to the left atrium unoxygenated. This phenomenon, a normal occurrence, is known as physiological shunting.

Disruptions in the transportation stage occur when there is an increase in the amount of unoxygenated blood returning to the left atrium. For every 4 liters of gas distributed in the lungs, 5 liters of blood are circulated in the pulmonary vasculature. This relationship is known as the ventilation-perfusion ratio. When this ratio is disturbed, a ventilation-perfusion inequality exists. Ventilation-perfusion inequalities occur when (1) venous blood bypasses alveoli that are collapsed or limited in their diffusion capabilities and therefore unable to receive oxygen, or (2) alveoli that are adequately ventilated do not receive adequate blood flow or hemoglobin for the oxygen to dissolve into and be transported.

Certain pulmonary diseases that cause regional overinflation of alveoli (asthma, bronchopulmonary dysplasia) also cause ventilation-perfusion inequalities because this overinflation results in a decreased blood flow to the region. In addition, acidosis and hypoxia, which cause vasoconstriction, contribute to ventilation-perfusion inequalities.

Some of the disease processes listed in Table 2-3 are associated with disruptions in more than one stage of respiration. Understanding the various stages also involves integrating them and realizing how interrelated the body systems are. Because no one system functions independently, no one disease process affects only one system.

BLOOD GAS TRANSPORT

Hemoglobin

The protein hemoglobin, which transports oxygen to the tissues and removes carbon dioxide from them, is the major component of red blood cells. Each hemoglobin molecule is composed of thousands of hydrogen, carbon, nitrogen, oxygen, and sulfur atoms, but it is its four iron atoms that enable it to carry oxygen.

The hemoglobin molecule consists of two parts, the heme portion and the globin portion. Heme is the result of a ferrous ion binding to a porphyrin ring. Each ferrous ion has six potential valence bonds, four of which attach to four nitrogen ions on the porphyrin ring (Fig. 2-1).

The protein globin results when four specific chains of amino acids (two alpha

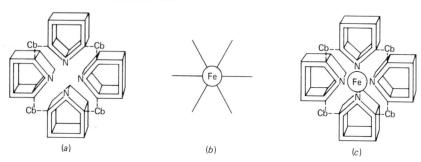

Figure 2-1. Chemical structure of heme. The binding of (A) a porphyrin ring with (B) a ferrous ion (Fe) results in (C) the heme portion of hemoglobin. The nitrogen ions (N) in the porphyrin ring combine with four of the six potential bonds of the ferrous ion. Cb, carbon. *Reprinted with permission from* Shapiro, B. A., R. A. Harrison, and J. R. Walton. 1977. Clinical Application of Blood Gases. Year Book Medical Publishers, Inc., Chicago. Second edition.

and two beta) are combined. The nitrogen in this resultant protein chain forms a bond with the ferrous ion. This bond constitutes the fifth potential bond of the ferrous ion. The sixth potential bond remains available for oxygen. Because the hemoglobin molecule is actually composed of four heme molecules attached to four globin chains, there are four atoms of iron in the hemoglobin molecule that can bind to oxygen (Fig. 2-2).

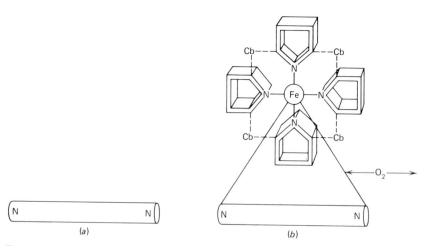

Figure 2-2. Chemical structure of hemoglobin. The binding of (A) the protein globin chain with the fifth potential bond of the ferrous ion (Fe) in the heme molecule forms (B) hemoglobin, and allows the sixth potential bond to be available for oxygen (O_2). (Hemoglobin is actually composed of four heme molecules and four globin chains, thus allowing four potential bonding sites for O_2.) Cb, carbon; N, nitrogen. *Reprinted with permission from* Shapiro, B. A., R. A. Harrison, and J. R. Walton. 1977. Clinical Application of Blood Gases. Year Book Medical Publishers, Inc., Chicago. Second edition.

When four molecules of oxygen bind to the four available atoms of iron, the hemoglobin is called oxyhemoglobin. This chemical bonding of oxygen to hemoglobin results in the red color of arterial blood. Reduced (nonoxygenated) hemoglobin has a purplish color.

Oxygen combines reversibly with hemoglobin. This enables hemoglobin to accept oxygen from the lungs and transport it to body tissues, where it is released. The actual delivery of oxygen, however, depends on oxygen affinity, which is the ability of the hemoglobin molecule to release or bind with an oxygen molecule. The concept of oxygen affinity and the factors affecting it are best explained by means of the oxyhemoglobin dissociation curve.

Oxyhemoglobin Dissociation Curve

For normal respiration and body metabolism to occur, oxygen must be delivered to all tissues. In order for oxygen to be successfully transported, an adequate concentration of hemoglobin must be available.

When blood is exposed to oxygen, the amount of oxygen that can be dissolved in the blood is proportional to the PO_2 (Henry's law). When oxygen enters the red cell, it attaches to a hemoglobin molecule. Gas diffusion continues to occur until the pressure gradient of the gas (oxygen) equals that of the solution (blood). At this point, hemoglobin is said to be equilibrated to the corresponding PO_2. If the PO_2 is increased, the oxyhemoglobin saturation will also increase, until a pressure gradient no longer exists. This relationship between the PO_2 and the percent saturation of hemoglobin is expressed by the oxyhemoglobin dissociation curve (Fig. 2-3).

This S-shaped (sigmoid) curve is steep between 10 and 50 mmHg of PO_2. A gentler rise is noted between 50 and 70 mmHg of PO_2 with the curve flattening out between 70 and 100 mmHg. The partial pressure of oxygen in normal arterial blood (PaO_2) is 97 mmHg, which corresponds to an oxyhemoglobin saturation of 97 percent.

The position of this curve is important, since it will vary with changes in pH, body temperature, and the partial pressure of arterial carbon dioxide ($PaCO_2$). In general, alkalosis, hypothermia, and hypocapnia will cause the curve to shift to the left. This shift implies that, for any given PO_2 there is an increased oxyhemoglobin saturation, which will increase the hemoglobin's oxygen-transport capabilities. However, because of hemoglobin's strong affinity for oxygen, it is now less able to release it, and this may cause a decrease in oxygenation of the tissues.

Conversely, the oxyhemoglobin dissociation curve is shifted to the right as a result of acidosis, fever, and hypercapnia. This shift implies that, for any given PO_2 there is a decreased amount of available oxyhemoglobin and, consequently, of oxygen-transport capabilities. Nevertheless, this shift will result in increased oxygen movement from the hemoglobin to the tissues because dissociation of oxygen from hemoglobin is easier at lower saturation levels (Fig. 2-4).

Severe acidosis or hypercapnia, however, may result in a sudden shift to the right. If this shift is extreme, it will decrease oxygen transport and the oxygen available to the tissues, despite easy dissociation of the oxygen from the hemoglobin.

Because of these variables, it is preferable to measure PaO_2 and oxygen saturation directly and independently rather than deriving one value from the other. If only one measurement can be obtained, the PaO_2 is a better guide to correct oxygen administration.

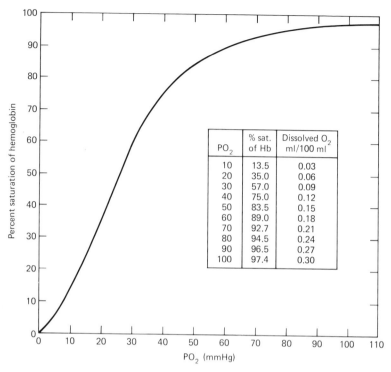

PO$_2$	% sat. of Hb	Dissolved O$_2$ ml/100 ml
10	13.5	0.03
20	35.0	0.06
30	57.0	0.09
40	75.0	0.12
50	83.5	0.15
60	89.0	0.18
70	92.7	0.21
80	94.5	0.24
90	96.5	0.27
100	97.4	0.30

Percent saturation of hemoglobin

PO$_2$ (mmHg)

Figure 2-3. Oxyhemoglobin dissociation curve. The percentage of hemoglobin (Hb) saturated with oxygen (O$_2$) is dependent on the partial pressure of oxygen (PO$_2$). This curve is applicable when the pH of the blood is 7.4 and the body temperature is 37°C (98.6°F). *Reprinted with permission from* Comroe, J. H., R. E. Forster, A. B. Dubois, W. A. Briscoe, and E. Carlsen. 1962. The Lung: Clinical Physiology and Pulmonary Function Tests. Year Book Medical Publishers, Inc., Chicago. Second edition.

Oxygen transport.   Oxygen is transported in the blood in two forms: (1) dissolved in the plasma and red cells and (2) bound to hemoglobin. Dissolved oxygen represents approximately 1 percent of the total amount of oxygen transported. This percentage is insignificant: it is hemoglobin that accounts for most of the oxygen carried to the tissues. When fully saturated, 1 gram of hemoglobin is capable of carrying 1.39 milliliters of oxygen.

As oxygenated blood flows into the systemic capillaries, oxygen diffuses into the tissues because of the gradient created by the PO$_2$. As the PO$_2$ decreases in the plasma, the dissolved oxygen in the red cell diffuses out, causing a decrease in the PO$_2$ in the red cell. This decrease causes oxyhemoglobin to dissociate into free oxygen. Thus, the degree of oxygen dissociation from hemoglobin is directly related to the PO$_2$. The hemoglobin is not completely desaturated as it circulates through the systemic capillaries. A large oxygen reserve is available for any increase in the needs of the tissues. Even in venous blood there is still a relatively large amount of oxygen bound to the hemoglobin.

Carbon dioxide transport.   Carbon dioxide is eliminated from the body through the lungs; it is transported from the tissues to the lungs via the blood. There are three

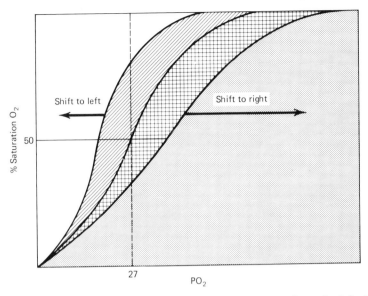

Figure 2-4. Affinity of hemoglobin for oxygen (O_2). The curve shifts to the left with alkalemia, hypothermia, and hypocapnia, meaning that there will be a higher O_2 content at any given partial pressure of oxygen (PO_2). The curve shifts to the right with acidemia, hyperthermia, and hypercapnia, meaning that there will be a lower O_2 content at any given PO_2. *Reprinted with permission from* Shapiro, B. A., R. A. Harrison, and J. R. Walton. 1977. Clinical Application of Blood Gases. Year Book Medical Publishers, Inc., Chicago. Second edition.

mechanisms for carbon dioxide transport in the blood: (1) physically dissolved carbon dioxide, (2) carbon dioxide chemically combined with amino acids, and (3) carbon dioxide converted to bicarbonate and hydrogen.

The physically dissolved carbon dioxide is responsible for only 10 percent of the carbon dioxide transported by hemoglobin.

Carbon dioxide chemically combined with hemoglobin is responsible for 20 to 30 percent of the carbon dioxide transported. (Unlike oxygen, the carbon dioxide molecule does not combine with the iron ion, but with the amino acids to form a carbamino compound, which is then transported in the blood in this form.)

Approximately 60 percent of the carbon dioxide transported in the blood is converted to bicarbonate and hydrogen. As blood flows through the systemic capillaries, carbon dioxide enters the plasma from the tissues. A small portion of carbon dioxide remains in the plasma, but most of it enters the red blood cell. Once the carbon dioxide is inside the cell, a small amount of it attaches to hemoglobin to form the carbamino-carbon dioxide compound. A larger amount of carbon dioxide is hydrated to form carbonic acid by the presence of the enzyme carbonic anhydrase. Carbonic acid is then dissociated into bicarbonate and hydrogen ions (Fig. 2-5).

The hydrogen ions are buffered by the hemoglobin. Because of the increasing carbon dioxide content of the red blood cell, the bicarbonate ions diffuse into the plasma. As the bicarbonate ion leaves the cell, it is exchanged for chloride. This is known as the chloride shift, because chloride levels decrease as a result of in-

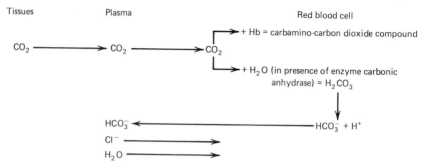

Figure 2-5. Carbon dioxide (CO_2) transport. See discussion on p. 31. Cl^-, chloride ion; H^+, hydrogen ion; Hb, hemoglobin; HCO_3^-, bicarbonate ion; H_2CO_3, carbonic acid; H_2O, water. *Adapted with permission from* Shapiro, B. A., R. A. Harrison, and J. R. Walton. 1977. Clinical Application of Blood Gases. Year Book Medical Publishers, Inc., Chicago. Second edition.

creasing bicarbonate concentration. As the carbon dioxide levels continue to rise in the red blood cell, water diffuses into the cell from the plasma. This diffusion of water causes the cells to expand as the arterial blood becomes venous blood.

Oxygenated hemoglobin is a stronger acid than reduced hemoglobin: when the oxyhemoglobin in arterial blood loses its oxygen to the cells it becomes a weak acid. This increases the blood's ability to allow carbon dioxide to bind with the hemoglobin for transport. As the blood passes through the lungs and oxygenation occurs, the hemoglobin becomes a strong acid and the bicarbonate and carbamino compounds are broken down, thereby enabling carbon dioxide to be expelled through the lungs. The relationship of oxygen to carbon dioxide transport is described by the Bohr effect and the Haldane effect. The Bohr effect states that the addition of carbon dioxide to the blood will encourage oxygen to be released from the hemoglobin. The Haldane effect states that the addition of oxygen to the blood will encourage the release of carbon dioxide from the hemoglobin molecule.

PRINCIPLES OF NURSING CARE

All individuals must have adequate ventilation and respiration to ensure optimal oxygenation to all body cells. The critical care nurse must be able to assess disruptions in normal ventilation that could potentially endanger the life of the seriously ill child. To assess adequately for disruptions and deliver complex nursing care, the critical care nurse needs an in-depth understanding of respiratory physiology and pathophysiology. The nurse then integrates this knowledge with the social and psychological needs of the child and family.

The most important principle of nursing care of the child with acute respiratory failure is to ensure the safety of the child's airway and prevent respiratory arrest. Airway obstruction in children can occur rapidly and from many causes. In infants, airway obstruction is frequently the result of incorrect head position. If the infant's head is hyperextended, the pliable tracheal cartilage can collapse. Airway obstruction in small children is often caused by the aspiration of foreign bodies and/or by infection. The small tracheal diameter in children is compromised easily by the inflammation and edema that result from infection. In children of all ages, airway obstruction is often the result of an inability to deal with increased secretions.

Close observation and assessment are necessary to ensure the safety of the child's airway. The patency of the airway is evaluated by assessment of the child's color and level of consciousness and by auscultation of breath sounds. This overall picture of the child's clinical condition, along with the results of diagnostic studies, provides the continuum for assessing the child's respiratory status, including airway patency and the prevention of respiratory arrest. Specific measures that maintain the patency of the airway include frequent suctioning, the maintenance of good body alignment, and, if necessary, insertion of an artificial airway.

A second principle of nursing care of the child with acute respiratory failure is to ease the child's respiratory effort. The first step in this process is the evaluation of the degree of fatigue and anxiety that the child is experiencing. The child in respiratory distress can be the victim of a vicious circle. As the child works harder at breathing to combat an existing hypoxia and/or hypercapnia, the child's anxiety increases. Initially, this anxiety exhibits itself as tachypnea. However, over a period of time, the child tires and respiratory effort diminishes. The child becomes increasingly hypoxic and/or hypercapnic, and, unless interrupted, this circle can terminate in respiratory arrest.

Along with protecting the natural airway of the child, elevating the head of the bed is a measure that eases the fatigue of the child's respiratory distress. This measure helps to promote optimal gas exchange by forcing down the diaphragm, thereby increasing lung expansion. Supplemental oxygen, administered to relieve hypoxia, also eases the work of breathing.

Additional measures to decrease the child's respiratory effort include the establishment of an artificial airway, the use of mechanical ventilation, chest physiotherapy, and neuromuscular blockade. All these measures are frightening, however, and can contribute to the child's feeling of helplessness, which, coupled with the fear of inadequate respiration and hypoxia, increases the child's level of anxiety.

Anxiety may be lessened by minimizing environmental stimuli and providing a calm, reassuring atmosphere. Imparting essential information to the family helps to decrease *their* anxiety. The family should be included in developing the child's plan of care, and their participation in effecting this plan should be encouraged.

All these measures are instrumental in maintaining a safe airway and easing the child's work of respiration. They should always be considered when providing care to the child with acute respiratory failure, regardless of the etiology and/or pathophysiology.

NURSING ASSESSMENT OF
THE RESPIRATORY SYSTEM

Assessment of a child's respiratory function begins with a physical examination that primarily involves inspection, observation, and auscultation. By observing the child's color, level of consciousness, and breathing effort, the nurse can determine if normal respiratory function has been compromised. Listening to breath sounds helps to identify how and where gas exchange has been disrupted.

This information can then be interpreted in conjunction with the results of various respiratory diagnostic studies. A plan of care can then be developed.

Physical Examination

Color.   Changes in skin color may be the earliest indicators of hypoxia. Color changes are most reliably assessed in those areas of the body where there is the least melanin production: sclera, conjunctiva, nail beds, lips, buccal mucosa, palms, and soles.[3] Oxygenated hemoglobin normally gives the skin a rosy color. Cyanosis, a significant observation that may indicate cardiopulmonary disease, results when there is an increased amount of deoxygenated hemoglobin circulating in the body. The following are the most common causes of cyanosis in children:[4]

1. Alveolar hypoventilation.
2. Uneven distribution of gas and blood throughout the lungs.
3. Anatomic right-to-left shunts of blood that occur in some forms of congenital heart disease.
4. Disruptions in alveolocapillary diffusion.

Central nervous system indicators.   As a child's oxygen tension decreases or $PaCO_2$ level increases, the nurse may observe changes in the level of consciousness. These changes can begin as restlessness, agitation, and irritability, and can progress to confusion, combativeness, and inappropriate behavior.

When oxygen deprivation affects tissues, metabolism changes from aerobic to anaerobic, thereby increasing the levels of lactic acid. When carbon dioxide levels rise, the central controls of respiration are stimulated to increase ventilation by hyperventilating. "Most of the autonomic effects associated with high $PaCO_2$ (e.g., increased pulmonary vascular resistance, bronchoconstriction, increased cardiac output, and increased ventilation) are secondary to the pH changes caused by hypercapnia."[5] The increased $PaCO_2$ and the anerobic metabolism result in both a respiratory and a metabolic acidosis. The child's system will attempt to preserve cerebral functioning by an alteration in vital signs, most significantly in the respiratory rate. However, if these conditions continue, and the brain is deprived of oxygen for longer than 4 minutes, irreversible damage can occur.

Respiratory function.   Observation of respiratory effort involves evaluation of respirations for rate, pattern, depth, and quality.

Rate: The child's rate of respiration will vary with age and development. (Table 2-4 lists the normal respiratory rates for different ages.)

The usual ratio of respirations to heart rate is 1:4. Critically ill children vary their respiratory rate to meet the needs of their bodies (as in, for example, septic shock, congestive heart failure, and central nervous system depression or injury).

Pattern: In the newborn, normal functions (i.e., crying, eating, and sleeping) can cause an irregular pattern of respiration. Respirations assume a more regular pattern after infancy. (The most common patterns of respiration are described in Table 2-5.)

Depth: The depth of respiration refers to the volume of air moving in and out of the lungs. (Changes in depth of respiration are described in Table 2-6.)

Quality: The quality of respiration should be automatic, effortless, and silent. During normal breathing, the diaphragm is used to initiate inspiration. Expiration

TABLE 2-4 Respiratory Rates of Children and Adults

Age	Normal range
	(breaths/min)
Newborn	30–50
1–6 months	20–45
6 months–2 years	20–40
2 years–6 years	20–30
6 years–12 years	12–30
Adult	12–20

occurs passively as these muscles relax. The ratio of inspiration to expiration is 1:1.5 in the younger child, and increases to 1:2 by adulthood.

Signs of respiratory compromise. Common signs of respiratory compromise are dyspnea, retractions, grunting, stridor, and nasal flaring. When these and other signs of respiratory distress occur on inspiration they are indicative of obstruction in the large airways (i.e., trachea, main-stem bronchi). Conversely, when they occur during expiration, they indicate obstruction in the smaller airways (i.e., bronchi and bronchioles).

Dyspnea: In the child, dyspnea (a sensation of shortness of breath) is usually accompanied by the use of accessory muscles. The dyspneic child uses accessory muscles of the shoulders, neck, and trunk to help in raising the ribs and compressing the diaphragm. In exhalation, the dyspneic child uses abdominal muscles to forcibly exhale by pushing up the relaxed diaphragm. (Costal breathing is consid-

TABLE 2-5 Patterns of Respirations

Type	Pattern	Description	Associated pathologies
Normal		Rapid and shallow	Stress, surgery, sepsis
Painful		Irregular pattern	Respiratory distress syndrome, increased intracranial pressure
Periodic			
Biot's		Increased depth and rate (each breath the same) with periods of apnea	Central nervous system problems, meningitis
Kussmaul's		Increased depth and rate	Metabolic acidosis, renal failure, diabetic ketoacidosis
Cheyne-Stokes		Gradual increase in depth and rate followed by periods of apnea	Decreased intracranial pressure, congestive heart failure, meningitis, drug overdose, renal failure

TABLE 2-6 Changes in Depth of Respiration

Type	Pattern	Description	Associated pathologies
Hypopnea	～～～	Decreased depth and normal rate (shallow respiration)	Metabolic alkalosis, pyloric stenosis, respiratory acidosis
Hyperpnea	∧∧∧∧	Increased depth and normal rate	Fever, severe anemia, salicylate overdose, diarrhea
Hypoventilation	⌣⌣⌣	Decreased depth and rate, (very shallow respirations)	Narcotic or barbiturate overdose, carbon dioxide narcosis, anesthesia
Hyperventilation	∧∧∧∧∧	Increased depth and rate (regular pattern)	Exertion, fever, pain, fear

ered normal in young children: these muscles stabilize the ribs so the diaphragm can function more efficiently.) When accompanied by retractions, dyspnea is an indication of increased respiratory effort.

Retractions: Retractions are the drawing in of the soft tissue around the thorax. They are identified and differentiated by their location, and are most frequently associated with obstructive and restrictive diseases.

Grunting: This is an abnormal sound produced upon expiration. It increases end-expiratory pressure by maintaining the patency of small airways and promoting gas exchange. Grunting is frequently heard in infants with respiratory distress syndrome, and in children who are in pain, in left-sided heart failure, or who have infections.

Stridor: Stridor is a harsh sound heard on inspiration. It is usually caused by laryngeal or tracheal obstruction.

Nasal flaring: Nasal flaring is another sign of respiratory compromise. It is seen in children of all ages and indicates an attempt to improve oxygen intake.

Auscultation of Breath Sounds

A stethoscope is used to assess the different sounds produced in the chest through the work of respiration. The diaphragm of the stethoscope is generally used for pulmonary auscultation because breath sounds are higher pitched than heart sounds. Auscultation of breath sounds is performed in a routine pattern by first listening to the anterior lobes and then to the lateral and posterior lobes. Listening to the areas of the lung field in this way allows for comparison of the sounds heard on corresponding sides. Breath sounds are best heard with the child in an upright position and taking deep breaths on command; however, this is rarely possible with the critically ill child, whose illness does not permit assuming this position or extending adequate cooperation.

Breath sounds, produced by the movement of air through the tracheobronchial tree, may be normal, abnormal, or adventitious.

TABLE 2-7 Normal Breath Sounds

Breath sound	Pitch	Intensity	Quality	Normal location
Bronchial	High	Expiration louder and longer than inspiration	Hollow (tubular)	Over trachea
Broncho-vesicular	Moderate	Inspiration and expiration equal	Harsh	Over manu-brium (bifur-cation of bronchi)
Vesicular	Low	Inspiration louder and longer than expiration	Soft, swishing	Over most of chest

Normal breath sounds. There are three kinds of normal breath sounds: bronchial, bronchovesicular, and vesicular. They are described according to pitch, intensity, quality, and normal locations (Table 2-7).

Abnormal breath sounds. When bronchial and bronchovesicular breath sounds are heard anywhere other than in their normal locations they are considered abnormal breath sounds. They occur when lung tissue becomes consolidated or compressed, as in pneumonia and atelectasis. Absent or diminished breath sounds in any portion of the respiratory tract may result from pleural effusion, pneumo- or hemothorax, atelectasis, bronchial obstruction, hypoventilation, or bronchopulmonary dysplasia.

Adventitious breath sounds. Adventitious breath sounds (Table 2-8) are superimposed on normal breath sounds and almost always indicate pathology. There are three kinds of adventitious breath sounds: rales, rhonchi, and pleural friction rubs. Rales and rhonchi are produced by the movement of air through a narrowed passageway. Pleural friction rubs occur when there is a disruption in the visceral and parietal linings of the pleura. The most common causes of adventitious breath sounds are fluid, secretions, edema, inflammation, exudate, bronchospasm, tumors, and foreign bodies.

Auscultation of breath sounds is an important aspect of nursing assessment of all critically ill children, and is crucial in the assessment of the child with an artificial airway. It is one of the most accurate methods for evaluating the position of an endotracheal or a tracheostomy tube. If bilateral breath sounds of equal intensity are not heard upon auscultation, it is quite probable that the tube is misplaced, especially in the presence of other corroborating clinical signs. The tip of an endotracheal tube should lie at the level of midtrachea. A tube that is too high will produce diminished breath sounds upon auscultation. If the tube is too

TABLE 2-8 Adventitious Breath Sounds

Type	Pitch	Sound	Intensity	Location
Rales (nonmusical, discontinuous)				
Fine	Low	Crackling	Loudest at the end of inspiration	Alveoli and small bronchioles
Medium	Moderate	Bubbling	Loudest halfway through inspiration	Larger passages of bronchioles and small bronchi
Coarse	High	Gurgling	Loudest early in inspiration	Trachea, bronchi
Rhonchi (musical, continuous)				
Sibilant	High	Wheezing	Louder on expiration	Smaller bronchi and bronchioles
Sonorous	Low	Snoring	Louder on expiration	Trachea, bronchi
Pleural friction rubs	Moderate	Grating	Heard on inspiration and expiration; louder at the end of expiration	Lower anterolateral chest wall

low, it will slide into the right or left main-stem bronchus and produce diminished breath sounds in the opposite chest. When a tracheostomy tube has been improperly inserted into the subcutaneous tissue, breath sounds will be absent.

The critically ill child requires frequent auscultation of breath sounds. They should be noted before and after chest physiotherapy and compared for any change. Some pulmonary changes can be identified by auscultation before they appear on chest x-rays. For example, fine rales may be auscultated in the child with pneumonia before any pulmonary changes are seen on the chest x-ray.

Diagnostic Studies for Respiratory Assessment

A number of diagnostic studies contribute valuable information for the assessment of the respiratory system. An understanding of these studies enables the critical care nurse to make decisions based on the information they provide, as well as to educate and assist the child undergoing the test. This discussion of the diagnostic tools used in respiratory assessment will include chest x-rays, arterial blood gases, mixed venous blood gases, end tidal carbon dioxide monitoring, and cutaneous oxygen monitoring.

Chest x-rays.   Chest x-rays can help identify lung pathology as well as indicate the position of an endotracheal tube. Chest x-rays are frequently taken in the intensive care unit to monitor the patient's progress.

The nurse of the critically ill child should have an understanding of the basic chest x-ray. This is particularly important because the nurse is often the first person to see the film. Basic x-ray interpretation depends on understanding density, contrast, and the technical concerns that affect the quality of the film.

Density: Density refers to the degree of blackness evident on a film. It is determined by the amount of x-ray energy reaching the film: the greater the energy reaching the film, the more exposed (or blacker) that portion of the film will be. X-rays are absorbed in varying degrees by the different body organs: the greater the amount absorbed by the body, the lighter that part of the film.

Four kinds of densities are seen in a chest film: air, water, fat, and bone or metal (Table 2-9). Air density appears in films of the normal lung, trachea, and bronchi. Because a minimal amount of x-ray is absorbed by these parts, they produce the darkest portion of the film. Water density occurs when x-ray energy passes through soft-tissue structures composed mainly of water. These include the heart, the great vessels, muscle, and blood, which all appear lighter than the structures characterized by air density. Fat density is lighter than water density and occurs

TABLE 2-9 X-ray Density

Density	Body structures	Degree of energy absorbtion	Resultant color in x-ray
Air	Lung, trachea, bronchi	Minimal	Black
Water	Heart, great vessels, muscle, blood		
Fat	Subcutaneous tissue		
Bone or metal	Ribs, clavicles, scapulae sternum, vertebrae	Maximum	White

when x-rays pass through subcutaneous tissue. Bone density results in the lightest part of the film and indicates the greatest amount of energy absorption. Bone density in a chest x-ray is produced by the ribs, clavicles, scapulae, sternum, and vertebrae.

Contrast: Structures are distinguished on x-ray by different or contrasting densities surrounding them. Under normal circumstances, x-rays are not discriminating enough to demonstrate the wall of a normal bronchus against the background of the normal lung because both structures are characterized by air density. The cardiac silhouette is easily discernible, however, because the water density of the heart and great vessels contrasts with the air density of the lung. It is necessary to know the normal densities of the chest x-ray in order to identify pathology.

Two terms related to contrast that are used in chest film interpretation are the *air bronchogram sign* and the *silhouette sign*. The air bronchogram sign is seen when lung tissue surrounding a bronchus becomes atelectatic or filled with fluid and thus acquires a water density. This tissue now contrasts with the air density of the bronchus and makes the normally invisible air-filled bronchus visible on x-ray. The *air bronchogram* sign identifies disease processes such as pneumonia and pulmonary edema. The *silhouette* sign appears when the edges of the heart are not clear and sharply distinguishable from the air density of the surrounding lungs. This occurs when atelectasis or pneumonia is present in that lung tissue. (Pneumothorax produces a darker-than-normal air density and is recognized when no lung markings are seen at the periphery.)

Technical concerns: In the intensive care setting, portable chest x-rays are most often used. Portable chest x-rays are inferior to those taken in the x-ray department because of the increased proximity of the x-ray machine. The recommended distance between machine and film is 6 feet. Portable films result in an increased magnification that may be mistaken for pathology. Because it is uncommon for a pathological change to be bilateral, the nurse should compare both sides of the chest film when the chest x-ray appears abnormal. If the same shadow appears on both sides, it is probably due to increased magnification.

Other factors that influence the quality of a chest x-ray include the position or the angle of the film, the phase of the child's respiration, and the motion or rotation of the child while the film is being taken. The child should be upright or flat in bed to provide a perpendicular angle between the x-ray beam and the child's body. (If an angle of less than 90 degrees is used, the lung fields appear foreshortened: this is referred to as a lordotic film.) In addition, a chest x-ray should be taken on inspiration because, if taken on expiration, the heart may appear enlarged and the lung fields cloudy. When a child is unable to remain flat and still against the x-ray plate, the resulting film often appears blurred and gives a false impression of mediastinal shift. Electrocardiogram (ECG) leads and wires on the child's chest should be removed to provide an accurate chest film. Nurses aware of these factors can reduce the incidence of poor films that must be repeated. A final but important consideration when chest x-rays are being taken is to ensure that lead shields are used to prevent unnecessary exposure to radiation.

Arterial blood gases.   Arterial blood gas (ABG) monitoring is a necessary component of evaluating the critically ill child. Because ABG measurements are commonly used to determine treatment and management, a knowledge of normal values is essential for the critical care nurse (Table 2-10). A change in these values provides the nurse with information on the functioning of the lungs and kidneys. In addition, the ABG analysis is often used to wean the patient from ventilatory support and to assess the child's readiness for extubation and/or decannulation.

TABLE 2-10   Normal Blood Gas Measurements in Children

Measurement	Definition	Normal arterial values	Normal venous values
pH	Hydrogen-ion concentration (reflects acid-base disturbances)	7.35–7.45 (7.40)	7.31–7.41 (7.36)
PO_2	Partial pressure of oxygen (O_2 tension)	75–100 mmHg	35–45 mmHg
PCO_2	Partial pressure of carbon dioxide (CO_2 tension)	35–45 mmHg	41–51 mmHg
O_2 sat	Oxygen saturation (percentage of hemoglobin carrying oxygen	95–98%	65–85%
HCO_3^-	Bicarbonate-ion concentration (reflects acid-base disturbances)	22–26 mEq/liter	22–26 mEq/liter

ABG measurements are extremely valuable in the management of the critically ill child because any alterations that disrupt normal body function (e.g., fever, sepsis, surgery, stress, shock, shivering, or seizures) will increase oxygen consumption and, therefore, increase oxygen demand. ABGs can also be useful for rapidly assessing the critically ill child's response to various treatments.

Analyzing ABGs should be done routinely by the critical care nurse. This analysis should begin by determining if the child's pH indicates acidosis or alkalosis. (It must be borne in mind that ABG measurements should always be used in conjuction with clinical assessment of the child.)

Respiratory acidosis: Respiratory acidosis occurs because of ventilatory failure, which decreases alveolar ventilation. This is reflected clinically by a rise in the PCO_2, which causes an increase in hydrogen-ion concentration and a decrease in the pH. Respiratory acidosis can be either an acute or a chronic problem.

There are three specific factors that can decrease alveolar ventilation: (1) depression of the respiratory center in the medulla from drugs or trauma, (2) decreased ventilation because of airway resistance from pulmonary disease (e.g., infection, asthma, or pneumonia), or (3) loss of structural chest wall and muscle tone because of a paralyzing disease (e.g., Guillain-Barré syndrome or poliomyelitis). When respiratory disturbances accompany any of these clinical problems, the PCO_2 rises and respiratory acidosis occurs.

The body attempts to meet this crisis by compensating. Compensation is a secondary physiological process that occurs in response to disturbances in acid-base balance. With respiratory acidosis, compensation is achieved in the kidneys by the retention of bicarbonate ions and the excretion of hydrogen ions. The pH of the excreted urine will thus be acidic. This compensatory mechanism is most evident in chronic respiratory acidosis because this form of acidosis allows the kidneys enough time to compensate.

TABLE 2-11 Clinical Signs and Symptoms of Respiratory Acidosis and Respiratory Alkalosis

	Respiratory acidosis	Respiratory alkalosis
Causes	Hypoventilation Central nervous system depressants Pulmonary diseases Asthma	Hyperventilation Brain tumors Anxiety Salicylate poisoning
Clinical signs	Decreased respiratory rate Dulled sensorium Tachycardia Coma, cyanosis (late signs)	Tachypnea Kussmaul's breathing Anxiousness Fear Light-headedness
Laboratory values	Decreased pH Normal PaO_2 Increased $PaCO_2$ Normal HCO_3^-	Increased pH Normal PaO_2 Decreased $PaCO_2$ Normal HCO_3^-
Compensated values	Normal or decreased pH Normal PaO_2 Increased $PaCO_2$ Increased HCO_3^-	Normal or increased pH Normal PaO_2 Decreased $PaCO_2$ Decreased HCO_3^-
Treatment	Treat underlying cause; provide airway; provide adequate ventilation	Treat underlying cause; employ rebreather mask

HCO_3^-, bicarbonate-ion concentration; $PaCO_2$, partial pressure of arterial carbon dioxide; PaO_2, partial pressure of arterial oxygen.

Respiratory alkalosis: Respiratory alkalosis results from an increase in alveolar ventilation, which decreases the PCO_2 levels. Some of the causes of respiratory alkalosis are (1) stimulation of the respiratory center in the medulla (e.g., by drug overdose with salicylates or amphetamines), (2) a protective reflex stimulation of the respiratory center by peripheral chemoreceptors (e.g., hypoxia at high altitudes), and (3) reflex stimulation of the respiratory center by intrathoracic stretch receptors (e.g., localized pulmonary edema).

Compensation for respiratory alkalosis is achieved by the kidneys. Hydrogen is emptied into the bloodstream in exchange for potassium. This causes a decrease in serum potassium. The kidneys then excrete bicarbonate with either a sodium or potassium ion to avoid losing the hydrogen ion. However, if the kidneys are depleting the body's supply of potassium or sodium, they will protect this supply first and the acid-base imbalance will continue. (Table 2-11 compares respiratory acidosis with respiratory alkalosis.)

Mixed venous blood gases. The co-oximeter is a laboratory instrument that analyzes hemoglobin in various forms. Total hemoglobin, reported in grams per 100 milliliters, can be used to calculate oxygen content, which is a measurement that is crucial to the care of the critically ill child because it indicates the extent to which tissues are perfused with oxygen and cleansed of carbon dioxide. Oxygen content is calculated according to the following formula:

$$CaO_2 = (1.39 \times Hb \times \text{arterial saturation}) + (PaO_2 \times 0.003).$$

This equation states that oxygen content (CaO_2) is calculated by multiplying 1.39 (the value that represents 1 gram of hemoglobin [Hb] fully saturated with oxygen) by the child's Hb and by the child's arterial oxygen saturation, and then adding this figure to the value obtained when 0.003 (a constant that represents the amount of oxygen dissolved in the plasma) is multiplied by the child's PaO_2.

Oxygen content is useful in determining whether the supply (cardiac output) or the demand (oxygen consumption) is responsible for impaired tissue oxygenation. This relationship, first expressed by Adolph Fick, is known as the Fick principle:

$$VO_2 = (CaO_2 - CvO_2) \times CO.$$

This equation states that the volume of oxygen consumption (or the demand of oxygen for body functions, VO_2) is equal to the amount of oxygen available to the body (oxygen content of arterial blood, CaO_2) minus the amount of oxygen returned by the body (oxygen content of venous blood, CvO_2) multiplied by the cardiac output (CO).

These formulas are essential to the care of the critically ill child because no mass spectrometer, co-oximeter, or other laboratory machine can calculate a child's oxygen consumption. In the clinical application of these complex formulas, it is necessary to understand that the tissues will extract the number of oxygen molecules needed to meet the demand. To determine how much oxygen is used by the tissues, an arterial and a mixed venous blood gas are obtained simultaneously. A true mixed venous oxygen tension may be measured only in the outflow tract of the right ventricle: the pulmonary artery.[6] This measurement is obtained by drawing a blood gas from the distal end of a pulmonary artery catheter. (The value obtained by subtracting the CvO_2 from the CaO_2 is often referred to as the arterial-venous oxygen difference [A-VDO_2]. Table 2-12 provides a list of normal values for mixed venous oxygen and A-VDO_2.)

In the care of the critically ill child, the measurement of cardiac output, CaO_2, and CvO_2 is a prerequisite for determining the child's oxygen consumption. With this knowledge, physiological changes can be used to predict cardiovascular changes, because changes in mixed venous blood gases often occur before arterial blood gases reflect them.

Capnography. Capnography (end-tidal carbon dioxide monitoring) is a noninvasive technique that is painless and harmless. In recent years, capnography has become popular as an additional diagnostic tool in the management of critically ill children with respiratory disorders. Capnography is the measurement and registration of the carbon dioxide content in respiratory gases by means of a direct,

TABLE 2-12   Normal Values of Mixed Venous Blood Gases

Mixed venous parameter	Normal values
PvO_2	40 mmHg
$PvCO_2$	44–46 mmHg
pH	7.34–7.36
A-VDO_2	5 vol%*

A-VDO_2, arterial-venous oxygen difference; $PvCO_2$, mixed venous carbon dioxide tension; PvO_2, mixed venous oxygen tension.

*5 ml/oxygen per 100 ml/blood.

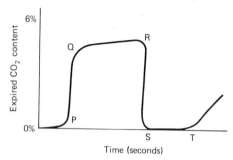

Figure 2-6.   Normal capnogram. At P, the expiration phase begins (carbon dioxide [CO_2] content rising); the Q–R "plateau" measures alveolar CO_2; at R, expiration ends and inspiration begins; at S-T, inspiration continues.

rapid analyzer.[7] The expired carbon dioxide content is recorded in the form of a wave (capnogram) and expressed numerically in percent or torr. (The normal capnogram wave for a single respiration is illustrated in Fig. 2-6.) The critical care nurse should be capable of interpreting either kind of recording.

Most analyzers record at two speeds in order to accommodate the recording of end-tidal carbon dioxide levels over a period of time as well as to demonstrate each respiration. Some models provide only a percentage reading. The end-tidal carbon dioxide measurement (in percent), when multiplied by 7.13 equates with the $PaCO_2$ in millimeters of mercury. (The value of 7.13 is based on the barometric pressure of 7.60, minus the water vapor pressure of 0.47.) For example, if the percentage reading is 5 percent (the normal value), the corresponding carbon dioxide value would be approximately 38 mmHg.

In the healthy individual, the end-tidal carbon dioxide closely approximates the arterial carbon dioxide. When a child has a respiratory disorder, however, mismatching of ventilation to perfusion interferes with normal delivery of carbon dioxide to the lungs. This results in an end-tidal carbon dioxide level that is lower than the arterial carbon dioxide. The difference between the two levels is known as the alveolar-arterial (A-a) gradient. Capnography is a useful diagnostic tool when used in addition to ABGs because it identifies the A-a gradient, which is an indicator of respiratory impairment. Comparison of periodic arterial carbon dioxide samples with end-tidal carbon dioxide readings provides an ongoing method of evaluating this gradient.

End-tidal carbon dioxide can be monitored over a long period of time, but is more often used intermittently to identify trends in the carbon dioxide levels without blood sampling. Although it has been established that the end-tidal carbon dioxide may be lower than the $PaCO_2$, the difference remains constant for many hours and is therefore a reliable indicator of carbon dioxide levels.[8]

Capnography is a recommended diagnostic tool for any child receiving respiratory support, particularly mechanical ventilation. The effectiveness of therapy can be readily identified without disturbing the child to obtain an arterial blood sample. When ventilation is inadequate, the end-tidal carbon dioxide will increase. Conversely, when a child is receiving excessive ventilation, the end-tidal carbon dioxide will fall. The appropriateness of increasing or decreasing ventilatory support can be determined by monitoring the end-tidal carbon dioxide and observing for abnormal increases or decreases after changes in settings.

It should be mentioned that the capnograph, in order to be a useful diagnostic tool, must be in optimal working condition. Proper maintenance and calibration of the machine are essential, along with the nurse's understanding of how the analyzer operates and of which mechanical problems will result in inaccurate or false readings.

Cutaneous oxygen monitoring.   Continuous estimation of the arterial oxygen tension (PaO_2) is now possible with the use of a cutaneous electrode. In 1973, Renate and Albert Huch refined the method for approximating PaO_2 noninvasively.[9,10] The electrode they devised contains a heating coil that dilates capillaries beneath the skin. The localized hyperemia facilitates a diffusion of oxygen through the skin, which is then measured by the electrode in millimeters of mercury. Cutaneous PO_2 readings are available in digital and graphic readouts. Cutaneous monitoring does not measure the exact PaO_2: it measures the amount of oxygen diffusing through the skin. Various studies, however, have demonstrated that there is a close correlation between cutanous readings and arterial blood samples, unless a condition of shock exists. The differences in the values are related to skin thickness and blood pressure, with variability increasing with age.

Cutaneous monitoring of PO_2 is extremely useful in the care of a child with a respiratory disorder because continuous monitoring identifies hypoxemia as it occurs. By means of this tool, nurses can observe for changes in the PO_2 associated with the child's care. Cutaneous PO_2 monitoring during suctioning, feeding, turning, and blood sampling has shown that all these procedures may be causes of hypoxemia. Immediate recognition of hypoxemia facilitates the nurse's response in correcting the PO_2. Better control of respiratory support systems is also possible with cutaneous PO_2 monitoring because the effects of adjustments in the fractional concentration of inspired oxygen (FIO_2), intermittent mandatory ventilation (IMV), and continuous positive airway pressure (CPAP) are available faster and without blood sampling. Cutaneous PO_2 monitoring is also useful in recognizing high levels of oxygen, which may result in oxygen toxicity.

The electrode is placed on the chest, and its position is changed every 2 hours to prevent the formation of blisters from the heating coil. As with the capnograph, the cutaneous PO_2 monitor needs proper maintenance and calibration to provide accurate readings, and the nursing staff must know how to operate and interpret data obtained from the monitor.

ACUTE RESPIRATORY FAILURE

Disruptions in the respiratory function of a child can lead to acute respiratory failure. This is a life-threatening situation that necessitates admission of the child to an intensive care unit. (*See* Table 2-3 for the many common diseases associated with respiratory failure in children.)

Pathophysiology

Acute respiratory failure occurs when the body is unable to maintain effective gas exchange. It is characterized by hypoxemia and/or hypercapnia. Although clinical recognition of hypoxemia and hypercapnia indicates acute respiratory failure, the diagnosis is determined by measurement of the pH, $PaCO_2$, and PaO_2. ABG values that indicate acute respiratory failure have been established as an arterial PO_2 level of less than 50 mmHg and an arterial PCO_2 level of greater than 50 mmHg.[11]

Critical Care Management

The goal of treatment in acute respiratory failure is the reestablishment of effective gas exchange. This is accomplished by coordinating medical management and nursing intervention. A team approach is necessary to continually plan, provide, and evaluate the child's care.

Clinical management. The clinical management of acute respiratory failure is based on correcting the disruption in respiratory function that has led to failure.

Airway management: Clinical management begins with the establishment of a patent airway to promote effective ventilation. When the natural airway is compromised, the insertion of an artificial airway is indicated. Intubation of a pediatric patient is initially achieved by means of an oral endotracheal tube because it can be accomplished faster. However, if the plan is for the child to remain intubated for longer than 12 hours, but less than 5 to 7 days, a nasal endotracheal tube is preferred. A properly placed nasal endotracheal tube provides stabler fixation, reduces the danger of accidental extubation, results in fewer oral and pharyngeal secretions, and permits care of the nose and mouth.[12] Cuffed endotracheal tubes are generally not used in children under the age of 9 years because the child's small tracheal diameter ensures a natural seal. In fact, tracheal irritation in children may be minimized by using an endotracheal tube that is smaller than the tracheal diameter and that allows for movement of air around it. The endotracheal tube that has a "leak" minimizes the trauma to the subglottic area. The leak is measured by attaching a manometer to the endotracheal tube and passively pressurizing the system while listening for air escaping around the tube. A properly fitted tube leaks at 20 to 30 centimeters of water. If a leak cannot be heard at pressures of less than 30 centimeters, the artificial airway may be damaging to the tracheal mucosa, and a smaller size endotracheal tube or a tracheostomy should be considered.

When long-term intubation is necessary for the management of acute respiratory failure, a tracheostomy may be performed. A tracheostomy is also indicated when airway edema or obstruction will not permit the passage of an endotracheal tube. The tracheostomy is usually performed in the operating room.

The child with a compromised airway requires nursing interventions to maintain its patency. Before an artificial airway is established, the child should be closely observed for signs of increased distress. Raising the head of the child's crib or bed can ease the work of respiration. If the child is unable to cough up secretions, oral and nasopharyngeal suctioning should be performed frequently.

When an artificial airway has been inserted, frequent suctioning is indicated because an artificial airway tends to increase the amount of secretions in the respiratory tract. Sterile technique is important in order to minimize the risk of infection. Because bradycardia and a rapid fall in PaO_2 can occur during suctioning, manual inflation with 100 percent oxygen should be performed before and after the procedure. Cutaneous PO_2 monitoring helps to identify children who become hypoxic during suctioning.

Maintaining the position of the artificial airway also depends on the nurse. Securing the endotracheal tube with tape, or the tracheostomy tube with ties, is often not enough to prevent the child from removing the airway. Some type of restraint may be necessary.

In addition, emergency equipment should be at the bedside in case there is an accidental extubation or decannulation. The nurse should know how to determine if the airway is in place. This is done by (1) auscultating for equal, bilateral breath sounds, (2) inspecting the chest x-ray for the position of the tube, and (3) being aware of the existing "leak" and recognizing any increase or decrease in it.

Oxygen therapy: Once the airway is established, delivery of gas to the lungs is made possible. Supplemental oxygen is often necessary to correct existing hypoxemia. The percentage of oxygen needed is determined by the blood gas values. Because prolonged exposure to high concentrations of oxygen is damaging to lung tissue, oxygen therapy must be closely supervised. The FiO_2 necessary to maintain a safe PaO_2 (between 80 and 100 mmHg) is determined by frequent ABG and FiO_2 measurements.

Positive airway pressure: When hypoxemia persists despite the administration of supplemental oxygen concentrations of 50 percent or greater, the use of positive airway pressure (PAP) is indicated. PAP maintains patency in the smaller airways and alveoli by providing a constant pressure to the lungs, which increases the functional residual capacity and promotes gas exchange throughout the respiratory cycle. When PAP is administered to the child who is breathing spontaneously, it is known as continuous positive airway pressure (CPAP). When PAP is administered to the child who is receiving mechanical ventilation, it is referred to as positive end-expiratory pressure (PEEP). The addition of PAP frequently increases the PaO_2 enough so that supplemental oxygen can be reduced to a less toxic level. Initially, the pressure is set at 5 to 10 centimeters of water, and subsequent increases or decreases are based on PaO_2 measurements. When higher levels of PAP are administered, it is important for the nurse to provide PAP manually during any time that the respiratory support systems must be disconnected (e.g., for turning or suctioning). The safest way to suction a child on high levels of PAP is for one nurse to suction while a second nurse manually hyperinflates the patient's lungs and maintains the PAP during passage of the suction catheter. The hand-ventilating system used for manual hyperinflation should contain a pressure gauge manometer to ensure that the proper amount of PAP is delivered by the second nurse. Sudden removal of PAP can cause rapid atelectasis of the alveoli.

Mechanical ventilation: Mechanical ventilation in the management of acute respiratory failure is indicated when there is (1) impairment of the respiratory center in the brain, (2) bellows dysfunction, or (3) a situation that does not improve with oxygen and PAP.

By assuming the role of respiratory center, the ventilator delivers the number of respirations needed for effective gas exchange. Gas is delivered to the lungs, which are forcibly inflated and passively deflated.

Since many children who develop respiratory failure continue to exhibit some spontaneous respirations, the type of mechanical ventilation that is used should allow for their continuation. IMV is a technique that allows the child to breathe spontaneously between delivered ventilations without the risk of rebreathing expired gas.

Respiratory equipment: The primary responsibility of the nurse caring for the child receiving additional respiratory support (oxygen therapy, CPAP, and mechanical ventilation) is to monitor its delivery. This includes analyzing oxygen concentration and maintaining correct CPAP and ventilator settings at all times. When changes are made in respiratory therapy, the nurse is responsible for evaluating the patient's responses to these changes. This evaluation includes assessing respiratory status and obtaining and interpreting ABGs.

Complications of PAP and mechanical ventilation.   The use of PAP and mechanical ventilation in the treatment of respiratory failure exposes the already ill child to some dangerous complications.

Decreased cardiac output: The use of CPAP will reduce cardiac output, especially if the child's circulatory volume is decreased. Central venous and pulmonary artery catheters are used to monitor cardiac response to positive pressure. In addition, vasopressor drug infusions are sometimes used to support the circulation.

Pneumothorax: A tension pneumothorax can develop from the high levels of positive pressure delivered by a PAP system or during mechanical ventilation. Pneumothorax is readily identifiable on chest x-ray. Clinical assessments associated with pneumothorax include (1) decreased or absent breath sounds on the affected side, (2) tracheal deviation toward the unaffected side, and (3) complaints of dyspnea. Pneumothorax is treated by the insertion of a chest tube into the pleural space.

Subcutaneous emphysema: High levels of PAP can result in leakage of air into the subcutaneous tissues. The air can travel upward and inflate the neck and eyelids, or downward into the abdomen and perineum. The child appears edematous, the skin is taut and shiny, and crepitation is easily palpable. The collection of air under the skin may eventually cause skin breakdown. Placing the child on a waterbed or an alternating pressure mattress can minimize the effects of this problem. Range-of-motion exercises are necessary to decrease the consequences of immobility because, as subcutaneous emphysema worsens, the child's joints stiffen.

Nutrition.   In the early stages of respiratory failure the child's nutritional and caloric needs are met by intravenous (IV) fluids. There are several reasons for this: (1) when the child is tachypneic, the possibility of aspiration increases when oral feedings are given; (2) the child often cannot spare the energy needed to ingest oral feedings; and (3) if an artificial airway has been established, enteral feeding should be delayed for several days. A 5 percent glucose solution with electrolytes is used initially. However, since this solution can provide only a fraction of the caloric needs, supplementary gastrointestinal feedings or IV hyperalimentation are initiated as soon as possible to prevent weight loss (*see* Chapter 8). IV fluid therapy must be monitored and administered accurately in children because fluid overload can occur easily. Daily weights should be recorded to identify any loss or gain.

Drug therapy.   Sodium bicarbonate is frequently used to correct the acidemia that occurs with acute respiratory failure (*see* p. 80).

Sedatives and/or neuromuscular blocking agents may be necessary to prevent the child's respiratory efforts from interfering with the delivery of mechanical ventilation. Morphine sulfate and diazepam (Valium) help to calm the child. Pancuronium bromide (Pavulon) can be administered in bolus doses or by continuous infusion to achieve total muscular blockage (*see* p. 227). Other drug therapy is dependent on the specific disease process that results in respiratory failure.

Emotional and psychological support.   Perhaps one of the biggest challenges for the nurse taking care of a child with respiratory failure is to establish a means of communication.

Communication: Most children find it extremely frightening and frustrating to lose their method of communication. Attaching bells to the side rails, using pen and paper, lipreading, asking questions that can be answered by nodding the head, and even teaching sign language to the child who needs long-term respiratory care become important ways to communicate. If a child is old enough to read, making an alphabet chart enables the child to spell words. It is also helpful to write out on the chart certain phrases of common needs, which the child may point to (e.g., "I'm tired," "I want my Mommy," or "I have to go to the bathroom").

Psychological care: The nurse can provide psychological support to the child and family in many ways. Careful explanation of all respiratory equipment can help the child feel more secure and comfortable in the hospital. Parents should be encouraged to bring in their child's favorite toy or blanket in order to lessen the trauma of being in a strange environment. Before any procedure is performed, it should be explained to the child and the parents in an honest and sincere manner: this helps to foster a trusting relationship. Involvement of the family in the planning and delivery of the child's care has two benefits: (1) it is often less frightening to the child for the parents to be present to deliver care or observe its delivery; and (2) when the child sees the parents accepting what the nurse is saying and doing, the child is more likely to accept the nurse.

Finally, the nurse should recognize the needs of the parents. They must be kept continually updated on the child's progress. Frequent visiting and participation in the child's care should be encouraged. Parents must often be reminded of their own need for food and rest while their child is in the intensive care unit. If feelings of trust are developed between the family and intensive care staff, the child's and family's needs can be met more easily.

CROUP

The term "croup" describes a complex of symptoms generally associated with upper airway disorders that result from swelling of the larynx. Croup is caused by a viral infection that attacks primarily the larynx. Three types of croup have been described, and their differentiation is based on clinical features and the degree of involvement of the lower airway.

Laryngotracheitis, the most common type of croup, is an inflammation confined to the larynx and trachea. It produces edema and exudate in the subglottic airway and promotes destruction of the tracheal epithelium.

Laryngotracheobronchitis (LTB) occurs when the virus attacks both the upper and lower airways. LTB usually originates in the larynx, but then progresses down to the trachea and frequently also involves the bronchi. This often results in a bacterial superinfection in the lower airway and alveoli.[13] The complications of such infections are less common now that antibiotics are available, but LTB nevertheless remains the most serious kind of croup. Involvement of the lower airway results in ventilation-perfusion inequalities and further increases respiratory effort.

Spasmodic croup occurs when there is edema, but no inflammation, in the subglottic area of the trachea. It has been claimed that the tracheal epithelium is not directly affected in spasmodic croup. This belief is supported by the relative simplicity of treatment.[13]

Pathophysiology

Croup is one of the major causes of laryngeal obstruction in children. The inflammatory edema narrows the diameter of the airway, particularly at the level of the cricoid cartilages, which are located at the narrowest portion of the airway (Fig. 2-

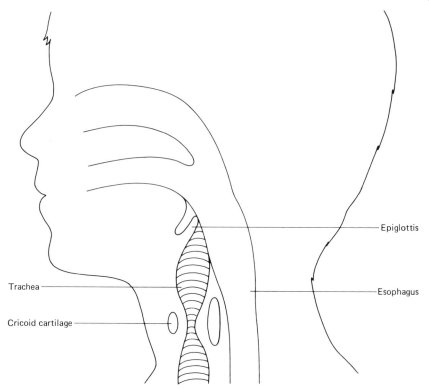

Figure 2-7. Airway obstruction with croup. Children with croup usually have a narrowed airway at the level of the cricoid cartilages.

7). The airway is further compromised by the presence of thick secretions that result from the inflammatory process.

Etiology

The principal viral agent responsible for croup is parainfluenza type 1.[14] Other croup viruses that have been isolated include parainfluenza types 2 and 3, respiratory syncytial virus, and various influenza viruses. The pathophysiology of viral infections helps explain the unpredictability of their severity: viral agents are intracellular and spread in a contiguous fashion; therefore, an infection of any part of the respiratory membrane can spread throughout the system.[15] The limiting factor in the viral spread is thought to be related to the child's age and development — a theory supported by the decreasing incidence of croup with increasing age.

History

Croup is seen most frequently in the pediatric age group of 3 months to 4 years, with a peak incidence in the second year of life. Infants and small children are more prone to developing croup for two reasons. First, the airway diameter of a child is much smaller than an adult's and becomes narrower more readily when inflamed. One millimeter of airway edema can compromise an infant's tracheal lumen by 50 percent.[16] Second, an infant does not have tracheal cartilage that is sufficiently developed to support the airway and maintain it in an open position at all times.

Clinical Presentation

The onset of LTB and laryngotracheitis is gradual, usually manifesting itself as an upper respiratory infection. It is initially characterized by mild fever (38 to 39°C [100.4° to 102.2°F]), hoarseness, a "barking" or "brassy" cough, rhinorrhea, and a sore throat. As subglottic edema narrows the airway, inspiratory stridor develops. The intensity of the stridor will increase as the airway obstruction increases. With severe obstruction, retractions occur, which may be accompanied by signs of hypoxemia (cyanosis, restlessness, anxiety, tachypnea, and tachycardia). Recognition and treatment of the increasing airway obstruction should take place before the signs of hypoxemia become evident.

Spasmodic croup occurs abruptly, and the onset is always at night.[13] The child awakens with sudden dyspnea, a croupy cough, inspiratory stridor, but no fever. Relief is provided by inhaling moist air, and hospitalization is rarely required.

Diagnostic Findings

The chest x-ray of a child with croup shows subglottic narrowing in the area of the cricoid cartilages. It is recommended that the diagnosis of croup by x-ray be made only after frontal and lateral films are taken on inspiration and expiration.[17] Multiple films of the airway better reveal the extent of the airway edema. Arterial blood sampling will generally indicate mild hypoxemia and hypercapnia, with a slight acidemia. The white blood count (WBC) is normal to slightly elevated, supporting a viral causative agent.

Critical Care Management

Only 5 to 10 percent of children with croup require hospitalization for significant laryngeal obstruction.[14] Those at risk for development of severe obstruction are (1) infants less than 12 months old, (2) children with congenital airway narrowing, (3) children who have recurrent croup, and (4) children who have required assisted ventilation with artificial airways. The primary reason for admission to the ICU is to observe for progressing laryngeal obstruction and to intervene before total obstruction.

Clinical management. Clinical management of croup involves airway management, the maintenance of temperature, the assignment of a croup score, and, if required, the establishment of an artificial airway.

Airway management: Initial therapy includes cardiac and respiratory monitoring to identify variations in rate and rhythm. Tachypnea and tachycardia are early signs of increasing respiratory effort. The child is positioned upright or in a semi-Fowler's position to avoid compromising the airway. Humidity, in the form of cool, misted air or oxygen, is provided to reduce the inflammation and edema of the airway, liquefy secretions, and ease respiration. For the young child, a mist tent is the most efficient way to provide humidification.

TABLE 2-13   Clinical Croup Score

Parameter	0	1	2
Inspiratory breath sounds	Normal	Harsh, with rhonchi	Delayed
Stridor	None	Inspiratory	Inspiratory and expiratory
Cough	None	Hoarse cry	Bark
Retractions and nasal flaring	None	Nasal flaring and suprasternal retractions	Nasal flaring, suprasternal retractions, and intercostal retractions
Cyanosis	None	In air	In 40% oxygen

Reprinted with permission from Downes, J. J., and R. C. Raphaely. 1975. Pediatric intensive care. Anesthesiology. **43**:238-250.

Maintaining temperature: Delivering cool misted air or oxygen to reduce the edema of the upper airway has long been a part of the treatment for croup. Initially, the cool mist is also helpful in reducing the mild fever generally seen in children with croup. Once the fever subsides, however, the cool mist can cause hypothermia, especially in the infant or very young child. Body temperature must be monitored frequently, and measures instituted to keep the child and bedding dry. Sometimes it is necessary to bundle the child with blankets to avoid a drop in body temperature. This should be done in a way that allows for continued close observation of the child.

Croup score: Downes and Raphaely[12] have developed a clinical scoring for croup that evaluates the child's respiratory status (Table 2-13). The clinical croup score, which can be used with all ages since it does not require verbal response, identifies the signs and symptoms commonly found in children with croup and serves as a guide for recognition of increasing respiratory distress. The croup score is taken as frequently as vital signs and before and after racemic epinephrine administration. A score of 4 or greater is suggestive of moderate airway obstruction, and would indicate the administration of racemic epinephrine. A continued rise in this score despite racemic epinephrine indicates impending respiratory failure, particularly if supported by ABGs demonstrating hypoxemia or hypercapnia. This should alert the critical care team to prepare for the insertion of an artificial airway.

Establishing an artificial airway: Nasotracheal intubation has become the preferred method of establishing an artificial airway in children with croup. Because the tracheal lumen is narrowed by edema, the endotracheal tube (ETT) should be at least two sizes smaller than indicated by the standard formula:[14] (*see* p. 79). However, if the airway diameter is greatly reduced, a tracheostomy is performed. Once the patency of the airway is reestablished, the respiratory distress is relieved, unless there is secondary compromise in the lower airway.

Management of the artificial airway includes frequent suctioning of secretions, and chest physiotherapy when the lower airway is atelectatic or infiltrated. The child may have to be restrained to prevent accidental removal of the ETT or the tracheostomy tube.

Drug therapy.   Drug therapy in the treatment of croup is a controversial subject. Various studies have attempted to determined the effectiveness of corticosteroids and racemic epinephrine.

TABLE 2-14   Recommended Dosages of Racemic Epinephrine

Weight	Dose*
kg	ml
20	0.25
20–40	0.50
40	0.75

*Milliliters in 3 to 5 ml of 9% pure sterile solution (PSS).

Corticosteroids: Some studies suggest that high doses (0.3 to 0.5 mg/kg) of dexamethasone (Decadron) significantly reduce the edema and exudate around the larynx and help maintain an adequate airway.[14] However, there is still no conclusive evidence that corticosteroids substantially alter the course of croup, and their use is not indicated in uncomplicated viral croup.[18]

Racemic epinephrine: The effectiveness of racemic epinephrine in croup is also not firmly established. When administered through a face mask, it works rapidly and has a vasoconstrictive effect on the inflamed airway. (Table 2-14 lists recommended doses.) Problems associated with racemic epinephrine are that it provides only transient relief and that the child develops a tolerance to it quickly. Thus, the time interval between doses must be decreased. When racemic epinephrine is needed for relief more frequently than every 2 hours, alternative therapies should be considered. The side effects of racemic epinephrine on the cardiovascular system (increased heart rate and blood pressure) should be monitored closely. It is contraindicated in children who have cardiac disease with muscular outflow obstruction.

Emotional and psychological support.   The child with an obstructed airway is extremely frustrated and apprehensive, and the same is often true of the parents. Allowing a parent to remain with the child often reduces anxiety. Maintaining a calm, quiet atmosphere at the bedside promotes rest and feelings of security. Thorough explanations of procedures and equipment will enhance the family's understanding of the treatment. Parental participation in calming the child can help to avoid use of restraints. Although it can initially be upsetting for the family to see the child with an ETT or tracheostomy, this reaction is accompanied by relief that the respiratory distress has been treated.

Ongoing management.   After the insertion of an artificial airway, the medical emergency has been resolved. The child remains in the ICU for continuing observation of respiratory status. Close supervision is needed to prevent accidental extubation or decannulation. Frequent suctioning is necessary to avoid blockage of the tube.

The child is evaluated daily for signs of decreased edema, which is evidenced by a continued increase in the air-leak, as well as by a normal body temperature, minimal tracheal secretions, and a normal ABG. In general, extubation is possible within 48 to 72 hours. Decannulation is performed after elective bronchoscopy in the operating room. After extubation or decannulation, the child is placed in a mist tent and is closely observed for at least 24 hours in the ICU. Oral feedings are withheld for 6 to 8 hours because, if the child shows any signs of respiratory distress, it may be necessary to reestablish the artificial airway. Racemic epinephrine is administered if the child exhibits increasing stridor, retractions, and a barking cough. Emergency equipment for reintubation is kept at the bedside, and

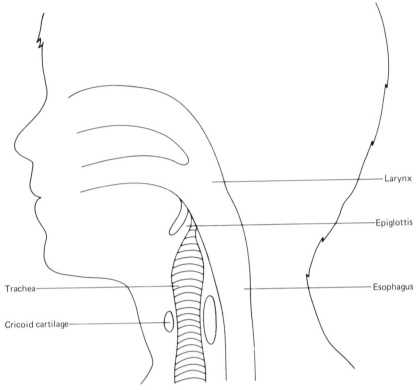

Figure 2-8. Airway obstruction with epiglottitis. The inflamed epiglottic cartilage causes obstruction in the supraglottic area of the larynx.

the croup score is used to assess for any continued distress. If the child tolerates extubation/decannulation, transfer out of the ICU occurs after 24 hours.

EPIGLOTTITIS

Epiglottitis is a disease of early childhood that can cause life-threatening upper airway obstruction. It is a rapidly progressing infectious process that responds quickly to medical intervention. Children with epiglottitis are admitted to the ICU for observation of increasing airway obstruction and for subsequent management of the artificial airway.

Pathophysiology

Epiglottitis is an inflammation of the supraglottic area of the larynx that directly affects the epiglottic cartilage (Fig. 2-8). Inflammation of this area produces edema of varying degrees that can rapidly obstruct the airway. The inflammation causes the epiglottis to curl posteriorly and inferiorly and to rest against the glottic orifice, resulting in progressive airway obstruction. Complete obstruction occurs when the epiglottis becomes further enlarged or when tenacious mucus occludes the already narrowed glottic orifice.

Etiology

Epiglottitis is most frequently caused by *Haemophilus influenzae* type B, although *Streptococcus* and *Staphylococcus* are sometimes implicated. The *H. influenzae* is more commonly isolated from the blood than from the larynx or trachea.[14]

Epiglottitis generally occurs in children between the ages of 3 and 7 years. It is seen more frequently in boys.

Clinical Presentation

The onset of epiglottitis is sudden, an important fact in distinguishing it from LTB and laryngotracheitis. Initial symptoms include a high fever (39 to 40°C [102.2 to 104°F]), sore throat, and mild dysphagia. It often follows a mild upper respiratory infection. Usually within 2 to 4 hours after onset, the disease produces lethargy, severe dysphagia with drooling, and an inability to swallow liquids. Speech becomes hoarse, and the child assumes an upright position with the chin thrust forward. As the supraglottic edema progresses, breathing becomes noisy and dyspneic, and suprasternal retractions are evident. Tachycardia, nasal flaring and cyanosis often develops. If inspiratory stridor is present, it is usually softer and much lower in pitch than that of croup, and accompanied by an expiratory snore.[14] At this stage of the disease, respiratory arrest can occur suddenly. Fatigue, septicemia, or inappropriate stimulation may precipitate acute obstruction and arrest.[14]

Diagnostic Findings

The diagnosis of epiglottitis is based on the history, clinical presentation, laboratory findings, and lateral neck x-ray. Because the causative agent of the disease is bacterial, a white blood cell count of greater than 16,000/mm^3 is common. Blood cultures are drawn immediately to identify the bacterial organism. Examination of the lateral neck film reveals the characteristic "thumb" sign. (The edema surrounding the glottic orifice changes the appearance of the epiglottis on x-ray from its normal "little finger" size to that of a "thumb.") In addition, the airway narrowing is evident on lateral neck x-ray.

Critical Care Management

Airway management. Immediately after the diagnosis of epiglottitis, an artificial airway is established to prevent the sudden respiratory arrest that can occur. Direct visualization of the epiglottis, which appears very swollen and cherry red, should never be attempted unless the examiner is prepared to intubate. The epiglottis is most safely visualized in the operating room under general anesthesia, immediately before placement of the artificial airway. The size of the ETT is usually two sizes smaller than would normally be used. After the establishment of the airway, the child is returned to the ICU. Intensive care monitoring is necessary for as long as the artificial airway is in place and for several hours after extubation. Placing the child in a mist tent for humidification allows the child more freedom of movement than with other closed systems available for delivery of gas. If, however, the ABG and the x-ray show signs of atelectasis and/or infiltration of the lower respiratory tract, oxygen and CPAP are indicated. Frequent suctioning of the airway is also important and should be performed at least every hour.

Isolation.   Respiratory isolation is recommended until antibiotic therapy has been administered for 24 hours. Many parents are frightened and stressed when informed that their child must be isolated. Suddenly being put in a room where everyone must wear a mask is also strange and confusing for the child. The job of maintaining the isolation and reinforcing the need for it belongs to the nurse. The nurse is also responsible for teaching the family how to follow the isolation instructions. Diversional activity helps the child adjust to being isolated and diverts attention from the ETT. Hand restraints may be necessary to prevent dislodgment of the ETT when the child is left alone.

Hydration.   The maintenance of an intravenous catheter is particularly important because it is needed for antibiotic administration and also because the child can have nothing by mouth (NPO) as long as the ETT is in place. The catheter should be secured and, if necessary, covered in order to prevent the child from playing with it.

Drug therapy.   Epiglottitis responds rapidly to antibiotic therapy with a resultant decrease in the supraglottic edema. The current recommendation of the Committee on Infectious Diseases of the American Academy of Pediatrics is to use both chloramphenicol sodium succinate 100 mg/kg/day and ampicillin 200 to 400 mg/kg/day intravenously until the antibiotic sensitivity tests are completed.[14] Ampicillin and chloramphenicol are antibiotics that are individually effective against *H. influenzae,* and for many years physicians selected one or the other drug to treat epiglottitis. Since 1974, however, an increasing number of medical centers are reporting ampicillin-resistant strains of *H. influenzae.* If the organism is found to be ampicillin-resistant, chloramphenicol is the only drug administered; if not, ampicillin is used solely. Antibiotic therapy is continued for 7 to 10 days.

When chloramphenicol is the drug of choice, it is important to monitor the complete blood count initially, and then twice a week during treatment, because this drug can produce blood dyscrasias.[19] The most serious toxic effect is depression of the bone marrow, which results in dyscrasias such as aplastic anemia and agranulocytosis. Chloral hydrate, 30 mg/kg/dose, is the drug of choice if a child requires sedation. If needed, this drug may be repeated in 1 hour at one half the dose.

Emotional and psychological support.   The loss of verbal communication, the isolation in a private room, and the ongoing administration of intravenous antibiotics are some of the reasons why hospitalization is stressful for the child with epiglottitis. If possible, the family should have 24-hour visitation privileges. The nurse should devise a communication system with the child that includes a method for summoning help when the child is alone. Play therapy involving isolation masks and syringes helps the child to act out feelings about treatment.

Ongoing management.   Once the airway is established and antibiotic therapy initiated, the management of epiglottitis consists of periodic evaluations of the ETT leak and daily laryngoscopic examinations to visualize the epiglottis. The laryngoscopic exam is done at the bedside after the child has been sedated and given a muscle relaxant. Direct visualization of the epiglottis allows the physician to assess the laryngeal edema and anticipate when extubation will be possible. An increase in the leak around the ETT is a sign that the edema is decreasing. The usual duration of intubation is 24 to 72 hours. After extubation, the child will remain in the ICU for observation and then be transferred to a regular unit.

Monitoring after extubation. Most children will remain in the ICU for a period of 12 to 24 hours for observation after extubation. Although children seem to tolerate an ETT better than adults, they are more prone to develop difficulties as a result of intubation. This is because of the smaller size of the airway and the tendency of the child to have more mucosal irritation from intubation.[20] After extubation, the child requires close observation for signs of subglottic edema, which include hoarseness, stridor, retractions, and cyanosis. Treatment of subglottic edema involves the administration of cool, humidified oxygen and racemic epinephrine (*see* p. 53). The child should remain NPO and should be hydrated intravenously. Continued distress despite this treatment indicates the need for reintubation. For this reason, emergency equipment for reintubation is kept at the bedside until the child's respiratory status stabilizes.

STATUS ASTHMATICUS

Asthma is a common respiratory disorder and one of the leading causes of chronic illness in children. It is a reversible obstructive process, characterized by heightened responsiveness of the large lower airways. Asthma is also a hypersensitive immune disorder that is mediated by immunoglobulin E (IgE) and other immunoglobulins.

Status asthmaticus is a clinical diagnosis that is made when the asthmatic child continues to have severe respiratory distress, despite the administration of three subcutaneous injections of epinephrine.

Pathophysiology

Airway obstruction in the asthmatic child occurs after exposure to an allergenic or a nonallergenic pathogen. The mechanisms responsible for obstruction are (1) edema of the mucous membranes, (2) increased accumulation of secretions from mucous glands, and (3) smooth-muscle spasm in bronchi and bronchioles. These mechanisms vary from patient to patient and from attack to attack (Fig. 2-9).

When a child suffers an asthmatic attack, immune and respiratory responses occur. The management and treatment of status asthmaticus is dependent on these two responses.

Immune response. A large number of asthmatic children have a strong predisposing allergic component in their genetic make-up. Many environmental factors are antigenic (capable of evoking an immune response): pollution, smoke, fumes, odors, pollen, etc. When the asthmatic is exposed to these irritants, sensitization occurs.

External antigens or allergens enter the body through any orifice or any weakened area of the skin or mucosa of the respiratory tract. Just beneath the skin or mucosa are plasma cells. Plasma cells are capable of producing IgE, an antibody formed in response to various allergens. As the antigen penetrates the skin or mucosa, it stimulates the plasma cell to produce IgE. As IgE leaves plasma cells, it attaches to mast cells. Mast cells are connective tissue cells containing

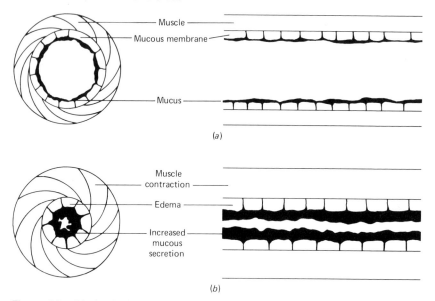

Figure 2-9. Mechanisms of obstruction in asthma. A, normal bronchus; B, asthmatic bronchus. *Reprinted with permission from* Whaley, L. F., and D. L. Wong. 1979. Nursing Care of Infants and Children. C. V. Mosby Co., St. Louis.

heparin and histamine that circulate with the white blood cells. They are important in cellular defense, especially during infection and injury. Once the IgE attaches to the mast cells, the person is said to be sensitized to the specific antigen (see Fig. 2-10).

After allergic sensitization has occurred and the child is again exposed to the same allergen, the antigen will enter the skin or mucosa and interact directly with the mast cell. As the antigen makes contact with the mast cell, it will bind to two IgE molecules. When this occurs, an enzymatic reaction is triggered, which causes the mast cells to release potent chemical mediators (Fig. 2-11). These mediators are histamine, slow-reacting substance of anaphylaxis (SRS-A), and eosinophil chemotactic factor of anaphylaxis (ECF-A). When this reaction occurs in the respiratory mucosa, the released mediators cause contraction of smooth muscle and increased mucus production from stimulation of the mucous glands.

The release of these mediators is regulated by receptors located along the surface of the mast cells: α- and β-adrenergic receptors, cholinergic receptors, and prostaglandin receptors. Stimulation of any of these receptors will regulate the release or retention of the cellular mediators.

Located within the mast cell are two cyclic nucleotides, cyclic 3′,5′-adenosine monophosphate (cAMP) and cyclic 3′,5′-guanosine monophosphate (cGMP). These nucleotides provide a second level of cellular response after the receptor sites are stimulated. Cellular mediators are thought to be regulated by the intracellular levels of cAMP or cGMP.[21] A rise in the cellular levels of cAMP inhibits the release of cellular mediators (mainly histamine) and causes smooth muscle relaxation. A rise in the cellular levels of cGMP stimulates the release of cellular mediators and causes smooth muscle contraction.

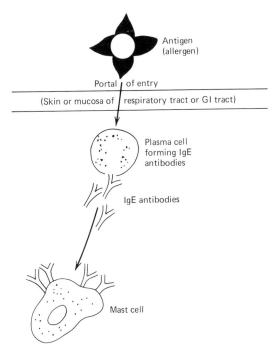

Figure 2-10. Normal Sensitization. See discussion on p. 57. GI, gastrointestinal; IgE, immunoglobulin E. *Reprinted with permission from* Levine, M. I. 1979. An introduction to modern allergy for the practicing pediatrician. *Pediatric Annals.* **8:**470–473.

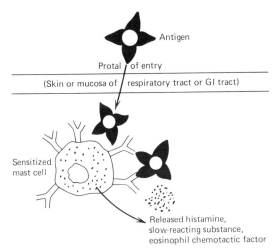

Figure 2-11. Sensitization after reexposure to an allergen. See discussion on p. 58. GI, gastrointestinal. *Reprinted with permission from* Levine, M. I. 1979. An introduction to modern allergy for the practicing pediatrician. *Pediatric Annals.* **8:**470–473.

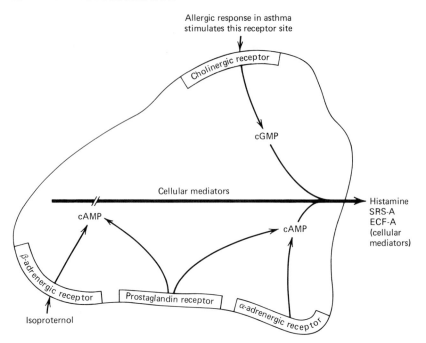

Figure 2-12. Immunologic release of cellular mediators. See discussion on p. 58. cAMP, cyclic 3',5'-adenosine monophosphate; cGMP, cyclic 3',5'-guanosine monophosphate; ECF-A, eosinophil chemotactic factor of anaphylaxis; IgE, immunoglobulin E; SRS-A, slow-reacting substance of anaphylaxis. *Adapted with permission from* Summers, R. J., and R. Evans. 1979. Autonomic mechanisms in asthma and other allergic diseases. *Pediatric Annals.* **8**:484–494.

An important characteristic of the mast cell in status asthmaticus is the location of the receptor site along the surface. This is helpful in understanding the action of isoproterenol (Isuprel) on the child in status asthmaticus. Isuprel acts on the β-adrenergic receptor sites, increasing cellular cAMP levels and decreasing the mediated cellular response (Fig. 2-12). Increased levels of cAMP promote bronchodilation and relaxation.

In status asthmaticus, the bronchial response results from the increased responsiveness of various allergens to the cholinergic receptor sites, or from a blockade to the adrenergic receptor sites. This blockade can be caused by infection, drugs, or a genetic predisposition. When this occurs, the cholinergic receptors become dominant, thereby increasing cellular levels of cGMP. The increase of cGMP causes a bronchial response of increased muscle spasm and vasoconstriction.

Respiratory response. While the immune process is occurring in the asthmatic child, respiratory impairment is also present. Respiratory impairment is the result of airway obstruction, which occurs because (1) severe bronchial constriction shortens and narrows the airway, thereby increasing air-flow resistance, and (2) increased secretions and mucosal edema further narrow the airway, promoting gas trapping at the end of expiration.

Gas trapping increases the residual volume, causing the asthmatic to breathe at

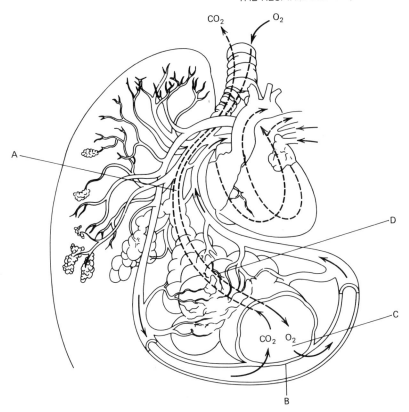

Figure 2-13. Respiratory changes in asthma. (A) Increased airway resistance resulting in gas trapping, (B) ventilation-perfusion disturbances resulting in hypoxemia, (C) alveolar hypoventilation resulting in hyperncapnia, (D) alveolar hyperinflation. CO_2, carbon dioxide; O_2, oxygen.

a higher lung volume. This interrupts normal ventilation and perfusion. Ventilation at high lung volumes is hard work, forcing the asthmatic to struggle to breathe. With this disruption in ventilation, the lungs become hyperinflated, an increased amount of oxygen is consumed, and large amounts of energy are expended. These disruptions cause hypoxemia, hypercapnia, and acidosis (Fig. 2-13). In response to low PaO_2 and severe acidosis, severe constriction of the pulmonary bed occurs. This creates a right-to-left shunt through the large vessels in the pulmonary vasculature, instead of through the small respiratory units (alveoli and capillaries) capable of ventilation and perfusion. This right-to-left shunt can cause right-sided heart failure in severe status asthmaticus.

The acidosis that occurs is both respiratory and metabolic. Respiratory acidosis exists because of the impairment in ventilation, which causes an increase in $PaCO_2$ levels. Metabolic acidosis exists because of the increased work of breathing and the decreased oxygen available for tissue metabolism, thereby increasing lactic acid levels.

History

On admission, it is essential that the following information be obtained: (1) onset or duration of the present asthmatic attack, (2) possible precipitating cause, (3) medications normally taken and medications taken during the attack, (4) fluid and caloric intake for the last 24 hours, and (5) past asthma history and measures necessary for treatment.

Clinical Presentation

The child in status asthmaticus will initially present with tachypnea, tachycardia, hypertension, and hyperthermia. These changes in vital signs are the result of the child's inability to inhale enough oxygen to meet the body's metabolic needs. The "air-hungry" child attempts to breathe faster to achieve adequate oxygenation. This increases the metabolic rate and causes an increase in the heart rate, blood pressure, and temperature from the exertion of breathing. Often, the child with asthma will sit leaning forward and use all intercostal, shoulder, and abdominal muscles to breathe. The use of abdominal muscles often causes the child with asthma to vomit and experience gastrointenstinal (GI) disturbances.

The child's $PaCO_2$ and PaO_2 levels initially fall, as the child hyperventilates and forcibly exhales. A normal $PaCO_2$ in a patient with severe asthma should be considered elevated, because carbon dioxide retention occurs late in the course of the illness.[22]

As the child's asthmatic attack progresses, ventilation becomes ineffective. The child works harder to breathe, causing a metabolic and respiratory acidosis. PaO_2 levels fall, while the $PaCO_2$ increases dramatically.

In an effort to standardize evaluation of respiratory failure in the asthmatic, a system for clinical scoring of asthma (Table 2-15) was developed by Downes and Raphaely: "The clinical asthma score attempts to evaluate oxygenation, gas exchange, work of breathing, airway obstruction, and cerebral function as affected by fatigue, hypoxia, or carbon dioxide narcosis."[12] This clinical score is designed to be used continuously throughout the child's asthmatic attack. However, it

TABLE 2-15 Clinical Asthma Score*

Parameter	0	1	2
PaO_2 (mmHg)	70–100 in air	70 in air	70 in 40% oxygen
Cyanosis	None	In air	In 40% oxygen
Inspiratory breath sounds	Normal	Unequal	Decreased to absent
Use of accessory muscles	None	Moderate	Maximal
Expiratory wheezing	None	Moderate	Marked
Cerebral function	Normal	Depressed or agitated	Coma

Reprinted with permission from Downes, J. J., and R. C. Raphaely. 1975. Pediatric intensive care. Anesthesiology. 43:238–250.

PaO_2, partial pressure of arterial oxygen.

*A total score of 5 or more indicates impending respiratory failure (obtain blood gases, notify anesthesia). A score of 6 may require transfer to intensive care unit (ICU). A score of 7 or more with a $PaCO_2$ (partial pressure of arterial carbon dioxide) of 65 mm Hg indicates existing respiratory failure.

should only be used in conjunction with ABG measurements and never in place of them.

Critical Care Management

Diagnostic findings. Diagnostic assessment of the asthmatic child includes chest x-ray, monitoring of ABGs, and laboratory work.

Chest x-ray: The chest x-ray of the asthmatic is usually hyperlucent because of the large amount of air trapping that occurs. The child's diaphragm becomes flattened (instead of domed) on x-ray as the child attempts to exhale forcibly and because of regional overexpansion and air trapping.

The x-ray of the asthmatic should always be assessed for the presence of atelectasis, pneumonia, pneumothorax, or pneumomediastinal shift.

ABGs: Frequent monitoring of ABGs is critical. Acidosis, hypoxemia, and hypercapnia require close observation and evaluation for rapid and accurate treatment. The increased airway resistance causes the $PaCO_2$ to increase and the PaO_2 to decrease correspondingly. If any atelectasis is present, blood shunted past the atelectatic alveoli will further compromise gas exchange.

Laboratory work: A complete blood count should be done to ensure adequate Hb for oxygen transport. The nurse should be aware of falsely elevated values secondary to dehydration. Nasopharyngeal and throat cultures should be sent for culture and sensitivity. A high concentration of eosinophils is suggestive of an allergic response. Serum electrolytes are often altered secondary to dehydration.

Clinical management. The clinical management of status asthmaticus involves primary and secondary respiratory support.

Primary respiratory support: Early critical care management of the child with status asthmaticus is as follows:

1. *Oxygen.* Supplemental oxygen is administered with high humidity to liquefy secretions, ease the work of respiration, and correct hypoxemia. Oxygen should be administered to achieve a PaO_2 of 150 mmHg.[23]

2. *Fluids.* Children presenting in status asthmaticus are dehydrated from large insensible fluid loss, inability to tolerate oral fluids, and possibly as a result of diuresis induced by theophylline (if administered). An IV infusion is started and isotonic fluids are administered at 2 to 2.5 times the normal maintenance rate until urine output is $\geq$ 2 ml/kg/hr. At that time, the normal maintenance rate is resumed.

3. *Sodium bicarbonate.* Any underlying acidosis is corrected with sodium bicarbonate administered every 4 to 6 hours at 1 to 3 mEq/kg for pH < 7.30. The primary indication for pharmacological treatment of metabolic acidosis is to increase the pH to greater than 7.35, at which levels antiasthmatic medications are most active.[24]

4. *Epinephrine.* When the asthmatic is first seen in the emergency room, subcutaneous epinephrine 1:1,000 is given at 0.01 mg/kg every 20 minutes to a maximum of three doses. If the child's respiratory distress does not improve, theophylline therapy is initiated.

5. *Theophylline.* The most frequently used derivative of theophylline is aminophylline, which is a methyl xanthine. The major action of aminophylline on the child in status asthmaticus is bronchodilation. Bronchodilation results

from aminophylline's inhibition of an intracellular enzyme, thereby preventing the breakdown of cAMP. This allows retention of cellular mediators (i.e., histamine and SRS-A) and the consequent relaxation of the bronchial tree. Aminophylline therapy is initiated with the administration of a bolus of 6 mg/kg, given intravenously over 20 minutes. This bolus is followed by an infusion at 1.1 mg/kg/hr for children weighing less than 40 kilograms or at 0.9 mg/kg/hr for children weighing more than 40 kilograms. The aminophylline infusion is mixed in 5 percent dextrose water in one quarter normal saline and is infused over the next 12 hours. The rate is increased in increments of 0.1 mg/kg/hr until the desired effects are seen and no toxicity is noted. The maximum dosage is 1.6 mg/kg/hr. It is important to monitor aminophylline blood levels; the first level should be drawn 12 hours after the beginning of the infusion. The therapeutic blood level of aminophylline is 10 to 20 µg/ml. The child receiving aminophylline should be monitored for potential side effects. Aminophylline toxicity is evidenced by hypertension, vomiting, cardiac irritability, GI discomfort, and central nervous system irritability. This frequently corresponds to blood levels greater than 20 µg/ml.

6. *Steroids.* Steroids are administered to modify or suppress the allergic response occurring in asthma. Stimulation of the β-adrenergic receptor site allows accumulation of cAMP, thereby decreasing bronchial edema. Methylprednisolone sodium succinate (Solu-Medrol) is the steroid of choice given at 4 to 5 mg/kg/day, in four divided doses. When the child has improved, Solu-Medrol should be discontinued slowly to avoid recurrence of airway edema. Hydrocortisone sodium succinate (Solu-Cortef) can also be used. However, because it has more salt-retaining properties, it is essential to monitor circulating blood volume and arterial blood pressure. When the child is in severe status asthmaticus, these additional fluid-retaining properties can increase the child's vulnerability to right-sided heart failure.

Secondary respiratory support: When the asthmatic fails to respond to primary respiratory support, secondary respiratory support is indicated. This is evidenced by a PCO$_2$ of 50, a clinical asthma score of 5 (*see* Table 2-15), and a past history of status asthmaticus requiring IV isoproterenol and/or mechanical ventilation. Assessing the need for additional respiratory support involves frequent monitoring of the child's vital signs, clinical condition, and blood gas determinations.

1. *Respiratory function.* Monitoring the child's clinical condition involves thorough assessment of the child's respiratory function. The child should be evaluated for the use of accessory muscles (i.e., sternal retraction, and the use of intercostal, shoulder, and abdominal muscles), nasal flaring, and level of consciousness (*see* p. 210–212). The head of the bed should be elevated at least 30 degrees. The nurse should assist the child in finding a comfortable position that is optimal for ventilation.

2. *Inspiratory: expiratory (I:E) time ratio.* Children in status asthmaticus have a prolonged expiratory phase, which alters their normal I:E ratio. This occurs when inhaled air is trapped in the alveoli, causing the lungs to become hyperinflated. Expiration becomes difficult, and is no longer a passive phase of respiration, but a forced purposeful phase. When expiration is forced through narrowed bronchi, a characteristic wheeze or sibilant rhonchus is heard. The I:E ratio is normally about 1:2; however, for the asthmatic, it can be 1:3 or even greater.

3. *Pulsus paradoxus.* This is a sign of impending respiratory failure that occurs with forced expiration. During inspiration there is normally a slight fall in the systolic arterial blood pressure of about 6 to 8 mmHg. In status asthmaticus the fall in pressure is much more significant, often 15 to 20 mmHg. This is due to increased compression of the great vessels of the heart, secondary to the pulmonary changes occurring in status asthmaticus. Pulsus paradoxus is confirmed by measuring the child's blood pressure during inspiration. The blood pressure cuff should be inflated to about 20 mmHg above the child's normal systolic pressure. As the cuff is slowly deflated, the first aberrant beat heard above the rhythmic systolic sounds should be noted, as well as the systolic value when the beat is heard. The difference in pressure at the first systolic sound and at the aberrant beat is the value of the pulsus paradoxus. The nurse should continually assess the child for a paradoxical pulse, and use it with other parameters in assessing respiratory failure.

4. *Arterial line.* Insertion of an indwelling arterial cannula provides a route for painless sampling of ABGs and constant monitoring of arterial blood pressure.

5. *Fluids.* In severe status asthmaticus, interstitial pulmonary edema may develop. This can occur as a result of fluid overload or secondary to intrapulmonary shunting. In this stage of the disease, fluids must be restricted. Fluid rates are adjusted individually after all parameters are evaluated (i.e., ABGs, x-ray, blood pressure, and urine output). If pulmonary edema is suspected or confirmed, furosemide (Lasix) is administered at 1 to 2 mg/kg IV.

6. *Isoproterenol.* Children with a clinical asthma score of 5 or higher, despite administration of oxygen, sodium bicarbonate, epinephrine, and aminophylline, and who have a $PaCO_2$ level of 55 mmHg or higher, warrant treatment with continuous isoproterenol (Isuprel).[12] Isuprel is begun at 0.1 µg/kg/min and increased in increments of 0.1 µg/kg/min every 15 to 20 minutes. The dose is continually increased until $PaCO_2$ levels fall below 50 mmHg or there is a 10 percent decrease in the $PaCO_2$ level from the preinfusion value. If the child's heart rate exceeds 200 beats/min or should a dysrhythmia occur, the infusion is discontinued immediately: "There is a significant association between heart rates of 180-200 beats/min. and a favorable clinical response."[25] Frequently, despite an initial reduction in the $PaCO_2$, the Isuprel infusion will still need to be increased for continued improvement. The infusion should be tapered only when the $PaCO_2$ level remains consistently below 45 mmHg and the clinical asthma score is less than 4. The infusion is decreased by 0.1 to 0.2 µg/kg/min each hour. When the $PaCO_2$ remains below 45 mmHg, the clinical asthma score is less than 3, and the infusion rate is 0.1 µg/kg/min or less for 2 hours, consideration can be given to discontinuing the infusion. Any increase in the $PaCO_2$ warrants returning to the previous setting. Throughout the Isuprel infusion, continuous ECG monitoring should be employed.

7. *Mechanical ventilation.* Failure to respond to Isuprel is indicated by (1) no decrease in clinical asthma score or a score of 7 or more; (2) an isoproterenol infusion rate of 3.5 µg/kg/min; (3) a $PaCO_2$ level of 65 mmHg; and (4) a decreased level of consciousness. These signs are indications for tracheal intubation, mechanical ventilation, and continuous neuromuscular blockage.[12] For the child in status asthmaticus, a volume ventilator is preferred because it delivers adequate inflating pressure and allows sufficient time for expiration to accommodate the asthmatic's prolonged expiratory phase. The child is initially given a large tidal volume that is set at 15 to 20 ml/kg and adjusted according to

ABG measurements.[25] During mechanical ventilation it is necessary to continually evaluate breath sounds because the child is at risk for developing pneumothorax. As the asthmatic attack begins to subside, rales are often noted. When this occurs, chest physiotherapy can be instituted. Mechanical ventilation continues until $PaCO_2$ levels fall below 50 mmHg, PaO_2 levels are above 100 mmHg, chest x-ray is improved, and no sibilant rhonchi are heard. The average time required for mechanical ventilation in the asthmatic child is 48 hours. Mechanical ventilation maintains respiratory function while the child's body slowly recovers from the immune and respiratory responses to the asthmatic attack.

8. *Neuromuscular blockade.* The asthmatic child generally requires neuromuscular blockade to ensure maximum alveolar ventilation at minimal tidal volumes and inflating pressures. Neuromuscular blockade is accomplished by continuous IV infusion of an agent such as pancuronium bromide (Pavulon). Continuous infusion of Pavulon prevents disruptions in ventilation caused by coughing or fighting the ventilator. (See p. 227 for dose of Pavulon infusion.) When the child is paralyzed, sedatives must be administered simultaneously. Morphine sulfate at 0.1 mg/kg or (diazepam) Valium at 0.2 mg/kg is frequently given. Sedation helps to decrease the fears and anxieties of the alert child who is unable to move. Continuous infusion of isoproterenol during mechanical ventilation will decrease bronchospasm and reduce the peak inflating pressure necessary for adequate ventilation. Weaning from the Isuprel infusion and the mechanical ventilation should be done simultaneously, based on the child's clinical condition and asthma score.

Emotional and psychological support.   The child who is admitted to the ICU in status asthmaticus is anxious, dyspneic, and fatigued from breathing effort and lack of sleep. The child's perception may also be distorted secondary to high $PaCO_2$ values.

It is important to place the child in a quiet area of the ICU to reduce the already heightened anxiety. The child should be addressed calmly and quietly. The nurse should explain all care and procedures to the child. It is imperative that the nurse be in control of the situation in order for the child to relax and completely trust the nurse.

Parents are frequently fatigued from the stress of watching their child struggle to breathe and from sleepless nights. They often need help in deciding when to leave the ICU and obtain well-needed sleep.

Behavioral problems are frequently seen in asthmatic children whose attacks began before 2 years of age or whose symptoms are prolonged and severe. It is unknown whether these behavioral problems result from the attack or are etiologic factors in the development of the attack.

A big factor in the child's adjustment to asthma is the family's commitment. The family's response can range from rejection to overprotection. Overprotection can encourage the child to become inactive for fear of participating in activities that will induce an asthmatic attack. Rejection of the child can cause the child to become manipulative of the environment. This can force the child to precipitate an attack in an attempt to receive parental attention. These behaviors can contribute to lack of self-confidence and alienation from peers. The family should thus do all in their power to encourage the child to engage in normal activities of daily living.

PNEUMOCYSTIS CARINII PNEUMONIA

Pneumocystis carinii is an organism believed by some to be a protozoan and by others to be a fungus. Because it has never been reproduced in vitro, the prevalence of *P. carinii* is a mystery. (*P. carinii* is probably ubiquitous.)

History

P. carinii was first identified in Brazil (1909) in the lungs of guinea pigs. However, it was not implicated as a human pathogen until World War II, when *P. carinii* reached epidemic levels in London. The affected population was debilitated premature infants. *P. carinii* has since become predominantly an opportunistic pulmonary infection (an infection caused by organisms that affect only an immunologically compromised host).

Epidemiology

P. carinii is an organism that rarely attacks healthy people (Table 2-16). As opposed to other pneumonias, there do not appear to be any seasonal or environmental factors that contribute to the occurrence of *P. carinii* pneumonia. It has been suggested that there may be a genetic predisposition to *P. carinii* and that families have an inheritable immunological defect that increases their susceptibility to *P. carinii*.

It is unknown how *P. carinii* is carried. It has been found in many animals (sheep, monkeys, goats, rats, rabbits, dogs, and certain other domestic animals).

The mode in which *P. carinii* is transmitted is unclear. It is known, however, that direct transmission of *P. carinii* can occur between two immunologically compromised patients. These patients should be isolated from each other if the possibility exists that one of them may have *P. carinii* pneumonia. In addition, normal healthy adults may also be carriers of *P. carinii*. This was determined by examining the titers of health care professionals caring for patients with *P. carinii* pneumonia. They were found to have higher than normal titers. It is therefore necessary for the patient with *P. carinii* pneumonia to be placed in respiratory isolation.

The most common portals of entry for *P. carinii* are the skin, the respiratory track, and the urinary tract (Table 2-17).

TABLE 2-16   Children at Risk for *Pneumocystis Carinii Pneumonia*

Group	Comments
Children with cancer	*P. carinii* occurs in approximately 5–6% of all children with cancer. It also occurs in a substantial number of children who are in remission from leukemia and are receiving maintenance therapy.
Debilitated infants	Premature infants are especially susceptible to *P. carinii*.
Organ recipients	Children who have been immunosuppressed to prevent rejection of an organ or graft become extremely susceptible to *P. carinii*.
Children with an immunological disorder	Protozoa, viruses, and fungi often affect patients with an underlying T cell deficiency.
Compromised hosts	Children who are being steroid suppressed are at risk for *P. carinii*.

TABLE 2-17   Portals of Entry for *Pneumocystis Carinii*

Location	Comments
Skin	The entry is usually through an intravenous line, other invasive lines, or breaks in the skin.
Respiratory tract	The entry is natural or via a nebulized solution (e.g., in oxygen or aerosol treatment).
Urinary tract	The entry is frequently via a Foley catheter.

The lung is the most common documented site for infection from *P. carinii*. *P. carinii* pneumonia accounts for 25 to 50 percent of all the infectious deaths of patients who have undergone immunosuppression.

Pathophysiology

P. carinii pneumonia is an interstitial pneumonia characterized by thickened alveolar walls. As the infection progresses, the alveoli become filled with a foamy, honeycomblike substance that causes the alveolar walls to distend to 5 to 10 times their normal thickness. It is presumed that this exudate results from the organism itself because the substance within the alveoli is composed largely of pockets of microorganisms. This exudate and the distended alveoli completely obliterate the alveolar space and cause an alveolocapillary blockage. The intensity of response evoked by *P. carinii* varies from host to host. *P. carinii* pneumonia is probably the most threatening infection for the bone-marrow transplant patient.

Clinical Presentation

The clinical presentation of *P. carinii* pneumonia depends on the age of the individual at risk. For debilitated infants, the onset is usually slow and insidious, progressing over 1 to 2 months. As is often the case with infants, these patients present with nonspecific signs and symptoms: restlessness, poor feeding, tachypnea, perioral and periorbital cyanosis that may develop gradually, a mild cough productive of a very sticky kind of mucus, and fever (usually low-grade). Auscultation of breath sounds reveals fine rales.

Beyond infancy, the onset of *P. carinii* pneumonia is abrupt, with a rapid, fulminating course. Approximately one third of all patients will have diarrhea and a preceding weight loss. A spiking fever, however, is the sign most consistently noted at first. Within a few days, tachypnea and a nonproductive cough develop. Despite the initial fever, tachypnea, and cough, the child may not appear to be in respiratory distress. However, intercostal and substernal retractions, nasal flaring, and color changes soon follow. If left untreated, *P. carinii* pneumonia can result in death within 1 to 2 weeks.

Critical Care Management

Diagnostic findings.   Early evaluation of the patient's ABGs is very helpful because these values are often the first indicators of respiratory compromise. It is not unusual for patients who appear to be in little or no distress to have ABGs indicative of borderline respiratory failure. The ABGs usually indicate hypoxemia and hypocapnia (as results of tachypnea).

The chest x-ray may initially be normal. However, as the infection worsens, the x-ray shows diffuse bilateral interstitial infiltrates. It resembles the chest x-ray of respiratory distress syndrome in its "ground-glass" appearance. Other routine laboratory data are usually of little value in diagnosing *P. carinii* pneumonia.

The definitive diagnosis of *P. carinii* pneumonia is made from direct examination of lung tissue or sputum smears. Sputum obtained from deep tracheal aspirates is frequently nonconclusive because it is often contaminated by many other organisms. Invasive measures are then necessary for the diagnosis. The methods most frequently used are open lung biopsy and needle aspiration.

Open lung biopsy is safely done in the controlled environment of the operating room. This is the preferred procedure because tissue samples obtained can be screened for both *P. carinii* and malignant tissue infiltrates. Needle aspiration is considered for the patient with marginal respiratory reserve who is considered a surgical and/or an anesthesia risk. Complications that can occur with either procedure are pneumothorax and intrapulmonary hemorrhage. Once obtained, the specimen is sent to the laboratory and stained with a silver nitrate stain for the definitive diagnosis.

Clinical management.   The clinical management of *P. carinii* pneumonia involves respiratory support, isolation, drug therapy, basic support, and education.

Respiratory support: Patients with a rapidly progressing respiratory infection frequently need assistance to maintain their respiratory balance. Supplemental oxygen may be provided noninvasively, but intubation is often necessary. Because of the involvement of the alveoli, PEEP is used to inflate available alveoli for oxygenation and perfusion. PEEP is increased rapidly in order to restore arterial PO_2 to an adequate level.

Maintaining high levels of PEEP is difficult. Any treatment that interrupts the delivery of PEEP (e.g., suctioning, or changing ventilatory tubing) should be performed by two nurses to ensure that the desired amounts of PEEP are continually delivered. PEEP may be accurately measured by connecting an airway manometer to the hand-ventilating or oxygen-bag system. The nurse must be alert for possible complications of high PEEP because this form of therapy places the child at risk for developing a pneumothorax or a pneumomediastinum. Frequent auscultation of breath sounds can provide early warning of possible complications. Daily chest x-rays should also be taken.

It is important to realize that the accepted airway "leak" normally maintained is not possible when high PEEP is required because the desired level of PEEP would continually escape through the airway leak (*see* p. 46). A cuffed ETT is often used with older children, whereas, for the infant and young child, an uncuffed ETT with a small leak is recommended.

Isolation: The patient with *P. carinii* pneumonia should be in respiratory isolation for the first 5 days of therapy and should not be assigned to the same room as a child who is immune or steroid suppressed. Also, if possible, these two patients should not be assigned to the same care giver. At all times, it is necessary to use strict aseptic technique, which will decrease the risk of any nosocomial infection to the patient.

Drug therapy: Pentamidine isethionate is the drug of choice in treating *P. carinii* pneumonia. This drug is dispensed only by the Parasitic Disease Drug Service of the Center for Disease Control in Atlanta. The dosage is 4 mg/kg/day, given as a single intramuscular injection for 10 to 15 days. If the patient improves after 5 days of therapy, the dosage can be decreased to 3 mg/kg/day. Intramuscular injections must be deep because there is a risk of fat necrosis at the injection site. (The fact that pentamidine is effective against *P. carinii* supports the theory that *P. carinii* is a protozoan.)

When *P. carinii* pneumonia is identified early and pentamidine therapy is initiated, the patient has a chance for cure. However, because the infection is difficult to diagnose, many patients do not live through the entire length of therapy.

The nurse should be aware of the side effects associated with pentamidine therapy (which occur in approximately one half of all patients treated): tachycardia, hypotension, nausea, vomiting, and facial flushing. Perhaps the most serious side effects are the development of severe hypoglycemia approximately 5 days into therapy, and the possibility of renal toxicity. Blood glucose should therefore be monitored every 4 to 6 hours after the initiation of pentamidine therapy. Continuous assessment of renal function is also required (*see* p. 335).

Recently, a combination of trimethoprim and sulfamethoxazole has been found to be effective against *P. carinii* without the side effects of pentamidine.

Basic support: During the intense period of respiratory compromise, the child with *P. carinii* pneumonia will need alternative fluid and nutritional support (i.e., nasogastric feedings or hyperalimentation). This should be provided according to the child's age and weight while the child is unable to tolerate feedings (*see* Chapter 8).

Skin care is critical because patients receiving high levels of PEEP begin to develop subcutaneous emphysema. These children should be placed on an alternating pressure mattress. Changing their position frequently and helping them perform range-of-motion exercises are helpful in preserving skin integrity.

Education: Because prevention and/or early management is essential with *P. carinii* pneumonia, critical care management should be first directed toward parental education. Parents of compromised children must be informed about the signs and symptoms of infection and about the need for early identification of these signs.

NEAR-DROWNING

Drowning is the third most common cause of death in children between 1 and 15 years of age. In recent years, more victims are surviving submersion in fluid. This is due to an improved understanding of the pathophysiology of drowning and to the increased training of the general public in cardiopulmonary resuscitation (CPR).

Pathophysiology

Drowning is defined as death from asphyxia resulting from submersion in fluid. Near-drowning is defined as survival, at least temporarily, after submersion in fluid. When a victim becomes submerged in fluid, the initial response is breath-holding. In 10 to 20 percent of victims, breath-holding will be followed by laryngospasm, which prevents aspiration of any fluid.[27] This is referred to as near-drowning without aspiration. If these victims are submerged for a longer period of time, however, unconsciousness from asphyxia will result. Once they are unconscious, the reflexes of the airway relax and fluid passively enters the lungs. In other cases of near-drowning, the initial breath-holding stage is followed by swallowing of fluid with subsequent aspiration into the lungs. This is referred to as near-drowning with aspiration. Regardless of whether fluid is aspirated, profound hypoxemia and metabolic acidosis result from asphyxia.

When water has been aspirated, it should be determined whether it was fresh or salt water. Salt water is hypertonic with respect to blood; its osmolality is three to four times greater than that of plasma. When salt water is aspirated, plasma is drawn from the circulation into the lungs to maintain osmotic equilibrium. The alveoli fill with fluid and become incapable of diffusing gas adequately. This results in ventilation-perfusion inequalities and hypoxemia. The shift of fluid from plasma into the lungs may also cause hypovolemia and increases in the serum concentrations of electrolytes, although humans rarely aspirate enough fluid to cause significant electrolyte disturbances. The hypovolemia, however, is often significant, and may necessitate fluid replacement.

Fresh water is hypotonic with respect to serum and has the opposite effect of salt water. Fresh water is rapidly absorbed from the alveoli into the vascular and interstitial spaces and can result in hypervolemia and decreases in serum electrolyte levels. Once again, the electrolyte changes are usually not significant, and the hypervolemic state is easily corrected if renal functioning is intact. The most damaging effect of fresh water is its altering of the surface tension of the alveoli by "washing out" surfactant. This alteration in surfactant activity causes alveolar collapse and atelectasis, ventilation-perfusion inequalities, and a decreased lung compliance.[28]

Clinical Presentation

Regardless of the amount and kind of fluid aspirated, the major problems in near-drowning are arterial hypoxemia and metabolic acidosis as a result of the intrapulmonary shunting of blood past nonventilated alveoli. Initially, there is a combined respiratory and metabolic acidosis, but the $PaCO_2$ is corrected once respiratory support is provided. Pulmonary edema occurs in aspiration of both fresh and salt water, although the mechanism for its development differs. In aspiration of salt water, the edema develops in the alveoli and is recognized in frothy, pink secretions. In aspiration of fresh water, the edema forms in the interstitial spaces and is not as readily apparent, although there may be subtle changes in the chest x-ray and in pulmonary compliance. Eventually, the interstitial edema will enter the alveoli and become clinically evident.[29]

Factors Affecting Survival

Survival after submersion is determined by a number of factors: (1) the age of the child, (2) the temperature of the water, (3) the submersion time, (4) the length of time between submersion and CPR, and (5) the child's condition upon arrival at the hospital. The younger the child, the greater the possibility for complete recovery.[30] This is due to the diving reflex and the child's response to cold water. The diving reflex is a neurogenic response that occurs when the face is submerged in cold water (less than 20°C [68°F]). It causes inhibition of the respiratory center and apnea, which prevent fluid from entering the lungs.[26] The reflex is potentiated by fear and is most active in young children. The reflex also shunts blood away from the nonessential organs and to the brain and heart. This is accompanied by severe bradycardia, decreased cardiac output, and decreased oxygen demand. All of these reactions serve to protect the body from the effects of submersion.

The child's body temperature while submerged also affects the chances for survival. Any person will experience a decrease in body temperature when submerged in cold water, but children, because of their larger body surface area per unit of weight and smaller amount of body fat for insulation, will exhibit a more rapid decrease. A decreasing body temperature causes a reduced basal metabolic rate, a decreased oxygen demand, and an increased tolerance of submersion. It also serves to prevent further injury to the hypoxic brain. Thus, the colder the water in which the child is submerged, the greater the chance for recovery. (However, if body temperature falls below 30°C [96°F], the risk of cardiac arrhythmias increases.)

A general statement cannot be made regarding a "safe" amount of time that a person can remain submerged and still recover. It is unknown how long a person can withstand hypoxia and survive normally. Studies have indicated complete recovery after submersion in warm water for 10 minutes and in extremely cold water for as long as 40 minutes.[29] However, it is generally agreed that irreversible neurological injury occurs within 4 to 5 minutes after submersion at normothermia.

Chances of survival after submersion are increased if CPR is provided promptly at the accident site. Although it is possible to reinstitute cardiac functioning after as long as 45 minutes of submersion, the brain is much more sensitive to hypoxia: each minute without CPR decreases the chances of cerebral recovery.[30]

There seems to be some correlation between complete recovery and the condition of the child upon arrival at a hospital. Modell and Boysen have classified patients (adults and children) according to their neurological status upon arrival at a hospital into three groups: (1) awake and alert; (2) displaying a blunted level of consciousness (lethargic, disoriented, confused, or agitated); and (3) comatose. Victims in group 1 had complete recovery 100 percent of the time. Group 2 victims had a 90 percent complete recovery rate. But victims of group 3 had a much lower rate of normal brain-function recovery (44 percent in children), with 17 percent surviving with incapacitating brain damage and 39 percent dying.

Critical Care Management

Once at the hospital, the near-drowning victim is admitted to the ICU for pulmonary and cardiovascular support.

Monitoring. Much of the care of the near-drowning victim involves monitoring. If the child was submerged in cold water, body temperature must be evaluated for signs of lingering hypothermia, and measures should be instituted either to maintain the hypothermal state (if cerebral edema is a concern) or to gradually rewarm the child to normothermia. Regulation of temperature is achieved by use of a temperature probe that provides a continuous readout of body temperature and a mattress that can cool or warm the child. Fever, which may indicate an infectious process resulting from the aspirated fluid, is treated with antibiotics and antipyretics. Cardiac monitoring is used to observe for bradycardia secondary to hypoxia and to identify dysrhythmias that occur from myocardial irritability or hypothermia. Respiratory monitoring is useful in identifying the need for respiratory support. If invasive catheters are in place, the nurse must ensure their patency and continually evaluate the oscilloscope wave forms and digital readouts for accuracy and for indications of cardiac stability.

Respiratory support. As soon as possible, blood samples are drawn to determine the degree of hypoxemia and acidosis. The degree of respiratory support needed can be identified by analysis of the pH, $PaCO_2$, PaO_2, and bicarbonate levels. This is facilitated by the insertion of an arterial catheter. An indwelling arterial catheter eliminates painful percutaneous blood-drawing and also provides a continuous blood pressure reading.

If CPR is instituted promptly, with restoration of circulation and ventilation, the child will probably only require supplemental oxygen and observation with cardiac and respiratory monitoring.

Intubation. Any child whose level of consciousness is blunted should be evaluated for elective intubation. Factors to consider are the child's ability to maintain a patent airway and the degree of pulmonary insufficiency. All comatose children should be intubated.[29]

PAP. In the past, various medications were used to treat the pulmonary edema that often accompanies fresh water and salt water aspiration. More recently, the use of PAP has found increasing favor. After salt water aspiration, CPAP expands the fluid-filled alveoli and often prevents the need for mechanical ventilation. After fresh water aspiration, PEEP and mechanical ventilation are usually necessary to treat the pulmonary edema because it is caused by the loss of functioning surfactant, which is necessary to maintain expanded alveoli. After the institution of PEEP, the functional residual capacity (FRC) increases, with a resulting decrease in ventilation-perfusion inequalities and an increase in PaO_2.[29] The amount of PAP used is titrated according to the ABGs and the clinical appearance of the child.

Respiratory care. Near-drowning victims who have aspirated fluid need frequent chest physiotherapy. Percussion, postural drainage, and vibration all serve to loosen and mobilize secretions in the alveoli. Frequent suctioning is necessary, and may require two nurses if high levels of PEEP must be maintained. Secretions should be inspected for signs of pulmonary edema and collected for laboratory cultures. ABGs are drawn frequently to evaluate the effectiveness of support.

Nasogastric tube. A nasogastric tube should be inserted as soon as possible to empty the stomach. If a large amount of fluid has been swallowed, the distended abdomen may impair respiratory effort. In addition, vomiting may occur, followed by aspiration.

Drug therapy. Almost every near-drowning victim will require some sodium bicarbonate therapy to correct the metabolic acidosis that follows hypoxia. The recommended dose is 1 to 3 mEq/kg initially, with subsequent doses determined by base deficits. Sodium bicarbonate should be administered slowly to children to prevent the side effects of its high osmolality.[26]

Cardiovascular support. Significant hypovolemia may occur after salt water aspiration. This may warrant insertion of a central venous catheter to monitor the child's central venous pressure. A low central venous pressure (normal in children is 5 to 15 mmHg) indicates the need for volume replacement. If high levels of PEEP are being administered, the insertion of a Swan-Ganz catheter may be considered in order to monitor the effects of high PEEP on the cardiac output. Occasionally, vasoactive drug infusions are used to support myocardial functioning and maintain blood pressure. In general, however, the circulatory effects of near-drowning are corrected by oxygen, bicarbonate, and fluid replacement.[29]

Neurological support. Frequent neurological assessment of the near-drowning victim must be performed (*see* p. 210–218). It is important to determine if the child can protect and maintain a patent airway. If cough and gag reflexes are absent, the child must be intubated. A depressed respiratory center impairs ventilation and indicates the need for respiratory support. Frequent neurological assessment is also important in identifying the hypoxic effect on the brain and any resultant cerebral edema.

There is some controversy over how much neurological support the comatose near-drowning victim should be given. It is generally agreed, however, that deliberate hyperventilation to reduce cerebral blood flow should be initiated and that corticosteroids should be administered to treat cerebral edema (*see* pp. 226–227).

Additional brain-protection therapy (hypothermia, barbiturate coma, and intracranial pressure monitoring *see* pp. 228–233) has not, however, significantly altered the outcome or survival rate of near-drowning victims and is now being performed only in some institutions.[29]

Emotional and psychological support.   It is unrealistic to suppose that the nurse alone can provide the emotional support that is necessary for the family of the near-drowning victim. In most cases, the family experiences almost inconsolable guilt. In the initial history-taking and during the bedside visits, the nurse should explore the existing family supports and contact additional professionals — social worker, clergyman, and psychiatrist — to help the family cope with the crisis. In attempting to alleviate their distress, however, the nurse should avoid making statements that give the family false hope.

Recovery.   The course of recovery from a near-drowning episode varies greatly. The child who is admitted awake and alert generally leaves the ICU within several days. Victims of fresh water aspiration generally need to be ventilated for 48 to 72 hours to allow time for resynthesization of surfactant. Any lowering of CPAP and PEEP levels should be done slowly to prevent additional alveolar collapse.[31] If invasive monitoring and respiratory support are required, recovery may take longer and the child will remain in the ICU until at least 24 hours after extubation. The recovery of the comatose child is difficult to predict and generally takes weeks to months.

CARDIOPULMONARY ARREST

Cardiopulmonary arrest (CPA) is defined as the sudden cessation of functional ventilation and circulation. The child who sustains a CPA requires immediate treatment to reestablish cardiac and respiratory functioning. Because pediatrics encompasses a wide range of patients, from the premature infant to the adultlike adolescent, this discussion will call attention to the differences in the CPR of infants, children, and adolescents. It will also focus on sequential management of airway, ventilation, circulation, and drugs and dosages used in the resuscitation of pediatric patients.

Pathophysiology

CPA in infants and children is usually precipitated by a primary respiratory arrest, which is most often the result of hypoxia. The primary respiratory arrest deprives the body of oxygen and sets off a chain of events that can culminate in sudden death. When hypoxia causes the heart to stop beating, the delivery of oxygen and energy substrates to the body cells is terminated. Body metabolism converts from the aerobic to the anaerobic route, producing lactic acid as its by-product. This results in a dramatic shift in pH and a combined acidosis: a respiratory acidosis from an increased PCO_2 and a metabolic acidosis from the increased lactic acid production. After a CPA, there is usually enough oxygen in the blood to sustain life for 2 to 4 minutes without brain damage. In the critically ill child, however, whose respiration is already compromised, this time limit is much shorter. The goal of resuscitation is to reestablish ventilation and adequate circulation as quickly as possible.

Etiology

The number of children who require resuscitation is small. Children in the critical care setting, however, are at risk for CPA because of life-threatening diseases or unstable physiological conditions. Children in the ICU most at risk for CPA are those with compromised respiratory, cardiovascular or neurological functioning. These children may require modification of the resuscitation procedure.

History

Identification of the event that precipitated the CPA is important for the treatment provided and the preventive measures instituted after resuscitation. Certain stressful procedures can also precipitate a CPA in the high-risk pediatric patient (Table 2-18).

TABLE 2-18 Stressful Procedures That Can Precipitate Cardiopulmonary Arrest

Procedure	Comments
Suctioning	This procedure can cause hypoxia, atelectasis, and reflex bradycardia.
Chest physiotherapy	This procedure can mobilize excessive secretions and block an artificial airway. It can also fatigue an already stressed child.
Lumbar punctures	In an infant with altered respiratory function, positioning for a lumbar puncture can totally occlude the airway. This procedure can also increase the child's intrathoracic pressure and cause bradycardia.
Vagal stimulation	Insertion of NG and NJ tubes can cause vagal stimulation and bradycardia.
Sedation	Administration of various sedatives can cause cough suppression and depression of the respiratory control center.
Respiratory support	Withdrawing or decreasing respiratory support can cause respiratory distress. Decreasing oxygen concentration, CPAP, or IMV can contribute to the deterioration of the child's respiratory status. Increasing these parameters (especially CPAP) can also compromise the child because of increased vulnerability to pneumothorax.

CPAP, continuous positive airway pressure; IMV, intermittent mandatory ventilation; NG, nasogastric; NJ, nasojejunal.

Critical Care Management

The critical care management of a CPA involves basic and advanced life support. Members of the critical care team should be certified in these areas according to the standards set by the American Heart Association.

Basic life support. The basic steps of CPR are the same whether the victim is an infant, child, or adult:

1. Establish unresponsiveness ("shake and shout").
2. Call for help.
3. Airway:
    a. open the airway.
    b. establish presence or absence of breathing ("look, listen, and feel").
4. Breathing:
    a. administer four quick staircase breaths.
    b. institute artificial breathing.
5. Circulation:
    a. establish presence or absence of pulse.
    b. apply external cardiac compression.

The differences in CPR for the infant and child are variations in technique based on the victim's size. Because airway obstruction is frequently a precipitating factor in CPA in children, great attention must be paid to establishing the patency of the airway and the adequacy of ventilation. Once unresponsiveness is established (by gentle shaking or tapping of the heal), the airway should be opened. This is done by placing the child's head in the "sniffing" position (Fig. 2-14). The sniffing position can be achieved by lifting the neck slightly and applying gentle

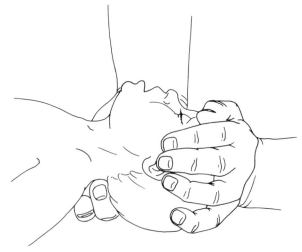

Figure 2-14. Sniffing position. When done correctly, the position should give the impression that the child is actually sniffing something.

pressure on the forehead to push the head back. (Because the trachea of the infant and young child lacks the firm, cartilaginous support of that of the adolescent, the neck of the infant or young child should never by hyperextended.) In addition, pulling the chin forward aids in opening the airway. If artificial ventilation is necessary, the infant's nose and mouth must be covered by the resuscitator's mouth. Inflation of the infant's lungs is accomplished by small, gentle breaths in the form of puffs from the resuscitator's mouth. In the child, the nose should be pinched closed and inflation of the lungs accomplished with expired gas from the resuscitator's lungs. The resuscitator can evaluate the adequacy of artificial ventilation by observing the rise and fall of the child's chest.

After the administration of four quick breaths, the presence of a heartbeat should be checked. The absence or presence of a pulse must be established after the administration of staircase ventilations to determine the need for cardiac compressions. The purpose of the four breaths is to provide sufficient oxygen to the lungs to allow time to check the pulse before continuing artificial ventilation. The pulse of a child can be felt over the carotid artery, in a manner similar to that in adult CPR technique. Palpation of a pulse in an infant is more difficult. Some infants with good cardiac activity may have a quiet precordium, which may lead to the erroneous impression that chest compression is indicated. Because of this difficulty, it is recommended that the brachial pulse be checked in infants.[32] This is done by placing the thumb on the outside of the infant's arm between the shoulder and elbow. The tips of the index and middle fingers are placed on the opposite side of the arm and pressed lightly toward the bone until the pulse is felt (Fig. 2-15). If a pulse is not palpable, combined artificial ventilation and cardiac compression must be provided (Table 2-19).

It is the technique for external cardiac compression that differs most between CPR in children and in adults. "Thumping" the chest, for example, is never used

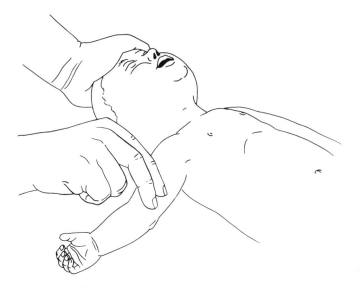

Figure 2-15. Palpation of brachial pulse.

TABLE 2-19   Ventilation-Compression Ratios

Group	Ventilations/min	Compressions/min
Infants	20	100
Children	16	80

with children. Other differences are related to the position of the heart within the chest, the small size of the chest, and the normally faster heart rate of children.

External cardiac compression should be done in a rhythmic fashion, with special attention given to hand placement (Table 2-20). Incorrect hand placement can easily result in damage to the young child's liver, which lies under the lower third of the sternum. With infants, the index and middle fingers of one hand should be used for cardiac compression while the other hand supports the infant's spine. Another method of cardiac compression often used with infants is the Thaler method (Fig. 2-16). With this technique, the infant's chest is encircled by the resuscitator's hands. The resuscitator's fingers support the infant's spine while the thumbs compress the sternum. With the Thaler method, chest excursion is limited by the span of the resuscitator's hands. For this reason, it should be used only with small infants.

Advanced life support.   Once basic life-support measures have been instituted, the critical care team should begin preparing to provide advanced life support. These measures include administering oxygen, establishing an artificial airway, inserting an IV line for fluid and drug administration, monitoring the ECG, and preparing for the possibility of defibrillation.

Oxygen: CPA interrupts normal ventilation and results in hypoxia and respiratory acidosis. Oxygen should be administered as quickly as possible and at 100 percent concentration. (Mouth-to-mouth resuscitation provides approximately 16 to 17 percent oxygen with a resultant PO_2 of 80 mmHg or less.)

Orlowski has written that "the amount of oxygen delivered to the tissues depends on the amount of oxygen carried by the blood (O_2 content) and on the ability of the heart to deliver the oxygen and blood to the tissues (cardiac output)."[33] Oxygen content is directly dependent on (1) the FiO_2, (2) the transfer of oxygen to the blood, and (3) the hemoglobin concentration. The cardiac output of a child in CPA is approximately 25 to 30 percent lower than normal, even when CPR is performed effectively.[33] Oxygen saturation of the tissues is thus severely compromised. ABGs should always be assessed to evaluate the child's oxygen requirements . (Good skin color and pink mucous membranes are indicators of adequate oxygenation and perfusion.)

Once the child is stable, the concentration of oxygen should be adjusted to maintain the PaO_2 between 60 and 90 mmHg. Although the hazard of oxygen

TABLE 2-20   Cardiac Compressions

Group	Site	Method	Depth
Infants	Midsternum (nipple line)	Two-finger method or Thaler method	½ inch
Children	Just below midsternum	One-hand method	1 inch

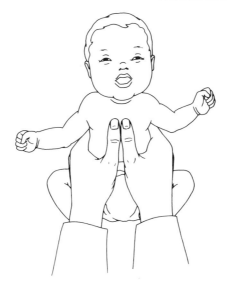

Figure 2-16. Cardiac compression (Thaler method).

toxicity at high concentrations must be kept in mind, a concentration of 100 percent oxygen should always be used during a CPA.

If endotracheal intubation is required, it should be performed by the most experienced member of the resuscitation team in order to minimize the length of time that CPR will be interrupted by this necessary procedure. The correct ETT size can be approximated by adding 16 to the patient's age and dividing that sum by four. For example, a child 2 years old will need an ETT of 4.5 millimeters:

$$\frac{2\,(\text{years}) + 16}{4} = 4.5\ (\text{mm ETT}).$$

Because this method provides only an approximation, it is recommended that the next smaller and larger size tubes also be available. When the ETT is in place and secured, a nasogastric tube is passed to empty the stomach of gastric contents and air.

While intubation is occurring, a second member of the team should be inserting IV catheters through which advanced life-support drugs may be administered. In an emergency the child's femoral vein is often the quickest and easiest vein to cannulate. This site provides quick access to the child's central circulation and does not interrupt CPR. (It is important to understand, however, that the femoral vein is not recommended for routine IV therapy.) If the child has a low circulating volume, it should be corrected before advanced life-support drugs are administered.

Sodium bicarbonate: When a CPA occurs, metabolic acidosis results. This is caused by an increase in lactic acid production from poor tissue perfusion. This state of metabolic acidosis increases the heart's vulnerability to ventricular fibrillation by decreasing the electrical threshold. This decrease in electrical threshold further decreases ventricular contractility. Cardiac output is thus decreased, and so is the heart's response to catecholamines.

The initial step in reversing acidosis is the administration of sodium bicarbonate, which increases the pH of the blood. This occurs when a bicarbonate ion (HCO_3^-) combines with a hydrogen ion (H^+) as illustrated in the following equation:

$$HCO_3^- + H^+ = H_2CO_3 = CO_2 + H_2O.$$

It is important that adequate ventilation be maintained during resuscitation because carbon dioxide is generated during this reaction.

Sodium bicarbonate is initially administered at a dose of 1 mEq/kg IV. It can also be administered continuously at 1 mEq/kg/min IV. Repeated administration of sodium bicarbonate should be calculated from the base deficit of the child's ABG. The following formula is helpful in calculating the correct amount of bicarbonate needed:

$$\text{bicarbonate (mEq)} = \frac{\text{base deficit (mEq/liter)} \times \text{child's weight (kg)} \times 0.4}{2}.$$

Caution is necessary in administrating sodium bicarbonate: overcorrection can result in a metabolic alkalosis. Metabolic alkalosis is difficult to correct and creates a stronger bond between the oxygen and the hemoglobin molecule, thereby decreasing oxygenation to the tissues. When sodium bicarbonate is administered to the child who is less than 6 months of age, it should always be diluted 1:1 with sterile water. The high osmolality of sodium bicarbonate in infants can result in a shift of free water into the vascular space. This can result in serious intracranial bleeding because of the fragility of the infant's cerebral blood vessels.

After the administration of sodium bicarbonate, it is necessary to clear the IV tubing thoroughly because the alkaline solution will inactivate calcium and catecholamines that may be needed during CPR.

Atropine sulfate: Atropine is a parasympathetic drug used to treat sinus bradycardia, which may be associated with hypotension, premature ventricular contractions, or changes in level of consciousness. It acts by decreasing vagal tone and increasing the rate of the sinoatrial node and the conduction to the atrioventricular node. It is also useful in the temporary treatment of second- and third-degree heart block. Atropine is administered at 0.01 mg/kg (minimum dose is 0.016 milligram). If no IV line is available, atropine can be administered via ETT or tracheostomy. Atropine is rapidly absorbed through the tracheal mucosa.

Epinephrine: Epinephrine is a sympathomimetic drug that has α- and β-adrenergic effects. Epinephrine increases the heart rate and the heart's force of contraction, thereby increasing cardiac output and cerebral perfusion. Epinephrine is also used to convert fine ventricular fibrillation to coarse ventricular fibrillation, which is more responsive to defibrillation. Administration of epinephrine with sodium bicarbonate can cause asystole to change to fibrillation, which, again, is responsive to defibrillation. Epinephrine is administered IV in a 1:10,000 solution at a dose of 0.1 ml/kg IV. (A 1:1,000 solution of epinephrine may be diluted by drawing up 1 milliliter of epinephrine 1:1,000 and diluting it with 9 milliliters of sterile water.) The half-life of epinephrine is about 5 minutes; therefore, repeated doses are necessary as resuscitation efforts continue. If IV access is not possible, epinephrine may also be administered by ETT or tracheostomy.

Calcium: Calcium is an essential electrolyte of the body. In the presence of a CPA, calcium increases myocardial contractility. Experimental evidence indicates that calcium ions may also enhance ventricular automaticity, and, therefore, the drug may be useful in restoring an electrical rhythm in the presence of ventricular standstill.

Calcium is available as calcium chloride and calcium gluconate. Because calcium chloride is extremely sclerotic, it should be administered only through a large-bore, deeply placed central line. (If only a peripheral IV line is available, calcium gluconate is the drug of choice.) Calcium chloride has a higher calcium ion content than calcium gluconate. Therefore, the dose of calcium chloride is approximately one third that of calcium gluconate. Calcium chloride should be given at 10 mg/kg, repeated at 10-minute intervals (depending on the plasma-ionized calcium level). The dose for calcium gluconate is 30 mg/kg. Calcium should be administered slowly because rapid injection can cause sinus bradycardia, prolonged myocardial contraction, or asystole. If the patient has been digitalized, calcium should be administered cautiously because it can potentiate dysrhythmias associated with digitalis.

Dextrose: In very small infants, CPA is accompanied by a fall in blood glucose. Therefore, 25 percent dextrose is slowly administered at 0.5 gm/kg IV. In older children, dextrose is used if the CPA is secondary to cerebral edema. Dextrose then acts as an osmotic diuretic to decrease intercranial pressure.

Lidocaine hydrochloride: Lidocaine is used to suppress ventricular ectopic or premature beats by raising the electrical threshold of the ventricles. Lidocaine is effective against both ventricular tachycardia and ventricular fibrillation. (Severe acidosis, hypoxemia, or electrolyte disturbances can be the cause of ventricular tachycardia or ventricular fibrillation and should be corrected before the administration of lidocaine.) Lidocaine is administered at 1 mg/kg, repeated three times at 5- to 10-minute intervals. Lidocaine's half-life is short; therefore, if the dysrhythmia persists, a lidocaine infusion should be initiated at 0.01 mg/kg/min.

Defibrillation: Another member of the team should assume responsibility for monitoring the ECG and defibrillating the patient. Dysrhythmias are a common cause of continued cardiovascular compromise and should be treated with oxygen, drug therapy, and, when indicated, defibrillation. The child should be prepared for defibrillation by the prior correction of any existing hypoxemia and acidosis.

The initial electrical charge administered to the child is 2 watt-seconds/kg. This level can be increased, in increments of 2 watt-seconds/kg, to a maximum of 8 watt-seconds/kg.

Before defibrillation is instituted, it is important to select paddles of the appropriate size. Paddles are available in infant and pediatric sizes. (Infant size is 4.5 centimeters in diameter, and pediatric size is 8 centimeters in diameter.) Conductive gel or correctly positioned 4″ × 4″ sponges dampened with normal saline should then be applied to the child's chest. It is important to understand that if too much gel or saline is applied, the electrical current delivered will be transmitted across the chest and not through to the heart. Paddles should be placed where a maximal amount of electrical current will be transmitted to the myocardium: "The standard placement is one paddle just to the right of the upper sternum and below the clavicle, the other paddle just to the left of the left nipple in the anterior axillary line."[32]

When correct position has been determined, the paddles should be given to the person designated to defibrillate. The correct electrical charge should then be set.

TABLE 2-21   Advanced Life Support Drugs and Defibrillation

Drug	Dose	Frequency
Sodium bicarbonate	1 mEq/kg	Every 5-10 min. May be repeated twice.
Atropine sulfate	0.01 mg/kg (0.016 mg minimum)	May be repeated once at double the initial dose.
Epinephrine (1:10,000)	0.1 ml/kg (0.01 mg/kg)	Every 3–5 min.
Calcium chloride	10 mg/kg	Every 2–5 min.
Calcium gluconate	30 mg/kg	Every 10 min.
Dextrose	0.5 gm/kg	May be repeated when indicated after blood glucose value is obtained.
Lidocaine	1 mg/kg	Every 5 min. (for 3 times).
Defibrillation	2 watt-seconds kg	If not effective, may be repeated in increments of 2 watt-seconds/kg to a maximum total dose of 8 watt-seconds/kg.

The designated person should then request that all resuscitators stand clear of the bed and should make certain that this request has been heeded. The paddles are then firmly placed against the chest, in correct position, and the charge is delivered. After defibrillation, the child's heart rate and ECG pattern should be reassessed in order to evaluate the effectiveness of the electrical shock. If defibrillation is unsuccessful, CPR should resume and the level of current should be increased. If higher levels continue to be unsuccessful, the child should be reevaluated for any underlying acidosis and/or alkalosis. Defibrillation is frequently successful in converting fine ventricular fibrillation to a coarse fibrillation and ventricular tachycardia to a safer rhythm. Before defibrillation is repeated, a dose of epinephrine and calcium should be given. (Table 2-21 lists appropriate doses and frequencies for all the drugs discussed.)

Organization of CPR.   It is essential that all members of the health care team in the ICU attend regular review sessions in CPR.

All resuscitation equipment and drugs should be checked for correct functioning and/or availability at the beginning of each shift.

When a CPA occurs, it is extremely important that the critical care team be organized to rapidly administer the care needed. The resuscitation team should include an anesthesiologist, a pediatric critical care specialist, a surgeon, a pediatrician, and available ICU nurses. Proper organization should include (1) a designated notification system for personnel needed for resuscitation (i.e., paging system or beeper system), (2) an emergency cart with resuscitation equipment (Table 2-22), and (3) a method for documentation of the resuscitation. Members of the team should be directed by the senior physician to coordinate basic and advanced life-support measures.

Emotional support of the family.   Throughout CPR, the major goal is the successful resuscitation of the child. The needs of the family, however, should not be forgotten. Because a simultaneous priority is continued reassessment of the child, an additional nurse may be needed to continue family-centered care. As soon as possible, the family should be provided with emotional support and factual infor-

TABLE 2-22 Emergency Resuscitation Equipment

Portable cart (with the following supplies)
Cardiac arrest boards (small and large)

Airway Equipment
Laryngoscope handle
Laryngoscope blades:
Miller 0, 1, 2, 3
MacIntosh 2, 3, 4
Wis-Hipple 1, 5
Flagg 2, 3
Oropharyngeal airways: Guedel sizes 00, 0, 1, 2, 3, 4
Nasopharyngeal airways: French sizes 12, 16, 20, 24, 28
Endotracheal tubes (I.D. sizes):
Uncuffed: 2.0 to 7.5
Cuffed: 5.0 to 9.0
Stylets: infant and adult
Magill forceps: child and adult
Extra batteries and laryngoscope lamps
Oxygen catheters: French sizes, 10, 14
Salem sump nasogastric tubes: French sizes 10, 14
Feeding tube: French size 8
Mapleson D circuit: sizes 0.5-, 1-, and 2-liter bags
Resuscitation masks: sizes infant through adult
Self-inflation resuscitation bags: sizes pediatric and adult

Circulation equipment
IV equipment: Butterfly sizes 19, 21, 23, 25
Quick Caths: sizes 16, 19, 20, 22
Waterproof tape: ½", 1", 2" in width
Alcohol swabs
4" × 4" sterile sponges
Tourniquet
Stopcocks
T-connectors
Armboards
Cutdown tray and equipment
Central venous pressure catheters: sizes 10, 11
Disposable syringes: sizes TB, 3 cc, 5 cc, 10 cc, 20 cc, 50 cc
Disposable needles: sizes 18, 20, 22, 25

Drugs
Pediatric Bristojets:
Epinephrine 1:10,000
Atropine 0.4 mg/0.5 ml
Sodium bicarbonate 7.5% (full strength)
4.2% (half strength)
Calcium gluconate
Lidocaine 1%
Dextrose 25%
Mannitol 20%
Vials
Calcium chloride 10%
Isoproterenol 0.2 mg/ml
Sterile water
Sterile sodium chloride

Miscellaneous equipment
ECG machine: ECG paper, gel, leads
Defibrillator:
Pediatric and adult paddles
Oscilloscope

ECG, electrocardiogram; I.D., internal diameter; IV, intravenous.

mation concerning the child's condition. Once the child's condition has been stabilized, the family should be encouraged to visit. The nurse should support the family and allow enough time for verbalization of their feelings regarding this frightening event.

REFERENCES

1. Vaughan et al. 924.
2. West. (1974) 24.
3. Whaley and Wong. 118.
4. Whaley and Wong. 1195.
5. Levin et al. 52.
6. Shapiro et al. 231.
7. Nuzzo.
8. Norton.
9. Huch and Huch.
10. Huch et al.
11. Emanuelsen and Densmore. 165.
12. Downes and Raphaely.
13. Cherry.
14. Barker.
15. Levin et al. 132.
16. Levin et al. 134.
17. Oliphant and Grossman.
18. Levin et al. 135.
19. Levin et al. 139.
20. Levin et al. 128.
21. Summers and Evans.
22. Levin et al. 121.
23. Levin et al. 122.
24. Levin et al. 123.
25. Levin et al. 124.
26. Goldfrank and Mayer.
27. Fandel and Bancalare.
28. Levin et al. 116.
29. Modell and Boysen. 10-22.
30. Conn et al.
31. Levin et al. 117.
32. Barclay.
33. Orlowski.

BIBLIOGRAPHY

Abels, L. F. 1979. Mosby's Manual of Intensive Care Nursing. C. V. Mosby Co., St. Louis, Mo.

Barclay, W. R. 1980. Standards and guidelines for cardiopulmonary resuscitation and emergency cardiac care. *(JAMA) Journal of the American Medical Association.* **244**:453-509.

Barker, G. 1979. Current management of croup and epiglottitis. *Pediatric Clinics of North America.* **26**:565-579.

Berger, A. J., R. A. Mitchell, and J. W. Severinghaus. 1977. Regulation of respiration. Part 1. *New England Journal of Medicine.* **297**:90-96.

Berger, A. J., R. A. Mitchell, and J. W. Severinghaus. 1977. Regulation of respiration. Part 2. *New England Journal of Medicine.* **297**:136-143.

Burke, B. A., and R. A. Good. 1973. *Pneumocystis carinii* infection. *Medicine.* **52**:23-51.

Bushnell, S. S. 1973. Respiratory Intensive Care Nursing: From Beth Israel Hospital, Boston. Little, Brown & Co., Boston.

Chai, H. 1975. Management of status asthmaticus in children. *Advances in Asthma and Allergy.* **2**:12.

Cherniack, N. S. 1976. The clinical assessment of the chemical regulation of ventilation. *Chest.* **70**:274-281.

Cherry, J. 1979. The treatment of croup: continued controversy due to failure of recognition of historic, ecologic, etiologic and clinical perspectives. *Journal of Pediatrics.* **94**:352-354.

Cohen, S. 1976. Blood-gas and acid-base concepts in respiratory care. *American Journal of Nursing.* **76** (6):24-54.

Commey, J. O., and H. Levison. 1976. Physical signs in childhood asthma. *Pediatrics.* **58**:537-541.

Comroe, J. H., R. E. Forster, A. B. Dubois, W. A. Briscoe, and E. Carlsen. 1962. The Lung: Clinical Physiology and Pulmonary Function Tests. Year Book Medical Publishers, Inc., Chicago. Second edition.

Conn, A. W., J. F. Edmonds, and G. A. Barker. 1978. Neardrowning in cold fresh water: current treatment regimen. *Canadian Anaesthetists' Society Journal.* **25**:259-264.

Cotton, E. K., and W. Parry. 1975. Treatment of status asthmaticus and respiratory failure. *Pediatric Clinics of North America.* **22**:163-173.

del Bueno, D. 1974. Making effective use of blood gas determinations. *RN.* **37**:40-43.

Dingle, R., M. D. Grady, J. Lee, and S. Paul. 1980. Continuous transcutaneous oxygen monitoring in the neonate. *American Journal of Nursing.* **80**:890-893.

Downes, J. J., and R. Godinez. 1980. Acute upper airway obstruction in children. American Society of Anesthesiologists Refresher Course Lectures in Anesthesiology. Vol. 8. 1-34.

Downes, J. J., and M. Heiser. Status asthmaticus in children. *In* Gregory, G., editor. Respiratory Failure in the Child. Churchill Livingstone, Inc., New York. (In press.)

Downes, J. J., and R. C. Raphaely. 1975. Pediatric intensive care. *Anesthesiology.* **43**:238-250.

Downes, J. J., D. W. Wood, T. W. Stroker, and J. C. Pittman. 1968. Arterial blood-gas and acid-base disorders in infants and children with status asthmaticus. *Pediatrics.* **42**:238-249.

Emanuelsen, K. L., and M. J. Densmore. 1981. Acute Respiratory Care. Fleschner Publishing Co., Bethany, Conn.

Fandel, I., and E. Bancalare. 1976. Neardrowning in children: clinical aspects. *Pediatrics.* **58**:573-579.

Feigin, R. D., and W. T. Shearer. 1975. Opportunistic infections in children. Part 1. *Journal of Pediatrics.* **87**:507-514.

Feigin, R. D., and W. T. Shearer. 1975. Opportunistic infections in children. Part 2. *Journal of Pediatrics.* **87**:677-694.

Feigin, R. D., and W. T. Shearer. 1975. Opportunistic infections in children. Part 3. *Journal of Pediatrics.* **87**:852-866.

Galant, S. P., C. E. Grancy, and K. C. Shaw. 1978. The value of pulsus paradoxus in assessing the child with status asthmaticus. *Pediatrics.* **61**:46-51.

Goldfrank, L., and G. Mayer. 1979. Salt and fresh water drowning. *Hospital Physician.* **15**:32-49 (July).

Greenman, R. L., P. T. Goodall, and D. King. 1975. Lung biopsy in immunocompromised hosts. *American Journal of Medicine.* **59**:488-496.

Gutgesill, H. P., and W. A. Tacker. 1976. Energy doses for ventricular defibrillation of children. *Pediatrics.* **58**:898-901.

Howry, L., R. Bindler, and Y. Tso. 1981. Pediatric Medications. J. B. Lippincott Co., Philadelphia.

Huch, A., and R. Huch. 1976. Transcutaneous non-invasive monitoring of PO_2. *Hospital Practice.* **11**:43-52 (June).

Huch, A., J. F. Lucey, and R. Huch. 1978. Oxygen noninvasive monitoring. *Perinatal Care.* **2**(18):25-30.

Hughes, W. T., S. Feldman, S. Chaudhary, M. J. Ossi, F. Cox, and S. K. Sanyal. 1978. Comparison of pentamidine isethionate and trimethoprim-sulfamethoxazole in the treatment of *Pneumocystis carinii* pneumonia. *Journal of Pediatrics.* **92**:285-291.

Hughes, W. T., S. Feldman, and S. K. Sanyal. 1975. Treatment of *Pneumocystis carinii* pneumonitis with trimethoprim-sulfamethoxazole. *Candian Medical Association Journal.* **112**(supple.):47S-50S.

Huges, W. T., S. Kuhn, and S. Chaudhary. 1977. Successful chemoprophylaxis for *Pneumocystis carinii* pneumonia. *New England Journal of Medicine.* **297**:1419-1426.

Hughes, W. T., R. A. Price, H. K. Kim, T. P. Coburn, D. Grigsby, and S. Feldman. 1973. *Pneumocystis carinii* pneumonitis in children with malignancies. *Journal of Pediatrics.* **82**:404-415.

Hunter, P. 1981. Bedside monitoring of respiratory function. *Nursing Clinics of North America.* **16**:211-224.

Johnson, T., W. M. Moore, and J. Jeffries. 1978. Children Are Different. Ross Laboratories, Columbus, Ohio.

Kassirer, J. P., and N. E. Madias. 1980. Respiratory acid-base disorders. *Hospital Practice.* **15**:57-71 (December).

Kempe, C. H., H. K. Silver, and D. O'Brien. 1980. Current Pediatric Diagnosis and Treatment. Lange Medical Publications, Los Altos, Calif. Sixth edition.

Kendig, E., and V. Chernick, editors. 1977. Disorders of the Respiratory Tract in Children. W. B. Saunders Co., Phildelphia. Third edition.

Kettrick, R. G., and S. Ludwig. 1981. Resuscitation in infants and children. *In* Current Topics in Emergency Medicine. Medical College of Pennsylvania. Vol. 1, No. 4. 1-4.

Keyes, J. 1974. Blood gases and blood gas transport. *Heart & Lung.* **3**:945-954.

Kim, H. K., and W. T. Hughes. 1973. Comparison of methods for identification of *Pneumocystis carinii* in pulmonary aspirates. *American Journal of Clinical Pathology.* **60**:462-466.

Lau, W. K., L. S. Young, and J. S. Remington. 1976. *Pneumocystis carinii* pneumonia. *(JAMA) Journal of the American Medical Association.* **236**:2399-2402.

Lee, C. A., V. R. Stroot, and C. A. Schaper. 1975. What to do when acid-base problems hang in the balance. *Nursing 75.* **5**:32-37 (August).

Levin, D. L., F. C. Morriss, and G. C. Moore. 1979. A Practical Guide to Pediatric Intensive Care. C. V. Mosby Co., St. Louis, Mo.

Levine, M. I. 1979. An introduction to modern allergy for the practicing pediatrician. *Pediatric Annals.* **8(8)**:470-473.

Levison, H., C. Collin-Williams, A. C. Bryan, B. J. Reilly, and R. P. Orange. 1974. Asthma: current concepts. *Pediatric Clinics of North America.* **21**:951-965.

Modell, J., and G. Boysen. 1981. Respiratory Crisis: State of the Art. Society for Critical Care Medicine, Fullerton, Calif.

Naumoff, M. D. 1977. A matter of life and breath. *In* Nursing Skillbook Series. 1977. Assessing Vital Functions Accurately. Intermed Communications, Inc., Horsham, Pa.

Neilsen, L. 1980. Mechanical ventilation: patient assessment and nursing care. *American Journal of Nursing.* **80**:2191-2217.

Norton, A. 1978. Introduction to Capnography. Beckman Instruments, Inc., Electronic Instruments Div., Schiller Park, Ill.

Nuzzo, P. 1978. Capnography in infants and children. *Perinatology/Neonatology.* Vol. 2.

Oakes, A., and H. Morrow. 1973. Understanding blood gases. *Nursing 73.* **3**:15-21 (September).

Oliphant, M., and H. Grossman. 1975. Acute upper airway obstruction: clinical radiologic approach. *Pediatric Annals.* **4**:650-662.

Orlowski, J. 1980. Cardiopulmonary resuscitation in children. *Pediatric Clinics of North America.* **27**:495-511.

Pavlin, E. G., and T. F. Horbun. 1978. The control of breathing. *Journal of the American Thoracic Society.* **7**:26-31 (November).

Pinney, M. 1981. Pneumonia. *American Journal of Nursing.* **81**:517-518.

Rokosky, J. S. 1981. Assessment of the individual with altered respiratory function. *Nursing Clinics of North America.* **16**:195-210.

Rosen, P. P., N. Martini, and D. Armstrong. 1975. *Pneumocystis carinii* pneumonia. *American Journal of Medicine.* **58**:794-802.

Shapiro, B. A., R. A. Harrison, and J. R. Walton. 1977. Clinical Application of Blood Gases. Year Book Medical Publishers, Inc., Chicago. Second edition.

Sherman, J. L., and S. K. Fields, editors. 1978. Guide to Patient Evaluation. Medical Examination Publishing Co., Inc., Garden City, N. Y. Third edition.

Sickles, E. A., V. M. Young, W. H. Greene, and P. H. Weirnik. 1973. Pneumonia in acute leukemia. *Annals of Internal Medicine.* **79**:528-534.

Simkins, R. 1981. Asthma. *American Journal of Nursing.* **81**:522-524.

Simkins, R. 1981. Croup and epiglottitis. *American Journal of Nursing.* **81**:519-520.

Summers, R. J., and R. Evans. 1979. Autonomic mechanisms in asthma and other allergic diseases. *Pediatric Annals.* **8(8)**:484-494.

Thaler, M. M., and H. C. Stobie. 1963. An improved technique of external cardiac compression in infants and young children. *New England Journal of Medicine.* **269**:606-610.

Tinker, J. 1976. Understanding chest x-rays. *American Journal of Nursing.* **76**:54-58.

Vaughan, V. C., R. J. McKay, and R. E. Behrman, editors. 1979. Nelson Textbook of Pediatrics. W. B. Saunders Co., Philadelphia. Eleventh edition.

Wade, J. F. 1981. Respiratory Nursing Care: Physiology and Technique. C. V. Mosby Co., St. Louis, Mo. Third edition.

Walzer, P. D., D. P. Perl, D. J. Krogstad, P. G. Rawson, and M. G. Schultz. 1974. *Pneumocystis carinii* pneumonia in the United States: epidemiologic, diagnostic and clinical features. *Annals of Internal Medicine* **80**:83-93.

West, J. B. 1974. Respiratory Physiology: The Essentials. Williams & Wilkins Co., Baltimore.

West, J. B. 1977. Ventilation/Blood flow and Gas Exchange. Blackwell Scientific Publications, Oxford. Third edition.

Whaley, L. F., and D. L. Wong. 1979. Nursing Care of Infants and Children. C. V. Mosby Co., St. Louis, Mo.

CHAPTER 3

THE CARDIOVASCULAR SYSTEM

Janis Bloedel Smith
with Mary Howell Giblin
and Janet A. Koehler

The pediatric critical care clinician will provide care to a large number of children who require close cardiovascular assessment and who may need cardiovascular support. Some of these children will have congenital heart defects. Congenital cardiac lesions (the focus of this chapter) are not the only cause of cardiovascular disease in children, but they are a more common critical care concern than the various forms of acquired heart disease. Much of the information in this chapter, however, is applicable to a variety of the children cared for in the pediatric intensive care unit (ICU).

This chapter begins with an overview of cardiovascular physiology that provides a foundation for understanding the sometimes complex pathophysiological changes seen in children with congenital heart defects. This overview is followed by a presentation of principles of nursing care that are applicable to all children with heart disease regardless of the specific nature of their individual defect. Nursing assessment of the cardiovascular system is then discussed. Though the focus is on techniques applicable to children with heart disease, many of them are crucial to the assessment of any critically ill child. The next sections detail the pathophysiology of all the common and many of the rarer congenital heart defects. The chapter ends with a section on the critical care management of the child with a cardiovascular disorder. Parts of this section are specifically applicable to the postoperative care of children who have had heart surgery, whereas others are applicable to all critically ill children with hemodynamic instability.

SELECTED ASPECTS OF CARDIOVASCULAR PHYSIOLOGY

Congenital cardiac defects result in alterations of normal cardiovascular hemodynamics caused by structural or anatomic anomalies. A clear understanding of the pathophysiology produced by a cardiac defect is best acquired by reviewing fetal circulation, the cardiovascular changes that occur at birth, and the normal hemodynamics of circulation. This section will conclude with a classification system of congenital heart defects that is based on the altered hemodynamics affecting children with congenital heart disease (CHD).

Fetal Circulation

The fetal heart and vascular system support intrauterine life and also permit a nearly instantaneous transition to extrauterine life at the time of birth. During fetal life, the placenta is the site of oxygenation (Fig. 3-1). Oxygenated blood flows from the placenta via the umbilical vein to the fetal liver. At this point, the flow is divided: some of the blood is directed into the hepatic circulation, whereas most of it is shunted through the ductus venosus to the inferior vena cava.

Blood entering the heart via the inferior vena cava is a mixture of more highly oxygenated blood (which has bypassed the liver) and of blood with a lower oxygen saturation (which has circulated through the abdominal viscera and lower extremities of the fetus). Most of the inferior vena cava blood is directed through the foramen ovale into the left atrium, bypassing the right ventricle and pulmonary circulation. Blood entering the left atrium via the foramen ovale is mixed with small amounts of blood returning from the pulmonary circulation via the pulmonary veins. This mixed blood has the highest oxygen saturation in fetal circulation. It is ejected from the left ventricle into the aorta and supplies the most crucial fetal structures: the heart and the developing brain.

Blood from the coronary arteries, the brain, and the upper extremities of the fetus returns to the right atrium via the superior vena cava. The brain and myocardium extract a great deal of oxygen from fetal circulation. Thus, this blood is low in oxygen content. Superior vena cava blood, mixed with some blood from the inferior vena cava, drains into the right ventricle. It is then ejected into the pulmonary artery, where the flow divides again. Some of this blood is directed to the lungs, but most of it flows through the ductus arteriosus and into the descending aorta. This blood, which is low in oxygen content, mixes with more highly saturated blood ejected into the aorta from the left ventricle. This supplies the lower extremities of the fetus and returns to the placenta for reoxygenation via the umbilical arteries.

Cardiovascular Changes at Birth

The main cardiovascular change that occurs at birth is the replacement of the placenta by the neonatal lung as the blood oxygenator (Fig. 3-2). Inflation of the lungs with air, combined with other factors (the presence of bradykinin enzymes, a higher partial pressure of arterial oxygen (PaO_2), and a higher pH), result in vasodilation of the pulmonary arteries and arterioles, thus permitting a large volume of blood to flow through the lungs. This rise in pulmonary blood flow increases the left atrial pressure and forces closure of the foramen ovale. The elevated PaO_2 of aortic blood and other factors produce spasm and constriction of the ductus arteriosus (see p. 124). Shunting through the ductus arteriosus may persist for 12 to 15 hours after birth; thereafter, there is complete closure of the ductus. (In addition, the ductus venosus closes, as do the umbilical arteries and vein, because they no longer transport blood. These events have less hemodynamic significance.) The neonate's heart also becomes more compliant and contractile than it was during fetal life. These last two factors permit regulation of cardiac output.

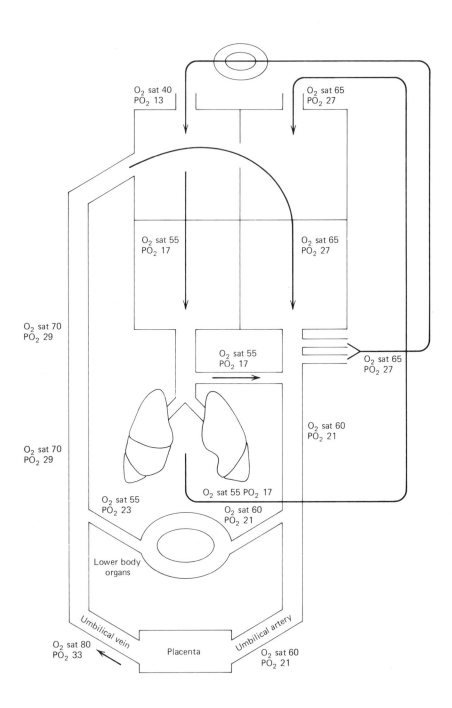

O₂ sat 40
PO₂ 13

O₂ sat 65
PO₂ 27

O₂ sat 55
PO₂ 17

O₂ sat 65
PO₂ 27

O₂ sat 70
PO₂ 29

O₂ sat 55
PO₂ 17

O₂ sat 65
PO₂ 27

O₂ sat 60
PO₂ 21

O₂ sat 70
PO₂ 29

O₂ sat 55
PO₂ 23

O₂ sat 55 PO₂ 17

O₂ sat 60
PO₂ 21

Lower body
organs

Umbilical vein

Umbilical artery

O₂ sat 80
PO₂ 33

Placenta

O₂ sat 60
PO₂ 21

Figure 3-1. Schematic representation of fetal circulation and oxygenation. Levels of oxygen saturation (O₂ sat) are given in percentages; levels of partial pressure of oxygen (PO₂) are given in millimeters of mercury.

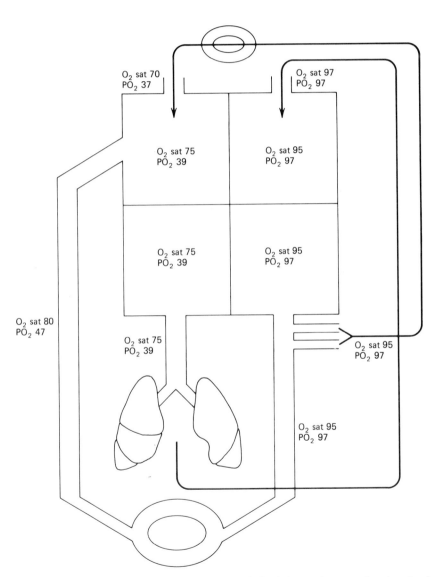

Figure 3-2. Schematic representation of postnatal circulation and oxygenation. Levels of oxygen saturation (O₂ sat) are given in percentages; levels of partial pressure of oxygen (PO₂) are given in millimeters of mercury.

Normal Hemodynamics

Blood flow through the vascular system is regulated by two variables: pressure and resistance. Blood, like any other fluid, always flows from an area of higher pressure to an area of lower pressure. Pressure is determined by a number of factors, including blood volume (preload) and resistance to flow (afterload).

Resistance results from the friction of blood against the walls of blood vessels. It is determined by the viscosity of the blood and the size of the blood vessels through which the blood flows. Resistance is directly proportional to the viscosity of blood and inversely proportional to the diameter of the vessels. This inverse relationship is especially important in understanding congenital cardiac defects.

The concepts of blood flow, pressure, and resistance are interrelated phenomena:

$$Pressure = resistance \times flow.$$

By means of simple computations, it is possible to identify how changes in either resistance or pressure will affect each other. In all circumstances in which either factor is altered, the body responds in a manner that attempts to maintain blood flow at normal levels. Therefore, if resistance is increased, pressure will also increase in order to maintain adequate blood flow. Conversely, if resistance is decreased, pressure will also decrease (*see* p. 415).

Pressure in the left side of the heart and in the systemic arteries is normally greater than pressure in the right heart and pulmonary vessels (Fig. 3-3).

Hemodynamics in CHD

Congenital heart defects result in abnormal blood flow caused by anatomic deviations from normal cardiovascular structure. Normal blood flow may be disrupted as the result of (1) an abnormal opening (or connection) between the systemic and pulmonary vascular systems, (2) an obstruction of the normal flow of blood through a heart chamber or blood vessel, or (3) a combination of 1 and 2. All of these disruptions are sensitive to the variables of pressure and resistance. Therefore, these variables provide the basis for the classification system used most frequently to describe congenital heart defects.

The initial determinant of the classification system is the presence or absence of cyanosis. This physical finding is confirmed by measurement of the PaO_2. The second determinant is the estimation of pulmonary blood flow (PBF) based on chest x-ray and careful physical examination. These two criteria permit the development of a relatively short list of possible diagnoses for a given child with suspected CHD and ensure a fairly high degree of accuracy (Table 3-1).[1] Of greater importance to the nurse is the fact that detection of cyanosis and/or abnormal PBF provides the foundation for deriving principles of nursing care for these children.

Acyanotic congenital heart defects with increased PBF. The first group of defects is that in which cyanosis is absent (acyanotic) and PBF is increased. In acyanotic cardiac defects there is no mixing of unoxygenated venous blood with oxygenated arterial blood in the systemic circulation. In these defects, an abnormal opening between the systemic and pulmonary circulations permits blood to flow between the two systems. Because blood flows from an area of higher pressure to one of lower pressure, the direction of the abnormal blood flow, or shunt, is from the left-

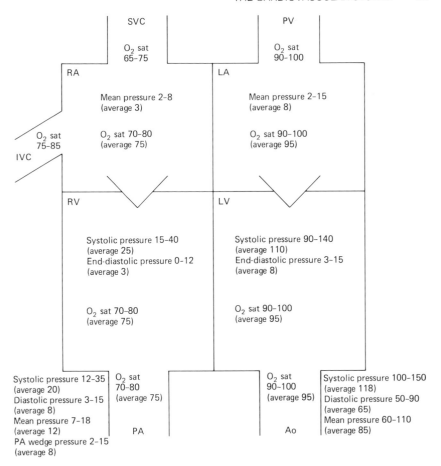

Figure 3-3. Schematic representation of pressures in the heart and great vessels (with normal oxygen saturation [O$_2$ sat] levels). Levels of O$_2$ are given in percentages; pressures are given in millimeters of mercury. Note: pressures in the left ventricle (LV) and aorta (Ao) vary with age. IVC, inferior vena cava; LA, left atrium; PA, pulmonary artery; PV, pulmonary vein; RA, right atrium; RV, right ventricle; SVC, superior vena cava.

sided (systemic) circulation to the right-sided (pulmonary) circulation, resulting in an increase in PBF and the absence of cyanosis. Atrial and ventricular septal defects, endocardial cushion defects, and patent ductus arteriosus are defects that are acyanotic with increased PBF due to a left-to-right shunt.

Acyanotic congenital heart defects with normal PBF. Congenital heart defects of the second group are acyanotic but evince no change in PBF. In these defects there is no opening between the systemic and pulmonary vascular systems; therefore, shunting of blood does not occur and PBF is normal. Abnormal blood flow, however, results from an increase in resistance to flow due to obstruction of a heart chamber or one of the great vessels. Cyanosis is absent because the obstruc-

TABLE 3-1 Classification of Congenital Defects

Type	PBF	Defect
Acyanotic	Increased	Patent ductus arteriosus Atrial septal defect Ventricular septal defect Endocardial cushion defect
	Normal	Coarctation of the aorta Aortic stenosis Pulmonic stenosis Mitral stenosis Endomyocardial disease
Cyanotic	Decreased	Tetralogy of Fallot Pulmonary atresia with intact ventricular septum Tricuspid atresia Truncus arteriosus with hypoplastic pulmonary arteries Transposition of the great arteries with pulmonic stenosis Ebstein's anomaly
	Increased	Transposition of the great arteries Total anomalous pulmonary venous return Truncus arteriosus Hypoplastic left-heart syndrome Single ventricle Double-outlet right ventricle

PBF, pulmonary blood flow.

tion does not interfere with pulmonary perfusion and because the oxygenation of venous blood occurs normally. Coarctation of the aorta, aortic stenosis, and pulmonic stenosis are the most common congenital heart defects that are acyanotic with normal PBF.

Cyanotic congenital heart defects with decreased PBF. In general, heart defects that result in cyanosis are more complex than acyanotic defects. In the first group of cyanotic defects, PBF is decreased because of obstruction at some point along the right heart. This increase in resistance to flow results in increased pressure in the right-heart chambers to the extent that right-heart pressures become greater than those in the left heart. Most of these obstructive defects are associated with an abnormal opening between the pulmonary and systemic circulations, or with the persistence of a fetal connection between the two systems (patent foramen ovale or patent ductus arteriosus). This permits shunting of blood from the right heart to the left heart. A right-to-left shunt always results in cyanosis because unoxygenated venous blood is mixed with oxygenated blood in the systemic circulation. The most common cyanotic defect with decreased PBF is tetralogy of Fallot. Others include severe pulmonic stenosis, pulmonary and tricuspid atresia, truncus arteriosus with hypoplastic pulmonary arteries, and transposition of the great arteries with pulmonic stenosis.

Cyanotic congenital heart defects with increased PBF. In cyanotic defects in which PBF is increased, there is no obstruction to PBF that results in cyanosis and right-to-left shunting of blood on this basis. Instead, there is mixing of arterial and venous blood at some point in the cardiovascular system because of the failure of the heart and great vessels to develop into distinct and separate systemic and pulmonary vascular systems prenatally. When communication between the two systems exists at any point in the cardiovascular system, both pressure and resistance may be altered. These changes result in shunts that mix arterial and venous blood in order to sustain adequate blood flow in both systems. Two of the more common cyanotic defects in which PBF is increased are transposition of the great arteries and total anomalous pulmonary venous return. Truncus arteriosus is a rare defect of this category.

PRINCIPLES OF NURSING CARE OF THE CHILD WITH CHD

Because of the large variety of congenital heart defects, the resultant alterations in cardiovascular hemodynamics range from those that are not immediately detectable to those that produce obvious and profound symptoms at birth or shortly thereafter. Approximately one third of all children with CHD will present within the first year of life with severe symptoms. These youngsters are defined as having critical CHD, which leads to cardiac catheterization, surgery, or death within the first year of life. Critical CHD is manifested most frequently by cyanosis and/or congestive heart failure (CHF). Heart defects with increased PBF all predispose the infant or child to CHF, regardless of the presence or absence of cyanosis. In addition, CHF can occur with defects that obstruct ventricular outflow, even when PBF is initially normal or even decreased. Decreased PBF also results in cyanosis, a progressive disorder that is responsible for the development of other significant physiological abnormalities. This section will discuss the principles of nursing care of infants and children with critical CHD who present with either CHF or cyanosis. The principles of care for children who do not develop either of these serious symptoms will also be presented.

CHF

The underlying principle of nursing care of the child with CHF is directed toward achieving two related goals: to preserve energy and to decrease metabolic demands on the failing myocardium. Specific management of the child is directed at reversing the CHF, whereas supportive care is based on conserving energy and minimizing demands on the cardiovascular system in order to lower the oxygen requirement of the tissues and, therefore, reduce the work load on the heart. The promotion of rest is thus of primary importance. The infant or child must be monitored closely and have physiological needs met in a way that allows for periods of undisturbed rest between care and treatment. If the child is unable to relax and rest because of extreme irritability or restlessness, sedation with morphine sulfate (10 µg/kg) may be necessary. After morphine is administered, it is very important to evaluate the child for signs of respiratory depression.

The work of respiration must be minimized in order to conserve energy and decrease metabolic demands on the heart. The pulmonary venous congestion characteristic of CHF in young children decreases lung compliance, thereby increasing the work of breathing. The increase in the work of respiration may be especially evident when the infant or child is lying in a supine position. In this position, fluid in the lungs is evenly distributed and reabsorbed in greater quantities, causing an increase in pulmonary blood volume. Therefore, the best position for these children is semi-Fowler's, which promotes the pooling of blood and fluid in the dependent portions of the lungs. This maneuver decreases the volume overload to the heart by limiting reabsorption of pulmonary fluid. Pulmonary congestion is also limited and, therefore, the work of breathing is eased. In addition, the enlarged liver is displaced in a downward position, which prevents it from impinging on the movement of the diaphragm. This eases respiration by permitting greater thoracic expansion. With infants, this position may best be maintained by placing them in an infant seat. Young children need to be adequately supported in semi-Fowler's position in order to prevent their sliding down or off to one side of the bed.

Humidified oxygen may be administered if tissue hypoxia is present. Oxygen is best administered by some noninvasive and nondisturbing route, such as a tent or oxygen hood, and is generally required only at relatively low levels (fractional concentration of inspired oxygen [FiO_2] of 25 to 40 percent). Supplementary oxygen decreases the work of respiration.

Suctioning of the naso-oropharynx may be necessary to maintain a patent airway. Unless needed, however, it should be avoided if the infant or child becomes excessively distressed during the procedure. Frequent, continuous assessment of the respiratory system is necessary to ensure adequate ventilation and distribution of oxygen.

During the acute state of CHF it is necessary to alter the child's feeding schedule in order to preserve energy. It may also be necessary to restrict fluid intake. Initially, the child's needs for fluids and electrolytes may best be met by the intravenous (IV) route. When oral feeding is resumed, it must be remembered that these children often become exhausted and very dyspneic during feeding. As a result, growth retardation is common among children with CHF. Nevertheless, the child's need for adequate caloric intake must be balanced against the need for rest and conservation of energy.

High-calorie formulas may be used to feed infants, and, as with all children with congenital heart defects, the emphasis must be on nutritional quality rather than quantity. These children generally eat better when fed small amounts frequently (every 2 or 3 hours) than when expected to consume a large amount of formula or food at one time. When feeding an infant, the nurse should choose a soft nipple that does not require the infant to suck vigorously. Because vomiting is not uncommon in these infants, they should be fed in a semiupright position and maintained in that position after feedings. If the infant or child is unable to tolerate oral feedings, alternative methods may be necessary to provide adequate caloric intake (*see* Chapter 8). The nurse must carefully calculate and document the child's intake. It is also important to be alert for signs and symptoms of hypoglycemia and hypocalcemia and to monitor the appropriate laboratory results.

A final consideration in the conservation of energy is the maintenance of normal body temperature. Maintaining the infant's or child's axillary temperature at 36.5°C (97.7°F) or rectal temperature at 37°C (98.6°F) decreases energy requirements and tissue demands for oxygen. Hypothermia and hyperthemia both require compensatory changes that the child with CHF may be unable to meet. An Isolette incubator or overbed warmer with Servocontrol is often necessary in order to avoid placing additional stress on the already failing cardiovascular system. Close monitoring of core temperature is essential.

The parents of young children with CHF are understandably anxious. The mere term "heart failure" can conjure up images of the heart stopping and death. In addition, parents of any acutely ill infant or child feel that they are unable to "help" their child in the complex ICU environment. It is critical that the ICU nurse support these parents by providing reliable information about their child and by specifically identifying what they can provide for their child that no other individual can (*see* p. 13).

Cyanosis

The underlying principle of nursing care of the cyanotic newborn or child is directed toward preventing stress. When these children are stressed, they demonstrate signs of severe hypoxia, air hunger, and, ultimately, severe cerebral hypoxia with loss of consciousness and seizures (or even sudden death). These complications are always attended by the possibility of irreversible central nervous system damage.

Temperature regulation is very important because hypothermia in the newborn intensifies hypoxia and acidosis and may lead to a vicious circle of these events. A radiant overbed heat source with Servocontrol maintains normal body temperature and permits accessibility to the infant.

The administration of relatively low concentrations of humidified oxygen serves to ease respiration and prevent additional stress, though arterial blood gas analysis will demonstrate minimal improvement, if any. Noninvasive, nondisturbing administration is preferred whenever feasible, but these critically ill infants may nevertheless require airway intubation and ventilatory support.

Oral feeding is discontinued during episodes of acute hypoxia because the energy required to feed is unavailable to these stressed infants. Maintenance of normal serum glucose and serum electrolytes must be achieved by the IV route. Fluid restriction is not usually necessary unless CHF is present.

Older children with persistent cyanosis develop progressive changes in the central nervous system, blood, heart, liver, and lungs (*see* p. 123). Whenever these children require hospitalization and intensive care, these changes must be thoroughly understood and incorporated into nursing care. Prevention of stress continues to be the underlying principle of care. Changes in the heart, lungs, blood, and liver severely limit the child's capacity to respond to stress. Changes in the central nervous system place the child at risk for serious complications. It is crucial that these changes be detected early in order to maximize the benefits of therapeutic intervention.

Normal Growth and Development

Although some children with congenital heart defects will be severely symptomatic within their first year of life, at least two-thirds of the children with CHD are not identified until later in their lives. Their symptoms are significantly milder and cause minimal physical limitation. Some of these children may evince mild growth retardation and a slightly limited capacity for vigorous, extended activity. They may also have a somewhat increased incidence of upper respiratory infections. Some will have no obvious clinical symptoms except those specific to the cardiac examination. The principle of nursing care of these children, as well as of those with more severe symptoms, is optimal promotion of normal physical and psychological growth and development.

The diagnosis of CHD evokes a great deal of fear within parents and children.

The heart is universally recognized as a vital organ and is also popularly associated with human love and emotion. Even when a child's defect is characterized by few risks and a low mortality rate, the child and family often fear that death will occur. Living on a daily basis with the threat of death makes it very difficult for a family to maintain normal relationships and promote the optimal development of each family member. A recent study demonstrated that between 30 and 60 percent of children with CHD suffer emotional disability. (This percentage is two to three times greater than that seen in physically normal children.) The emotional problems of these children were primarily related to how their families responded to the children. In addition, this study reported that emotional disability was often more severe in children with less complex forms of CHD.[2]

Promoting healthy family relationships in spite of the stress related to the real or imagined threat of death is an important role for all nurses caring for these families. Family members should be encouraged to discuss their feelings about each other. Parents need assistance and encouragement in order to maintain equal expectations for all siblings, to provide consistent discipline to the child with a heart defect and to understand the eventual difficulties of fostering overdependency. The child should be encouraged to participate in social experiences and to pursue age-appropriate goals in order to achieve optimal development.

There must also be provision for adequate physical growth. Children with congenital heart defects that produce severe symptoms are often physically underdeveloped. Nutritional assessment and counseling is important (*see* p. 467). The nurse should also provide information for parents on how children learn early to manipulate them through behaviors related to eating. This kind of behavior is often found in children, but may be exaggerated when parents are understandably more anxious about adequate food intake.

Physical exercise should be encouraged. In general, children with heart disease are able to limit their own activities by responding to how they feel. Overzealous limiting of active play is not required and may delay normal development.

The ICU nurse may have limited interaction with families of children with CHD and may not feel that there are many opportunities for teaching parents about issues related to normal growth and development. However, most parents of these infants and children indicate that, except for the period of time when they first learned of their child's diagnosis, the child's hospitalization is the time of greatest crisis for the family. Individuals in crisis are especially open about their feelings and concerns when approached with sincere interest, and they are also uniquely open to teaching. The ICU nurse has a special opportunity to interact with these individuals.

NURSING ASSESSMENT OF THE CARDIOVASCULAR SYSTEM

Thorough examination of the heart and circulatory system is essential in pediatric critical care nursing. The child's cardiovascular system responds quickly to the stress of illness (and to other types of stress) as is evident on even a cursory physical examination. However, continued adequate cardiovascular response to critical or life-threatening illness or injury may require external support. Therefore, detailed and accurate assessment of the cardiovascular system must be performed routinely on all critically ill children. This section will provide a guide to the physical assessment of the heart and circulatory system that is applicable to any child in the pediatric ICU. The specific findings that may be expected in a child with CHD will be discussed. There will also be a review of the additional information available to the critical care nurse via the invasive monitoring of cardiovascular pressures and hemodynamics. The section ends with the diagnostic tools and studies used to evaluate the cardiovascular system.

Cardiovascular Assessment

General health and appearance.   The status of the cardiovascular system is usually reflected in a child's general health and appearance. However, the connection between them is not always present and cannot be assumed. For example, a child whose growth has been limited and who has poor appetite and little energy may have a serious disorder, but it may not be of cardiovascular origin. On the other hand, anorexia in a child with known CHD may be among the first symptoms of CHF. Similarly, a child who has frequent chest colds does not necessarily have heart disease, although this finding is related to increased PBF in children with congenital heart defects. It is obvious that the presence of cardiovascular disease or an accurate assessment of cardiovascular status cannot be established on the basis of the child's general appearance and health alone. However, careful questioning of the parents and child (if old enough and able to participate) may elicit information that leads to further investigation and provides broad evidence of cardiovascular adequacy. The following areas relate closely to the cardiovascular system and should be assessed or investigated with the family to provide the foundation for more specific cardiovascular assessment:

1. *Physical growth:* Height and weight should be measured and plotted on a standard growth chart.
2. *Appetite:* Intake of fluid and food should be assessed. Sources of dietary iron should especially be noted because anemia can increase breathlessness and exercise intolerance in children, with or without concomitant cardiac disease.
3. *Exercise tolerance:* An estimate of the functional limitation imposed by a disease should be obtained. In addition, the occurrence of any chest pain with exertion should be clearly noted because this indicates severe obstruction with increased pressure in a ventricle.
4. *Frequency of colds or other infections:* Frequent chest colds are related to increased PBF in children with CHD. Colds and other infections may also be more serious in the child with a heart defect.
5. *Breathing pattern:* Tachypnea and dyspnea are symptoms of pulmonary vascular congestion and should be noted. Children with cyanotic heart defects with limited PBF may experience paroxysmal hyperpnea.

In addition, the family should be asked about any medications the child takes. Careful inquiry should be made as to dosage and frequency of administration of medications. Finally, parents can be asked if there is any other concern or question that they have about their child. Because parents have the greatest amount of experience with their own child, they often make astute observations about characteristics of the child that are important to investigate further.

Vital signs.   The measurement of heart rate and blood pressure is a familiar and important technique in evaluating the cardiovascular system. Table 3-2 presents

TABLE 3-2 Normal Range of Heart Rate in Children at Rest

Age/sex*	Normal range	Average
Newborn	70–170	120
1–12 months	80–160	120
2 years	80–130	110
4 years	80–120	100
6 years	75–115	100
8 years	70–110	90
10 years	70–110	90
12 years		
Female	70–110	90
Male	65–105	85
14 years		
Female	65–105	85
Male	60–100	80
16 years		
Female	60–100	80
Male	55–95	75
18 years		
Female	55–95	75
Male	50–90	70

*Differences in heart rate begin to be linked to differences in sex only at puberty.

the normal range of heart rate for children of various ages. The heart rate in children is particularly variable, increasing rapidly in response to excitement, stress, activity, or fever. With fever, a child's heart rate increases approximately 15 to 20 beats/min for each centigrade degree of temperature rise above normal. Because of the great variability in children's heart rates, tachycardia is especially significant if it persists during sleep. The heart rate can be counted satisfactorily in the radial pulse of healthy children over 2 years of age. However, in critically ill children of any age, heart rate is most accurately ascertained by auscultating and counting the apical pulse.

Careful measurement of blood pressure in every critically ill child is of great importance and can be achieved by several different techniques: palpation, flush method, auscultation, ultrasonic transducer, or electronic monitoring device. Auscultation of blood pressure or use of an ultrasonic transducer necessitates judicious selection of an appropriately sized blood pressure cuff. The width of the cuff should be 20 to 25 percent greater than the diameter of the upper arm (or thigh), and the inflatable bladder within the cuff should completely encircle the extremity (see p. 370). A blood pressure cuff that is too narrow will cause a falsely elevated systolic reading; a cuff that is too wide will underestimate the true systolic reading, although this margin of error is less than that associated with an excessively narrow cuff. A blood pressure cuff may be folded in order to achieve the needed size without influencing the accuracy of the blood pressure measurement to any great extent. (The preferred method of measuring cuff blood pressure is described on p. 371.)

Auscultation of thigh blood pressure may be necessary for a variety of reasons and is always indicated if hypertension is detected in the arm blood pressure measurement. The same considerations for cuff size are applicable when determining leg blood pressure. The systolic blood pressure in the thigh is equal to arm pressure in infants and very young children. After 1 year of age, the leg systolic pressure is 10 to 20 mmHg higher than that obtained in the arm. Lower systolic pressure in the leg than in the arm is indicative of coarctation of the aorta. Diastolic pressure in the leg is approximately equal to that obtained in the arm.

If blood pressure cannot be auscultated and ultrasonic blood pressure equipment is not available, blood pressure may be estimated by two other methods. Palpation of the radial pulse while an arm blood pressure cuff is deflated will provide a figure that approximates the systolic pressure. The flush method approximates the mean arterial blood pressure at the reading obtained when the color returns to a blanched extremity as the blood pressure cuff is deflated (*see* p. 372). Auscultation of blood pressure or use of ultrasonic equipment is clearly preferable to these techniques because it provides systolic, diastolic, and pulse pressure measurements instead of a single value.

A final aspect of vital sign assessment is the respiratory rate. The cardiovascular and respiratory systems are inseparably linked, and both must be fully assessed in the critically ill child (*see* p. 33).

Inspection.   Examination of the cardiovascular system proceeds with inspection, which begins with evaluation of the child's color. It is important, whenever possible, to assess color in natural lighting. The child's peripheral color is influenced by vasoconstriction due to cold, pain, or fear, and is not an accurate reflection of arterial oxygen saturation. Vasoconstriction is also caused by CHF, but other signs and symptoms such as tachycardia, tachypnea, diaphoresis, and hepatomegaly are also evidenced in such a case.

Assessment of the child's color in the most highly vascularized areas of the head and neck, the earlobes, and mucous membranes provides a better indication of true color. Nowhere, however, does skin actually derive its color from arterial blood. Therefore, this bedside assessment is only an indirect means of judging arterial saturation and requires additional confirmation. Changes in skin color should be apparent to the nurse who has continuously and carefully assessed a critically ill child and should be investigated further by arterial blood gas analysis or transcutaneous PO_2 determination.

Two color changes are of particular cardiovascular significance: pallor and cyanosis. Pallor may be related to anemia, but also results from mild vasoconstriction. When central cyanosis is detected, confirmation of a corresponding low PaO_2 by blood gas analysis is desirable. Other findings accompany cyanosis that has persisted for longer than a few weeks. Clubbing of the fingernails and toenails occurs, and dry skin and dry, brittle hair are evidence of nutritional deficiencies related to inadequate oxygenation. Persistent cyanosis also results in polycythemia. Although determination of hemoglobin and hematocrit levels, like blood gas analysis, is not a part of the physical examination per se, increased levels of hemoglobin and hematocrit corroborate the finding of cyanosis.

A second general aspect of inspection of the cardiovascular system is the detection of any visible edema. Edema is rare in children, even in those with chronic CHF, with the exception of children with nephrotic syndrome. Periorbital edema, however, and, very rarely, ankle or tibial edema may be detected in infants and very young children with CHF.

A third general aspect of inspection is related to the child's sensorium. Level of consciousness is dependent on adequate cardiac output. In addition, the child's general appearance of comfort and of ease in activity indicates adequate cardiac output.

Specific inspection of the cardiovascular system includes the notation of visible pulsations or of venous distention in the neck and chest. The jugular veins are normally distended and visible when a child is in the supine position. However, they should no longer be visible if the child sits up or if the head of the bed is elevated 35 to 45 degrees. Persistent neck vein distention is seen in CHF or when the vascular system has been overloaded with volume. Carotid pulsations may also be visible in the supine position.

When the chest is inspected, both sides of the rib cage are compared. Any obvious bulging over the precordium is due to chronic cardiac enlargement related to a volume overload such as a large left-to-right shunt. In young children who have thin chest walls or in very thin children of any age, the apical pulse may be visible as a precordial impulse. The visible pulsation normally corresponds to the area at which the point of maximal impulse (PMI) is palpated. This is usually the apex of the heart and is located at the left midclavicular line (or 1 to 2 centimeters to the right of it) in the fifth intercostal space in children who are 8 years of age or older. In infants and younger children, the heart is normally positioned more horizontally and the apex is higher (at the third or fourth intercostal space and to the left of the midclavicular line). The visible precordial impulse is generally a normal finding, but, if it becomes apparent in a child in whom it was previously undetected, it may indicate that the left ventricle is either volume- or pressure-overloaded. Finally, the visible precordial impulse must be differentiated from a precordial lift or heave. These abnormal findings involve the actual movement of a portion of the chest wall with contraction of the underlying cardiac muscle. Cardiac enlargement is generally the cause of a precordial lift or heave.

Palpation. Even in children in whom the impulse produced by left ventricular contraction cannot be seen, the impulse can generally be palpated by placing the fingers over the apical area. (Its position is as described above. Other positions may indicate cardiac enlargement.) The impulse should be felt as a single pulsation. Double or paradoxical impulses may indicate CHF. If the impulse is very prominent, it may be associated with CHF or with increased pressure in the left ventricle. In addition to the PMI palpable at the apex, a slight, brief pulsation may be felt as a normal finding in the pulmonic area in a child who has a thin chest. It may also be detected upon exertion, or in children with fever or anemia. A strong pulsation in this area may indicate hypertension or mitral stenosis.

A cardiac lift or heave can best be palpated by placing the palm of the hand over the entire precordial area. Right ventricular enlargement or increased pressure in the right ventricle may produce a heave in the sternum or very near it. Enlargement of, or increased pressure in, the left ventricle produces a lift or heave at the apex or even more laterally. Each of the valve areas should also be palpated for lifts or heaves (Fig. 3-4).

During palpation, the cardiac area of the chest wall is also assessed for thrills, which are palpable cardiac murmurs that result from abnormally turbulent blood flow. They can be compared to the vibrations felt when a cat purrs or to those felt over the larynx when the sound of *m* is produced. Thrills are generally best palpated at the valve areas and should be described in terms of duration, intensity, and as to whether or not the vibrations radiate to any other location in the chest or neck. Table 3-3 describes the thrills palpated at specific locations as determined by the congenital heart defect that produces them.

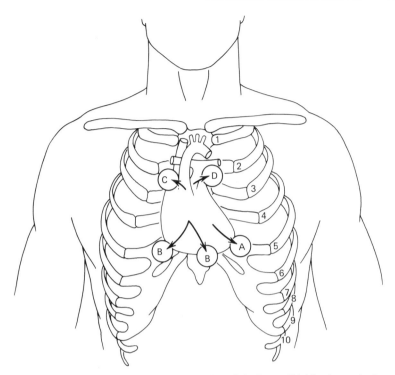

Figure 3-4. Areas for auscultation and palpation of the heart. (A) Mitral or apical area, where the first heart sound is loudest and where the third and fourth heart sounds may be heard, (B) tricuspid area, where a split in the first heart sound may be heard, (C) aortic area, where the second heart sound is heard well, (D) pulmonic area, where a split in the second heart sound may be heard.

A pericardial friction rub may be palpated as a scratchy or grating sensation over the precordium. Unlike a pleural friction rub, it does not vary with respiration. It is always an abnormal finding, indicating pathology within the pericardium.

Palpation of the abdomen provides information relative to the presence and status of CHF in infants and young children. The liver cannot usually be palpated in adolescents or adults because it is above the right costal margin. In the normal infant, however, the liver edge may be as much as 3 centimeters below the costal margin in the midclavicular line. The size of the liver relative to the child's size decreases with age. At 1 year of age, the liver edge is palpable at 2 centimeters below the costal margin, and, by 4 or 5 years of age, it can be located 1 centimeter below the costal margin. Palpation of a normal liver reveals a sharp edge, as opposed to the blunted edge of the liver that is distended as the result of CHF. In addition, the distended liver is usually tender.

The final elements to be evaluated by palpation are the peripheral pulses, which are evaluated for intensity. Intensity is rated on a scale from 0 to +4. An absent pulse receives 0; a pulse that is palpable, but weak and easily obliterated by

TABLE 3-3 Palpable Cardiac Thrills Associated with Congenital Heart Defects

Defect	Description of associated thrill
Patent ductus arteriosus	Palpable throughout cardiac cycle at left sternal border in 2nd and 3rd ICS.
Ventricular septal defect	Palpable during systole at left sternal border in 4th, 5th, and 6th ICS. May radiate to axillary line.
Aortic stenosis	Palpable during systole at right sternal border in 2nd ICS. May radiate to right neck.
Pulmonic stenosis	Palpable during systole at the left sternal border in 2nd ICS. May radiate to left neck.

ICS, intercostal space.

fingertip pressure, receives a + 1; an average or normal pulse that can be palpated with ease and cannot be obliterated is assigned a + 2; a full pulse receives a + 3; and a full and bounding pulse that may be visible is assigned a + 4 (Table 3-4). The carotid, brachial, radial, and femoral pulses occur simultaneously. The brachial and femoral pulses are approximately equal in intensity. These evaluations are important for determining the presence of obstruction to aortic blood flow. In addition, pulses on each side of the body (e.g., both radial pulses) are compared for equality.

Percussion. Percussion of the cardiovascular system is limited to determining the size of the heart by locating its borders within the thorax. Heart size is determined by either the direct or indirect method of percussion, beginning at the lateral aspect of the chest wall and percussing medially. The percussion note elicited changes from a resonant note to one that is dull at the cardiac border. The right cardiac border is normally percussed just to the right of the sternum, and, at its lower edge, the dullness percussed extends into the dullness percussed over the adjacent liver. The left border of cardiac dullness extends to the midclavicular line at the lower sternal border. Deviation from the norm may indicate cardiac enlargement or displacement and warrants further investigation. The chest x-ray provides definitive information about cardiac size, shape, and position.

TABLE 3-4 Intensity of Peripheral Pulses

Pulse	Normal intensity*
Temporal	+2
Carotid	+2
Brachial	+2
Radial	+1 to +2‡
Femoral	+2
Popliteal	+1 to +2‡
Posterior tibial	+1
Dorsalis pedis	+1

*See p. 103 for a discussion of intensity gradations.

‡Depending on age.

Auscultation. The final aspect of cardiovascular physical assessment is auscultation of the heart sounds. The familiar "lub-dub" of the heart are sounds produced by closure of the heart valves. These sounds are, therefore, associated with mechanical events occurring during the cardiac cycle. Briefly, these events and the associated sounds are as follows:

1. Systemic and pulmonary venous blood returning to the right and left atria, respectively, flows directly into the relaxed right and left ventricles. At this point in the cardiac cycle, the ventricles are in diastole, and the mitral and tricuspid valves (atrioventricular valves) are open.

2. After atrial electrical stimulation and the resultant muscular contraction, pressure in both ventricles rises as they fill with blood. This rapid increase in ventricular pressure causes the atrioventricular valves to close immediately before ventricular systole, thereby preventing regurgitation of blood into the atria.

3. Closure of the mitral and tricuspid valves occurs almost simultaneously and is usually heard as a single sound. This is the first heart sound (S_1), or the "lub" of "lub-dub." In some individuals, the mitral valve may close slightly before the tricuspid valve so that the S_1 sound is slightly split.

4. After closure of the atrioventricular valves, ventricular electrical stimulation takes place, which results in muscular contraction of the ventricles. The aortic and pulmonic valves are forced open, and blood fills the aorta and pulmonary artery.

5. When the ventricles have emptied, high pressure in the aorta and pulmonary artery causes the aortic and pulmonic valves to close, thereby preventing backflow of blood into the ventricles.

6. Closure of the aortic and pulmonic valves is heard as the second heart sound (S_2), or the "dub" of "lub-dub." The aortic and pulmonic components of S_2 often differ in intensity and do not occur simultaneously in children and young adults. The split of S_2 is generally more pronounced on inspiration than expiration.

Each heart sound is reflected to a specific area of the chest wall and can be best heard in that area (*see* Fig. 3-4). The mitral component of S_1 is best heard in the area near the position of the PMI. In children of at least 8 years of age, this is the fifth left intercostal space (ICS), near the midclavicular line. In younger children, mitral S_1 may be heart better in a higher and more lateral position (*see* p. 102). The tricuspid component of S_1 is best heard in the fifth right ICS, or sometimes in the midline below the sternum or just to the left of it. A split S_1 is best heard in one of these positions. The aortic component of S_2 is best heard at the second right ICS. The pulmonic component of S_2 is best heard in the second left ICS. A split S_2 is also most clearly audible in this position. In general, S_1 is slightly longer in duration than S_2 and is also somewhat lower in pitch.

Both S_1 and S_2 are usually heard as single sounds. However, a split S_2 is not uncommon in children and does not necessarily indicate pathology. A "normally" split S_2 is wider on inspiration than expiration. Therefore, if the width of the split does not vary with respiration (a "fixed" split) or is wider on expiration than inspiration (a "paradoxical" split), the sound is generally considered abnormal and warrants further investigation. A split S_1 may also be detected in a child without cardiovascular abnormality. It is not common, however, and is indicative of pathology more frequently than an S_2 split. It therefore warrants additional investigation.

As each component of S_1 and S_2 is auscultated, the other heart sounds remain audible. The clinician must become skilled at listening to only one aspect of each heart sound at a time. This skill requires concentration, can only be developed by serious practice, and is at least partially dependent on establishing a routine method of auscultating heart sounds and on following it faithfully. A suggested routine is as follows:

1. Listen to the mitral component of S_1.
2. Listen to the tricuspid component of S_1.
3. Listen to the aortic component of S_2.
4. Listen to the pulmonic component of S_2.

This routine is based on the sequence of mechanical events occurring during the cardiac cycle and, therefore, seems logical; but others are also acceptable. The important point is that the clinician listen to heart sounds in the same way each time in order to develop the skill necessary to distinguish normal from abnormal sounds.

Extra heart sounds: After a careful evaluation of S_1 and S_2, auscultation proceeds to the detection of extra heart sounds. A third heart sound (S_3) is sometimes heard. This sound is produced by the rapid entry of blood into an empty or dilated ventricle and is referred to as a "ventricular flow sound." S_3 is a dull, low-pitched sound best heard at the apex early in diastole, just after S_2. Although it can indicate decreased left-ventricular compliance and is heard in both adults and children with CHF, S_3 is often normal in children and in athletic adults. Careful auscultation differentiates the abnormal S_3 gallop rhythm associated with CHF from the isolated and normal S_3.

A fourth heart sound (S_4) may be produced by atrial contraction. This mechanical event, which occurs at the very end of ventricular diastole, is normally inaudible. Like S_3, S_4 is a dull, low-pitched sound that is best heard at the apex. It is distinguished from S_3 by its timing during the cardiac cycle, being heard just before S_1. S_4 is almost never a normal finding, and is usually indicative of CHF, anemia, hypertension, or other diseases.

Murmurs: Cardiac murmurs are the result of abnormally turbulent blood flow within the heart, at the heart valves, or within the great arteries. The location at which a murmur is best heard depends, like other characteristics of the murmur (timing, duration, intensity), on the specific defect that results in the abnormal blood flow. The location of the murmur, as well as its radiation to any other area, should be recorded.

The timing of a murmur is related to S_1 and S_2. Systolic murmurs occur between S_1 and S_2 during ventricular systole. Diastolic murmurs are heard after S_2 during ventricular diastole. Continuous murmurs are heard throughout the cardiac cycle during both systole and diastole.

Murmurs are also evaluated in terms of their intensity (Table 3-5). Grade I murmurs are the faintest audible murmurs, and grade VI murmurs are the loudest. A grade VI murmur continues to be audible even when the clinician lifts the stethoscope away from the child's chest. The assigning of a specific gradation to a murmur is subject to individual interpretation, and there are often discrepancies in the responses of different observers. When a single individual continues to assess

THE CARDIOVASCULAR SYSTEM

TABLE 3-5   Intensity of Cardiac Murmurs

Grade	Description
I	Faintest murmur audible; often not discovered initially.
II	Faint, but heard without difficulty.
III	Soft, but louder than II.
IV	Loud, but not as loud as V; associated with a palpable thrill.
V	Loud; still audible when stethoscope is lifted partially off the chest; associated with a cardiac thrill.
VI	Loudest murmur; still audible when stethoscope is lifted away from the chest.

a child with a cardiac murmur, however, any changes in the intensity of that murmur should be further evaluated for their significance.

The intensity of a murmur is also assessed for variation. The following is a brief list of the most common variations:

1. Ejection murmur (usually systolic ejection murmur): loudest at midsystole or middiastole.
2. Holosystolic or holodiastolic murmur (usually systolic, since holodiastolic murmurs are rare): heard throughout systole or diastole in equal intensity.
3. Crescendo murmur: marked by increasing intensity during systole or diastole.
4. Decrescendo murmur: marked by decreasing intensity during systole or diastole.
5. Crescendo-decrescendo murmur: marked by increasing, then by decreasing, intensity during systole or diastole.

Heart murmurs that are produced by cardiac defects are referred to as organic murmurs. A number of children who do not have heart disease have innocent, or functional, heart murmurs. Functional murmurs are generally quiet (grade I/VI or II/VI), systolic murmurs of short duration that are best heard at the pulmonic area and that do not radiate or transmit sound to other areas. These murmurs are heard in children with normal growth and development. The murmurs heard with specific congenital heart defects are described later in this chapter.

Other abnormal sounds: Several additional unusual sounds may be heard during cardiac auscultation. *Ejection clicks* are crisp sounds that are well localized to either the pulmonic or the aortic area. Pulmonary and aortic ejection clicks are heard most frequently in early systole. A pulmonary ejection click may diminish in intensity with inspiration. It is associated with pulmonic stenosis or pulmonary hypertension. An aortic ejection click does not vary with respiration, and it is associated with aortic valve stenosis, coarctation of the aorta, or aortic aneurysm. (Mitral valve prolapse produces a *midsystolic click*. This is not an uncommon finding in the general population, and, though not a critical care problem, it may be detected in children or adolescents in the ICU.)

A low-pitched hum may be audible throughout the cardiac cycle, often increasing in intensity during diastole. This sound, called a *venous hum*, is often detected at the second or third ICS on either or both sides of the sternum, but it is loudest over the clavicles. The sound can be obliterated by occluding the child's carotid artery or by turning the child's head to one side. A venous hum is almost always normal, but may be associated with anemia.

A *pericardial friction rub* is a high-pitched, variable, grating sound heard over the lower sternum. It is not usually related to systole or diastole or to phase of respiration. This sound is never normal. It is heard after open heart surgery because the pericardium has been incised, and it may also be audible in children with pericarditis.

Cardiovascular Assessment of the Critically Ill Child

In a seriously ill child, peripheral tissue metabolic and oxygen demands may be greater than normal. The cardiovascular system must perform optimally, because any compromise in performance may be profoundly detrimental to the child. Close monitoring of the efficiency of the cardiovascular system is therefore imperative in order to ensure adequate tissue perfusion. In addition to thorough cardiovascular physical examination, the clinician in the ICU makes use of a variety of electronic monitoring devices and diagnostic studies to completely assess the functioning of the cardiovascular system.

Electrocardiography. The electrocardiogram (ECG) of the seriously ill child is generally recorded continuously by three chest leads that often also serve to record the child's respiratory rate. Because the placement of leads is not standardized, the bedside ECG is not considered a totally accurate diagnostic tool, but is utilized primarily to count heart rate and provide a base-line assessment of cardiac rhythm. Suspected arrhythmias require additional investigation and documentation with a 12-lead ECG. The heart rate of an ill child is often more rapid than that of a healthy child of the same age. Tachycardia, necessary to achieve and maintain an effective cardiac output, is, even when prolonged, generally well tolerated by children.

Hemodynamic monitoring. Hemodynamic monitoring of cardiovascular pressures requires the conversion of a biophysical event into an electrical signal that can be displayed, recorded, and quantified. This conversion is accomplished by the use of a transducer. The most popular external transducer is the strain gauge type, in which blood pressure is reflected by changes in the tension on wires beneath the metal diaphragm of the transducer. Changes in tension on these wires result in changes in the current (voltage) present. These voltage changes constitute electrical signals that can be amplified and displayed on the oscilloscope of a monitor or recorded on moving chart paper and quantified and displayed as a digital readout of blood pressure.

The continuous monitoring of pressures permits the detection of subtle, trend-setting changes in the cardiovascular system. A variety of right and left heart pressures (systemic arterial pressure, central venous or right atrial pressures, pulmonary artery pressure, and left atrial pressure) can be measured via a catheter inserted into a vein, artery, or heart chamber and connected to a calibrated pressure transducer. Figure 3-5 depicts a typical monitor that is capable of recording ECG, respirations, and a number of cardiovascular pressures.

Whenever a vascular catheter is in place, it is recommended that catheter patency be maintained by a constant, slow-infusion flush system rather than by intermittent manual flushing with a syringe. This latter practice is associated with the risk of a clot or air bubble being embolized into the central circulation. De-

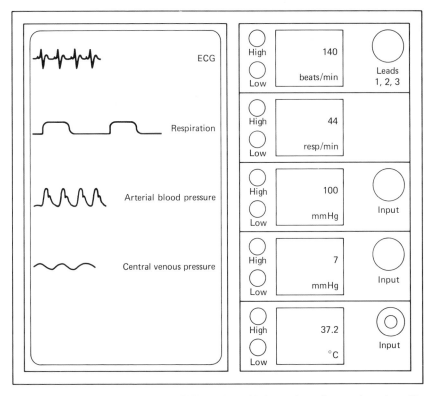

Figure 3-5. Electrocardiogram (ECG) monitor with hemodynamic panels and oscilloscope display.

vices that permit continuous irrigation of the catheter as well as simultaneous monitoring and recording of pressure are readily available (Fig. 3-6). In addition, such a system allows for accurate measurement of the fluid intake absorbed from this route and minimizes the danger of unintentional volume overload.

Systemic arterial blood pressure: Although arterial blood pressure measurement alone is inadequate for determining the efficiency of the cardiovascular system, it is nevertheless an important index of its status. Pressure pulses within the arterial system are a direct result of the intermittent ejection of blood into the aorta as the ventricles contract in systole. Systolic arterial pressure partially reflects the maximal pressure with which blood is ejected from the left ventricle. Because the pressure measured in a peripheral artery is amplified through the arterial system, however, the systolic pressure measurement obtained is actually higher than pressure in the aorta. Diastolic pressure is the lowest pressure in the arterial system, occurring just prior to ventricular contraction. Diastolic pressure reflects the rapidity of blood flow through the arterial system and the elasticity of the arterial walls. Mean arterial pressure indicates the functional pressure that exists in the arterial system during all phases of the cardiac cycle. This pressure is indicative of the pressure with which body tissues are perfused.

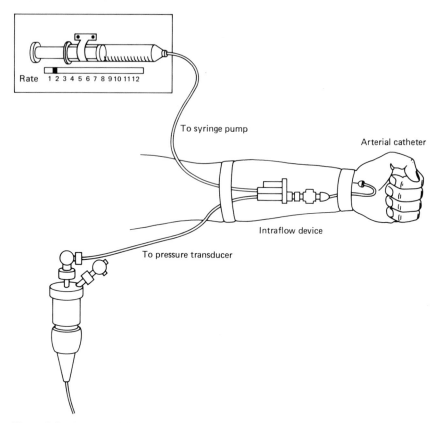

Figure 3-6. Intra-arterial catheter attached to monitoring and flushing systems. Use of the intraflow device permits simultaneous recording and monitoring of pressure while the system is being continuously flushed. The syringe infusion pump is recommended for accurate measurement and control of fluid intake.

Mean arterial pressure is not exactly equal to the arithmetic average of systolic and diastolic pressure because diastole generally lasts about twice as long as systole. Diastolic pressure persists for approximately two-thirds of the cardiac cycle, making mean pressure closer to the diastolic value than to the systolic. Mean arterial pressure can be closely approximated by two formulas (all units are in mmHg):

$$MAP = \frac{SAP + 2(DAP)}{3}, \text{ or}$$

$$MAP = \frac{DAP + PP}{3},$$

where MAP is mean arterial pressure, SAP is systolic arterial pressure, DAP is diastolic arterial pressure, and PP is pulse pressure. The electronic equipment used to monitor arterial pressures performs these calculations automatically and provides the clinician with readouts of the systolic, diastolic, and mean arterial pressures.

Arterial pressure is monitored via a catheter inserted into a peripheral artery. The radial artery is often the vessel of choice. The dorsalis pedis or temporal arteries may also be used, as may the femoral or brachial vessels, although these larger vessels are selected less frequently because the risk of embolization is greater in vessels closer to the central circulation. In newborn infants, the umbilical artery can be cannulated during the first 3 to 4 days of life, before it becomes obliterated. Insertion is achieved by either percutaneous or cutdown technique.

The wave form produced by arterial pressure is characterized by a steep upstroke that corresponds to ventricular systole and the QRS complex of the ECG. Systolic blood pressure is measured at the peak of the upstroke, which is followed by a more gradual downstroke to the diastolic pressure. The downstroke correlates with the gradual decrease in pressure within the arterial system until the next systole. A characteristic notch on the downstroke, called the dicrotic notch, represents closure of the aortic valve. Figure 3-7 illustrates the typical arterial wave form.

When monitoring systemic arterial pressure in the critically ill child, the clinician records systolic, diastolic, and mean pressures, and also notes pulse pressure and the configuration of the wave form. A decrease in the slope of the arterial pressure upstroke reflects a decrease in the velocity with which blood is ejected

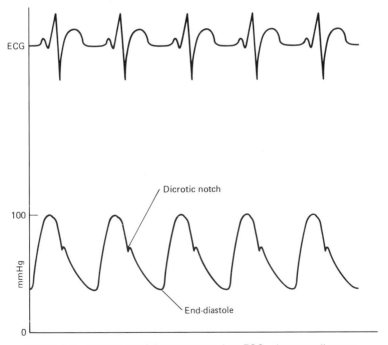

Figure 3-7. Normal arterial pressure tracing. ECG, electrocardiogram.

from the left ventricle and a concomitant decrease in myocardial contractility. Ventricular outflow obstruction, as produced by aortic stenosis or pericardial tamponade, also decreases the slope of the arterial pressure upstroke. A rapid, exaggerated upstroke and little area under the pulse contour suggest decreased stroke volume and increased vascular resistance, even when systolic pressure is normal. When a child requires positive pressure ventilation, its effects on the pressure wave form should be noted. If the arterial pressure decreases with mechanical inspiration, excessive use of positive pressure ventilation and/or relative hypovolemia may be indicated.

Central venous or right atrial pressure: Central venous pressure (CVP) or right atrial pressure (RAP) are referred to as right heart filling pressures. Because the central veins drain directly into the right atrium, CVP is dependent, in part, on RAP. RAP, in turn, is dependent on the volume of venous blood returned to the atrium and on the ability of the atrium to pump that volume into the right ventricle effectively. Both CVP and RAP provide a measure of intravascular volume and right heart contractility. Normal CVP is 4 to 12 mmHg; normal RAP is 0 to 4 mmHg. These measures would be reduced in hypovolemic states (such as those related to burns and acute fluid and electrolyte loss) or after major abdominal surgery. CVP and RAP are increased in CHF or fluid overload.

A CVP or RAP catheter can be inserted by percutaneous or cutdown technique from a number of large veins in the antecubital fossa or via the internal or external jugular vein or the subclavian vein.

The wave form produced by CVP or RAP is characterized by three positive and two negative deflections arbitrarily labeled a, c, v, x, and y (Fig. 3-8). These

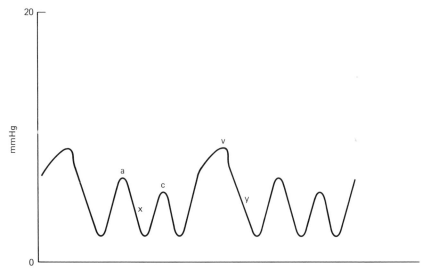

Figure 3-8. Right atrial central venous pressure tracing, showing a, c, and v waves and x and y descents. (*See* text for discussion.) The a wave corresponds to the P wave on the electrocardiogram.

waves and descents correspond to the following mechanical events in the cardiac cycle:

a wave: atrial systole
c wave: start of ventricular systole, with resulting increased pressure on the atrioventricular valves
v wave: atrial filling
x descent: between a and c waves; relaxation of the base of the atria during ventricular contraction
y descent: rapid decrease in atrial pressure as the ventricles fill with blood

In the monitoring of CVP and RAP, only the mean pressure is displayed and recorded. It is sometimes difficult to interpret the numerical value of this reading without additional information about the particular child from whom the data is obtained. For example, a child with CHF may present with an elevated CVP despite hypovolemia. In addition, whenever a child requires positive pressure ventilation, especially with the addition of end-expiratory pressure, the numerical value cannot be strictly interpreted. In such instances, the clinician must note changes in the trend of CVP or RAP readings. Finally, the clinician must remember that CVP and/or RAP may not accurately reflect left-heart filling pressure or functioning.

Right ventricular pressure: Right ventricular pressure (RVP) is not usually monitored in the ICU setting. However, the possibility of the displacement of either a central venous, right atrial, or pulmonary artery catheter into the right ventricle is present when any of these catheters is used. Therefore, the critical care nurse must be familiar with the normal RVP wave form (Fig. 3-9) and normal RVP (20 to 30 mmHg systolic/ < 5 mmHg diastolic) in order to detect this phenomenon, should it occur.

Pulmonary artery pressure: Pulmonary artery catheterization, best done with a quadrilumen catheter (pulmonary artery, right atrial, thermistor tip, and balloon lumens; Fig. 3-10), provides information about left ventricular filling pressure and left ventricular functioning. Repeated measurements of cardiac output can be obtained by thermodilution (*see* p. 117), as can appropriately mixed venous blood for intrapulmonary shunt and arteriovenous oxygen difference determinations (*see* p. 42).

Systolic pulmonary artery pressure (SPAP) corresponds directly to RVP, and should be equal to the systolic RVP in individuals with a normal pulmonary valve. Diastolic pulmonary artery pressure (DPAP) is the lowest pressure in the pulmonary artery just before the next right ventricular systole. Given the continuity of fluid in the pulmonary vascular system between the catheter tip and the left heart, the DPAP indicates the left ventricular end-diastolic pressure (LVEDP) in individuals with normal lungs and a normal mitral valve. LVEDP is determined by the compliance of the left ventricle, i.e., its ability to relax and accept blood from the left atrium during diastole. Therefore, DPAP is a measure of left ventricular functioning and diastolic filling pressure. Mean pulmonary artery pressure (MPAP) is also calculated. It is a measure of the average pressure in the pulmonary artery.

A final measurement of pulmonary artery pressure is made by inflating the balloon at the distal end of the catheter. This maneuver occludes the pulmonary

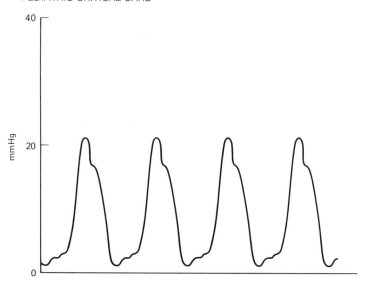

Figure 3-9. Normal right ventricular pressure tracing.

artery, obstructing blood flow from the right ventricle so that the catheter tip is exposed only to pressures reflected retrograde through the pulmonary vasculature from the left atrium. Therefore, the pulmonary artery occluded pressure (PAOP) corresponds closely to the left atrial pressure and provides the most accurate information about left-heart filling pressures. The following are normal values (in mmHg) for the various pressures recorded in the pulmonary artery:

SPAP: 20 to 30
DPAP: < 10
MPAP: < 20
PAOP: 4 to 12

A pulmonary artery catheter is inserted by percutaneous or cutdown technique via a large vein in the antecubital fossa or via the saphenous vein. The catheter is directed into the right atrium and right ventricle, where the balloon tip is inflated. The catheter is then directed by normal blood flow into the pulmonary artery until it cannot be advanced farther (Fig. 3-11). The progress of the catheter through the right atrium, right ventricle, and pulmonary artery is followed by fluoroscopy and by monitoring the pressure wave form displayed on the oscilloscope of the cardiovascular monitor (Fig. 3-12). The ECG is also continually assessed during the insertion procedure because there is a great risk of arrhythmias, especially premature contractions, as the catheter passes through the right ventricle.

The pulmonary artery pressure wave form (Fig. 3-13) resembles that of systemic arterial pressure. It is characterized by a steep upstroke during right ventricular systole and ejection of blood into the pulmonary artery. The upstroke is followed by a more gradual descent, while blood continues to be ejected from the ventricle, until closure of the pulmonic valve. This event results in a notch on the

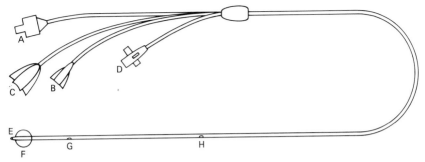

Figure 3-10. Quadrilumen pulmonary artery catheter. (A) Thermistor port connects to cardiac output computer to measure temperature change in pulmonary artery; (B) proximal lumen port monitors right atrial pressure and receives flush solution to maintain catheter patency and calculate cardiac output; (C) distal lumen port monitors pulmonary artery pressure and pulmonary artery occluded pressure and receives flush solution to maintain patency; (D) balloon inflation port receives gas used to inflate balloon and occlude the pulmonary artery; (E) distal lumen in pulmonary artery; (F) balloon occludes pulmonary artery, leaving distal lumen open; (G) thermistor; (H) proximal lumen in right atrium.

downstroke and continued decreasing pressure until the next right ventricular systole. The base line of the pulmonary artery wave form may vary with respiration because of changes in intrathoracic pressure.

When monitoring pulmonary artery pressure, the clinician records systolic, diastolic, mean, and occluded pressures. When the balloon tip is inflated to obtain the PAOP, it should be inflated in small increments and only enough to obtain the desired wave form. The wave form must be observed continuously for confirmation of occlusion (Fig. 3-14). Balloon overinflation produces a progressive elevation of the occluded wave form and a concomitant increase in the PAOP readout (Fig. 3-15). Overinflation can result in rupture of the balloon with risk of air embolization or rupture of the pulmonary artery.

The effects of positive pressure ventilation on the left atrium and pulmonary capillaries, and hence on the PAOP reading, are not known with certainty. Many other variables may influence the relationship between left atrial pressure, LVEDP, and left ventricular end-diastolic volume, and these variables may also alter the measurement of these relationships. The clinician must be aware that all measurements must be continuously assessed, evaluated, and interpreted in light of the given child's clinical condition.

Left atrial pressure: Measurement of left atrial pressure (LAP) is accomplished by means of a catheter placed directly into the left atrium, usually during the course of a thoracotomy. This pressure reading provides the most sensitive index of left-heart filling pressure and left-heart functioning. In addition, it is an extremely sensitive indicator of cardiovascular fluid balance.

Because of the location of the catheter — directly in the left heart — introduction of an embolus has serious implications. This is especially true of air emboli, regardless of the amount of air introduced.

Normal LAP is 4 to 12 mmHg. The LAP wave form (Fig. 3-16) is comparatively flat, like the CVP, RAP, or PAOP wave form. It also consists of the same positive and negative deflections that are seen in the CVP or RAP wave form. A left atrial

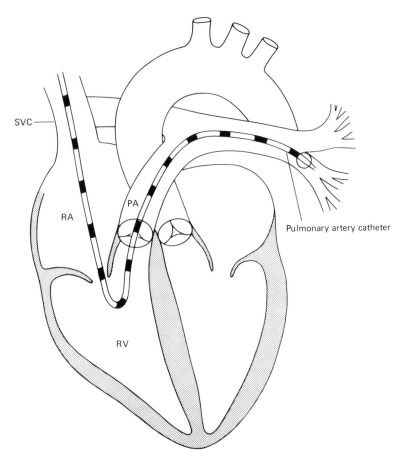

Figure 3-11. Pulmonary artery catheterization. PA, pulmonary artery; RA, right atrium; RV, right ventricle; SVC, superior vena cava.

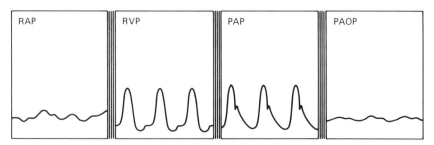

Figure 3-12. Oscilloscope monitoring of pulmonary artery catheter placement. PAOP, pulmonary artery occluded pressure; PAP, pulmonary artery pressure; RAP, right atrial pressure; RVP; right ventricular pressure.

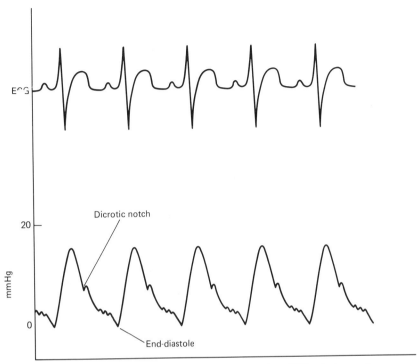

Figure 3-13. Normal pulmonary artery pressure tracing. ECG, electrocardiogram.

line may be displaced through the mitral valve into the left ventricle. The consequent change in pressure wave form and readout is a marked one (Fig. 3-17). The clinician must carefully observe the LAP wave form and record the pressure readout.

Cardiac output determination.   The volume of blood circulated by the heart in 1 minute is determined by the volume of blood ejected with a single heart beat

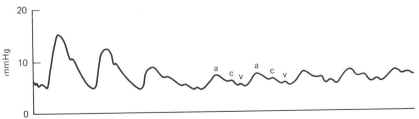

Figure 3-14. Normal pulmonary artery occluded pressure (PAOP) tracing. Note dampening of pulmonary artery pressure tracing as balloon is inflated to obtain PAOP.

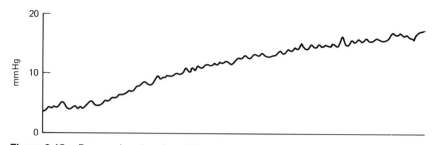

Figure 3-15. Progressive elevation of the pulmonary artery occluded pressure wave form because of overinflation of the catheter balloon.

(stroke volume) and by the heart rate. The value determined is cardiac output (CO), which is calculated by the following formula:

$$\text{CO (liters/min)} = \text{SV (liters/beat)} \times \text{HR (beats/min)},$$

where SV is stroke volume and HR is heart rate. CO can be measured in the critically ill child by using the thermodilution technique. This procedure is accomplished by injecting a thermal indicator (usually cool normal saline or 5 percent dextrose solution) into a central venous or right atrial catheter, and then measuring the resultant change in temperature with a sensitive thermistor downstream in the pulmonary artery. The cold thermal indicator injected in the right atrium is mixed with body-temperature blood in the right atrium and ventricle. When the mixture of indicator and blood flows past the pulmonary artery thermistor, the dilution of the thermal indicator is measured by the change in its temperature. This information is received by the CO computer, and a temperature-time curve is produced. The computer calculates the area under the curve and provides a digital readout of CO in liters/min.

In general, CO determination by the thermodilution technique is accomplished by using a quadrilumen pulmonary artery catheter. However, a right atrial catheter and pulmonary artery thermistor may be placed during cardiac surgery.

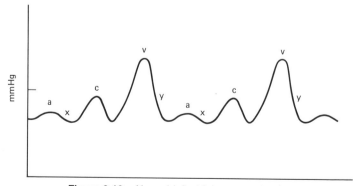

Figure 3-16. Normal left atrial pressure tracing.

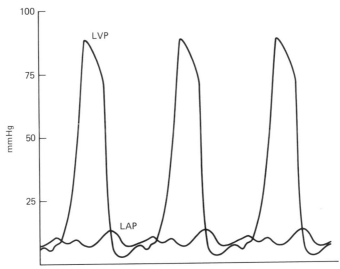

Figure 3-17. Comparison of left atrial pressure (LAP) and left ventricular pressure (LVP) tracings.

The normal volume of blood measured by CO is 4 to 7 liters/min in an individual at rest. This measurement, however, does not take body size into account. Thus, when CO is divided by body surface area (BSA), a more precise measurement is obtained. The resultant value is cardiac index (CI), which is calculated by the following formula:

$$CI \ (liters/min/m^2) = \frac{CO \ (liters/min)}{BSA \ (m^2)}.$$

Normal CI is 2.5 to 4.4 liters/min/m^2.

Diagnostic Studies for Cardiovascular Assessment

A number of diagnostic studies are necessary for complete evaluation of the cardiovascular system. Many of these techniques are used only if the child is suspected or known to have CHD, whereas others are applicable to a variety of children who are critically ill.

Electrocardiography. The conventional 12-lead ECG provides a great deal of reliable information about disorders of cardiac rhythm, disturbances of conduction, and chamber size and work. Always a part of the diagnostic evaluation of the child with CHD, the ECG, by itself, is nonspecific and does not diagnose heart disease: many critically ill children have their ECGs evaluated.

Although it is beyond the scope of this text to review the clinical evaluation and interpretation of the ECG, these skills are nevertheless important and necessary for the ICU clinician. There are a number of excellent and readily available texts specific to this topic.

Chest x-ray.   Chest x-ray is another nonspecific tool for cardiovascular assessment. It is crucial to the evaluation of heart size, detection of enlargement of specific chambers, and determination of the normalness of PBF. Most of the information needed can be obtained from a standard posteroanterior chest film, although lateral and oblique views are helpful in the detection of specific changes in cardiac shape and size.[3]

The skeletal aspects of the chest x-ray are examined because of the association of congenital heart defects with other congenital anomalies (including vertebral and other skeletal abnormalities). Rib notching is a specific finding of coarctation of the aorta in the older child.

The pulmonary parenchyma is inspected because pneumonia is a common problem in children with large left-to-right shunts and high pulmonary venous pressure, such as are seen in ventricular septal defect or a large patent ductus arteriosus. Atelectasis may also occur in these children, especially in the period after cardiac surgery.

Detection of cardiac enlargement is an important goal of chest x-ray. Often, this determination is made by measuring the transverse diameter of the heart and comparing it with the width of the thorax. Cardiomegaly is defined as heart size greater than one half the chest width. This measurement technique, however, does not reliably detect right ventricular enlargement. Whereas left ventricular enlargement can be easily detected on the conventional posteroanterior chest x-ray, right ventricular enlargement is best seen on the lateral chest film.

The second major goal of x-ray diagnosis is the assessment of the pulmonary vasculature. Children with significant left-to-right shunts have an increase in PBF, which results in increased size of the pulmonary vessels well into the peripheral lung fields. Children with decreased PBF will have diminished vascular markings in the lung fields.

The chest x-ray also demonstrates on which side of the thorax the aorta descends. A right-sided aortic arch and descending aorta are associated with certain congenital heart defects. Approximately three-quarters of the children with this finding have tetralogy of Fallot. Truncus arteriosus and tricuspid atresia are also associated with a right-sided aortic arch.

Echocardiography.   Echocardiography is a new but well-accepted tool in the diagnosis of infants and children with CHD. Echocardiography makes use of high-frequency sound waves (ultrasound) to provide important anatomic and functional information about the heart, which could previously be obtained only by cardiac catheterization. Because the echocardiogram is noninvasive, it has a distinct advantage over catheterization in terms of safety.

Ultrasound studies of the heart permit identification and measurement of all four heart valves, both ventricles, the ventricular septum, the left atrium, and the great vessels. A number of congenital heart defects can be identified by echocardiography, including patent ductus arteriosus, transposition of the great arteries, aortic stenosis, hypoplastic left heart syndrome, tricuspid atresia, pulmonary atresia, tetralogy of Fallot, and truncus arteriosus.

Children with myocarditis, postoperative cardiac patients, and patients with direct trauma to the chest may develop pericardial effusion. Because echocardiography is a sensitive technique that can detect even small amounts of fluid, pericardial effusion can be diagnosed by cardiac ultrasound.

Application of echocardiography to the assessment of hemodynamics and cardiac performance is gaining popularity as increased experience provides more reliable results.[4,5] The effects of volume or pressure overload on the heart can be evaluated in terms of chamber enlargement or wall thickening. Motion of the cardiac walls may be useful in estimating left ventricular stroke volume and other measures of ventricular functioning. The degree of left-to-right shunting through a patent ductus arteriosus can also be estimated.

Cardiac catheterization. Cardiac catheterization is an invasive procedure that provides definitive information about the heart and great vessels. A catheter is introduced into a peripheral vein or artery by either cutdown or percutaneous technique and advanced through the vascular system to the heart. In children, the saphenous or femoral veins are most frequently selected for access to the right heart. The left heart may be catheterized from the right heart via the atrial septum or retrograde from the femoral or brachial artery.

The following measures may be obtained during cardiac catheterization:

Hemodynamic indices

1. Pressures in the heart chambers, great vessels, and across the cardiac valves (*see* Fig. 3-3)
2. Blood oxygen saturation in the heart chambers, great vessels, and across shunts (*see* Fig. 3-3)
3. Blood-flow calculations of CO, CI, shunt volume, and regurgitant flows
4. Cardiac performance

Visual indices

1. Chamber size and functioning
2. Valvular functioning
3. Septal patency
4. Vessel patency and origin

In addition, the conduction system can be identified and mapped through the heart. Electrophysiologic studies clarify rhythm or conduction disturbances so that appropriate pharmacological or surgical treatment can be provided.

Finally, several palliative and corrective procedures for specific congenital heart defects are possible during cardiac catheterization. Balloon septostomy can be a life-saving procedure for the newborn with transposition of the great arteries (*see* p. 167). Nonoperative closure of atrial septal defects by means of an umbrella patch inserted through a cardiac catheter has been achieved (*see* p. 130). Catheter closure of patent ductus arteriosus has also been successful (*see* p. 125).

PATHOPHYSIOLOGY

The bulk of this section is devoted to specific information on the more common congenital heart defects. It is prefaced, however, by a brief discussion of CHF and cyanosis because these phenomena are applicable to many cardiac defects.

CHF

CHD is not the only cause of CHF in infancy and childhood, but it is one of the most common. In general, CHF associated with CHD will develop initially during the first 3 or 4 months of life. Thereafter, the incidence of CHF decreases markedly: it is rare as an initial event in children older than 1 year of age.

CHF is a syndrome in which the heart is unable to sustain a sufficient CO to meet the metabolic demands of the body. CHF may result from volume overload, pressure overload, or an inadequately functioning myocardium. Congenital heart defects most commonly result in either volume or pressure overloading. Volume overloading may occur whenever there is an abnormal connection between the systemic and pulmonary vascular systems (resulting in a large left-to-right shunt and increased PBF) or as the result of valvular regurgitation. Pressure overloading may occur when the normal circulation of blood is obstructed.

Regardless of the cause, CHF results in a decrease in CO, an increase in end-diastolic pressure in the ventricles, and a corresponding rise in the atrial, pulmonary venous, and systemic venous pressures. Infants and young children usually present with biventricular (*i.e.*, both right and left) CHF. Right-sided failure results from, and is almost always associated with, left-sided failure.

The manifestations of CHF include the following physical signs:

1. *Tachycardia:* Increased heart rate above the normal level for age is indicative of a stressed cardiac state.

2. *Tachypnea:* Increased respiratory rate without retractions is indicative of early CHF with interstitial pulmonary edema.

3. *Dyspnea:* Increased breathing effort is evident in retractions, grunting, and nasal flaring, and is indicative of more severe CHF.

4. *Coughing, wheezing:* Airway obstruction due to airway edema caused by left atrial hypertension or by pulmonary hypertension and distended pulmonary arteries in children with large left-to-right shunts is indicative of increasingly severe CHF.

5. *Rales:* Pulmonary edema in the alveolar spaces is indicative of severe CHF.

6. *Precordial bulge, hyperactive precordium:* Increased PBF results in an increased volume load and cardiac enlargement.

7. *Hepatomegaly:* An enlarged and tender liver is a sign of systemic venous congestion and indicates CHF of varying degrees by the relative increase in organ size. Hepatomegaly contrasts with peripheral edema, which (with the exception of periorbital edema) is an unusual finding in infants and young children, but is common in older individuals with CHF.

8. *Gallop rhythm:* The presence of an S_3 gallop rhythm is frequently associated with CHF, but an isolated S_3 may be heard in individuals without cardiac disease and in infants or children with cardiac defects that result in increased flow across the mitral or tricuspid valve or in large left-to-right shunts when CHF is absent. An S_4 gallop, never considered normal, indicates CHF.

9. *Narrow pulse pressure:* Poor CO is manifested by narrow pulse pressure, weak peripheral pulses, cold extremities, and decreased urine output. These signs are indicative of severe CHF.

10. *Pulsus paradoxus, pulsus alternans:* Alterations in systolic blood pressure related to phase of respiration or despite normal cardiac rhythm are indicative of severe myocardial dysfunction and CHF.

Cyanosis

Cyanotic infants often present a confusing diagnostic picture. In addition to the difficult task of differentiating cardiac disease from pulmonary disease in these infants, there is the further complication that cyanotic congenital heart defects are associated with either increased or decreased PBF. Defects that result in decreased PBF are characterized by obstruction of the right-heart chambers or vessels. These defects are manifested by the following physical signs and symptoms:

1. *Cyanosis:* Cyanosis is severe (i.e. central cyanosis) and unrelated to immature vasomotor status. The cyanosis may be episodic and is intensified by crying. It is not relieved by the administration of oxygen, even at high concentrations.
2. *Tachypnea:* Extremely rapid respirations that are not accompanied by dyspnea, retractions, grunting, or nasal flaring (which are associated with pulmonary disease or pulmonary edema) are indicative of cyanotic CHD with decreased PBF.

When cyanotic CHD is associated with increased PBF, the following signs and symptoms are generally present:

1. *Cyanosis:* With the exception of transposition of the great arteries (in which cyanosis is severe and present within the first few hours or days of life), the cyanosis tends to be mild to moderately severe. Rubor (ruddiness) may be detected as an early sign of mild arterial desaturation.
2. *Precordial bulge, hyperactive precordium.*
3. *Additional signs and symptoms of CHF (see p. 122).*

Young children with cyanotic CHD are at risk for the development of sudden, severe hypoxic spells if right-ventricular outflow stenosis is part of the diagnosis (*see* p. 154). In other children, this life-threatening event is less of a problem. Chronic cyanosis and hypoxia, however, have deleterious effects on many body systems. These effects include changes in the following tissues and organs:[6]

1. *Central nervous system:* Chronic hypoxia may cause cerebral underperfusion and a diffuse, inflammationlike vascular reaction. Acute insults may result, with episodes of syncope and seizures and the possibility of death. Chronic complications include cerebral thrombosis and tissue infarction. In addition to the risk of stroke, these children are at risk for increased incidence of meningitis while young and for brain abscess when older. These can occur because venous bacteria are shunted into the systemic circulation without undergoing the normal filtering process in the lungs.
2. *Blood:* Chronic hypoxia stimulates overproduction of red blood cells in the bone marrow, which results in polycythemia. When polycythemia is severe, the increased viscosity of the blood impairs circulation to body tissues. Polycythemia also results in thrombocytopenia and impaired platelet aggregation. Reduction of clotting factors (V, VIII, and II, VII, X [the prothrombin complex]) may occur. These hematologic changes, uncommon in infancy, are usually found in older children and can lead to bleeding disorders.
3. *Heart:* Hypoxia evokes cardiac compensatory changes, including coronary vasodilation and the development of myocardial collateral circulation. Despite these changes, the myocardium is depressed, and these children have a severely limited capacity for exertion. In addition, hypoxia has a deleterious

effect on the heart's conduction system, and arrhythmias or conduction defects may occur.

4. *Liver:* Chronic hypoxia results in depletion of the liver's glycogen stores. Hypoglycemia is the obvious consequence. (Depletion of clotting factors has been described.)

5. *Lungs:* Acidosis and hypoxia may lead to increased pulmonary vascular resistance by pulmonary vasoconstriction. Increased pulmonary vascular resistance increases the right-to-left shunting seen in these children, which exacerbates the hypoxia and acidosis and leads to the possibility of a vicious circle.

ACYANOTIC CONGENITAL HEART DEFECTS WITH INCREASED PBF

Congenital heart defects that produce a left-to-right shunt at varying points in the heart lead to an increase in blood flow to the lungs. The most common lesions that create this alteration in hemodynamics are patent ductus arteriosus, atrial septal defect, ventricular septal defect, and endocardial cushion defect. (Table 3-6 summarizes the findings on cardiac examination, ECG, and chest x-ray of children with these defects.)

Patent Ductus Arteriosus

Patent ductus arteriosus (PDA) is a fairly common congenital heart defect, accounting for approximately 10 percent of the total number of cardiac defects. (CHD, in any of its forms, occurs in approximately 8 out of every 1,000 births.) PDA occurs more frequently in females, and is commonly found in offspring of women who have been exposed to rubella during the first trimester of pregnancy. Approximately 15 percent of all children with PDA have an associated anomaly such as ventricular septal defect or coarctation of the aorta.

Etiology. The ductus arteriosus is formed during the fifth to seventh week of gestation. It connects the pulmonary artery at its bifurcation to the aorta, thereby causing blood to bypass the lungs in fetal circulation. The ductus is approximately 1 centimeter in length, slightly less than 1 centimeter in diameter, and has a sphincterlike muscle in its wall. The ductus begins to close within 10 to 15 hours of birth, and closure is usually completed in 2 to 3 weeks. Although a ductus can close spontaneously at any time other than the newborn period, this is very unlikely after the age of 1 year because specific physiological occurrences contribute to its closure.

At birth, concomitant with the onset of respiration, pulmonary vascular resistance decreases as the pulmonary arterioles dilate, causing a rise in PaO_2. In addition, vasoactive substances are released. The combination of the rising PaO_2 and the circulating humoral substances causes the ductus to contract. Eventually, the ductus becomes fibrous. If these processes do not occur, however, a PDA is the result. Factors known to cause a ductus to remain open are prematurity, hypoxia, and scarring of the ductus during fetal life from rubella.

Alteration in hemodynamics. When a patent ductus is present, alteration in normal blood flow through the heart and lungs occurs. Because the pressure in the aorta is higher than that in the pulmonary artery, blood is shunted continuously from the aorta across the patent ductus to the pulmonary artery and the lungs, only to return again to the left heart (Fig. 3-18). This creates an increased volume load on the left side of the heart. Clinical findings vary directly with the amount of shunting from the aorta to the pulmonary artery.

Clinical presentation. Most children with PDA are asymptomatic: they present on routine physical examination with a murmur classically known as a "machinery" murmur, a loud, continuous murmur that is heard throughout systole and diastole and that may obscure S_2. It is best heard at the left upper sternal border and under the left clavicle. In the presence of a large patent ductus, a palpable cardiac thrill at the left sternal border and a prominent left ventricular impulse may be present. Peripheral pulses may be bounding, and a widened pulse pressure may be detected on measurement of blood pressure. Mild symptoms of heart disease may be present, such as some physical underdevelopment, fatigability, and an increased number of respiratory infections.

Chest x-ray usually reveals increased pulmonary vascularity, prominent pulmonary arteries, and enlargement of the left ventricle and aorta with the presence of a significant shunt. ECG findings vary directly with the degree of increased work load on the left heart, the amount of time the increased work load has been present, and the age of the patient. Left ventricular hypertrophy may be present. Often the ECG is normal. An echocardiogram detects the presence, and may help to estimate the size, of a PDA. Definitive diagnosis is usually made by cardiac catheterization.

In contrast to this typical clinical presentation, the premature infant with PDA may present with CHF and may require immediate intervention (*see* p. 122). Hepatomegaly and splenomegaly are usually present, as are bounding posterior tibial and dorsalis pedis pulses.

If definitive diagnosis and correction of PDA are not made, two serious complications can occur. Because of the persistent increased blood flow across the ductus to the lungs, progressive changes in the pulmonary arteries may occur and cause pulmonary hypertension. In addition, the ductus remains a constant potential site of bacterial endocarditis.

Medical management. Medical management of children without serious symptoms related to PDA is conservative. These children do not require exercise restriction if pulmonary artery hypertension is not present. Protection against infective endocarditis is necessary when dental work or any surgical procedure is performed.

Medical management of the small or premature infant with a PDA requires more complex care. This consists of treating the CHF with fluid restriction, diuretics, and digitalization (*see* p. 175). If, however, CHF cannot be controlled by these measures within 48 to 72 hours, surgical intervention is recommended.

Two new developments in the medical care of children have been used to treat PDA. The first is catheter closure of the ductus. During cardiac catheterization, a "plug" is deposited in the ductus by a catheter. This procedure is most prevalent in Japan and Germany. It is not a widely accepted practice in the United States. The second method of ductus closure is by the administration of a pharmacological agent, indomethacin, used primarily with premature infants. Indomethacin, an acetylsalicylic acid, is a prostaglandin inhibitor. Prostaglandin in utero is known to induce active dilation of the ductus arteriosus. With the onset of birth, prostaglandin production is thought to cease. However, the exact mechanism of

TABLE 3-6 Acyanotic Congenital Heart Defects with Increased Pulmonary Blood Flow

Defect	Cardiac examination	Electrocardiogram	Chest x-ray
PDA	"Machinery" murmur heard throughout systole and diastole; best heard at left upper sternal border and under left clavicle. Palpable cardiac thrill (with large PDA) at left sternal border.	May be normal or demonstrate left ventricular hypertrophy.	Increased pulmonary vascularity, prominent pulmonary arteries, enlargement of the left ventricle and aorta.
ASD Ostium Secundum and sinus venosus Ostium Primum	Normal S_1. Soft systolic ejection murmur best heard at 2nd left ICS, fixed and widely split S_2.	May be normal, but right axis deviation, right ventricular hypertrophy, and right BBB are detected in some. Left axis deviation, right BBB.	Increased pulmonary vasculature, enlargement of right atrium, right ventricle, and pulmonary artery; aorta smaller than normal
VSD Small, muscular	Loud, harsh systolic murmur localized to left sternal border. Associated cardiac thrill.	Normal.	Normal heart size and PBF
Moderate to large	Rumbling murmur heard best at lower left sternal border; radiates across the left chest sometimes as far as the midaxillary line. Pulmonic component of S_2 loud and widely split.	Left ventricular dominance and left ventricular hypertrophy.	Cardiomegaly, enlarged left atrium, enlarged left ventricle, prominent pulmonary vascular markings.
Eisenmenger's complex	Quieter heart murmur. S_2 loud and booming.	Dominant right ventricular hypertrophy.	Enlarged right atrium, right ventricle, and pulmonary artery; small distal pulmonary vessels; variability in size of left atrium and left ventricle.

ECD			
Incomplete; competent mitral valve	Same as for ASD.	Same as for ostium secundum ASD.	Same as for ASD.
Mitral insufficiency	Systolic murmur best heard apically; radiates to the axilla.	Left ventricular hypertrophy.	Enlargement of left ventricle and left atrium.
Complete	Combination of ASD, VSD, and atrioventricular valve insufficiency murmurs. No murmur may be present. With pulmonary artery hypertension, S_2 is loud and widely split.	Left axis deviation and biventricular hypertrophy.	Cardiomegaly and increased pulmonary vascular markings.

ASD, atrial septal defect; BBB, bundle-branch block; ECD, endocardial cushion defect; ICS, intercostal space; PBF, pulmonary blood flow; PDA, patent ductus arteriosus; S_1, first heart sound; S_2, second heart sound; VSD, ventricular septal defect.

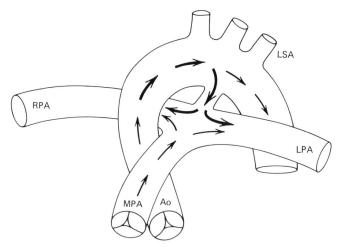

Figure 3-18. Patent ductus ateriosus. Ao, aorta; LPA, left pulmonary artery; LSA, left subclavian artery; MPA, main pulmonary artery; RPA, right pulmonary artery.

cessation of prostaglandin production is not yet clearly understood. Based on the theory that prostaglandins may still be working to maintain dilation of the ductus, indomethacin therapy is used to promote closure of the ductus. Indomethacin is usually given at a dose of 0.2 mg/kg orally or intravenously in a single dose and, if necessary, repeated after 8 hours and 16 hours. Because indomethacin is an acetylsalicylic acid, it cannot be given to the infant with poor renal functioning, necrotizing enterocolitis, bleeding dyscrasias, hyperbilirubinemia, or internal bleeding. When this drug is administered, close assessment for signs and symptoms of abnormal bleeding is crucial. (Studies to determine the safety and effectiveness of indomethacin administration to secure ductal closure are still in progress. Indomethacin therapy is not universally accepted as the treatment of choice.)

Definitive surgical correction. Surgical correction of PDA is the optimal treatment. It is recommended for all infants who present with CHF and for any child with a PDA over the age of 1 year. Children who do not present with any problems directly related to the PDA usually undergo surgical correction during the preschool years. The surgery is performed through a posterolateral incision in the fourth left ICS. In the infant, the ductus is usually ligated with heavy ligature. In the older child, the ductus is divided between clamps, and the severed ends are closed by suture. Postoperative complications are rare except in the premature infant, for whom other factors, such as respiratory distress, complicate recovery.

Atrial Septal Defect

Atrial septal defect (ASD) is a fairly common congenital heart defect, accounting for approximately 10 percent of the total number of cardiac defects. It occurs more frequently in females. An ASD exists when there is a communication between the left and right atrium that persists beyond the perinatal period.

Etiology. During fetal life, the atrial septum is formed during the fourth to sixth week of gestation. An opening, however, called the foramen ovale, persists in the atrial septum throughout intrauterine existence. This opening permits blood to bypass the lungs. After birth, with an increase in LAP, the foramen ovale closes. In the growth of the atrial septum during fetal life, failure of the septal layers to fuse completely results in an ASD.

Alteration in hemodynamics. Defects in the atrial septum, which can occur in different locations, are identified by where they occur. The most common site is at the center of the atrial septum at the level of the foramen ovale. This defect is called an ostium secundum ASD. If the defect occurs high in the atrial septum, it is called a sinus venosus ASD. This defect, located near the junction of the superior vena cava and the right atrium, is often associated with abnormal drainage of the pulmonary veins. When the defect occurs low in the septum, it is identified as an ostium primum ASD (Fig. 3-19). This defect is more complex, and is often associated with abnormalities of the atrioventricular valves. Ostium primum ASDs are less common than ostium secundum or sinus venosus ASDs.

Because of higher pressure in the left atrium, and because the right atrium and

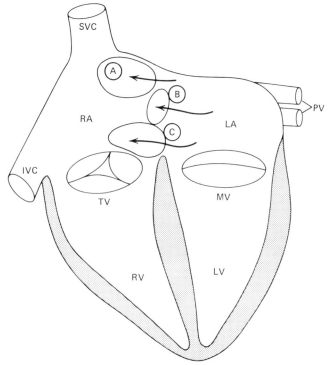

Figure 3-19. Three kinds of atrial septal defect (ASD). (A) Sinus venousus ASD, (B) ostium secundum ASD, (C) ostium primum ASD. IVC, inferior vena cava; LA, left atrium; LV, left ventricle; MV, mitral valve; PV, pulmonary vein; RA, right atrium; RV, right ventricle; SVC, superior vena cava; TV, tricuspid valve.

right ventricle are more compliant, blood is shunted from the left atrium across the ASD into the right atrium, thereby altering normal blood flow through the heart. This creates a burden on the right side of the heart. However, significant shunting across the ASD may not occur until early childhood due to the relative noncompliance of the right atrium in infancy. This explains why many ASDs are not detected until early childhood.

Clinical presentation. Children with ASDs are generally in a normal state of health. Their growth and development is normal, and, usually, so is their exercise tolerance. Some children may experience tiredness on extreme exertion, and, sometimes, there may be a history of more frequent respiratory infections, but most children with ASDs are only identified when a previously undetected heart murmur is heard during a routine physical examination. As with any shunting within the heart, symptoms vary according to the size of the shunt. However, children with ostium primum ASDs with associated atrioventricular valve abnormalities may present with CHF in infancy or early childhood.

On cardiac examination, S_1 is normal, but there is a soft systolic ejection murmur best heard at the second left ICS and a fixed, widely split S_2. The fixed splitting of S_2 is a classic sign of ASD and very useful in diagnosis.

On chest x-ray, pulmonary vasculature is increased; the right atrium, right ventricle, and pulmonary artery are enlarged; and the aorta may appear smaller than normal. The ECG varies according to the type of ASD present. With ostium secundum ASD and sinus venosus ASD, the ECG may be normal, or it may show right axis deviation, right ventricular hypertrophy, and, often, right bundle-branch block. With ostium primum ASD, the ECG is usually abnormal. Left axis deviation and right bundle-branch block are present. By means of an echocardiogram, a more definitive diagnosis can be made by location of the defect, assessment of size of the shunt, and detection of right ventricular enlargement. Cardiac catheterization confirms a definitive diagnosis, provides differential diagnosis of ostium primum as opposed to ostium secundum ASD, and quantifies the shunt volume.

Failure to diagnose an ASD in children usually does not cause any irreversible damage to the cardiac or pulmonary system. However, if ASD remains undetected until adulthood is reached, CHF and pulmonary vascular disease may occur in those over 30 years of age. There is also a risk of subacute bacterial endocarditis in older individuals with an ASD.

Medical management. Medical management of the child with an ASD is conservative because the majority of children are asymptomatic. Children with an ostium primum ASD with associated atrioventricular valve abnormalities who present with CHF are treated with digoxin, fluid limitation, and diuretics (*see* p. 175).

Nonoperative closure of ASDs has been achieved by means of an umbrella technique performed via a cardiac catheter. A patch is folded like an umbrella within a special catheter. It is then opened within the left atrium and drawn against the atrial septum. This technique, although regarded as experimental, has been successful in a number of children.[7]

Definitive surgical correction. Surgical repair of the ASD is recommended. Because most of the children are in a normal state of health, elective surgery is usually performed in the preschool or early school years. Surgical correction is performed by means of a midline sternotomy incision. The child is placed on cardiopulmonary bypass. The ASD is then either closed by suture, or a Dacron patch is sutured in place. With sinus venosus ASD, the patch is placed so as to close the ASD and to direct any anomalous pulmonary venous drainage into the left atrium. Because the atrioventricular bundle of His is close to the area being sutured, care must be used during suturing. Interference in conduction during surgery occurs more in ostium primum ASD than in ostium secundum and sinus venosus ASDs. Postoperative complications may include transient pulmonary edema in patients with pulmonary hypertension and heart block.

Ventricular Septal Defect

Ventricular septal defects are the most common congenital heart defects, accounting for 20 percent of the total number of cardiac defects. A ventricular septal defect (VSD) is a communication between the ventricles that permits blood to flow freely between them. This defect occurs more frequently in males; the precise etiology is unknown. VSD is seen in infants with Down's syndrome and other autosomal trisomies, and is associated with renal anomalies. VSDs are also seen in conjunction with a variety of other congenital heart defects, especially coarctation of the aorta, PDA, and transposition of the great arteries.

Etiology. The ventricular septum is established in fetal life during the fourth to eighth week of gestation. The ventricular septum is formed from muscular and membranous tissues that fuse with the endocardial cushions and bulbus cordis. If inadequate development of these tissues occurs in fetal life, a VSD will result. The size of a VSD varies from that of a pinpoint to the absence of the entire septum. A VSD may occur in either the membranous or the muscular portion of the ventricular septum (Fig. 3-20).

Alteration in hemodynamics. At birth, a VSD does not alter flow of blood through the heart because pressure in the right and left ventricle is essentially equal. As the infant matures, resistance in the lungs decreases, RVP drops, pressure in the left ventricle becomes greater than in the right, and blood is shunted from left to right. This explains why the diagnosis of VSD is most frequently made at an infant's 6-week checkup.

After 6 weeks of age, VSD is often responsible for significant left-to-right shunting. However, the size of the shunt is determined by the size and location of the VSD, and it directly influences the child's initial clinical presentation and the effect of this excessive blood flow on the pulmonary vasculature. A sizable left-to-right shunt causes significant changes in the pulmonary vascular bed. In response to the abnormally high flow of blood that is under increased pressure, the pulmonary vessels hypertrophy and actually undergo histological changes of the intima. As a result of these changes, an increase in pulmonary vascular resistance occurs, which further serves to increase pulmonary pressure and RVP. When pressure in the right ventricle is equal to or greater than left ventricular pressure, shunting across the VSD is eliminated or may occur in the opposite direction.

These hemodynamic changes are the result of pulmonary artery hypertension, but do not occur in every child with VSD. Most children with VSD have small defects in the muscular portion of the ventricular septum. These are common defects that usually close spontaneously within the first 4 to 6 years of life and are not associated with large shunts.

Moderate to large VSDs occur most commonly in the membranous portion of the septum, in proximity to the bundle of His and below the aortic and pulmonic valves. The size of the shunt in moderate to large VSDs varies directly with the size of the defect and the proximity of the pulmonic valve.

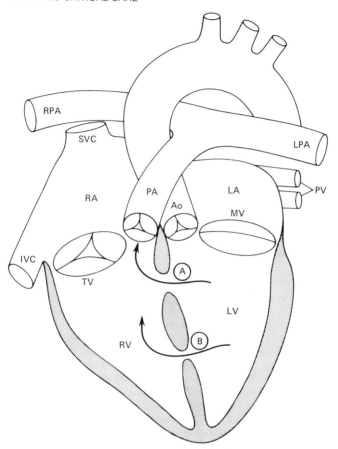

Figure 3-20. Two kinds of ventricular septal defect (VSD). (A) Membranous VSD, (B) muscular VSD. Ao, aorta; IVC, inferior vena cava; LA, left atrium; LPA, left pulmonary artery; LV, left ventricle; MV, mitral valve; PA, pulmonary artery; PV, pulmonary vein; RA, right atrium; RPA, right pulmonary artery; RV, right ventricle; SVC, superior vena cava; TV, tricuspid valve.

Clinical presentation. The child's initial clinical appearance is determined directly by the size of the VSD and the amount of shunting that occurs. When shunting is prolonged and pulmonary vascular changes result, these changes also affect the child's appearance and clinical findings. Children with small, muscular VSDs appear healthy and normal. They have a loud, harsh, systolic murmur that is well localized to the left sternal border, and they often have an associated cardiac thrill. The ECG is normal, and heart size and PBF appear normal on chest x-ray. Most defects in this category are diagnosed clinically and do not require cardiac catheterization.

Children with moderate-sized defects may be asymptomatic except for a proneness to tire more easily than their peers. Children in this category are also more prone to upper and lower respiratory infections.

Children with large VSDs are usually very thin. Their anterior chest wall may be prominent because it develops around an enlarged heart. The heart murmur in moderate to large VSDs is best heard at the lower left sternal border, and it sometimes radiates across the left chest as far as the midaxillary line. It is usually less harsh than the murmur of a small VSD and has a rumbling quality. The pulmonic component of S_2 is loud. Peripheral pulses and perfusion are normal. On ECG, left ventricular dominance and left ventricular hypertrophy may be seen. Cardiomegaly, enlarged left atrium, enlarged left ventricle, and prominent pulmonary vascular markings are noted on chest x-ray. By means of an echocardiogram, the quantity of shunting can be estimated. Cardiac catheterization can demonstrate the exact size and location of the VSD and the quantity of shunting. Pressures within the ventricles, pulmonary artery, and aorta can be measured to determine if pulmonary hypertension is present. These determinations are vital if surgery is to be performed.

Infants with large defects do not tolerate the increased PBF well. They are often diaphoretic, tachypneic, and tachycardiac. They have difficulty with feeding and do not gain the expected amount of weight in their first weeks or months of life. CHF may occur and is usually manifested in the first several months of life (*see* p. 122).

Children who develop pulmonary artery hypertension from a large, prolonged left-to-right shunt present with a very different clinical picture. If pulmonary hypertension has reached a level at which right ventricular pressure has increased and is equal to left ventricular pressure, no shunting will take place across the VSD. Therefore, no murmur will be heard. If the pulmonary hypertension has caused RVP to become greater than left ventricular pressure, the shunt will reverse and become a right-to-left shunt. This alteration in shunt direction is called Eisenmenger's complex. Children with shunt reversal are cyanotic and may develop clubbing of the nail beds. Their heart murmur becomes quieter, but S_2 becomes loud and booming. The chest x-ray reveals an enlarged right atrium, enlarged right ventricle, enlarged pulmonary artery, prominent proximal pulmonary vessels, small distal pulmonary vessels, and variability in the size of the left atrium and ventricle. Dominant right ventricular hypertrophy is evident on ECG.

Medical management.   Medical management of children with small VSDs is conservative. Because these children are asymptomatic, and because spontaneous closure of the defect often occurs, intervention is rarely necessary. Even if spontaneous closure does not occur, surgery is generally not recommended. With a small defect, life expectancy is normal, and the risk of operating is deemed greater than the risk of not operating.

Children and infants with moderate to large VSDs require close medical assessment. Their heart murmur must be evaluated frequently for an increase in shunt size and for possible development of pulmonary hypertension. Signs and symptoms of pulmonary hypertension are also monitored by chest x-ray, ECG, and echocardiogram. These children are also monitored closely for signs and symptoms of CHF, and they are often maintained on digoxin and diuretics. They are also assessed closely for signs and symptoms of pneumonia, which they are prone to develop and which can be a life-threatening illness, especially in infants. Children with large VSDs are at significant risk for the development of subacute bacterial endocarditis.

Palliative surgical management.   In infants, surgery is necessary if CHF cannot be managed. The surgery may be either palliative or corrective. Palliative surgery for a VSD, known as pulmonary artery banding, decreases the amount of PBF to the lungs. This is accomplished by placing a segment of Teflon tape around the pulmonary artery. Sutures are then placed through the tape to the desired degree of constriction. This procedure is generally performed via a left posterolateral incision. Most institutions, however, favor corrective surgery in the infant (unless severe pulmonary disease is present or unless VSD is complicated by other heart defects) because pulmonary artery banding drastically complicates later definitive surgery.

Definitive surgical correction.   Corrective surgery is recommended for children with moderate to large VSDs. The timing of surgery is dependent on the presence or absence of complicating factors. In children who are asymptomatic, surgery is recommended in the preschool years. If growth and development are impeded by chronic respiratory infections or CHF as well as by the presence of pulmonary hypertension, surgery is recommended at an earlier age.

Corrective repair of VSD is achieved via a midline sternotomy incision. Cardiopulmonary bypass and deep hypothermia are required. The defect is closed by sutures or a patch. Because of the proximity of these defects to the bundle of His, extra care is taken to prevent conduction problems postoperatively. Postoperative complications may include hemorrhage and heart block as well as cyanosis, dyspnea, and hypotension in patients with pulmonary hypertension. Aortic insufficiency also develops in a few children, and it is identified by the presence of a widened pulse pressure and a diastolic murmur.

Endocardial Cushion Defect

Endocardial cushion defects (atrioventricular canals) account for approximately 5 percent of the total number of congenital heart defects. An endocardial cushion defect (ECD) exists when there is an abnormal communication between the atria or the ventricles, or when there is communication between the atria and ventricles as well as an insufficiency of the atrioventricular valves. ECDs occur slightly more frequently in females. The precise etiology of this defect is unknown. Children with Down's syndrome, however, have a high incidence of ECDs.

Etiology.   During fetal life, the endocardial cushions are responsible for the development of components of the mitral and tricuspid valves, the upper ventricular septum, and the lower atrial septum. The cushions also play a role in the placement of the atrioventricular conduction system. These developments occur between the fourth and eighth week of gestation. Inadequate development of the cushions may result in varying combinations of defects in any of these specified parts of the heart. It is for this reason that ECDs are classified as either incomplete, transitional, or complete.

Because transitional ECDs encompass multiple variations of abnormalities in the atrial and ventricular septa and the atrioventricular valves, it is impossible to accurately present a clear clinical picture to the reader. Therefore, incomplete and complete ECDs will be the primary focuses of the following section.

Alteration in hemodynamics

Incomplete ECD: The child with an incomplete ECD presents with an ostium primum ASD as well as a variable degree of mitral valve abnormality, generally a cleft mitral valve (Fig. 3-21). If the mitral valve is competent, despite an abnormality in its structure, alteration in hemodynamics is the same as in the child with an ostium primum ASD (*see* p. 129). The presence of an insufficient mitral valve in

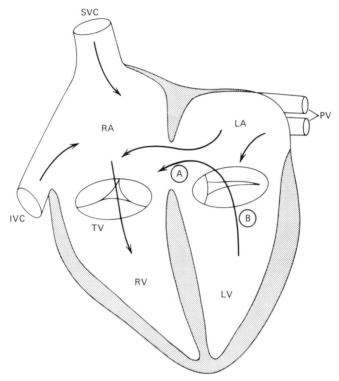

Figure 3-21. Incomplete endocardial cushion defect. (A) Site of ostium primum atrial septal defect, (B) site of cleft mitral valve. IVC, inferior vena cava; LA, left atrium; LV, left ventricle; PV, pulmonary vein; RA, right atrium; RV, right ventricle; SVC, superior vena cava; TV, tricuspid valve.

addition to an ASD will further increase the burden on the right side of the heart. If the ASD is small, however, any mitral insufficiency will increase the burden on the left side of the heart.

Complete ECD: In the complete form of ECD, an ostium primum ASD, a VSD in the upper ventricular septum, and a common atrioventricular valve are present (Fig. 3-22). The end result is free communication between all chambers of the heart. Shunting occurs at the atrial and ventricular levels in a left-to-right direction. (It is important to note that the ventricular shunt may become a right-to-left shunt in the presence of pulmonary artery hypertension.) In addition, the right atrium receives blood from two other sources within the heart. During systole, the right atrium can receive blood from the left ventricle via the insufficient mitral valve and the ASD. Blood can also enter the right atrium from the right ventricle via the incompetent tricuspid valve. It is for these reasons that there is an excessive volume load on the right side of the heart and the pulmonary vasculature. Pulmonary hypertension is a frequent complication because of this increased volume load. The left side of the heart is also stressed, thereby compromising normal heart functioning even further. Because of the presence of a VSD and

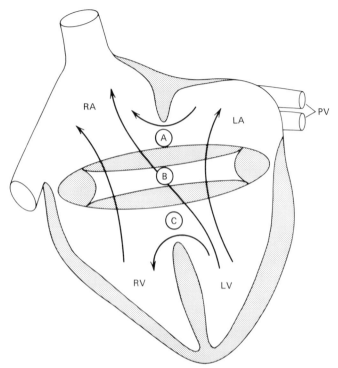

Figure 3-22. Complete endocardial cushion defect. (A) Site of ostium primum atrial septal defect, (B) site of common atrioventricular valve, (C) site of ventricular septal defect. LA, left atrium; LV, left ventricle; PV, pulmonary vein; RA, right atrium; RV, right ventricle.

mitral insufficiency, the left atrium and left ventricle receive excess volume. However, the increased volume in the left atrium is relieved by means of the ASD. With regard to the alternate paths of flow, certain factors play an important role in determining the degree of shunting. These are pulmonary resistance, systemic resistance, left ventricular pressure, RVP, and the compliance of all heart chambers.

Clinical Presentation

Incomplete ECD: The clinical presentation of the child with an incomplete ECD varies directly with the degree of insufficiency of the mitral valve and the size of the ASD. If the mitral valve is competent, despite an abnormality in its structure, the child will appear healthy and will present with the same clinical picture as the child with an ASD (*see* p. 130). If the mitral valve is insufficient, the clinical presentation will be altered in direct relation to the alterations in blood flow that result.

When a large ASD and an insufficient mitral valve are present, the child presents with the same clinical picture as the child with a large ASD except that the symptoms are more severe and begin earlier. On cardiac examination, the murmur is the same as that of ASD with the addition of the murmur of mitral insufficiency. A classic mitral murmur is systolic and apical, and it characteristically radiates to the axilla. ECG and x-ray findings are consistent with the findings seen in an ASD.

When a small ASD and an insufficient mitral valve are present, the child's clinical presentation is as follows. Left-sided CHF may develop in infancy, or it may be delayed, with only mild dyspnea and fatigue being experienced by the young child. On cardiac examination, the classic mitral insufficiency murmur is heard. The ECG frequently demonstrates left ventricular hypertrophy. Left ventricular and atrial enlargement are seen on chest x-ray.

Complete ECD: The clinical presentation of the infant or child with a complete ECD is as follows. CHF generally becomes a problem early in life, physical growth is poor, and respiratory infections are a common problem. The infant may be compromised by tachypnea, tachycardia, and difficulty with feeding. A prominent left chest may be evident due to cardiomegaly.

On cardiac examination, peripheral pulses are normal. The cardiac murmurs in these children may consist of a combination of ASD, VSD, and atrioventricular valve insufficiency murmurs. Because of the complicated shunting, however, a balance in hemodynamics may occur so that no murmur results. If pulmonary hypertension is present, S_2 is loud. Arterial blood gas will demonstrate desaturation.

On chest x-ray, gross cardiomegaly and increased pulmonary vascular markings are seen. Left axis deviation and biventricular hypertrophy are evident on ECG. The echocardiogram provides useful information regarding atrioventricular valve insufficiency. Cardiac catheterization provides definitive diagnosis and essential preoperative information such as chamber pressures and oxygen saturations.

Medical management

Incomplete ECD: The infant or child with an incomplete ECD is treated in the same way as children with ASD (*see* p. 130). However, precautions against infective endocarditis are necessary because of mitral valve insufficiency. If mitral insufficiency causes CHF to develop, the child is treated with digitalization and diuretics (*see* p. 175). Close assessment of these children is vital.

Complete ECD: A complete ECD generally requires close assessment and aggressive intervention because of the frequency with which CHF occurs. Digoxin and diuretics are again the treatment of choice. These children are also watched closely for signs and symptoms of pneumonia. Monitoring of heart murmurs is vital to the prognosis of these children. Auscultatory evidence of pulmonary artery hypertension is specifically assessed for. If pulmonary artery hypertension is a problem, exercise may be restricted.

Palliative surgical management. Surgery is recommended immediately for those children whose CHF cannot be controlled medically. Pulmonary artery banding (*see* p. 133) is the palliative surgical intervention for ECD. However, this measure is generally not recommended because it increases the mortality rate for later surgical correction.

Definitive surgical correction. Surgical correction of an ECD is generally performed during the preschool years. Corrective surgery is performed via a midline sternotomy incision. Deep hypothermia and cardiopulmonary bypass are required. An incomplete ECD is repaired with a patch of the ASD and by suturing the cleft in the mitral valve. Corrective repair of a complete ECD involves patch repair of the ASD and VSD and repair of the mitral and tricuspid valves. Mitral valve replacement with a porcine valve may be necessary. Close care is taken during suturing to prevent heart block. Postoperative complications may include heart block and persistence of atrioventricular valve insufficiency. Precautions against endocarditis are necessary both preoperatively and postoperatively.

ACYANOTIC CONGENITAL HEART DEFECTS WITH NORMAL PBF

Coarctation of the aorta and aortic stenosis are two common cardiac lesions that result in increased heart work and that especially affect the left ventricle. However, because there is no abnormal connection between the systemic and pulmonary vascular systems, shunting of blood does not occur and PBF is normal. These defects do not cause alteration in the oxygen saturation of arterial blood. Therefore, children with these defects are acyanotic. Pulmonic stenosis, unless very severe, is a third common defect that does not produce either cyanosis or altered PBF despite obstruction and the increased work of the right heart. (Table 3-7 summarizes the findings on cardiac examination, ECG, and chest x-ray of children with these defects.)

Coarctation of the Aorta

Coarctation of the aorta is a common congenital heart defect, accounting for approximately 10 percent of the total number of cardiac defects. It occurs more frequently in males. A coarctation, or narrowing, of the aorta usually occurs beyond the left subclavian artery at the area of the ductus insertion. However, coarctation of the abdominal aorta may also be seen, though infrequently. Other forms of CHD may occur with a coarctation. Of all the children with a coarctation, 50 percent have a bicuspid aortic valve.

Etiology.   Between the fifth and eighth week of gestation, development of the aortic arch occurs. If the arch develops improperly a restricted opening or lumen in the aorta results. This occurs most commonly in the area of the aorta near the ductus arteriosus, and it may be proximal or distal to the insertion of the ductus. It is for this reason that coarctation is classified as preductal or postductal. Differentiation between a preductal and postductal coarctation is made by the presence or absence of a patent ductus. If the ductus remains open, the coarctation is classified as preductal. If the ductus is very small or totally obliterated, the coarctation is classified as postductal. Preductal coarctation is often associated with severe cardiac defects such as hypoplastic left heart syndrome and VSD. Postductal coarctation is associated with VSD and aortic stenosis, but these associated defects are seen less frequently and are generally not as severe as the defects associated with preductal coarctation.

Alteration in hemodynamics

Preductal coarctation: A preductal coarctation results in abnormal blood flow from the left and right heart. Blood leaving the left ventricle will enter the ascending aorta and flow to the site of the coarctation. Below the coarctation, blood will enter the descending aorta from the pulmonary artery via the ductus (Fig. 3-23). (*see* p. 142). Therefore, because of the position of the coarctation, the upper half of the body will be saturated by blood from the left ventricle and the lower half of the body will be saturated by blood from the right ventricle. This alteration in hemodynamics causes an enlarged right ventricle, enlarged pulmonary artery, and a prominent descending aorta.

Postductal coarctation: A postductal coarctation causes alteration in normal blood flow but in a pattern entirely different from that of preductal coarctation. This coarctation is distal to the insertion of the ductus and requires the development of collateral circulation to the lower half of the body (Fig. 3-24). (*see* p. 143). This process begins in fetal life because the greater portion of right ventricular outflow empties into the ascending aorta via the ductus.

Because of the high pressure that develops in the ascending and descending aorta from the narrowed portion, increased stress is placed on the left atrium and ventricle. This causes enlargement of both these chambers, though left ventricular enlargement is more pronounced.

Clinical presentation

Preductal coarctation: The infant with preductal coarctation presents early in life with CHF. Hypertension is present in the upper extremities, as opposed to low pressure in the lower extremities. Femoral pulses are present but weaker than brachial and radial pulses, and, in comparison with the radial pulse, their onset is delayed. In addition, because the lower half of the body receives its blood flow from the right ventricle via the ductus, arterial desaturation exists in the lower extremities. Cyanosis of the lower extremities, however, can rarely be visualized.

On cardiac examination, no murmur is heard because of the absence of collateral vessel formation. An enlarged right ventricle, enlarged pulmonary artery, and a prominent descending aorta develop from the alteration in hemodynamics. However, chest x-ray may show only cardiomegaly because this type of coarctation almost always presents in the newborn period, when specific chamber enlargement is difficult to discern. The ECG consistently demonstrates right ventricular hypertrophy.

Postductal coarctation: Most children and infants with postductal coarctation follow one of two courses: they may present with CHF in the first 3 months of life, or they may grow normally without any symptomatology. The latter is more often the case. Most coarctations are detected on routine physical examination. The clinical findings depend on the age of the child at the time of presentation and may vary. Some children may complain of headaches, nosebleeds, fatigue, or "cool feet."

On physical examination, these children are generally pink. Blood pressure in the upper extremities is higher than in the lower extremities. Pulses in the upper extremities are full, in contrast to weak or absent pulses in the lower extremities. In fact, by accurate assessment of pulses, the location of the coarctation can be estimated. For example, if pulses are absent in the left arm and the legs but present in the right arm, the coarctation is either at the site of, or proximal to the site of, the left subclavian artery. Cardiac catheterization is required for definitive diagnosis.

On cardiac examination, heart sounds are generally normal. However, if the coarctation is severe, a loud S_2 will be heard. In addition, if collateral flow is large, a continuous systolic murmur will be heard, especially over the child's back. An enlarged left atrium, enlarged left ventricle, and a dilated ascending aorta are generally evident on chest x-ray. Rib notching from collateral circulation may also be seen but is usually not evident in children under 8 years of age. Varying degrees of left ventricular hypertrophy are demonstrated on ECG.

If a coarctation remains undetected, damage to the aorta may occur. The ascending aorta, in response to persistent high pressure, becomes thin, friable, and, eventually, calcified. In addition, aneurysms frequently develop in the intercostal arteries.

Medical management. Medical management of children with coarctation depends on the clinical presentation. The infant who presents with CHF is treated with

TABLE 3-7 Acyanotic Congenital Heart Defects with Normal Pulmonary Blood Flow

Defect	Cardiac examination	Electrocardiogram	Chest-x-ray
Coarctation of the aorta			
Preductal	Normal heart sounds.	Right ventricular hypertrophy.	Cardiomegaly.
Postductal	Normal heart sounds, but S_2 may be accentuated with severe coarctation. With large collateral flow, continuous systolic murmurs develop.	Varying degrees of left ventricular hypertrophy.	Enlarged left atrium and left ventricle; dilated ascending aorta. Rib notching in children over 8 years of age with extensive collateral circulation.
AS			
Valvular (Mild to moderate)	Ejection click best heard at the 4th ICS to the left of the sternum. Rough, harsh murmur best heard at base of the heart to the right of the sternal border.	Left ventricular hypertrophy, or may be normal.	May appear normal. Possible left ventricular enlargement and dilated ascending aorta.
(Moderate to severe)	Palpable thrill best felt at the suprasternal notch and at the 2nd right ICS. Diminished S_2.	Left ventricular hypertrophy; possible S-T and T wave changes, or may be normal.	Same as for mild to moderate AS. Pulmonary congestion may be seen.
IHSS	Midsystolic ejection murmur best heard near the apex; palpable thrill may be present. Normal S_2	Left ventricular hypertrophy.	Left ventricular enlargement and cardiomegaly.
Subvalvular	Similar to valvular AS, with absence of ejection click.	Same as for valvular AS.	Similar to valvular AS, but dilation of aorta absent.
Supravalvular	Normal S_1; absent ejection click; ejection systolic murmur; palpable thrill may be present.	Same as for valvular AS.	Ascending aorta smaller than normal; descending aorta normal in size.

	Auscultation/Physical findings		Radiographic findings
PS			
Valvular (Mild to moderate)	Ejection click after S_1, followed by systolic ejection murmur best heard at upper left sternal border and radiating widely. Palpable thrill at 2nd left ICS. S_2 widely split, with diminished pulmonic component. Right ventricular lift.	Right ventricular hypertrophy.	Right ventricular and main pulmonary artery enlargement. Normal left heart and pulmonary vascular markings.
(Severe)	Murmur increased in duration and intensity, obscuring S_2. No ejection click audible.	Right ventricular and right atrial hypertrophy.	Same as above, with right atrial enlargement.
Infundibular (Fibrous ring)	Similar to valvular PS, but no ejection click or change in intensity of S_2, which is widely split.	Same as for valvular PS.	Right ventricular enlargement. Normal pulmonary artery, left heart, and pulmonary vascular markings.
(Muscular)	No ejection click. Short systolic murmur ending before S_2, best heard at 3rd or 4th left ICS. Palpable thrill with severe stenosis. Widely split S_2. Bulging of lower precordium; right ventricular heave.	Same as for valvular PS.	Same as for fibrous ring infundibular PS.
Subinfundibular	Similar to muscular infundibular PS.	Same as for muscular infundibular PS.	Same as for muscular infundibular PS.
Supravalvular	Systolic ejection murmur heard over sites of obstruction, radiating through pulmonary vasculature. Occasional continuous murmur. Normal S_1 and S_2; no ejection click.	Variable increased right heart work.	Variable enlargement of right heart chambers and main pulmonary artery. Variable changes in pulmonary vascular markings.

AS, aortic stenosis; ICS, intercostal space; IHSS, idiopathic hypertrophic subaortic stenosis; PS, pulmonic stenosis; S_1, first heart sound; S_2, second heart sound.

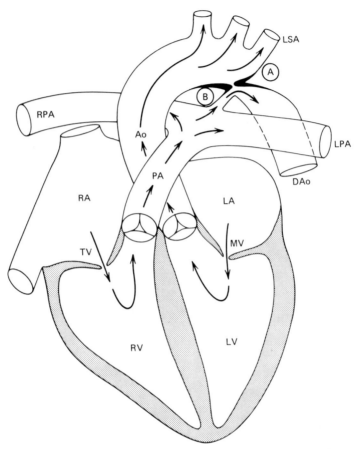

Figure 3-23. Preductal coarctation of the aorta (Ao). (A) Site of coarctation, (B) patent ductus arteriosus. DAo, descending Ao; LA, left atrium; LPA, left pulmonary artery; LSA, left subclavian artery; LV, left ventricle; MV, mitral valve; PA, pulmonary artery; RA, right atrium; RPA, right pulmonary artery; RV, right ventricle; TV, tricuspid valve.

digitalization and diuretics (*see* p. 175). Surgery is recommended only if medical management is unsuccessful.

The older child whose coarctation is detected on routine physical examination requires close assessment of blood pressure. Significant hypertension may require the use of antihypertensives preoperatively (*see* p. 375). If significant hypertension is present at rest, exercise restriction may be recommended. Antibiotic prophylaxis against bacterial endocarditis is recommended preoperatively and postoperatively because of the high risk of this serious infection in children with a bicuspid aortic valve with coarctation.

Definitive surgical correction. Elective surgery is recommended between the ages of 4 and 8 years. During this age span, the child's aorta is close in size to that of an

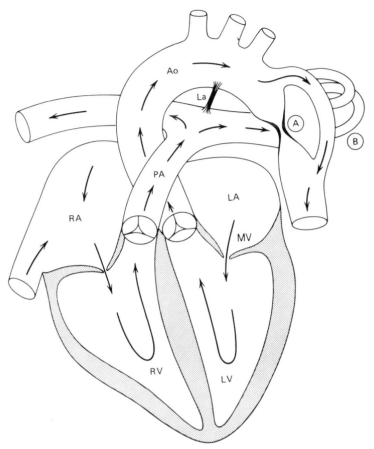

Figure 3-24. Postductal coarctation of the aorta (Ao). (A) Site of coarctation, (B) site of development of collateral circulation. LA, left atrium; La, ligamentum arteriosum; LV, left ventricle; MV, mitral valve; PA, pulmonary artery; RA, right atrium; RV, right ventricle; TV, tricuspid valve.

adult, and hypertension is generally reversible. Surgery is performed via a posterolateral thoracotomy incision. The aorta is temporarily clamped while an end-to-end anastomosis is performed. Occasionally, a graft is necessary to bridge the space made by the segment of coarcted tissue that is removed. If inadequate collateral circulation is present, hypothermia, a temporary shunt, or partial cardiopulmonary bypass is recommended to prevent ischemia to the spinal cord. If a PDA is present, as with preductal coarctation, division of the PDA is performed in addition to coarctation repair (*see* p. 128).

Although end-to-end anastomosis and graft insertion have been the conventional methods used to correct coarctation, an alternative procedure known as subclavian-flap aortoplasty may be performed on the infant with preductal coarctation. The left subclavian artery is ligated distally. The area of coarctation is then incised to the point of origin of the subclavian artery. The subclavian artery, having been incised lengthwise to form a flap, is sutured in place over the opening created in the aorta. The advantages of this procedure are seen to be the following: the time required for cross-clamping the aorta is generally shorter, the suture lines undergo less tension than in an end-to-end anastomosis, and the flap tissue will continue to grow with the child.

Postoperative complications of coarctation repair may include paraplegia, hemorrhage, and gangrenous bowel attributable to paradoxical hypertension of the abdominal arteries. These complications rarely occur, but some patients do experience abdominal pain postoperatively from paradoxical hypertension. It is important to note that hypertension does not necessarily resolve itself after repair of a coarctation.

Postoperative management is aimed at controlling hypertension, because it is imperative to avoid any undue stress on the suture line. This is achieved by the use of one of two vasodilators, sodium nitroprusside (Nipride) (*see* p. 191) or trimethaphan camsylate (Arfonad). Arfonad, the shortest-acting α-adrenergic blocker, can, when used as a vasodilator, increase the size of the vascular bed. Arfonad is administered by continuous IV infusion, 500 milligrams in 500 milliliters of IV fluid. The dose is then titrated to maintain blood pressure at the appropriate level.

Maintenance of an appropriate blood pressure also requires control of postoperative pain (*see* p. 191).

Aortic Stenosis

Aortic stenosis (AS) accounts for approximately 5 to 10 percent of the total number of congenital heart defects. It occurs more frequently in males. AS is defined as a lesion that creates obstruction of blood flow out of the left ventricle. This obstruction may occur at, above, or below the aortic valve.

Etiology. The aortic valve is formed during the sixth to ninth week of gestation, when the pulmonary artery and the aorta are formed from the division of the truncus arteriosus. The cusps of the aortic valve arise from three tubercles that proliferate within the aorta. Failure of the cusps to separate, creating a fusion, causes *valvular AS*, the most common form of this defect. Most often, the valve is bicuspid. This lesion may occur with endocardial fibroelastosis, PDA, coarctation of the aorta, VSD, and pulmonic stenosis.

However, since AS is defined as an obstruction at, above, or below the valve, it is evident that failure of the cusps to separate is not the only cause of AS. Stenotic muscle formation around the valve also contributes to the development of AS. AS is thus further classified according to location as idiopathic hypertrophic subaortic stenosis (IHSS), subvalvular AS and supravalvular AS (Fig. 3-25).

Left ventricular outflow obstruction in *IHSS* occurs from an enlargement of the left side of the ventricular septum and from possible anomalous placement of the anterior leaflet of the mitral valve in the hypertrophied septum. This is a progressive muscular hypertrophy. A normal aortic valve is usually present.

Subvalvular AS is caused by the formation of a fibrous ring below the aortic valve. Aortic insufficiency is a common finding with this lesion.

Supravalvular AS causes obstruction to left ventricular outflow by the presence of a fibrous membrane, by hypoplasia of the ascending aorta, or by an "hourglass" deformity of the aorta. This lesion is frequently found in children with

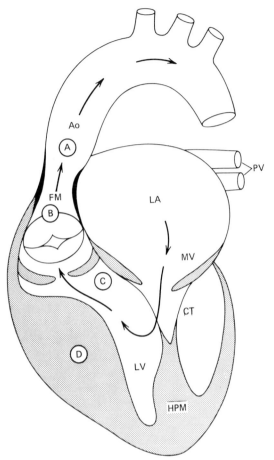

Figure 3-25. Four kinds of aortic stenosis (AS). (A) Supravalvular AS; (B) valvular AS (bicuspid valve with fused or stenotic cusps); (C) subvalvular AS caused by formation of a fibrous ring; (D) idiopathic hypertrophic subaortic stenosis caused by hypertrophic sub- aortic muscle. Ao, aorta; CT, chordae tendineae; FM, fibrotic membrane; HPM, hyper- trophic papillary muscle; LA, left atrium; LV, left ventricle; MV, mitral valve; PV, pulmonary vein.

Williams's syndrome, who have characteristic faces (elfin), developmental delay, and personality changes. Hypercalcemia and peripheral pulmonary stenosis may also be present. Supravalvular AS occurs less frequently than all other forms of AS.

Alteration in hemodynamics

Valvular AS: Obstruction at the valvular level creates increased stress on the left ventricle and ascending aorta. The left ventricle must exert increased pressure to overcome the resistance to blood flow at the stenotic valve. This increased work load on the left ventricle causes muscular hypertrophy. Because blood is ejected from the left ventricle under increased pressure, the turbulence of its flow stresses the ascending aorta, causing it to dilate.

IHSS: Obstruction to left ventricular outflow in this lesion occurs within the ventricle, below the valve. Once again, the left ventricle must exert an increased pressure to overcome the resistance of the stenotic muscle. In response to this stress, the left ventricle hypertrophies. If the stress is very great, the left atrium may also enlarge to compensate for the stress occurring in the ventricle.

Subvalvular AS: Obstruction below the aortic valve creates an increased stress on the left ventricle. However, since the aortic valve is normal, no excess stress is placed on the ascending aorta. The increased stress on the left ventricle results in hypertrophy.

Supravalvular AS: This form of obstruction creates the same stress on the heart as valvular AS (see above).

Clinical presentation.   Children with AS present either in infancy or the early months of life with florid CHF, or otherwise much later in childhood. The majority fall in the latter category. These children grow and develop normally, and most are asymptomatic. However, if significant stenosis is present, chest pain, light-headedness, and syncope will be experienced with exercise. On physical and cardiac examination, findings vary with the type of stenosis present and the degree of obstruction caused by the stenosis.

Valvular AS: On cardiac examination, S_1 is normal. An ejection click will be heard because of the impaired mobility of the aortic valve leaflets. This is best heard at the fourth left ICS. The murmur of AS, best heard at the base of the heart to the right of the sternal border, is rough and harsh. With moderate to severe AS, a palpable thrill will be present. This is best felt at the suprasternal notch and at the second right ICS. The aortic component of S_2 is diminished. Splitting of S_2 progressively narrows as the degree of stenosis increases. A left ventricular thrust can be felt because of hypertrophy of the left ventricle. A narrow pulse pressure detected by blood pressure measurement will characteristically be present.

The chest x-ray may appear normal, but left ventricular hypertrophy and dilation of the ascending aorta are often seen. With severe stenosis, pulmonary congestion may be observed. Cardiomegaly is generally not present. The ECG will demonstrate left ventricular hypertrophy in most cases. If S-T and T wave changes are present on the ECG, significant obstruction is present. However, because children with significant AS have been known to present with a normal ECG, this test cannot be relied on for a definitive diagnosis. The echocardiogram is very helpful in the evaluation of children with AS. The level of the lesion can be identified, and a good quantitative analysis of left ventricular pressure is possible. Definitive diagnosis is made by cardiac catheterization.

IHSS: On cardiac examination, a midsystolic ejection murmur, best heard near the apex, will be detected. A thrill may be present if the obstruction is of sufficient intensity. An ejection click is not heard, and S_2 and pulse pressure are normal.

On chest x-ray, left ventricular enlargement will be seen. The ascending aorta is normal, however, as is the right side of the heart. Cardiomegaly will usually not be seen. The ECG will demonstrate left ventricular hypertrophy. The echocardiogram may demonstrate the abnormal placement of the anterior mitral valve leaflet in the septum. Definitive diagnosis is made by cardiac catheterization.

Sudden death is known to occur with IHSS. Most patients with IHSS, a familial disorder, do not live beyond the age of 50 years.

Subvalvular AS: On cardiac and physical examination, the findings are similar to those of valvular AS, with a few variations. Because the aortic valve is normal, the ejection click is absent and the aorta is protected from excessive ejection pressure. This prevents dilation of the aorta. If aortic insufficiency is present, a diastolic murmur will be heard to the left of the sternum in the third and fourth ICS.

Supravalvular AS: The cardiac and physical findings are very similar to those of valvular AS. S_1 is normal, but an ejection click is not heard. An ejection systolic murmur is present. A thrill may be palpable, depending on the intensity of the murmur.

Differential diagnosis from valvular AS can be made by close assessment of peripheral blood pressures and pulses. A discrepancy between left and right arm blood pressures is generally found in supravalvular AS.

Medical management. The infant with critical AS who develops CHF is medically managed with digitalization and diuretics (*see* p. 175). If these measures prove unsuccessful, surgery is recommended.

Medical management of the older child with AS is directed toward detection of stenosis that interferes with meeting the demands placed on the heart during exercise. It is important to note that AS is known to be a progressive disease that requires serial evaluation. Competitive athletics and sustained activities that provide no opportunity for rest are not recommended for the child with moderate or severe AS.

The older child who presents with IHSS with symptomatology of fatigue, syncope, angina, and dyspnea on exertion is treated with propranolol hydrochloride (Inderal) to alleviate symptoms. Digitalis, isoproterenol, and nitroglycerin are never used with these patients because these medications result in increased muscular hypertrophy.

Of vital importance in medical management are the maintenance of good dental hygiene and the taking of protective measures against infective endocarditis.

Definitive surgical correction. Surgery is recommended for children who are symptomatic, have ECG changes, or have a pressure gradient of more than 70 to 80 mmHg between the left ventricle and the aorta.

Surgery is performed via a midline sternotomy incision. Cardiopulmonary bypass is used for all patients except the small infant with valvular AS, in whom surgery may be performed under inflow occlusion.

Valvular AS is corrected by a commissurotomy. In this procedure, the valve is dilated and the commissures of the valve are incised. On surgical visualization, the valve may not be suitable for commissurotomy. In cases in which a commissurotomy would create significant aortic insufficiency, a valve replacement may be necessary. Surgical correction of IHSS is recommended not only for those who are symptomatic but also for any asymptomatic patient with a parent or siblings who died suddenly from this disease. Surgical correction is performed by resection of hypertrophied muscle in the interventricular septum. Subvalvular AS is corrected by one of two methods: the fibrous membrane may be excised, or the whole length of the fibrous area may be incised. Supravalvular AS is surgically corrected by vertical incision of the stenosed area. A large patch is then placed in the area incised in order to enlarge the aortic diameter.

Postoperative complications may include persistent stenosis, restenosis of the aortic lumen, and insufficiency of the aortic valve. These problems may become evident long after surgery, as the child matures. Aortic valve replacement may be required in adulthood.

Pulmonic Stenosis

Pulmonic stenosis (PS) is the result of an obstructive lesion that interferes with blood flow from the right ventricle. Like AS, this lesion can occur at a number of locations in the right ventricular outflow tract. PS accounts for approximately 10 percent of the total number of congenital heart defects. It is only slightly more common in males than in females. One variation of PS is seen with increased frequency in infants with rubella syndrome or Williams's syndrome.

Etiology.   The pulmonic valve develops between the sixth and ninth weeks of gestation, at the same time as the development of the pulmonary artery and the aorta from the truncus arteriosus. It is formed by the proliferation of three tubercles within the lumen of the pulmonary artery, which later thin by tissue resorption to form the three cusps of the pulmonic valve. Failure of this process to occur results in abnormality of the valve. Such an abnormality may present as a bicuspid valve that is fused at the commissures of its two leaflets, or as a tricuspid valve with thickened leaflets that may be partially or completely fused at the commissures. In either case, *valvular PS* results, which severely restricts valve motion and impedes blood flow from the right ventricle. Valvular PS occurs in approximately 95 percent of the children with PS.

The infundibulum of the right ventricle is formed during the fifth to seventh week of gestation, slightly before the development of the pulmonic valve. The infundibulum develops from resorption of tissue in the bulbus cordis. If this tissue is not resorbed adequately, an area of infundibular hypertrophy results, which causes *infundibular PS*. Alternatively, abnormal bands of muscle may form within the chamber of the right ventricle. The result is *subinfundibular PS*, a rare defect. Both of these variations may be classified as *subvalvular PS*.

At approximately the same time as the development of the right ventricular infundibulum, the branch pulmonary arteries differentiate. These vessels grow to anastomose proximally with the main pulmonary artery and distally with the smaller pulmonary arteries. The development of these branch and peripheral arteries may be interfered with, and the vessels may not become sufficiently hollow. The result, *supravalvular PS*, can occur within the main pulmonary artery or within any of its branches (Fig. 3-26). Often, multiple areas of stenosis exist throughout the pulmonary vasculature. Supravalvular PS is also a rare defect.

Alteration in hemodynamics.   Regardless of the specific location of the lesion in PS, the hemodynamic result is obstruction of blood ejected from the right ventricle in systole. This obstruction places a pressure burden on the right ventricle.

Valvular PS: Obstruction to ventricular emptying and the resultant increase in RVP from valvular PS cause right ventricular and main pulmonary artery enlargement. The right ventricle enlarges as its muscular wall hypertrophies in response to the increased pressure work load that it must overcome. The main pulmonary artery enlargement is characteristic of a poststenotic dilation. However, pressure in the pulmonary trunk is normal or lower than normal, and, therefore, the peripheral pulmonary vasculature and the left heart are unaffected. When severe valvular PS is present, RAP may also increase with resultant enlargement of the right atrial chamber.

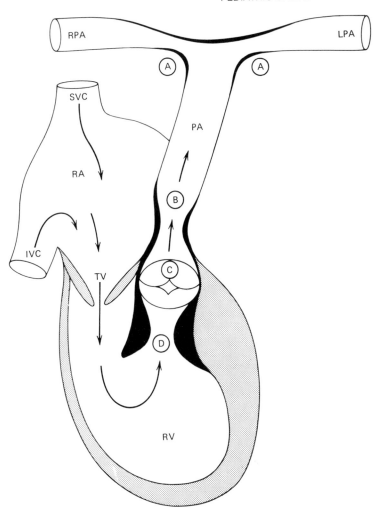

Figure 3-26.   Four kinds of pulmonic stenosis (PS). (A) Supravalvular PS of the branches of the pulmonary artery (PA); (B) supravalvular PS of the main PA; (C) valvular PS caused by either a bicuspid pulmonic valve or by a tricuspid pulmonic valve with thickened or fused commissures; (D) subvalvular PS caused by either infundibular hypertrophy or by a fibrous ring. IVC, inferior vena cava; LPA, left PA; RA, right atrium; RPA, right PA; RV, right ventricle; SVC, superior vena cava; TV, tricuspid valve.

Subvalvular PS: Both infundibular and subinfundibular PS are characterized by right ventricular hypertrophy that develops in response to the increased blood pressure in the ventricle as it pumps against an obstruction. However, the increased force is dissipated over an area of obstruction that is larger than that of valvular PS, and, as a result, the main pulmonary artery remains normal in size. Pressure in the main pulmonary artery is normal or reduced.

Supravalvular PS: Unlike the other forms of PS, supravalvular lesions produce hypertension in the main pulmonary artery as well as in the right ventricle. However, ventricular and pulmonary artery enlargement vary with the severity and location of the lesions.

Clinical presentation. Murmurs of PS are frequently detected early. Parents are likely to know that their child has a congenital heart defect before discharge from the newborn nursery. However, children with PS are generally healthy, grow well, and experience only minimal exercise intolerance. Only occasionally, in the case of branch or supravalvular PS, are poor growth and abnormal development demonstrated. These children often have rubella syndrome or Williams's syndrome. Rarely, cyanosis and right-sided CHF develop fulminantly in the infant between the neonatal period and age 6 months. These babies have very severe valvular PS and present much like the infant with pulmonary atresia (*see* p. 158).

Valvular PS: Children with valvular PS appear normally healthy. Cyanosis is absent, and pulse and blood pressure are normal. A systolic thrill is detected in the second left ICS and may also be present in the suprasternal notch. On auscultation, a normal S_1 is heard, followed by an ejection or a crescendo-decrescendo systolic murmur. The murmur may be soft in mild obstruction or extremely loud in severe obstruction. Moderate obstruction generally produces a grade III/VI or IV/VI murmur. These murmurs are well localized at the upper left sternal border and may be transmitted to the back and widely across the left chest. An ejection click is often heard after S_1 and before the systolic murmur, but is absent in severe stenosis. S_2 is widely split, and the pulmonic component is diminished. A loud murmur may obscure the pulmonic component of S_2 so that the split is not audible by auscultation. A right ventricle lift can usually be palpated.

The ECG demonstrates right ventricular hypertrophy. Right atrial hypertrophy is also seen if the stenosis is severe. The chest x-ray shows right ventricular and main pulmonary artery enlargement, as well as normal pulmonary vasculature and a normal left heart. The echocardiogram may detect thickness and decreased motion of the pulmonic valve, but is not definitive. Cardiac catheterization confirms the diagnosis by identifying the nature of the stenotic valve and by determining the severity of the stenosis.

Occasionally, children with very severe PS experience chest pain (angina), dizziness, and dyspnea on exertion. Fatigue may also be a problem. Some of these children die suddenly, but this is rare.

Infundibular PS: Either a discrete fibrous ring just below the pulmonic valve or thickened, hypertrophied muscle tissue can be responsible for infundibular PS. If a fibrous ring is the cause, clinical findings are quite similar to those seen in children with valvular PS. However, because the valve itself is normal, the ejection click is absent and the pulmonic component of S_2 is normal in intensity. It is delayed, however, so that S_2 is widely split.

Muscular infundibular PS is characterized by absence of an ejection click (because the pulmonic valve is normal) and by a murmur that is briefer than that of valvular PS, ending before S_2. The murmur is heard lower on the chest, at the third or fourth ICS to the left of the sternum. The intensity of the murmur varies with the severity of the stenosis from grade II/VI to IV/VI. A thrill is palpable with a murmur of grade IV/VI. With severe infundibular PS, the right ventricle hypertrophies greatly and may produce a bulging of the lower portion of the precordium and a right ventricular heave. S_2 is widely split because of delayed closure of the pulmonic valve, but the pulmonic component of S_2 is of normal intensity.

The ECG demonstrates abnormal right heart work in both forms of infundibular PS. The chest x-ray reveals right ventricular enlargement, but the pulmonary artery is not dilated. Cardiac catheterization is necessary to differentiate these forms of PS from other forms of right ventricular obstruction.

Subinfundibular PS: The findings of the clinical examination of the child with subinfundibular PS are very similar to those of infundibular PS. Cardiac catheterization is generally required for differentiation.

Supravalvular PS: Children with supravalvular PS are more often affected by a syndrome such as rubella or Williams's. As a result, their growth and development are less likely to be normal than those of children with the other forms of PS. The cardiac examination of children with single or multiple, localized or diffuse stenoses in the main pulmonary artery, its branches, or in peripheral vessels detects a murmur that results from turbulent blood flow through the obstruction. The murmur is transmitted distal to the obstruction throughout the pulmonary vasculature. In general, a systolic ejection murmur is heard, although turbulence may persist through systole and diastole and generate a murmur similar to that of PDA (*see* p. 125). An ejection click is not heard.

Medical management.   Children with PS are followed closely in order to detect, as early as possible, progression of their stenoses with growth. Although progression is less likely in children with PS than in those with AS, it is detected by changes in the murmur (increased intensity, loss of ejection click, the development of a palpable thrill), increased right ventricular hypertrophy on ECG, or increased clinical symptoms. Exercise restriction is generally not required, although sustained competitive athletics are to be avoided by children with severe stenoses. Children with PS have a low risk of developing infective endocarditis, but antibiotic prophylaxis with dental work or other surgical procedures is generally provided.

Definitive surgical correction.   Complete repair of PS is generally recommended for children who have a pressure gradient of 60 mmHg or more across the pulmonic valve. Cardiopulmonary bypass is used, and an incision is made in the pulmonary artery. Valvular stenosis is relieved by incising the fused commissures as widely as possible. The right ventricular infundibulum is palpated through the newly enlarged pulmonic valve to detect localized muscular or fibrotic obstruction. Severe subvalvular stenosis is excised widely by means of a right atriotomy.

Postoperatively, children who have had repair of valvular PS may have some degree of pulmonary regurgitation, but this is generally not significant. Patients who had significant right ventricular hypertension and hypertrophy may develop some degree of right-sided CHF postoperatively and may require digoxin and/or diuretic therapy for variable periods of time. Most children recover uneventfully and continue to grow and develop normally. No limitation of activity is required.

CYANOTIC CONGENITAL HEART DEFECTS WITH DECREASED PBF

Heart defects that produce both cyanosis and decreased PBF are characterized by obstruction at some point in the right heart. This obstruction always results in a lower than normal flow of blood to the lungs. These obstructive defects are also associated with an abnormal opening between the pulmonary and systemic circulations or with the persistence of a fetal connection between the two systems. This permits shunting of blood from the right heart to the left heart and results in cyanosis. Tetralogy of Fallot is the most common cyanotic CHD with decreased PBF. Pulmonary atresia with intact ventricular septum and tricuspid atresia are rare defects that result in the same alteration in hemodynamics. (Table 3-8 summarizes the findings on cardiac examination, ECG, and chest x-ray of children with these defects.)

Tetralogy of Fallot

Tetralogy of Fallot (TOF) is a fairly common congenital heart defect, accounting for 6 to 10 percent of the total number of cardiac defects. The child with TOF has (1) a VSD; (2) PS that is usually infundibular, but may be valvular, supravalvular, or combined; (3) right ventricular hypertrophy on ECG as a result of the increased RVP caused by the obstruction of blood flow from the ventricle; and (4) varying degrees of overriding (dextroposition) of the aorta (Fig. 3-27). Although these last two factors are consistently anatomically present, they do not significantly influence the physiological alterations seen in the child with TOF. Instead, the pathophysiological results of TOF are determined by the size of the VSD and the severity of the PS. Table 3-9 depicts the possible variations. Classic TOF, characterized by a large VSD and severe PS, will be discussed in the present section.

Etiology.   Between the fourth and eighth week of intrauterine life, the single ventricular chamber is divided in two (*see* p. 131). During the sixth to ninth week of gestation, formation of the pulmonic valve occurs, with the right ventricular infundibulum (outflow tract) developing slightly earlier than the valve (*see* p. 148). Failure of these events to occur results in the variable defects seen in TOF. The exact mechanism responsible is thought to be either an abnormality in septation of the truncus arteriosus or an abnormality in development of the infundibular area of the right ventricle. Sex distribution of TOF is about equal, with only slightly more males affected.

Alteration in hemodynamics.   Because of the coexisting VSD and the obstruction to blood flow from the right ventricle, children with TOF have decreased blood flow to the lungs and increased blood flow to the body. Blood flow to the lungs is diminished because of the PS, whereas blood flow in the systemic circulation is increased because of the addition of venous blood (which flows across the VSD) to the systemic volume normally present in the left ventricle. The obstruction to right heart emptying results in increased pressure in the right ventricular chamber, permitting the right-to-left shunt.

The effect on the heart of these changes in hemodynamics includes an increase in the size and work of the right ventricle. The right atrium is usually unaffected. There is an increased volume load on the left ventricle, but this problem is generally reflected in enlargement of the aorta only, and the left ventricle remains normally compliant.

Clinical presentation.   The most characteristic presentation seen in the child with TOF is that of development of cyanosis after several months of age. Cyanosis may be present in the neonatal period, but, as a rule, it becomes obvious by 3 to 6 months of age. This occurs because the infundibular PS characteristic of TOF is progressive, increasing with the age of the child. As a result, the right-to-left shunt through the VSD also increases, thereby increasing cyanosis. Consequently, most

TABLE 3-8   Cyanotic Congenital Heart Defects with Decreased Pulmonary Blood Flow

Defect	Cardiac examination	Electrocardiogram	Chest x-ray
TOF	Loud systolic murmur with palpable thrill along the entire left sternal border. Pulmonic S_2 diminished or inaudible. Prominent inferior sternum and right ventricular impulse.	Right axis deviation and right ventricular hypertrophy. Occasional right atrial hypertrophy.	Normal cardiac size with concavity in main pulmonary artery area. Decreased pulmonary vascular markings. Boot-shaped heart silhouette. Right aortic arch common.
Pulmonary atresia with intact ventricular septum	Heart murmur may be absent; when detected, usually holosystolic blowing murmur of tricuspid regurgitation and continuous, "machinery" murmur of PDA. No pulmonic S_2, S_3, or S_4	Absence of or decrease in right ventricular forces. Left ventricular dominance.	Type 1: Similar to TOF. Type 2: Cardiomegaly with significant right atrial enlargement. Decreased pulmonary vascular markings.
Tricuspid atresia	No tricuspid S_1. S_2 also often a single sound: no pulmonic S_2. Variable systolic (VSD and PS) murmurs or diastolic (mitral flow) murmur. Often, no murmur is audible.	Left axis deviation. Left ventricular, left atrial, and right atrial hypertrophy. No right ventricular forces.	Normal overall heart size with concavity in main pulmonary artery area. Right atrial, left atrial, left ventricular, and aortic enlargement. Decreased pulmonary vascular markings.

PDA, patent ductus arteriosus; PS, pulmonic stenosis; S_1, first heart sound; S_2, second heart sound; S_3, third heart sound; S_4, fourth heart sound; TOF, tetralogy of Fallot; VSD, ventricular septal defect.

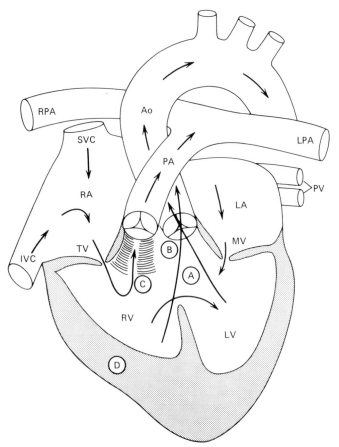

Figure 3-27.   Tetralogy of Fallot. (A) Ventricular septal defect (VSD); (B) aorta (Ao) over-riding the VSD; (C) pulmonic stenosis; (D) right ventricular hypertrophy. IVC, inferior vena cava; LA, left atrium; LPA, left pulmonary artery; LV, left ventricle; MV, mitral valve; PA, pulmonary artery; PV, pulmonary vein; RA, right atrium; RPA, right PA; RV, right ventricle; SVC, superior vena cava; TV, tricuspid valve.

children with TOF are deeply cyanotic by 5 to 8 years of age. During this time, persistent cyanosis results in the clubbing of the nail beds of the fingers and toes, polycythemia, and exercise intolerance (*see* p. 123). Activity, straining, or crying causes increased cyanosis and dyspnea.

Children with TOF may squat spontaneously to rest from activity. Although it is not clear exactly how squatting exerts beneficial effects, it nevertheless serves to alleviate dyspnea and the feeling of faintness that often accompany activity by diminishing the hypoxia experienced by these children on exertion.

Some children with TOF experience episodes of dramatically increased cyanosis that may progress to limpness, loss of consciousness, or seizures. These episodes are referred to by a number of designations, including tet, cardiac, or

TABLE 3-9   Variations in Tetralogy of Fallot

Type	Characteristics
Large VSD	Mild to moderate PS ("acyanotic" tetralogy)
	Severe PS ("classic" tetralogy)
	Complete PS (tetralogy with pulmonary atresia)
Small VSD	Mild PS
	Severe PS

PS, pulmonic stenosis; VSD, ventricular septal defect.

hypoxic spells and paroxysmal hyperpnea. These crises can lead to brain damage or even death. Tet spells are most common in the first 6 months of life and are often associated with crying, feeding, or a bowel movement, especially if these activities occur when the infant has just awakened. Spells begin with moderate but progressive dyspnea, and they culminate in hyperpnea and syncope. The precise mechanism responsible for the tet spell has not been completely identified, but a vulnerable respiratory control center, tachycardia, and infundibular contraction are thought to contribute.[8] The result is an increase in right-to-left shunting and a sharp fall in PBF, causing severely decreased levels of systemic PaO_2 and pH and a rise in the partial pressure of arterial carbon dioxide ($PaCO_2$). The child who suffers a tet spell requires emergency treatment and continued medical management (*see* p. 156). Palliative or definitive surgical intervention may be indicated.

The newborn with TOF appears normally grown. Chronic cyanosis prevents continued adequate growth, however, so that children with TOF are small in size and physically underdeveloped.

The cardiac examination of the child with TOF reveals a loud systolic murmur (associated with a palpable thrill) that is audible along the entire left sternal border. The murmur may vary from the lower to the upper sternal border. The S_1 is normal, but the pulmonic component of S_2 is diminished or inaudible because it may be obscured by the loud murmur. As a result of restricted PBF, collateral circulation through bronchial vessels or through other aorto-pulmonary communications develops in some children with TOF. The development of collateral circulation can be detected by the presence of audible continuous murmurs, generally heard over the child's back. The increased work of the right ventricle is evinced by a heave at the inferior part of the sternum or by a prominent right ventricular impulse.

Chest x-ray of children with TOF reveals normal cardiac size, decreased PBF, a concavity in the left heart border at the area of the main pulmonary artery, and small branch pulmonary arteries. Hypertrophy of the right ventricle pushes the apex of the heart upward and, in combination with the concavity in the left heart border, gives the heart a classic, boot-shaped silhouette. A right aortic arch may be present.

The ECG demonstrates right axis deviation and right ventricular hypertrophy. Occasionally, right atrial hypertrophy is detected. The echocardiogram demonstrates the VSD and PS characteristic of TOF. Cardiac catheterization is used to confirm the diagnosis, to measure the size of the VSD as well as the pressures in the pulmonary artery and both ventricles, and to calculate the volume of the right-to-left shunt.

CHF is extremely rare in children with TOF, and its presence suggests a CHD other than TOF.

Medical management. Before surgical correction, children with TOF require close monitoring of their degree of hypoxia because it poses a variety of long-term problems (*see* p. 123). Avoidance of tet spells is a primary objective. Propranolol hydrochloride (Inderal), in doses of 0.5 to 2 mg/kg/day, has been useful in controlling tet spells in young children with TOF. If a tet spell occurs the infant or child is placed in a knee-chest position to mimic the squatting position spontaneously assumed by these youngsters, and oxygen is immediately administered along with morphine sulfate, 0.1 mg/kg IV. Morphine relaxes the right ventricular infundibulum, thereby increasing PBF and decreasing the right-to-left shunt. Vital signs are monitored with care. Bradycardia, which may be associated with a tet spell, necessitates immediate intervention. Metabolic acidosis, which frequently results from the severe hypoxia characteristic of the spell, requires correction with sodium bicarbonate (*see* p. 180). Tet spells are often considered an indication for either palliative or corrective surgery.

Children with long-standing cyanosis are at risk for the development of serious problems. The risk of serious bacterial infections necessitates antibiotic prophylaxis for any minor surgical or dental procedures. Polycythemia places these children at risk for bleeding abnormalities and dehydration. Polycythemia is also an indication for surgery. The constant presence of a right-to-left shunt makes the likelihood of cerebral embolism far greater in these children. Whenever hospitalization is required, all personnel caring for the child must be acutely aware of the implications of the child's shunt and treat IV lines with appropriate care. Any infusion of air or any clearing of a plugged IV catheter could result in cerebral embolization.

Exercise restriction is generally not necessary for children with TOF because these youngsters tend to limit their own activity on the basis of their hypoxia. Severe hypoxia that impairs the child's quality of life is a final indication for surgical palliation or repair of this defect.

Palliative surgical management. Palliative surgical intervention is sometimes preferred for infants less than 3 to 6 months of age who present with either severe hypoxia, hematocrit greater than 60 percent, tet spells, or impaired quality of life. The risks of total correction in these infants may often be deemed greater than those associated with palliation and later corrective surgery.

A number of palliative shunt procedures are available for the treatment of these children. The Blalock-Taussig subclavian-pulmonary artery anastomosis (Fig. 3-28) is the procedure that is generally recommended. The right or left subclavian artery is selected, depending on the direction of the aortic arch. (The vessel on the opposite side of the arch is selected.) The artery is ligated and divided, and then turned to anastomose with the branch pulmonary artery on the same side. It is possible to construct very small shunts that are unlikely to cause pulmonary congestion but that maintain patency and successfully increase PBF. An additional advantage to the Blalock-Taussig shunt is the ease with which it is removed at the time of definitive repair.

Other palliative shunts are possible, and all serve to increase PBF: (1) the Waterston shunt, in which the ascending aorta and right pulmonary artery are anastomosed; (2) the Potts-Smith-Gibson operation, which consists of connecting the descending aorta and the left pulmonary artery; and (3) the Glenn procedure, in which the right pulmonary artery is connected to the side of the superior vena

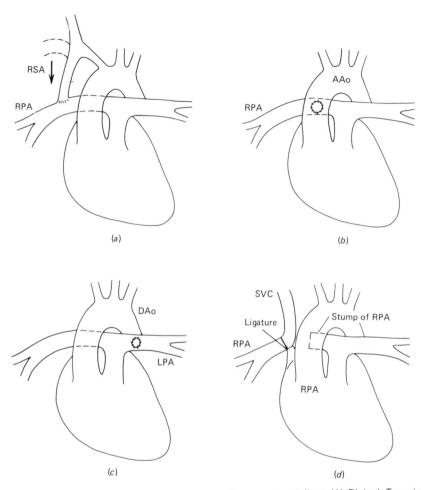

Figure 3-28. Palliative shunts to increase pulmonary blood flow. (A) Blalock-Taussig anastomosis, (B) Waterston anastomosis, (C) Potts-Smith-Gibson anastomosis, (D) Glenn anastomosis. (*See* discussion in text.) AAo, ascending aorta; DAo, descending aorta; LPA, left pulmonary artery; RPA, right pulmonary artery; RSA, right subclavian artery; SVC, superior vena cava.

cava (Fig. 3-28). All of these procedures, however, are associated with difficult repair at the time of corrective surgery. In addition, the Waterston shunt presents difficulty with control of the volume of flow through the anastomosis, too frequently resulting in pulmonary congestion.

Definitive surgical correction. Total correction of TOF is performed during cardiopulmonary bypass. In infants and young children, deep hypothermia and circulatory arrest may be used. After early infancy, the child's age is less of a consideration in timing definitive correction than is the child's clinical condition.

Indications for corrective surgery are severe hypoxia, hematocrit greater than 60 percent, tet spells, or impaired quality of life. During corrective repair, any previously constructed palliative shunt is closed immediately before the initiation of cardiopulmonary bypass. Then, the right ventricular outflow obstruction is excised in order to create an unobstructed channel to the pulmonic valve. If the pulmonic valve is also stenotic, it is incised. A patch of Dacron or pericardium may be used to enlarge the ventricular outflow tract in infants or very small children. Finally, the VSD is closed with a patch.

Postoperatively, almost all children who have had total correction of TOF will demonstrate a right bundle-branch block on ECG. Some transient CHF is not uncommon, and this development requires digoxin and/or diuretics for several weeks or months postoperatively. Serious problems include persistent right ventricular failure and more complete forms of heart block. Pulmonic valve regurgitation occurs in some children. Antibiotic prophylaxis against endocarditis must be continued with dental work or surgical procedures. Some children will continue to have exercise limitations.

Pulmonary Atresia with Intact Ventricular Septum

Pulmonary atresia with intact ventricular septum (Fig. 3-29) is a rare congenital heart defect, accounting for only 1 percent of the total number of cardiac defects. It is the extreme form of valvular PS.

Etiology. Failure of the pulmonic valve to develop between the sixth and ninth week of gestation (*see* p. 148) results in a valve that is small and imperforate. Development of the right ventricle is also affected. Children with one form of this serious defect (designated type 1) have a hypoplastic or rudimentary right ventricle, whereas others have a normal or dilated right ventricle associated with an incompetent tricuspid valve (type 2). In both types, the distal pulmonary arteries are patent.

Alteration in hemodynamics. Children with type 1 pulmonary atresia are physiologically similar to those with tricuspid atresia (*see* p. 160). Those with type 2 have slightly different hemodynamics. Systemic venous blood that enters the right atrium drains immediately into the right ventricle because of the incompetent tricuspid valve. Because no exit from the ventricle exists, it is subject to both volume and pressure overload, and blood is regurgitated into the right atrium. Pressure in the right atrium is greater than that in the left, resulting in a right-to-left shunt at the atrial level via the foramen ovale (or sometimes an ASD) that is present. Blood flow to the lungs is accomplished by a left-to-right shunt across a PDA. Occasionally, other aortobronchial collaterals develop as well, although this does not occur early. Therefore, blood in the left heart and the systemic circulation is a mixture of desaturated, systemic venous blood and fully saturated, pulmonary venous blood.

Clinical presentation. Children with pulmonary atresia with intact ventricular septum present as newborns with severe cyanosis, hypoxia, and metabolic acidosis. CHF is rare, but, when it occurs, it also is often severe. A heart murmur, which may or may not be detected, is most often characteristic of tricuspid regurgitation (a grade II/VI or III/VI holosystolic, blowing murmur) and of the loud, continuous, machinery murmur of PDA. S_2 is single, with no pulmonic component, and an S_3 or S_4 gallop sound can be detected.

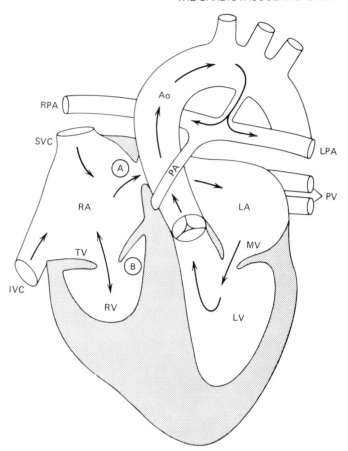

Figure 3-29. Pulmonary atresia with intact ventricular septum and hypoplastic pulmonary artery (PA) and branches. (A) Atrial septal defect, (B) atretic pulmonic valve. Ao, aorta; IVC, inferior vena cava; LA, left atrium; LPA, left PA; LV, left ventricle; MV, mitral valve; PV, pulmonary vein; RA, right atrium; RPA, right PA; RV, right ventricle; SVC, superior vena cava; TV, tricuspid valve.

The ECG usually demonstrates the absence of, or a decrease in, normal right ventricular forces. Left ventricular dominance is characteristic. The chest x-ray resembles that of classic TOF (*see* p. 155) in type 1 pulmonary atresia with intact ventricular septum. When a larger right ventricle and a significant tricuspid regurgitation volume are present (type 2), heart size on chest x-ray is larger than normal because of a markedly dilated right atrium. The echocardiogram detects ductal flow, absence of the pulmonic valve, and lack of shunting at the ventricular level. Cardiac catheterization is necessary to determine the exact cardiac and pulmonary anatomy. These factors determine the options that are available in the treatment of a particular infant.

Medical management. Medical management of these critically ill infants is directed toward stabilization of their condition by control of hypoxia and correction of metabolic acidosis (*see* p. 180). CHF, when present, also requires aggressive intervention (*see* p. 175). In some infants, the ductus arteriosus will close suddenly, despite its necessity for PBF, causing sudden death. Ductal patency may be maintained by continuous IV infusion of prostaglandin E, which is known to maintain ductal patency during fetal existence. This technique is quite new, but it has been demonstrated to relax the ductus and delay its closure.[9] In infants with pulmonary atresia with intact ventricular septum, prostaglandin infusion increases PaO_2, thereby permitting stabilization of their condition. Cardiac catheterization is necessary to establish a definitive diagnosis so that appropriate surgical intervention can be planned. Operability is dependent on the size of the right ventricle and the pulmonary arteries.

Palliative surgical management. The objective of palliative surgery in these infants is to increase PBF, thereby lessening cyanosis, hypoxia, and acidosis. Either a Waterston or a Blalock-Taussig anastomosis is generally used (*see* p. 156–157). During the operation, a pulmonary valvulotomy may be performed in infants with a patent main pulmonary artery and a small right ventricle. This procedure may induce growth of the right ventricle, thus improving the infant's outlook for later definitive correction.

Postoperatively, infants who have undergone a systemic-pulmonary artery shunt have a persistent right-to-left shunt at the atrial level, and they are, therefore, at risk for the same potential problems with this shunt as children with TOF (*see* p. 156). Cyanosis may persist, necessitating early reoperation. CHF secondary to pulmonary overcirculation can occur with large palliative shunts.

Definitive surgical correction. The aim of definitive surgical repair of pulmonary atresia with intact ventricular septum is to establish continuity between the right ventricle and the main pulmonary artery. A reasonably well-developed right ventricle and a tricuspid valve that is not too badly malformed are necessary to permit definitive correction of this defect. Cardiopulmonary bypass is used, and deep hypothermia with circulatory arrest may be necessary in small children. Continuity between the ventricle and the pulmonary artery is established with a valved conduit. Plastic repair of the tricuspid valve is performed.

Tricuspid Atresia

Tricuspid atresia occurs in 1 to 2 percent of children with a congenital heart defect. It consists of an absent or imperforate tricuspid valve, which results in a complete right-to-left shunt at the atrial level and in variable degrees of right ventricular hypoplasia. There is no sex differentiation with this defect.

Etiology. The tricuspid valve is formed at about the fifth week of gestation as a result of the blending of endocardial cushion tissue, a portion of the ventricular septum, and ventricular muscle itself. A disruption in the formation of this valve can result in the utter lack of valve tissue and the consequent lack of a communication between the right atrium and the right ventricle.

Like many other kinds of congenital heart defects, tricuspid atresia exists in a number of forms. These vary, depending on the relationship of the great arteries (normally positioned or transposed), the nature of the ventricular septum (intact or VSD), and the nature of the pulmonic valve (normal, pulmonary atresia, or PS). These variations combine in a number of ways. Most commonly, the infant with tricuspid atresia has normally positioned great arteries, a small VSD, and hypoplastic right ventricle, pulmonic valve, and pulmonary vessels (Fig. 3-30).

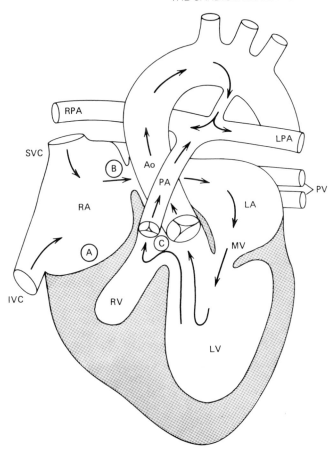

Figure 3-30. Tricuspid atresia with a small ventricular septal defect and hypoplastic pulmonary artery (PA), and branches. (A) Atretic tricuspid valve, (B) atrial septal defect, (C) ventricular septal defect. Ao, aorta; IVC, inferior vena cava; LA, left atrium; LPA, left PA; LV, left ventricle; MV, mitral valve; PV, pulmonary vein; RA, right atrium; RPA, right PA; right ventricle (RV); SVC, superior vena cava.

Alteration in hemodynamics. Regardless of the various defects associated with tricuspid atresia, blood flow through the heart is essentially the same. Systemic venous return in these children flows across the atrial septum from the right to the left atrium via a patent foramen ovale or an ASD (if present). This shunt is obligatory because there is no other exit from the right atrium, and it results in complete mixing of desaturated systemic venous blood and fully saturated pulmonary venous blood. This mixed blood is then ejected by the left ventricle. Most of it flows out the aorta, where a portion shunts left to right across a PDA. Some flows through the VSD into the right ventricle, but this volume is small because of the high RVP relative to the small chamber size and because of the relative stenosis of the pulmonic valve and pulmonary vessels. Essentially, the left ventricle pumps blood into both great vessels. As a result, there is an increase in left heart work from volume overload.

Clinical presentation.   Infants with tricuspid atresia typically present very early in life with cyanosis. CHF is rare, but can occur if a nonrestricting VSD, right ventricle, and pulmonary circuit exist. (These children will have minimal cyanosis.) Because most infants have reduced PBF, cyanosis is severe and accompanied by tachypnea, hypoxia, and metabolic acidosis.

The cardiac examination reveals a single S_1 because the tricuspid portion is missing. S_2 is also usually a single sound with an absent pulmonic component. Variable systolic murmurs (of VSD and PS, if present) or a diastolic murmur (because of increased flow across the mitral valve) may be heard. Most often, however, no murmur is heard. The ECG demonstrates left axis deviation and left ventricular and left and right atrial hypertrophy. Right ventricular forces are lacking. The chest x-ray typically shows normal overall heart size and decreased pulmonary vascular markings. A concavity is detected in the pulmonary artery region, as are an enlarged right and left atrium, left ventricle, and aorta. The echocardiogram detects absence of the tricuspid valve, a small right ventricle, and a large left ventricle and ascending aorta. Other defects such as VSD may be detected. Cardiac catheterization is necessary to confirm the diagnosis and delineate the specific anatomy of the defect.

Medical management.   Before cardiac catheterization, these sick infants require stabilization and correction of acidosis (*see* p. 179). Hypoxia may be controlled or decreased in some by the use of IV prostaglandin E to maintain ductal patency (*see* p. 160). At cardiac catheterization, balloon atrial septostomy may be necessary to maintain unrestricted flow across the atrial septum (*see* p. 167). Because some kind of palliative surgical intervention is generally necessitated early, medical care is directed toward control of hypoxia or CHF (*see* p. 175).

Palliative surgical management.   Because the majority of children with tricuspid atresia have decreased PBF, palliative shunts to improve PBF are frequently performed in early infancy. The Blalock-Taussig, Waterston, Potts-Smith-Gibson, and Glenn anastomoses have all been used to palliate this serious defect (*see* p. 156). The Blalock-Taussig anastomosis is preferred because, with the others, PBF is often too great and also because these other anastomoses are more difficult to resect at a later operation. However, the Blalock Taussig shunt can be too small, or it may be outgrown, in both of which cases there is a worsening of cyanosis.

Definitive surgical correction.   A fairly new operation that creates a connection between the right atrium and the pulmonary arteries with a valved conduit has been devised by Fontan.[10] In this operation, which necessitates cardiopulmonary bypass, all the systemic venous return reaching the right atrium flows through the conduit into the pulmonary arteries. The ASD is closed in order to achieve this, and previous palliative shunts are resected. The right ventricle is completely bypassed in this procedure; therefore, the right atrium is used as the pumping chamber for the pulmonary circuit. This operation has a high mortality rate, and its long-term effectiveness is questionable. CHF is a significant problem postoperatively.

CYANOTIC CONGENITAL HEART DEFECTS WITH INCREASED PBF

The prenatal failure of the heart and blood vessels to differentiate into distinct systemic and pulmonary vascular systems gives rise to defects that mix arterial and venous blood. The result is cyanosis. The lack of obstruction to blood flow to the lungs results in increased PBF. This is usually the case with these complex defects, although variations exist. Transposition of the great arteries is the most common defect in this category. Total anomalous pulmonary venous return and truncus arteriosus are rare defects of this type. (Table 3-10 summarizes the findings on cardiac examination, ECG, and chest x-ray of children with these defects.)

Transposition of the Great Arteries

Transposition of the great arteries (TGA) accounts for approximately 5 percent of the total number of congenital heart defects. It occurs more frequently in males. TGA exists when the pulmonary artery arises from the left ventricle and the aorta arises from the right ventricle. The pulmonary artery arises from the left ventricle, posterior to the aorta. The aorta arises from the right ventricle at a higher level than, and, anterior to, the pulmonary artery. Coexisting lesions occur frequently with TGA. The most common are PDA, VSD, VSD with PS, and a combination of these defects. When a coexisting lesion is present, TGA is often referred to as complicated TGA.

Two types of TGA exist: D-TGA and L-TGA. D-TGA is the defect that produces cyanosis and is the focus of this section. L-TGA, also known as corrected transposition, exists when the right and left ventricles are displaced, in addition to displacement of the aorta and pulmonary artery. Because of the ventricular displacement, the pulmonary artery arises from the physiological venous ventricle, and the aorta arises from the physiological arterial ventricle. Therefore, venous and arterial flow leave the heart in the correct vessels, and cyanosis is not present.

Etiology.   Between the third and fourth week of gestation, the truncus arteriosus is divided into the pulmonary artery and the aorta. This results from spiral growth of the truncoconal ridges. Failure of the truncoconal ridges to spiral or rotate completely results in displacement of the aorta and the pulmonary artery on the ventricles.

Alteration in hemodynamics

Uncomplicated TGA: The child with uncomplicated TGA essentially has two independent parallel circuits of circulation (Fig. 3-31). Venous blood from the body enters the right atrium, moves into the right ventricle, flows out of the aorta to the body, and returns again to the right atrium. Oxygenated blood from the lungs enters the left atrium, moves into the left ventricle, flows out of the pulmonary artery to the lungs, and returns again to the left atrium. Intermixing of these two circuits of blood occurs at the foramen ovale and ductus arteriosus. At the level of the foramen ovale, blood is shunted from the left atrium to the right atrium or from the pulmonary circuit to the systemic circuit. Blood is shunted across the ductus arteriosus in the opposite direction, from the aorta to the pulmonary artery. This alteration in hemodynamics creates a stress on the right atrium, the right ventricle, and the pulmonary vessels because of the increased volume of blood they continuously receive. Pulmonary artery hypertension is likely to develop from this increase in blood flow (*see* p. 131). An additional stress is placed on the right ventricle because it must function as the systemic ventricle.

Complicated TGA: The child with TGA complicated by the presence of a VSD has two communicating circuits of circulation. The two circuits mix via the VSD. Blood from the right ventricle generally is shunted to the left ventricle because pressure in the pulmonary circuit is less than that in the systemic circuit. This

TABLE 3-10 Cyanotic Congenital Heart Defects with Increased Pulmonary Blood Flow

Defect	Cardiac examination	Electrocardiogram	Chest x-ray
TGA			
Uncomplicated	Murmur may not be present. S_2 louder than normal and accentuated.	Right ventricular hypertrophy, possible right atrial hypertrophy, right axis deviation. May be normal in newborn.	Cardiomegaly, narrow mediastinum, increased pulmonary vascular markings. May be normal in newborn.
Complicated (with VSD)	Loud S_2. Holosytolic murmur best heard at 4th ICS to left of sternum. Thrill may be present.	Right ventricular hypertrophy.	Cardiomegaly, narrow mediastinum, increased pulmonary vascular markings.
Complicated (with VSD and PS)	Loud S_2. Holosystolic murmur. Ejection systolic murmur best heard along left sternal border.	Right ventricular hypertrophy.	Cardiomegaly, narrow mediastinum, decreased pulmonary vascular markings.
TAPVR			
With obstruction	Cardiac murmurs minimal or absent.	Right ventricular hypertrophy.	Increased pulmonary vascular markings. Normal-sized heart.
Without obstruction	Systolic ejection murmur best heard high in the left chest. Mid-diastolic murmur best heard low in the left chest. Widely split S_2	Right axis deviation, right atrial hypertrophy, right ventricular hypertrophy.	Supracardiac: "Figure eight" or "snowman" configuration. All defects: Enlarged right atrium, right ventricle, and main pulmonary artery. Increased pulmonary vascular markings.
Truncus arteriosus	Normal S_1, single S_2, ejection click. Loud, continuous (PDA type) murmur with unrestricted PBF. Murmur shortened and softened by decreasing PBF.	Left ventricular hypertrophy; biventricular hypertrophy seen occasionally.	Nonspecific except for alteration in pulmonary vascular markings. May detect right-sided aortic arch, and pulmonary vessels may arise abnormally high in the chest.

ICS, intercostal space; PBF, pulmonary blood flow; PDA, patent ductus arteriosus; PS, pulmonic stenosis; S_1, first heart sound; S_2, second heart sound; TAPVR, total anomalous pulmonary venous return; TGA, transposition of the great arteries; VSD, ventricular septal defect.

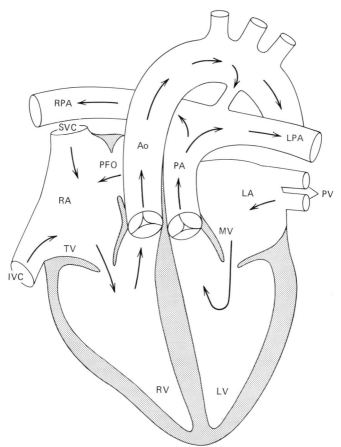

Figure 3-31. Uncomplicated D-transposition of the great arteries. Ao, aorta; IVC, inferior vena cava; LA, left atrium; LPA, left pulmonary artery; LV, left ventricle; MV, mitral valve; PA, pulmonary artery; PFO, patent foramen ovale; PV, pulmonary vein; RA, right atrium; RPA, right PA; RV, right ventricle; SVC, superior vena cava; TV, tricuspid valve.

shunting may not occur at birth because pulmonary resistance is equal to systemic resistance at this time (*see* p. 131). Pulmonary resistance decreases with maturation. Because an increased volume of blood is returned to the pulmonary circuit via the VSD, the left atrium receives an enlarged volume from the lungs. This causes the pressure in the left atrium to be higher than that in the right atrium. Blood, therefore, will be shunted from the left atrium to the right atrium via the foramen ovale. Enlargement of the right ventricle, left atrium, left ventricle, main pulmonary artery, and pulmonary vessels develops from these alterations.

The presence of PS as well as of a VSD alters hemodynamics even further. PS decreases blood flow to the lungs and increases left ventricular pressure. As a result of the increased left ventricular pressure, a greater amount of blood is shunted to the right ventricle and subsequently sent out of the aorta. Therefore, more oxygenated blood is delivered to the body. However, as the degree of PS increases, the resistance of flow to the lungs increases, causing a substantial decrease in PBF. LAP decreases, and blood is shunted from the right atrium to the left atrium. This causes further desaturation of blood delivered to the right ventricle and the aorta via the VSD. This further alteration in hemodynamics creates enlargement of the right atrium, right ventricle, and left ventricle and a decrease in size of the main pulmonary artery and the pulmonary vessels.

Clinical presentation

Uncomplicated TGA: The clinical picture seen in a child with uncomplicated TGA depends on the age at presentation. Generally, the child with uncomplicated TGA presents early in infancy. The infant's weight is usually normal or greater than normal. Marked cyanosis and tachypnea are present because of the lack of sufficient mixing of venous and oxygenated blood. Metabolic acidosis can occur rapidly from this hypoxic state and can ultimately lead to death. Rapid deterioration may result from physiological closure of the ductus arteriosus in the newborn. CHF is an early problem because of the increased work load on the heart and the overload of blood in the pulmonary circuit.

After the newborn period, cyanosis, clubbing of the nail beds, and polycythemia are evident as the child grows, dyspnea is present, and exercise tolerance is decreased. It is important to note that intellectual deficit does not occur in these children despite the chronic hypoxia.

On cardiac examination, a murmur may not be detected because of the low volume of blood that is shunted across the ductus arteriosus and the foramen ovale. S_2, which signifies aortic closure, is louder than normal and accentuated. If pulmonary artery hypertension is present, S_2 is altered (*see* p. 133). Arterial blood gases demonstrate desaturation. Polycythemia develops from this chronic arterial desaturation. Right ventricular hypertrophy, possible right atrial hypertrophy, and right axis deviation are seen on ECG; however, the ECG may be normal in the first few days of life.

Hepatomegaly is present in those children with CHF. The chest x-ray demonstrates cardiomegaly, a narrow mediastinum because of the displacement of the major vessels, and increased pulmonary vascular markings. The chest x-ray may appear normal in the first few days of life. Definitive diagnosis is established by cardiac catheterization.

Complicated TGA: The clinical picture of this child is, except for a few variables, very similar to that of the child with uncomplicated TGA. Tachypnea, CHF, and cyanosis generally occur at a later age. If good mixing results from a coexisting lesion, such as a large VSD, cyanosis may be quite mild. However, if severe PS is present, cyanosis may be more pronounced than that of uncomplicated TGA or of TGA with VSD alone. In addition, the presence of infundibular PS may cause the child to have cardiac spells (*see* p. 154).

On cardiac examination, the child with TGA and a VSD has a loud S_2 and a holosystolic murmur created by the VSD that is best heard at the fourth left ICS. A thrill may be present with a significant murmur. If pulmonary artery hypertension is present, S_2 will be altered (*see* p. 133). The chest x-ray demonstrates cardiomegaly, a narrow mediastinum, and increased pulmonary vascular markings. Right ventricular hypertrophy is evident on ECG.

The child with TGA, VSD, and PS has a loud S_2, a holosystolic murmur, and an ejection systolic murmur (best heard along the left sternal border) as a result of the PS. Decreased pulmonary vascular markings, cardiomegaly, and a narrow mediastinum are seen on chest x-ray. Right ventricular hypertrophy is evident on ECG.

Medical management.   Medical management in the newborn is aimed at controlling CHF, correcting metabolic acidosis, and increasing arterial oxygenation. CHF is controlled by the use of digitalization and diuretics (*see* p. 175). Metabolic acidosis is corrected by the use of sodium bicarbonate. Further metabolic acidosis is prevented by maintaining normal body temperature and normal serum glucose (*see* p. 179). Arterial oxygenation is increased by performing a balloon atrial septostomy during cardiac catheterization or by administering prostaglandins to maintain patency of the ductus arteriosus (*see* p. 160).

Balloon atrial septostomy, also known as the Rashkind procedure, is performed during cardiac catheterization. A catheter with a balloon tip is inserted into the saphenofemoral vein or the umbilical vein. The catheter is then threaded into the right atrium and guided across the foramen ovale into the left atrium. The balloon is then inflated and pulled in a left-to-right direction through the foramen ovale in order to increase its size. Complications, which are rare, include cardiac perforation, damage to the inferior vena cava, inability to deflate the balloon, and damage to the atrioventricular valves. In addition, inadequate atrial mixing may persist despite successful completion of an atrioseptostomy.

Prostaglandins may be administered to the child with severe PS who is totally dependent on ductal flow to the lungs or in whom atrioseptostomy does not provide adequate arterial oxygenation. It is important to note that prostaglandins are used only as a temporary measure to decrease the stress on the infant until further palliative measures can be taken (*see* p. 160).

Medical management of the older infant and child is aimed at controlling CHF and at close monitoring for signs of the development of pulmonary hypertension and increasing polycythemia.

Palliative surgical management.   Blalock-Hanlon atrioseptectomy, pulmonary artery banding, Blalock-Taussig shunt, and Waterston shunt (*see* p. 156) are palliative measures for TGA. These measures allow stabilization of cardiac and respiratory status until corrective surgery can be performed at an optimal age. Some institutions do not use palliative measures, but recommend early definitive repair instead. This, however, is not a generally accepted practice.[11]

In the infant with persistent arterial desaturation and metabolic acidosis despite medical intervention, an atrioseptectomy (Blalock-Hanlon procedure) may be performed. The atrial septum is surgically excised to permit additional shunting between the atria. This technique may be used in the young infant when definitive surgical repair would be too great a risk. It is generally performed in children with uncomplicated TGA.

Pulmonary artery banding (*see* p. 133) may be performed in the young infant who has TGA with a large VSD. This procedure will decrease CHF and the risk of developing pulmonary artery hypertension. An atrioseptectomy may be performed at the same time to increase arterial saturation.

Blalock-Taussig and Waterston shunts are generally performed in the infant with TGA, VSD, and severe PS. A Blalock-Taussig shunt is performed by anastomosing the subclavian artery to the pulmonary artery. In a Waterston shunt, the right pulmonary artery is anastomosed to the ascending aorta. Both of these procedures serve to increase PBF. An atrioseptectomy may also be performed at the same time in order to further improve arterial oxygenation.

Definitive surgical correction.   Elective surgical correction is generally performed in children at the age of 1 year. However, the presence of high pulmonary artery pressures, persistent cyanosis, and CHF may necessitate surgery at an earlier age. Definitive surgical correction is most often achieved by either a Mustard repair or a Senning repair. The presence of a VSD, PS, or both further complicates the surgery.

Surgery is performed via a midline sternotomy incision. Cardiopulmonary bypass and hypothermia are required. Deep hypothermia with total circulatory arrest may be used.

A Mustard repair is performed in the following manner. The atrial septum (excluding the anterior portion that contains the conduction pathway) is excised. A pericardial or Dacron patch is then used to form a baffle or tunnel. The baffle is placed within the atrium to direct systemic venous blood flow through the mitral valve into the left ventricle. Pulmonary venous blood is directed into the right ventricle via the tricuspid valve. The baffle is sutured to the anterior atrial septum, around the openings of the superior and inferior venae cavae, and around the pulmonary vessels. Systemic venous blood flows posteriorly to the baffle. Pulmonary venous blood flows anteriorly to the baffle. The coronary sinus will generally drain into the left ventricle. PS and VSD, if present, are also corrected at this time.

If irreversible pulmonary vascular disease from pulmonary artery hypertension is present (generally related to the presence of a VSD), a palliative Mustard repair is done. A baffle is inserted to redirect blood flow at the atrial level, but the VSD is left open. This allows a greater flow of blood to the lungs, which is needed to overcome the irreversible vascular changes that result from prolonged and severe pulmonary artery hypertension.

The Senning repair is very similar to the Mustard repair. The primary difference is the use of the right atrial wall and the interatrial septum as the baffle, as opposed to the use of either pericardium or a Dacron patch. The atrial septum is incised to form a trapezoid flap. If the atrial septum is too small because of the presence of an ASD, a Dacron patch is added to the septum to form the flap. The foramen ovale is closed by suture or patch. The flap is then sutured in place as in the Mustard repair. The advantages of this repair over the Mustard repair are seen to be the following: baffle obstruction is less likely to occur, and baffle tissue has the capacity to grow with the child.

Postoperative complications may include hemorrhage; conduction problems; arrhythmias; obstruction of the superior vena cava, inferior vena cava or pulmonary veins by the baffle; and baffle leaks. Baffle caval obstruction is manifested by edema (especially facial) and by prominence of the superficial venous collateral circulation. Pulmonary venous hypertension results if the pulmonary veins are obstructed. This can greatly alter the postoperative prognosis. A baffle leak will permit shunting of blood at the atrial level in either direction. An additional concern with both the Mustard and the Senning procedures involves the as yet unanswered question of how long the right ventricle can function effectively as a systemic pump. At present, the life-span of these children is unknown.

Total Anomalous Pulmonary
Venous Return

Total anomalous pulmonary venous return (TAPVR) accounts for only approximately 1 percent of the total number of congenital heart defects. TAPVR is

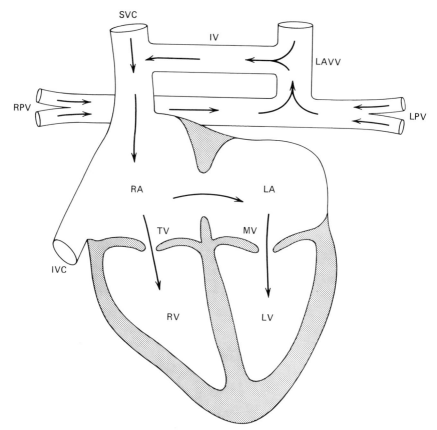

Figure 3-32. Total anomalous pulmonary venous return (TAPVR). This figure illustrates the supracardiac form of TAPVR, in which the venous return occurs via the superior vena cava (SVC). IV, innominate vein; IVC, inferior vena cava; LA, left atrium; LAVV, left anomalous vertical vein; LPV, left pulmonary vein; LV, left ventricle; MV, mitral valve; RA, right atrium; RPV, right pulmonary vein; RV, right ventricle; TV, tricuspid valve.

defined as a failure of pulmonary venous blood to return to the left atrium because the pulmonary veins enter either the right atrium or another site in the systemic venous vasculature. The anomalous pulmonary vein pathway may occur at four different levels: (1) supracardiac via the superior vena cava (Fig. 3-32); (2) cardiac via the coronary sinus; (3) cardiac via direct flow to the right atrium (Fig. 3-33); and (4) infradiaphragmatic via the inferior vena cava and the portal vein or ductus venosus (Fig. 3-34). Most common is supracardiac TAPVR. An ASD, a vital component of this lesion, is always present.

TAPVR may occur with or without obstruction in the pulmonary venous pathway. TAPVR with obstruction occurs predominantly in the infradiaphragmatic type. Obstruction may occur from constriction of the vein as it passes through the diaphragm or from obstruction of flow as it passes through the ductus venosus and the liver. In general, supracardiac and cardiac TAPVR are not obstructed. The

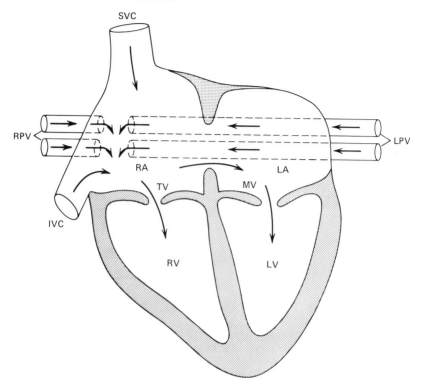

Figure 3-33.   Total anomalous pulmonary venous return directly into the right atrium (RA). IVC, inferior vena cava; LA, left atrium; LPV, left pulmonary vein; LV, left ventricle; MV, mitral valve; RPV, right pulmonary vein; RV, right ventricle; SVC, superior vena cava; TV, tricuspid valve.

clinical presentation varies remarkably according to the presence or absence of obstruction.

TAPVR without obstruction occurs equally in males and females. TAPVR with obstruction, however, occurs more frequently in males.

Etiology.   The pulmonary venous system develops at about the third week of gestation. The splanchnic plexus, which is connected to the umbilical vitelline veins and the cardinal veins, is in direct communication with the lung buds. The common pulmonary vein, which arises in the common atrium, grows to join the splanchnic plexus. Once the common pulmonary vein and the splanchnic plexus are joined, the cardinal veins and vitelline veins are no longer connected to the splanchnic plexus. The pulmonary veins then drain into the left atrium via the common pulmonary vein. Gradually, the common pulmonary vein is absorbed into the body of the left atrium, and four distinct pulmonary veins draining into the left atrium persist. Failure in any of these steps leading to the formation of the four pulmonary veins results in TAPVR and explains why many types of TAPVR exist.

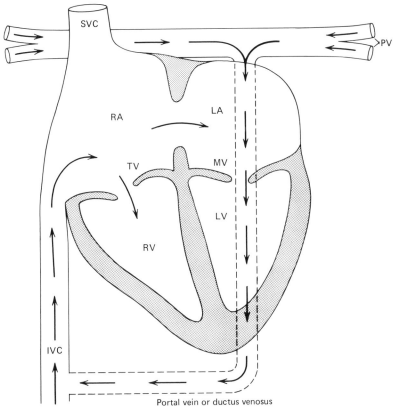

Figure 3-34. Total anomalous pulmonary venous return (TAPVR). This figure illustrates the infradiaphragmatic form of TAPVR, in which the venous return occurs via the inferior vena cava (IVC). LA, left atrium; LV, left ventricle; MV, mitral valve; PV, pulmonary vein; RA, right atrium; RV, right ventricle; SVC, superior vena cava; TV, tricuspid valve.

Alteration in hemodynamics

TAPVR with obstruction: Blood from both the pulmonary and the systemic venous systems returns to the right atrium. However, because of the presence of an obstruction in the pulmonary venous pathway, the volume of blood that returns to the right atrium is not greatly increased. The right atrium remains normal in size, and the left atrium and ventricle are small. Because of higher pressure in the right than in the left atrium, blood is shunted in a right-to-left direction across the ASD.

Because of the obstruction in pulmonary venous flow, pulmonary venous pressure is high, causing a rise in pulmonary vascular resistance. This leads to pulmonary artery hypertension and, in turn, puts stress on the right ventricle.

TAPVR without obstruction: Blood from both the pulmonary and the systemic venous systems returns to the right atrium. This results in an increased volume of blood to the right heart. Blood is shunted across the ASD to the left atrium. The right atrium, right ventricle, pulmonary artery, and pulmonary vessels enlarge to compensate for the increased volume. The left atrium and ventricle may be small because of the decreased volume of blood they receive.

Clinical presentation

TAPVR with obstruction: The clinical presentation of these children depends on the degree of obstruction and the amount of blood that is able to flow past the obstruction. In general, these children present early in infancy with CHF, dyspnea from pulmonary edema, and hypoxia. They are generally cyanotic; and deterioration may occur rapidly.

On cardiac examination, a murmur may be minimal or absent because the venous return to the right atrium is not considerably increased. Arterial blood gases are desaturated. Blood pressure and peripheral pulses are normal. The ECG demonstrates right ventricular hypertrophy, and the chest x-ray reveals a normal-sized heart and the presence of increased pulmonary vascular markings.

TAPVR without obstruction: Children with this lesion generally appear normal in early infancy. In the first few months of life, tachypnea, irritability, feeding problems, and failure to gain weight develop. Cyanosis becomes evident, increasing with crying and increased activity. CHF and recurrent pulmonary infections may occur by 6 months of age. However, some children may present with symptoms similar to those for a large ASD, except for the presence of cyanosis.

On cardiac examination, a systolic ejection murmur best heard high in the left chest, a mid-diastolic murmur best heard low in the left chest, and a widely split S_2 are present. If pulmonary artery hypertension develops from the increased flow to the pulmonary vasculature, the splitting of S_2 will narrow. The left chest is prominent. Arterial blood gases are desaturated. The ECG demonstrates right axis deviation and right atrial and right ventricular hypertrophy.

The chest x-ray of a child with cardiac TAPVR via the coronary sinus will appear similar to that of a child with an ASD (*see* p. 130). The chest x-ray of supracardiac TAPVR via the superior vena cava will demonstrate a classic "figure eight" or "snowman" configuration. The heart forms the lower portion of the snowman, and the upper portion of the snowman's body results from the widening of the common pulmonary vein on the left of the mediastinum and of the superior vena cava on the right of the mediastinum. The right atrium, right ventricle, and main pulmonary artery are enlarged in both of these defects. Pulmonary vascular markings are increased.

Medical management. The infant with obstructed TAPVR who presents with florid CHF, tachypnea, dyspnea, and pulmonary edema requires rapid and aggressive intervention. Stabilization of cardiovascular status by decreasing CHF (*see* p. 175) and pulmonary edema is mandatory. When definitive diagnosis is made by cardiac catheterization, immediate surgery is recommended.

Management of the child with TAPVR without obstruction is aimed at controlling CHF and failure to thrive and at treating any respiratory infections. Close assessment of heart sounds to detect the onset of pulmonary artery hypertension is vital. The development of any of these problems warrants surgical intervention. Surgery can be optimally performed at any age.

Definitive surgical correction. Surgical correction is performed via a midline sternotomy incision. Cardiopulmonary bypass and hypothermia are required. The common pulmonary vein is anastomosed to the left atrium. The connecting vein to the systemic venous circulation is then ligated, and the ASD is closed. In cardiac

TAPVR via the coronary sinus, a patch is placed in the atrial septum to direct coronary sinus and pulmonary venous return into the left atrium. Postoperative complications may include hemorrhage and acute pulmonary failure. Heart block may occur with cardiac TAPVR.

Truncus Arteriosus

Truncus arteriosus is a rare congenital heart defect, accounting for less than 1 percent of the total number of cardiac defects. It represents failure of the primitive arterial trunk (the truncus arteriosus) to septate and divide into a distinct aorta and pulmonary artery. Instead, a single large vessel leaves the heart, giving rise to the coronary arteries, aorta, and pulmonary arteries, and containing only one set of semilunar valves. The truncus arteriosus lies over a VSD that is always seen in conjunction with this defect and that is an integral part of its pathophysiology (Fig. 3-35).

Etiology. The aorta and the pulmonary artery normally develop from the common truncus arteriosus at the end of the third week and during the fourth week of gestation. This occurs by virtue of the unique development of truncoconal ridges, which separate and position the great arteries. Failure of septation of the common trunk results in the persistence of a single vessel that receives blood from both the right and the left ventricles. Because the truncal septum is involved in the complete closure of the ventricular septum, failure of truncal septation always results in a VSD.

Truncus arteriosus exists in four distinct anatomic varieties. Variation occurs with respect to the size and site of origin of the pulmonary arteries. The truncus in all children with this defect features a dominant aorta. Most often, the pulmonary arteries arise from the ascending truncus arteriosus and are well developed.

Alteration in hemodynamics. All children with truncus arteriosus have a common outlet for right and left ventricular blood. However, the amount of blood flow to the lungs varies greatly, depending on the nature of the pulmonary arteries. Most children have well-developed pulmonary arteries and receive several times more blood in their pulmonary circulation than is normal; others have somewhat hypoplastic pulmonary vessels. Some, in whom the pulmonary arteries arise from the descending truncus arteriosus, have significantly reduced PBF.

Clinical presentation. The physical findings in children with truncus arteriosus vary with the degree of PBF: from severe cyanosis because of markedly decreased PBF to mild cyanosis with markedly increased PBF. Hypoxia is the primary problem for those with severe cyanosis, and CHF is the primary problem for those with unrestricted PBF.

On cardiac examination, all childen with truncus arteriosus have a normal S_1, but there is usually a single S_2 and an ejection click. With unrestricted PBF, a loud, continuous murmur like that of PDA is heard. As pulmonary resistance increases, the murmur is shortened and softened. The child with little PBF may have only a very soft, nonspecific murmur.

The chest x-ray is rather nonspecific except for alteration in pulmonary vascular markings. A right-sided aortic arch is present in some children. The pulmonary vessels may appear to arise abnormally high in the chest. The ECG generally shows left ventricular hypertrophy or biventricular hypertrophy. The echocardiogram detects the single large vessel overriding the ventricular septum but does not

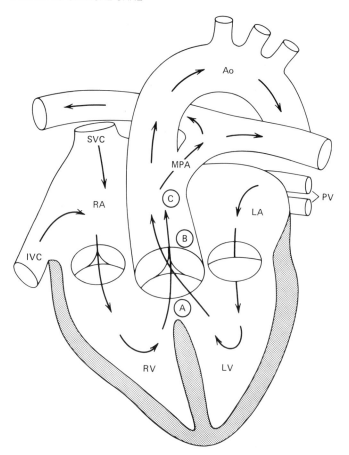

Figure 3-35. Type I truncus arteriosus. (A) Ventricular septal defect, (B) truncal valve; (C) common truncus arteriosus. Ao, aorta; IVC, inferior vena cava; LA, left atrium; LV, left ventricle; MPA, main pulmonary artery; PV, pulmonary vein; RA, right atrium; RV, right ventricle; SVC, superior vena cava.

provide a definitive diagnosis. The relationship of the pulmonary arteries to the truncus arteriosus may be detected. Cardiac catheterization is necessary for a definitive demonstration of the anatomy and physiology of the defect.

Medical management.   Medical management is determined by the clinical presentation of the particular child with truncus arteriosus. Most often, CHF must be controlled (*see* p. 175). Severe restriction of PBF may be ameliorated by correction of acidosis and by palliative surgery (but not complete repair).

Palliative surgical management.   In the past, for lack of a better alternative, children with truncus arteriosus who had unrestricted PBF, which caused CHF that was resistant to medical management, were treated surgically by palliation with pulmonary artery banding (*see* p. 133). Now that reparative intervention is possible, palliative banding is no longer recommended, although there remains the risk of pulmonary vascular disease. Children who are severely cyanotic because of decreased PBF may be helped by one of the systemic-pulmonary shunts that increase PBF (*see* p. 156).

Definitive surgical correction. Children with increased PBF are candidates for corrective surgical repair of truncus arteriosus. Cardiopulmonary bypass, deep hypothermia, and circulatory arrest are necessitated. The pulmonary arteries are excised from the common truncus arteriosus and anastomosed to a valved conduit from the right ventricle. The VSD is patched in a manner that locates the truncus arteriosus to the left of the septum, where it functions as the aorta only.

With a prosthetic conduit and valve in place, these children require lifelong prophylaxis against infective endocarditis. No limitations of physical activity are necessary. Surgery may have to be repeated if the conduit malfunctions or if the child outgrows it.

CRITICAL CARE MANAGEMENT OF THE CHILD WITH A CARDIOVASCULAR DISORDER

Critical care management of the infant or child with a congenital heart defect may involve care before and during diagnosis, in the medical management of the child, or after either palliative or corrective surgery. Children with cardiovascular disorders are characterized by extreme hemodynamic instability and an extensive potential for complications. Their care is dependent on the ability of the critical care clinician to simultaneously assess and evaluate their status and to intervene as necessary. In general, the aim of the critical care management of these children is to maintain adequate CO, upon which life itself is dependent.

This section will detail the critical care management of infants or children with CHF, of children who are severely cyanotic, and of those who have had cardiovascular surgery. There will also be a brief description of cardiopulmonary bypass techniques in order to facilitate understanding of postoperative management.

CHF

The presence of CHF necessitates a number of diagnostic studies. Chest x-ray is performed to assess the extent of cardiac enlargement and the degree of pulmonary congestion. The ECG detects myocardial hypertrophy and any dysrhythmias. Though it does not actually determine the presence of CHF, a base line is nevertheless established. Echocardiography is frequently performed, principally to determine the anatomic diagnosis rather than to confirm the presence of CHF. Myocardial functioning, however, can be evaluated by the echocardiogram.

Arterial blood gases are measured. Because CHF causes decreased CO, the child's metabolic needs are not met and acidosis develops. Metabolic acidosis is of particular concern in the child with CHF because it further impairs myocardial functioning. When CHF and pulmonary congestion are severe, the resultant ventilation-perfusion abnormalities may lead to respiratory acidosis, hypercapnia, and some degree of hypoxia.

Because glucose is the primary metabolic energy source for the myocardium, serum glucose determination is important. Hypoglycemia often accompanies CHF, and blood glucose may fall precipitously in infants with CHF — especially in neonates with scanty glycogen stores.

A normal serum calcium level is essential for adequate myocardial contractility. Serum calcium may be low in the neonatal period, especially in infants of diabetic mothers.

Hyponatremia may be present in the infant or child with CHF secondary to water retention. Myocardial contractility is decreased by hyponatremia. Myocardial functioning and response to digoxin therapy are related to serum potassium levels. Serum potassium levels may increase with the decreased urine output associated with severe CHF. Hypokalemia, which potentiates the action of digoxin on myocardial cells, must be corrected before the initiation of digoxin therapy.

Hematologic studies may indicate a relative anemia (because of water retention), which, if severe, may interfere with oxygen delivery. The white blood cell count may be increased in CHF. Although this finding does not necessarily indicate bacterial infection, the clinician must be alert to other signs and symptoms of infection if leukocytosis is present.

When renal blood flow is decreased because of CHF, the results are oliguria, albuminuria, hematuria, and an increased urine specific gravity. Accurate calculation of intake and output is essential. As CO improves with successful treatment of CHF, renal blood flow and urine output increase dramatically.

Specific management of CHF includes digitalization, administration of diuretic agents, and fluid restriction. Digitalization is accomplished over 24 hours. (Lanoxin, a brand name of digoxin, is the specific digitalis preparation recommended for use with infants and children.) Digoxin is generally administered by the IV route. The infant or child with CHF may vomit, and thus be unable to tolerate oral preparations of digoxin. In addition, CHF is associated with significant bowel wall edema, which may interfere with the absorption of the medication in its oral form. The intramuscular route is not suggested because CHF causes peripheral vasoconstriction and venous pooling, which render intramuscular absorption unreliable.

Digitalization is accomplished by the initial administration of large doses, followed by lower maintenance doses. Because digoxin is readily absorbed by all body tissues, comparatively large initial doses are needed to achieve organ saturation and an adequate serum level. The recommended dosage for digitalization and maintenance, listed in Table 3-11, is dependent on both the child's age and weight. Premature infants require a lower dose per kilogram of body weight because their renal function is immature and, thus, comparatively less of the drug is excreted. Young children (from birth to 2 years of age) require a relatively higher dose per kilogram of body weight because children of this age-group have proportionally larger organ mass in comparison to total body weight and because they also have a rapid turnover of body water.

Digitalization is generally accomplished by initially administering one half of the total digitalizing dose (TDD). Administration of a large initial dose promotes rapid action of the drug and permits observation for untoward side effects before the administration of further doses. The second dose of digoxin is administered 6 to 8 hours after the first, and it constitutes one quarter of the calculated TDD. The third digitalizing dose is also one quarter of the TDD, and it is administered 6 to 8 hours after the second dose. A maintenance dose of one eighth the TDD is ad-

TABLE 3-11   Recommended Lanoxin* Dosage in Infants and Children

Age of child	TDD†
Premature Infant	
500–1,000 g	20 μg or 0.02 mg/kg
1,000–1,500 g	20–30 μg or 0.02–0.03 mg/kg
1,500–2,000 g	30 μg or 0.03 mg/kg
2,000–2,500 g	30–40 μg or 0.03–0.04 mg/kg
Term infant to 1 month	60 μg or 0.06 mg/kg
1 month to 2 years	60–80 μg or 0.06–0.08 mg/kg
2 years to 10 or 12 years‡	40–60 μg or 0.04–0.06 mg/kg
Over 10 to 12 years‡	15–20 μg or 0.015–0.020 mg/kg

*Brand name of digoxin manufactured by Burroughs Wellcome Co. (Research Triangle Park, N.C.).
†The TDD is for intramuscular or oral administration; the intravenous dose is 75 percent of the oral or intramuscular dose. The maintenance dose is one eighth of the TDD, repeated every 12 hr.
‡Or until the child's weight results in a TDD of greater than 1.0 to 1.5 mg.
TDD, total digitalizing dose.

ministered 12 hours after the third digitalizing dose, and it is repeated every 12 hours thereafter. Adequate digitalization is assured by measurement of the serum digoxin level. The desired therapeutic level is 1.2 to 2.2 mg/100 ml.

The recommended dose of digoxin may be altered in children in whom renal function is impaired or in the presence of myocardial dysfunction. In addition, it is imperative that the nurse review results of laboratory measurement of serum electrolytes. Electrolyte imbalance may necessitate alteration of the recommended dose. Increased serum calcium and decreased serum potassium or magnesium increase the myocardial absorption of digoxin and potentiate its cardiac action.

The desired effects of digitalization include reduction of tachycardia, improvement of blood pressure, and increased urine output. It is important that the clinician assess the infant or child for these changes. In addition, knowledge of untoward side effects and careful observation for their development are crucial aspects of critical care. Digoxin toxicity results in cardiac rhythm disturbances; gastrointestinal side effects, including anorexia, nausea, and vomiting; and neurological effects such as lethargy and irritability. Accurate assessment of digoxin toxicity is complicated by the fact that both the early gastrointestinal and neurological side effects are difficult to differentiate from the pathophysiological effects of CHF.

The extent of digoxin toxicity is determined by measurement of the serum digoxin level. This measurement, however, is often unreliable in children. Furthermore, in the case of children who are also being administered spironolactone (Aldactone), it is known that this medication interferes with accurate measurement of the serum digoxin level. In general, when digoxin toxicity is suspected, the medication is discontinued and the child is closely evaluated. Physical signs and symptoms may be classified in relation to mild, moderate, or severe digoxin toxicity. Table 3-12 presents the clinical symptoms that the nurse might expect to observe with varying degrees of digoxin toxicity.

In conjunction with digitalization, the specific management of CHF in infants and children with critical CHD includes diuretic therapy and fluid restriction. Diuretics serve to eliminate excess accumulated water in order to reduce volume overload and, as a result, the mechanical work load on the heart. Furosemide is

TABLE 3-12   Clinical Symptoms of Digoxin Toxicity in Children

Degree of toxicity	Gastro-intestinal system	Central nervous system	Cardiac rhythm
Mild	Anorexia Nausea	Lethargy	Sinus bradycardia
Moderate	Nausea Vomiting	Irritability	Sinus arrest with nodal escape beats Second-degree atrioventricular heart block Premature atrial or nodal contractions Wandering atrial pacemaker Wenckeback phenomenon
Severe	Vomiting (may be absent)	Irritability Seizures	Third-degree atrioventricular block Paroxysmal atrial tachycardia Atrial fibrillation or flutter Nodal tachycardia Ventricular arrhythmias Asystole

generally the diuretic of choice during periods of acute CHF. Initially, it is best administered intravenously in order to ensure maximum response. The recommended dose is 1 to 2 mg/kg IV, which may be repeated in 6 to 12 hours. Diuretic therapy may be necessary over prolonged periods in order to prevent recurrent episodes of CHF. Oral preparations of furosemide ([Lasix] 2 to 3 mg/kg/day), chlorothiazide ([Diuril] 40 mg/kg/day), or spironolactone ([Aldactone] 0.7 to 1.0 mg/kg/day) may be used alone or in conjunction with each other for maintenance therapy.

During episodes of acute CHF, fluid intake may be restricted to two-thirds or three-quarters of the maintenance level. Restriction of fluid intake, in conjunction with diuretic therapy and digitalization, serves to eliminate the volume overload present with CHF.

Nursing intervention is a crucial aspect of the specific management of the infant or child with CHF. During digitalization, accurate calculation and measurement of the ordered medication are paramount. In order to avoid errors, many institutions require that digoxin be ordered both in micrograms (or milligrams) and in the milliliter equivalent and that the dosage calculation and measurement be verified by two licensed professionals before its administration.

Before digoxin is administered, heart rate and rhythm are carefully assessed. In most children, if the heart rate is less than 100 beats/min, or if the rhythm is abnormal, the nurse should not proceed with the administration of digoxin. Consultation with the physician and further evaluation of the child are necessary to determine whether the medication should be administered. The nurse must be knowledgeable about the therapeutic and toxic effects of digoxin, as well as about its interaction with serum electrolytes. Because there is no antidote to digoxin, its safe administration requires astute nursing assessment.

Evaluation of the effectiveness of digoxin and diuretic therapy requires accurate recording of intake and output. In addition, depending on the severity of the CHF, these children may be weighed every 8 or 12 hours or on a daily basis. Serum electrolytes must also be monitored closely because hyponatremia and hypokalemia can result from either diuretic therapy or fluid and sodium restriction. Careful physical assessment to detect systemic and pulmonary venous congestion is very important.

Cyanosis

As is the case with CHF, CHD is not the only cause of cyanosis in infants and children. The other major cause of cyanosis in children is pulmonary disease. This is an important distinction to make, especially in the care of newborns. In the first few hours of life, the normal newborn may have acrocyanosis (peripheral cyanosis) because of instability of the vasomotor system and the resultant capillary stasis of blood. Central cyanosis, however, is pathological at any age. It is best detected by examining the mucous membranes in natural light (*see* p. 101). This is especially important when cyanosis is not generalized or severe, which makes recognition more difficult.

When cyanosis is detected in the infant, the first objective of critical care management is to determine whether its origin is pulmonary or cardiac in nature. With regard to the medical history, obtaining answers to the following questions may be important. When was the onset of cyanosis first detected — at birth or within the first few weeks or months of life? (Onset of cyanosis at birth or shortly thereafter is characteristic of both pulmonary and cardiac disease, whereas later onset is more indicative of cardiac disease.) Is the cyanosis continuous or episodic? Does it occur in spells? Does it worsen with activity and crying? Episodic cyanosis ("cyanotic spells") is characteristic of cardiac disease. During the newborn period, cyanosis related to pulmonary disease tends to decrease with crying, whereas cyanosis attributable to cardiac disease intensifies.

The chest x-ray is often helpful in detecting pulmonary diseases (such as respiratory distress syndrome of the newborn) and various aspiration syndromes, including meconium aspiration. However, it is not always conclusive. In addition, the chest x-ray of the newborn with cyanotic CHD may be normal or very similar to that of the newborn with transient pulmonary artery hypertension (persistent fetal circulation).

Arterial blood gas analysis may reveal some helpful differential findings. In lung disease, the $PaCO_2$ tends to be elevated, whereas in cardiac disease it is normal, or even lower than normal, because of tachypnea and consequent overexcretion of carbon dioxide. The hyperoxia test is a useful tool in further differentiation of cardiac from pulmonary disease. A high concentration of oxygen (preferably 100 percent) is administered via a tight-fitting face mask for 10 minutes. In cardiac disease there is no significant change in PaO_2, whereas in pulmonary disease an appreciable change can be effected. This change, or lack of change, can best be assessed if PaO_2 is measured in the right radial or temporal arteries, which arise from the aortic arch before the level of the ductus arteriosus. Right-to-left shunting of desaturated blood at the ductal level is characteristic of transient pulmonary artery hypertension.

Further diagnostic studies reveal additional data. The chest x-ray of the cyanotic infant without signs of CHF usually reveals normal heart size and diminished pulmonary vascular markings. The shape of the heart may be typical of specific defects. When PBF is increased, the pulmonary vascular markings are prominent and the heart size is usually large. The ECG usually indicates right atrial and/or right ventricular hypertrophy in defects with diminished PBF, but it is quite variable in lesions with increased PBF. Echocardiography may determine an exact anatomic diagnosis.

Arterial blood gases reveal marked hypoxia and normal and subnormal $PaCO_2$ (as described above). Acid-base balance is initially maintained, but severe cyanosis results in increased anaerobic metabolism and in excess production and accumulation of lactic and other organic acids.

Hematologic evaluation is important because oxygen can only be transported in the body by hemoglobin. Visible cyanosis is dependent on the amount of hemoglobin and the degree of arterial desaturation. Therefore, an anemic infant or child may not appear as cyanotic as would be the case if the level of hemoglobin were normal. In addition, persistent hypoxia stimulates red blood cell production with resultant polycythemia. Both anemia and polycythemia can interfere with adequate oxygen transport to body tissues, thereby aggravating tisue hypoxia and acidosis.

Cyanosis generally does not cause alteration in serum electrolytes. Serum glucose, however, must be monitored closely because the stress of cyanosis causes depletion of liver stores of glycogen. Serum calcium must also be monitored.

Specific management of these infants and children is usually directed toward establishing a definitive diagnosis. Sudden, severe, hypoxic episodes may result in rapid deterioration and death in infants with decreased PBF. Therefore, palliative or corrective surgery may be necessitated on an emergency basis. Cyanotic infants with increased PBF are generally less hypoxic, but may have fulminating CHF. Because the clinical presentation of these infants varies with the degree of PBF, the specific management also varies.

The cyanotic infant with increased PBF requires urgent management of CHF and supportive care that conserves energy and decreases metabolic demands on the cardiovascular system. The cyanotic infant with decreased PBF is characterized by severe hypoxia that may result in metabolic acidosis. Monitoring and correcting any acid-base imbalance are the first objectives of specific management. Sodium bicarbonate is administered by IV infusion to correct acidosis. The dose of sodium bicarbonate (in milliequivalents) is calculated by means of the following computation:

$$0.3 \times \text{body weight (kg)} \times \text{base deficit (mEq/liter).}$$

One half of the full dose required is administered over 30 minutes; the remainder is administered over the next 4 hours. Because small infants are unable to tolerate large solute loads, sodium bicarbonate may be diluted to a 50 percent concentration before administration. Whenever sodium bicarbonate is administered, serum electrolytes must be closely evaluated for development of hypernatremia.

Morphine sulfate may be required to interrupt a severe hypoxic spell. Morphine is administered in a dose of 10 to 20 µg/kg IV or intramuscularly. If necessary, the dose may be repeated once or twice at 30- to 60-minute intervals. Further administration may cause severe respiratory depression and is contraindicated unless the child is receiving ventilatory support. Vigilant respiratory assessment is required whenever morphine is administered to these children.

After stabilization of the hypoxic infant's condition, definitive diagnosis is established by cardiac catheterization. Palliation may be possible at catheterization (balloon atrial septostomy), or palliative or corrective surgery may be indicated immediately. Supportive care of these infants is directed at avoiding any additional stress.

Cardiopulmonary Bypass

Cardiovascular surgery may involve the complete correction of congenital defects; the improvement of circulatory functioning without the complete restoration of normal circulatory patterns or the achievement of complete cure; or the replacement of missing tissue with synthetic patches, artificial valves, or conduits in order to enhance circulatory functioning. Palliative procedures are often used to either increase or decrease PBF.

Cardiovascular operations are referred to as either closed heart or open heart procedures. *Closed heart surgery* may be safely performed without the use of cardiopulmonary bypass (extracorporeal circulation). Closed heart surgery includes PDA ligation, correction of coarctation, the shunt procedures that are used to increase PBF, and pulmonary artery banding (*see* p. 128). These procedures are all extracardiac in nature. *Open heart surgery* requires the use of cardiopulmonary bypass to correct or improve intracardiac lesions.

Bypass equipment and procedures. The function of cardiopulmonary bypass is to assume the roles of the heart and lungs during open heart operations. Venous blood is directed to the bypass circuit by means of cannulas placed in the superior and inferior venae cavae or in the right atrium. The blood is then oxygenated and returned to the arterial system by means of an aortic cannula. The total bypass circuit includes a pump, oxygenator, heat exchanger, filter, tubing, and intracardiac suction apparatus.

The pump most often used is a roller pump. The rotary movement of the rollers occludes the tubing in varying degrees to move blood along in a unidirectional, nonpulsatile manner. The oxygenator not only aerates the blood but allows for the elimination of carbon dioxide. Three kinds of oxygenators are in current use: bubble, film, and membrane. Heat exchangers aid in the control of body temperature by cooling the body (and thereby reducing metabolic demands) and then rewarming the body at the close of the surgical procedure. Filters aid in the prevention of embolization. Intracardiac suction is used to keep the operative field bloodless. Priming solutions for the bypass circuit include 5 percent dextrose and electrolytes, with additional salt-poor albumin or whole blood to prevent excessive hemodilution.

Complete or partial bypass may be used during cardiac surgery. Partial bypass involves only a partial diversion of venous drainage through the bypass circuit, while the remaining portion of venous drainage is pumped by the heart to the pulmonary circulation. Complete or total bypass involves the total diversion of all venous blood to the pump and also provides arterial return to the body by means of cannulas placed in the aorta. The rate and amount of blood flow are based on the child's resting CI, the degree of hypothermia used in conjunction with bypass, the degree of hemodilution, the arterial resistance, and the contractile tone of the veins.

Hypothermia: Moderate (28 to 32°C [82.4 to 89.6°F]) or deep (18 to 22°C [64.4 to 71.6F]) hypothermia may be used in conjunction with bypass or complete circulatory arrest in order to provide periods of safe, low perfusion during an operative procedure. Hypothermia is initiated through surface cooling of the child's body with ice packs and hypothermia blankets. Cooling is completed by the initiation of bypass with blood cooled to the desired temperature.

Careful use of anesthesia and hypercapnia aids in preventing the onset of cardiac arrhythmias during the cooling process. At 18 to 22°C (64.4 to 71.6°F), circulation can be interrupted safely in infants for 50 minutes, during the correction of complex cardiac anomalies, without the danger of cerebral ischemia. The risk of permanent neurological complications is less than 4 percent during circulatory arrest and deep hypothermia in infants.[12]

Heparinization: Complete heparinization is achieved before the insertion of the venous and aortic cannulas. Heparin (3 mg/kg IV) renders the blood incoagulable, thus preventing clotting along the bypass circuit with the serious consequence of embolization.

Monitoring: Various physiological parameters are closely monitored during extracorporeal circulation. Mean arterial blood pressure should be assessed carefully. A brief period of hypotension often occurs at the onset of perfusion; however, when equilibration is reestablished, the mean arterial blood pressure is maintained at physiological levels by adjusting the perfusion flow rate and/or by the administration of additional fluids or blood. CVP should be measured closely, and the ECG should be monitored continuously. Electroencephalographic monitoring is occasionally instituted during deep hypothermia. Close surveillance of core temperature via esophageal and/or rectal probes aids in maintaining constant body temperature. Blood studies are drawn frequently to monitor acid-base balance and electrolyte and hematocrit levels. Urine output is measured routinely to assess the adequacy of perfusion to the renal vasculature.

Discontinuation of bypass: At the close of surgery, partial perfusion is reinstated. Before withdrawal of bypass, the rate of perfusion is decreased gradually, and perfusion rewarming is begun. In general, as the child in hypothermia is rewarmed, the heart begins beating spontaneously. In some cases, electrical cardioversion is required. Once the child's circulating blood volume, RAP, and LAP are adequate, extracorporeal circulation is completely withdrawn. The venous and aortic cannulas are removed after air evacuation from the cardiac chambers. Blood coagulability is restored through the administration of protamine sulfate (3 mg/kg IV).

Complications associated with cardiopulmonary bypass. The use of cardiopulmonary bypass has enabled surgeons to effectively perform cardiovascular surgery for longer periods of time — in some instances up to 6 hours, although the average time of perfusion during most cardiovascular operations is 1 hour. The greater the length of time that a child requires bypass, the greater are the chances for complications. In addition, because the digoxin in body tissues is leached during cardiopulmonary bypass, with digoxin toxicity as a potential result, digoxin is discontinued before open heart surgery. The major complications of cardiopulmonary bypass may be categorized as metabolic, hematologic, pulmonary, renal, and neurological. The following list outlines the more common complications, discussed in the sections below:

Metabolic
  Acidosis
  Hypoglycemia
  Hyperglycemia
  Hypokalemia
  Hypocalcemia
Hematologic
  Hemolysis

Coagulation abnormalities
Disseminated intravascular coagulopathy
Thrombocytopenia
Hypotension
Pulmonary
Atelectasis
Pulmonary edema
Renal
Hemoglobinuria
Acute renal failure
Neurological
Cerebral ischemia

Metabolic complications: Metabolic and/or respiratory acidosis may result from oxygen deficits when pump perfusion flow rates are too low, when rewarming after hypothermia occurs too rapidly or when carbon dioxide elimination is inadequate. Temporary hypoglycemia may occur when the priming solution is low in glucose. Secondary hyperglycemia may occur as a result of decreased insulin production during hypothermia. Hypokalemia may be induced as a result of increased urine output and increased urinary potassium excretion associated with hemodilution during bypass, or it may be related to respiratory alkalosis.

Coagulation: Bypass may cause alterations in the blood: protein denaturation, thrombocytopenia, destruction of red and white blood cells, and coagulation defects. Severe bleeding postoperatively is often related to abnormal fibrinolytic activity. If complete heparinization does not take place before the full initiation of bypass, there is the danger of intravascular coagulation and capillary obstruction by microthrombi. Incomplete reversal of heparinization by the administration of protamine sulfate at the close of surgery may lead to prolonged bleeding and the danger of cardiac tamponade and/or hypovolemic shock. If abnormal coagulation develops postoperatively, thrombocytopenia may also occur as platelets are deposited and incorporated in the clotting process (*see* p. 431). Severe metabolic acidosis related to inadequate perfusion may also lead to continued oozing of blood from operative sites.

Hypotension: Hypotension occurring at the initiation and termination of bypass is usually a result of hypovolemia. Volume may be replaced by means of priming solutions, blood products, or albumin. If hypotension persists despite normal blood volume, inotropic agents such as dopamine hydrochloride or epinephrine may be considered (*see* p. 437).

Respiratory compromise: The major pulmonary consequences of bypass perfusion are reduced lung compliance and reduced ventilation: perfusion ratios. These changes can lead to atelectasis, pulmonary edema, and hypoxia. The extent of pulmonary compromise is dependent on preexisting pulmonary disease and the length of time that the child requires bypass.

Atelectasis is related to loss of surfactant during bypass and to the consequent alteration in alveolar surface tension. Interstitial edema, to a limited degree, results from lung manipulation during the thoracotomy. Pulmonary edema is most often the result of left ventricular dysfunction.

Renal injury: The kidneys may sustain either transient or permanent injury during cardiopulmonary bypass. Hemolysis may result in significant hemoglobinuria. Renal failure may be associated with severe hemolysis or may be the result of poor perfusion during bypass related to hypotension and/or hypovolemia.

Neurological injury: Cerebral ischemia is a serious potential complication of cardiopulmonary bypass. The primary causes of central nervous system insult are hypoxia, low perfusion, and embolization. Uncompensated or uncorrected acid-base imbalance also affects cerebral perfusion and oxygen delivery.

Postoperative Management of the Cardiac Patient

The period after open or closed heart surgery is a crucial one, during which a child may require many simultaneous assessments and interventions. Supportive care is aimed at maintaining an adequate CO and avoiding complications. The child must be monitored continuously and extensively because of hemodynamic instability and the wide range of possible complications, Knowledge of the child's preoperative status and intraoperative course, of the duration of cardiopulmonary bypass, and of the normal growth and physiological parameters of the pediatric patient is imperative in providing optimal supportive care.

The child will return from the operating room with a variety of invasive monitoring lines to facilitate the monitoring of hemodynamic parameters. The child's ECG and the appropriate physiological parameters: CVP, RAP and/or LAP, arterial pressure, and pulmonary artery pressure, will be monitored. A Foley Catheter will be inserted to facilitate assessment of fluid status and renal functioning. Often, the child initially requires some form of respiratory support, which may vary from supplemental oxygen to full ventilatory support. Chest tubes (pleural and/or mediastinal) allow for fluid drainage and for restoration of negative intrathoracic pressure. In addition, temporary pacing wires are inserted in the atria, the ventricles, or both during open heart surgery, in the event that external pacing should become necessary during the postoperative period.

Caring for the child after cardiovascular surgery requires that the ICU clinician possess keen observational skills and make accurate assessments. Observation and assessment are guided by an understanding of the specific potential complications associated with various cardiovascular operations. These vary depending on the specific defect that is palliated or repaired (Table 3-13). In addition, the child having cardiovascular surgery is subject to all the risks that any individual requiring an operative procedure experiences (e.g., fever and infection, paralytic ileus, wound dehiscence, etc.). The prevention and/or early detection of complications by thorough assessment of the child and integration of assessment data relative to all body systems is of paramount importance. The next section provides a framework from which the clinician can plan the assessments and interventions required during the postoperative management of the child who has had cardiovascular surgery.

Management of cardiac functioning. A successful postoperative course is dependent on the adequate functioning of the heart as a pump to maintain an optimal CO and on an intact vascular system to distribute it. If there is compromised functioning of either the pump or the vascular system, the child will be less able to respond adequately to the stress of the postoperative period.

CO can be assessed by means of clinical observations. The following are the assessment criteria: heart rate; blood pressure; CVP; LAP and RAP (the left- and right-heart filling pressures); peripheral perfusion; renal, respiratory, and neurological functioning; and blood pH determinations.

TABLE 3-13   Potential Complications After Corrective Cardiac Surgery According to Specific Defects

Defect	Complications
PDA	Phrenic nerve injury, chylothorax
ASD	Transient pulmonary edema, heart block, hemorrhage.
VSD	PS secondary to pulmonary artery banding; heart block; residual shunt; aortic insufficiency with widened pulse pressures; cyanosis, dyspnea, and hypotension associated with preoperative pulmonary hypertension.
Complete ECD	Persistent atrioventricular valve insufficiency; complete heart block; residual shunts.
CAo	Hypertension; paraplegia; hemorrhage; restenosis; mesenteric arteritis secondary to paradoxical hypertension; phrenic nerve injury; chylothorax; injury to the left recurrent laryngeal nerve (infrequent).
AS	Persistent stenosis; restenosis of the aortic lumen; aortic valve insufficiency; low CO secondary to left ventricular malfunction.
PS	Pulmonary regurgitation of variable degrees; right-sided CHF; transient arrhythmias; respiratory compromise; neurological injuries; hemorrhage.
TOF	Persistent right ventricular failure; heart block; ventricular arrhythmias; pulmonary regurgitation; low CO states.
TAPVR	Hemorrhage, acute pulmonary failure secondary to pulmonary venous obstruction; heart block.
TGA	Baffle obstruction of the superior and inferior venae cavae and of the pulmonary veins; baffle leaks causing residual shunts; atrial dysrhythmias; pulmonary venous hypertension; tricuspid regurgitation; hemorrhage; failure of the right ventricle as a pump for the systemic circulation.

AS, aortic stenosis; ASD, atrial septal defect; CAo, coarctation of the aorta; CHF, congestive heart failure; CO, cardiac output; ECD, endocardial cushion defect; PDA, patent ductus arteriosus; PS, pulmonic stenosis; TAPVR, total anomalous pulmonary venous return; TGA, transposition of the great arteries; TOF, tetralogy of Fallot; VSD, ventricular septal defect.

CO can be measured directly by the thermodilution technique with a Swan-Ganz catheter or by dye dilution (*see* p. 117). The range of normal CI, which can be evaluated from the CO (*see* p. 119), is 2.5 to 4.4 liters/min/m^2 (mean 3.5). A CI of less than 2.5 liters/min/m^2 requires investigation for cause and initiation of appropriate treatment. If the CI falls as low as 1 liter/min/m^2, the child is not likely to survive.[13]

CO is determined by a number of factors: (1) preload (ventricular filling pressure); (2) myocardial contractility; (3) heart rate; and (4) afterload (resistance to outflow). To some extent, all of these factors can be manipulated during the postoperative period. The desired goal of altering any of these factors is increased CO — achieved either by increased heart rate or by increased stroke volume (as produced by more efficient filling and emptying of the ventricles).

Heart rate: ECG changes are common in children after open heart surgery. Some of these changes are innocuous and do not require treatment, whereas other dysrhythmias may lead to low CO and are life-threatening. The underlying cause of the rhythm disturbance must be identified and treated. Dysrhythmias are usually the result of surgical trauma, hypoxia, acid-base imbalance (acidosis), electrolyte imbalance (hypo- or hyperkalemia), or digoxin toxicity (*see* p. 177). When dysrhythmias occur, the child should be observed for the frequency of the abnormal rhythm(s) and for hypotension, changes in peripheral circulation, and changes in sensorium as indicators of compromised CO. Blood studies are required in order to determine blood pH, serum electrolyte concentration, and digoxin level (if applicable). Emergency medications must be readily accessible in the event of a life-threatening dysrhythmia.

The child is placed on a continuous ECG monitor when admitted to the ICU. An initial 12-lead ECG is obtained for base-line information and repeated as indicated. The abnormal rhythms often seen by children after cardiovascular surgery are discussed below.

Sinus tachycardia may not require specific drug treatment, but its cause must be investigated. Common causes are anxiety, pain, fever, and anemia, but it may also be an indicator of atelectasis or cardiac tamponade. Hypotension may result with heart rates of greater than 160 beats/min in a child or 180 beats/min in an infant if the tachycardia is especially prolonged.[14] In general, a rapid heart rate is well tolerated by children.

Junctional (nodal) rhythms may be the result of digoxin toxicity, hypoxia, hypercalcemia, hyperkalemia, or surgical trauma. CO may be less than adequate because the heart rate is sometimes too slow and because the ventricles do not receive the benefit of synchronized atrial contraction. Pacing may be necessary to provide a more rapid heart rate.[14]

Right bundle-branch block is common after a right ventriculotomy. Left bundle-branch block may be associated with beginning left heart failure, and its detection on ECG requires close observation for other signs of CHF.

Supraventricular tachycardia will decrease CO because synchronized atrial contraction is lost and the ventricular rate is too rapid.[15] Vagal stimulation may convert paroxysmal atrial tachycardia to a slower sinus rhythm. Rapid atrial pacing may capture the pacemaker control and interrupt the arrhythmia. Digoxin is the drug of choice (*see* p. 176) in treatment of supraventricular tachycardia. Atrial fibrillation or flutter may require prompt cardioversion.

Premature ventricular contractions (PVCs) may precede the onset of ventricular tachycardia or fibrillation, depending on the frequency of the PVCs and on their location with respect to the T wave. PVCs may also be indicators of hypoxia or acidosis. Lidocaine is the treatment of choice (1 mg/kg IV). Phenytoin ([Dilantin] 5 to 10 mg/kg IV) may also be effective. Some PVCs do not require treatment. Isolated, univocal PVCs that do not result in a hemodynamic change or PVCs that represent a continuation of preoperative cardiac rhythm are generally not treated.

Bradyarrhythmias generally do not require treatment unless hypotension or decreased CO is present. Sinus bradycardia may be associated with sedative overdose or hypothermia in infants.

First-degree heart block is rarely a problem postoperatively. Second- and third-degree heart blocks require temporary or permanent artificial pacing. Drugs that may be useful in individualized doses are atropine, glycopyrollate, isoproterenol, and epinephrine. Detection of a conduction block always necessitates investigation of potential digoxin toxicity.

Alteration of the heart rate to maintain an adequate CO may be achieved by the use of pacemaker therapy and/or drug therapy. Epicardial pacemaker wires are routinely inserted in the right atrium, right ventricle, or left ventricle after open heart surgery. Slowed ventricular rates or instances of decreased CO because of

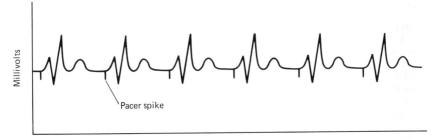

Figure 3-36. Typical pacemaker electrocardiogram (epidural pacer in left ventricle).

tachyarrhythmias or heart block are indications for pacing. When pacing is mandated, either a demand pacer or an atrioventricular sequential pacemaker is used in children. The optimal heart rate required will vary according to the age of the child, the defect corrected, and the presence of residual shunts. In general, higher rates are beneficial for younger children in the presence of low ventricular compliance, valvular insufficiency, and volume overload secondary to residual shunts. Lower rates may be indicated in older children and in children with residual stenosis after cardiovascular surgery.

When a child is admitted to the ICU after open heart surgery, a temporary external pacemaker and additional batteries must be available at the bedside at all times. Epicardial wires that are not in use are placed within rubber finger cots and taped to the child's surgical dressing in order to avoid the dangers of electric shock. The wires are generally left in place until the child's sutures are removed or until just before discharge.

When temporary pacing is necessitated, pacemaker functioning must be continuously ensured by assessment of the ECG (Fig. 3-36) and the child's clinical status. The pacemaker may lose power or be insufficiently powered to maintain firing, sensing, or capture. Competition from the child's innate heart rhythm is also possible. Complications related to inadequate or improper pacemaker functioning can be avoided by close observation of its functioning.

Preload, afterload, and myocardial contractility: Control of preload and afterload is also essential in providing a maximized CO in the postoperative period. Ventricular filling pressures can be augmented by increasing the preload with the use of volume expanders (e.g., colloid, plasma, whole blood), which raise the RAP and LAP. Stroke volume is consequently increased, and CO is improved, as evidenced by increased systemic blood pressure, warm extremities, strong peripheral pulses, adequate renal perfusion, and reversal of any existing acidosis.

Improved stroke volume and CO benefit myocardial contractility by improving myocardial perfusion. Myocardial contractility may also be improved by the administration of digoxin, calcium, and catecholamines.

Afterload may affect CO by increasing or decreasing the resistance to ventricular emptying, thereby affecting stroke volume. Vasoconstriction may seriously increase afterload, necessitating the administration of vasodilators (e.g., sodium nitroprusside) to counteract the vasoconstriction (*see* p. 374, 384).

Hypovolemia: Hypovolemia, a common postoperative problem, decreases preload and myocardial contractile force. As a compensatory response, systemic vascular resistance (afterload) increases, as vasoconstriction occurs in an attempt to sustain CO and maintain blood flow to critical organs.

Hypovolemia is evidenced by a CI of less than 2.5 liters/min/m^2, tachycardia, low LAP (less than 4 mmHg), narrowed pulse pressure, low systemic blood pressure, decreased urine output (less than 0.5 ml/kg/hr), and the presence of vasoconstriction. Volume replacement is prescribed initially to raise the LAP to 14 to 15 mmHg. Whole blood or packed red blood cells (if the patient's hemoglobin is less than 15 grams), fresh frozen plasma, or colloid may be transfused. If raising the LAP alone is not successful, inotropic agents such as isoproterenol (0.1 to 1.0 μg/kg/min) or dopamine hydrochloride ([Intropin] 10 to 15 μg/kg/min) may be administered (*see* p. 437).

Agents that reduce afterload, such as nitroprusside in low doses (1 to 2 μg/kg/min), may be required in conjunction with catecholamines in order to decrease peripheral vasoconstriction (*see* pp. 439, 684). Whenever nitroprusside is administered, the blood pressure and the LAP must be monitored closely for sudden decreases attributable to vasodilation. Additional volume expanders may be required.

The cause of hypovolemia must be investigated while the child's blood pressure is stabilized. The cause may simply be volume underload; a more serious cause is hemorrhage. With hemorrhage, the additional complication of cardiac tamponade may result.

Bleeding: Postoperative bleeding may be due to either a coagulopathy or to surgical bleeding. Coagulation studies should be evaluated immediately upon the child's admission to the ICU. These studies include platelet count, prothrombin time, partial thromboplastin time, and activated clotting time. Protamine sulfate (0.25 to 0.50 mg/kg/dose) is required when the partial thromboplastin time and the activated clotting time are prolonged in order to complete heparin reversal after bypass. Platelets (1 U/10 kg) are required if the platelet count is less than 50,000/mm^3. Fresh frozen plasma (20 ml/kg) may be needed when the prothrombin time and the partial thromboplastin time are abnormal.

Surgical bleeding can exist in the presence of abnormal or normal coagulation studies. The common sites of surgical bleeding are the bypass cannulation sites, vascular anastomoses, small vessel bleeding, and thoracic or pericardial adhesions from previous operations. Chest tube drainage must be closely monitored not only for amount and character, but also for the rate of drainage. Blood loss of 10 percent of the child's total blood volume per hour necessitates further surgical exploration in the operating room. When cardiac tamponade is suspected, a bedside thoracotomy in the ICU may be required.

Cardiac tamponade: Cardiac tamponade causes compression of the atria, restricting their filling and, thus, decreasing ventricular output. The chest x-ray reveals a widened mediastinal shadow. Clinically, tamponade may be evidenced by a sudden rise in a previously stable CVP or RAP, increasing heart rate with a falling blood pressure, and pale, slightly cyanotic skin with slowed capillary refill. A pulmonary artery occluded pressure equal to the RAP strongly suggests tamponade. Heart sounds become muffled and distant. Compression of the superior vena cava is evidenced by facial and nuchal edema. A pulsus paradoxus of greater than 10 to 15 mmHg with each inspiration suggests tamponade. Prompt emergency treatment is essential and involves the reopening of the mediastinal thoracotomy site. The maneuver will relieve the high intrathoracic pressure and cardiac compression. If necessary, volume replacement and catecholamine support are used concurrently. Surgical reexploration and repair are required after emergency treatment.

Cardiogenic shock: Cardiogenic shock exists when there is decreased CO with either normo- or hypovolemia. The cause may be increased afterload, decreased preload, or cardiac muscle dysfunction. Treatment with vasoactive agents is directed toward resolution of the CHF and pulmonary edema that result from cardiogenic shock. The primary agents used for enhancing myocardial contractility are epinephrine, isoproterenol, dopamine, and nitroprusside.

Adrenergic receptors in the myocardium are the site of action of the catecholamines. The receptors respond by increasing sinus heart rate, atrioventricular conduction rate, the force of myocardial contraction, vasoconstriction of most blood vessels, and vasodilation of nutrient blood vessels (see p. 437).

Epinephrine increases heart rate, myocardial contractility, arteriolar resistance, and pulmonary vascular resistance (see p. 439). An adverse effect that occurs at high doses is severe peripheral vasoconstriction, which may worsen an existing metabolic acidosis. The dosage varies, but continuous infusion is started at 0.1 μg/kg/min, with a maximum dose of 1.5 μg/kg/min.

Isoproterenol (Isuprel) may be used to treat cardiogenic shock (see p. 439). The strong chronotropic effect of isoproterenol causes increased oxygen consumption by the myocardium and may produce hypoxic damage as well as dysrhythmias. An advantage to the use of isoproterenol, however, is its effect of peripheral vasodilation. When administered, the minimum dose that will result in increased CO is used. The starting dose is 0.1 μg/kg/min, with a maximum of 1.5 μg/kg/min.

Dopamine (Intropin) (see p. 437) has become the drug of choice in the treatment of low CO states associated with cardiogenic shock. At low doses (5 μg/kg/min), dopamine decreases pulmonary and systemic vascular resistance. Dopamine also has the advantage of diminishing renal vascular resistance, thereby increasing renal blood flow. Dopamine increases myocardial contractility without significantly increasing heart rate. The usual dosage range of dopamine is 1 to 10 μg/kg/min, with a maximum of 30 μg/kg/min.

Nitroprusside decreases systemic and pulmonary vascular resistance through vasodilation and, thus, improves CO by decreasing afterload. The usual range is 0.5 to 4.0 μg/kg/min (see pp. 439, 684). Afterload-reducing agents may be required when catecholamines are needed to maintain CO.

Pulmonary edema is a consequence of left heart failure or cardiogenic shock. With an ineffective left ventricular pump, the LAP increases, causing an increase in the mean pulmonary capillary pressure. This results in the movement of fluid from the capillaries to the pulmonary interstitial spaces and interferes with gas exchange. Evaluation of breath sounds is vital in the care of the child with pulmonary edema because atelectasis is often an associated condition. Diuretic therapy, most frequently with furosemide (1 to 2 mg/kg/dose), and continuous positive airway pressure (CPAP) are commonly employed. Arterial blood gases and chest x-ray must be monitored closely to evaluate the effectiveness of management.

The ICU nurse is instrumental in the assessment of the child's postoperative cardiovascular functioning. Through accurate observation and integration of assessments, appropriate interventions can be made. The identification of trends and changes in vital signs, ECG rhythms, peripheral circulation, urine output, chest drainage, and sensorium is vital in the management of the child. Changes in any of these parameters could be an indication of a low CO state, warranting further investigation.

Management of respiratory functioning.   Maintenance of pulmonary gas transfer and the prevention of pulmonary complications are the two main objectives of respiratory management in the child who has undergone cardiovascular surgery. After open heart surgery, the pulmonary system is already compromised by two primary mechanisms: (1) the loss of surfactant during cardiopulmonary bypass, which may lead to atelectasis; and (2) the invasion of the chest cage by the surgical thoracotomy. In addition, the alteration of plasma proteins during the use of bypass can disrupt the balance of pulmonary water, which will move into the interstitial and alveolar spaces. Postoperative cardiac insufficiency can further compromise pulmonary functioning. Left heart dysfunction causes an increase in transcapillary pressure in the pulmonary venous system. This, too, causes a shifting of pulmonary water into the interstitial and alveolar spaces. The end result will be a "stiff lung," with ventilation-perfusion inequality and pulmonary edema.

Correction of specific heart defects produces dramatic pulmonary circulatory changes. For example, in patients with large left-to-right shunts (e.g., VSD), the increased PBF results in increased pulmonary vascular resistance and decreased lung compliance (*see* p. 131). Postoperative respiratory problems include pulmonary edema and poor lung compliance, which result in hypoventilation. Children with decreased PBF (e.g., TOF) must adapt to increased PBF after cardiovascular surgery. The objective of care of these children is to maintain arterial gas tensions that will provide the lowest pulmonary vascular resistance. Those children whose blood flow through the heart has been redirected (e.g., TGA) will experience a rise in pulmonary venous pressure postoperatively, often requiring months of adaptation to the new hemodynamics.

Respiratory support: Postoperative respiratory support may be provided by a variety of techniques. Most children who have had closed heart surgery require only humidified oxygen by mask, oxyhood, mist tent, or nasal cannula for 12 to 24 hours. Postoperative airway intubation is indicated for children who have had prolonged surgery or who have sustained lung trauma intraoperatively, for those with limited respiratory reserve, and for those who require frequent administration of analgesics. Three levels of support may be used after intubation: CPAP, intermittent mandatory ventilation, and controlled ventilation (*see* p. 47). The type of support required depends on the child's postoperative course. CPAP is generally required only at low levels to increase functional residual volume and PaO_2, to prevent atelectasis, and to decrease the required FIO_2.

High CPAP, which may be required in the presence of pulmonary edema, can have a deleterious effect on cardiac performance while having a beneficial pulmonary effect. High CPAP can result in decreased CO as a result of the increased intrathoracic pressures. This transmission of elevated airway and alveolar pressures can also cause increased pulmonary vascular resistance, thereby increasing cardiac work. With the use of high CPAP, the pulmonary artery pressure and LAP must be monitored closely, as must the clinical signs of diminished CO. High CPAP can also be responsible for spontaneous pneumothorax (*see* p. 48).

Arterial blood gases: Arterial blood gases must be monitored frequently in the postoperative period, especially for changes in the PaO_2, $PaCO_2$, and pH. In the evelution of postoperative blood gases, the child's preoperative and intraoperative blood gas values must be taken into consideration. The PaO_2 is at least partially dependent on the presence of residual shunts and the type of correction or palliation achieved with surgery. Postoperative PaO_2 and $PaCO_2$ are considered in conjunction with clinical signs of excessive respiratory work. They determine the need for, and the kind of, respiratory support, and they also indicate the effectiveness of respiratory support changes. Clinical signs of excessive respiratory work include nasal flaring, subcostal retractions, restlessness, unequal chest excursion, bradycardia, and cyanosis.

Acid-base imbalance, which can influence cardiac performance, requires frequent assessment. Respiratory alkalosis is caused by hyperventilation. The effects of hypocapnia can lead to decreased CO and coronary blood flow, diminished cerebral blood flow, a shift to the left in the oxyhemoglobin dissociation curve (see p. 29), and increased potassium excretion, which may, in turn, contribute to digoxin toxicity and dysrhythmias. The correction of hypocapnia usually necessitates a change in the ventilatory rate and/or volume on the ventilator. Respiratory acidosis is usually an indication for assisted ventilation. Severe acidosis has a depressive effect on the myocardium.

Weaning from ventilatory support and extubation are performed when the child's CO, circulatory dynamics, and arterial blood gases are stable. Before extubation, it is generally desirable that the child's oxygen requirement be no greater than 40 percent. After extubation, the child may continue to receive supplemental oxygen through some noninvasive means and is gradually weaned to room air. Arterial blood gases must be monitored closely during weaning from respiratory support. If respiratory acidosis or respiratory distress develops, reintubation is indicated.

Respiratory care: The potential pulmonary complications of hypoventilation, hypoxia secondary to airway obstruction or atelectasis, and pneumonia can be prevented through meticulous airway maintenance and thorough assessment of the child's respiratory status.

The tracheobronchial tree must be kept free of secretions through oropharngeal or endotracheal suctioning every 2 hours or as indicated by the child's respiratory status. Before suctioning, intubated children should be manually hyperinflated with 100 percent oxygen in order to minimize hypoxia during suction (see p. 46). Special care must be taken to avoid evoking pulmonary arteriospasm in those children with pulmonary artery smooth muscle hypertrophy secondary to a large, long-standing left-to-right shunt. Hypoxia and acidosis can stimulate this problem, which is manifested by severe cyanosis, a rise in pulmonary artery pressure, and a fall in systemic blood pressure and CO. The risks of arteriospasm are greatest during endotracheal suctioning because it causes a rapid drop in the PaO_2. Hyperoxygenation is extremely important, as is the avoidance of overzealous, overlong suctioning, in preventing pulmonary arteriospasm.

Position changes and the early institution of vibration and percussion will aid in the prevention of atelectasis, fluid pooling, and pneumonia. The use of blow bottles or incentive inspirometers is helpful in caring for the child who is not intubated, as are coughing and deep-breathing exercises. Careful assessment of breath sounds is needed to ensure airway patency and to detect any potential complication early.

Management of pain: Pain management is part of respiratory management because of the direct effect of pain on ventilation. A thoracotomy incision causes pain that will lead to splinting of the chest wall and diminished excursion of the diaphragm. This altered ability to move air in and out of the lungs results in a decreased tidal volume and alveolar hypoventilation. As a compensatory response, the child will increase the respiratory rate.

Pain also prevents the child from taking deep breaths, thereby increasing the risk of atelectasis. If atelectasis develops, the lungs become stiff, decreasing the functional residual volume and causing ventilation-perfusion inequality. The end result is hypoventilation and a decline in PaO_2.

The inhibition of the cough reflex because of pain leads to secretion retention and bronchoconstriction, with collapse of the small airways and alveoli. Immobility because of pain also has an adverse effect on pulmonary functioning because it causes elevation of capillary hydrostatic pressure in the dependent areas of the lungs. The end result is excessive fluid accumulation in the interstitial spaces, which decreases lung compliance and increases small airway resistance.

The appropriate administration of analgesics is a fundamental part of respiratory care. The child's tolerance of pain must be assessed, and analgesics must be administered accordingly. Morphine sulfate (0.1 mg/kg) or diazepam ([Valium] 0.1 mg/kg) can be administered by the (IV) route. The child must be observed closely for hypotension and/or hypoventilation after the administration of either medication. Decreasing the child's pain with analgesics not only eases respiration, but can also facilitate acceptance of respiratory care procedures and mitigate the massive anxiety associated with the postoperative period.

Management of renal functioning and fluid balance. Adequate renal functioning is maintained by an optimal CO. The desired minimal output of urine is 0.5 to 1.0 ml/kg/hr, and is best measured through the use of a Foley catheter. Weighing of diapers may be adequate in the younger child whose condition is stable. Measurement of urine specific gravity and evaluation of urine characteristics with Labstix are suggested every 2 to 3 hours. Hemoglobinuria secondary to hemolysis may be present after cardiopulmonary bypass for open heart surgery. Mannitol (0.5 g/kg IV) may be administered to facilitate hemoglobin clearance. A urine specimen should be obtained for microscopic examination with continued hematuria.

Acute renal failure is a serious complication after open heart surgery. Renal failure is most often associated with prolonged periods of hypovolemia and/or severe hemolysis after bypass. Early signs of acute renal failure include decreasing hourly urine output despite normovolemia, rising blood urea nitrogen and creatinine levels, hyperkalemia, and increased urine osmolality (*see* p. 386). The use of loop diuretics such as furosemide (1 to 2 mg/kg IV) or ethacrynic acid (1 to 2 mg/kg IV) has proven to be helpful in lowering the incidence of postoperative renal failure. Dopamine is often used to support renal functioning (*see* p. 437).

Measurements of extracellular fluid volume after open heart surgery have demonstrated a 5 to 33 percent increase in volume although blood volume is considerably reduced. After cardiopulmonary bypass, the ability of the kidneys to eliminate water and salt is limited because of increased secretion of antidiuretic hormone (ADH) and aldosterone in response to major surgery and to changes in hemodynamics. As a result, the urine excreted in the early postoperative period is often very concentrated.

In the early postoperative course, hyponatremia and hypo-osmolality may develop secondary to hemodilution or intracellular sodium shifting, rather than from a sodium deficit. The management goal is to encourage water loss and thus increase plasma sodium and osmotic concentration. Careful management is especially important when a child develops CHF and the concomitant inability to excrete salt and/or water in adequate amounts.

Fluid and electrolyte requirements: IV fluid maintenance requirements are limited to approximately three-quarters of full maintenance volume in an attempt to make use of the already existing expanded volume of extracellular fluid. During the first 24 hours, fluids are limited to 1,000 ml/m^2, then increased to 1,500 ml/m^2. Additional fluid may be necessary when radiant warmers are used to maintain normothermia in infants and small children because insensible water loss is increased. Daily measurement of the child's weight is helpful in the early detection of fluid overload and impending CHF.

Sodium requirements are low after cardiovascular surgery and cardiopulmonary bypass. Sodium intake should be limited to 1 mEq/kg/day. A 5 percent dextrose solution with 0.2 percent sodium chloride will fulfill this requirement.

Potassium loss is increased after cardiopulmonary bypass. Potassium is added to the IV solution in a maximum concentration of 40 mEq/liter, provided that the child is not oliguric. Serum potassium levels must be monitored frequently to ensure that a serum concentration of above 3.5 mEq/liter is maintained. Hyperkalemia (greater than 5 mEq/liter) may be an early indication of renal failure when oliguria is present. ECG changes associated with hyperkalemia must be observed for (see p. 395). Hypokalemia may increase the risk of digoxin toxicity (see p. 177).

Calcium requirements are usually met by the addition of 2 g/liter of calcium gluconate to the maintenance IV fluids. Calcium deficits result in decreased myocardial contractility. The use of acid-citrate-dextrose or citrate-phosphate-dextrose bank blood during surgery decreases the available ionized calcium because of its chelating effect on calcium. Calcium chloride (maximum of 20 mEq/kg) is a primary source of ionized calcium, but must be administered slowly through a central vein because of its sclerosing effect on peripheral blood vessels.

Calories are supplied through the use of dextrose solutions. In general, 10 percent dextrose solutions are recommended for infants because they are more prone to hypoglycemia. Minimum caloric requirements are met by a 5 percent dextrose solution in children weighing more than 10 kilograms. The Dextrostix should be checked every 2 to 4 hours on infants, and serum glucose levels should be measured as indicated. Parenteral nutrition support may be required by children with a prolonged and complicated postoperative course (see p. 494).

Acid-base management: Metabolic acidosis (base deficit) may be caused by prolonged periods of poor tissue perfusion by either the heart or during cardiopulmonary bypass. Mild degrees of acidosis (indicated by base deficits of -3 to -4) do not usually require treatment. However, more severe acidosis depresses CO, reduces cerebral blood flow, and increases pulmonary vascular resistance. A base deficit of greater than -4 mEq/liter and a pH of less than 7.4 necessitate correction by administration of a buffer. Sodium bicarbonate is the buffer of choice. The base deficit is generally not corrected fully at once, but by increments of one quarter to one half of the total bicarbonate needed (see p. 180). The child's serum sodium and osmolality must be evaluated frequently during bicarbonate replacement because they have a tendency to rise rapidly. Excessive sodium or serum osmolality can cause mental obtundation, coma, and cerebral insult.

Metabolic alkalosis (base excess) occurs quite frequently in infants after open heart surgery. The base excess may be caused by the frequent administration of buffers to correct the acidosis that results from the use of bank blood during surgery. Acidic urine prohibits the excretion of bicarbonate, and the increased aldosterone secretion after surgery decreases urinary bicarbonate loss. Severe metabolic alkalosis decreases CO, increases urinary potassium loss, and affects brain perfusion and oxygen delivery. Mortality is high when the base excess exceeds $+15$ mEq/liter. Base excess is treated with ammonium chloride when the pH is greater than 7.58 and the base excess is greater than $+5$ mEq/liter. Total correction is not advisable; one half correction is suggested with frequent serum pH analysis. Urine pH analysis will detect early trends toward excessive urine acidity.

Infection control.   Children are at increased risk for acquiring an infection after cardiovascular surgery. In addition, they often have a predisposition to bacterial endocarditis secondary to valve replacement and to the presence of synthetic patches and intracardiac shunts. The chances of acquiring an infection are increased with the use of bypass, which alters blood protein components and antibodies. After bypass, there is also a decreased number of white blood cells and decreased phagocytic activity. The potential for infection also increases with the use of multiple invasive monitoring lines, catheters, and endotracheal tubes, and with the presence of surgical incisions.

Strict asepsis is imperative during the postoperative period. Thorough hand washing is a basic but critical aspect of maintaining asepsis. Routine dressing changes and Foley catheter care may vary in institutions, but the maintenance of asepsis is invariable. Prophylactic antibiotics are routinely ordered. Gentamicin sulfate (2 mg/kg every 8 hours IV) and oxacillin sodium (25 mg/kg every 6 hours IV) are recommended for 5 to 10 days postoperatively. Erythromycin (6 mg/kg every 6 hours) can be used in penicillin-sensitive children.

Fever (a body temperature of greater than 38.5°C [99.3°F]) must be regarded with suspicion and its cause investigated. Fever may be indicatve of atelectasis, pneumonia, and sepsis, or it may be secondary to the presence of blood or fluid in the pleural or mediastinal spaces. Such a collection of blood is an excellent medium for bacterial growth. Chest tubes must be kept patent to decrease the accumulation of intrathoracic fluid.

Fever can be treated with acetaminophen (10 mg/kg every 4 hours). Blood should be drawn for culture and placed in aerobic and anaerobic culture media. Aspiration of tracheal secretions for Gram staining and culture is necessary to rule out pulmonary infection. A urine culture is necessary to detect urinary tract infection. The tips of invasive monitoring and/or IV lines may also be sent to the laboratory for culture. All indwelling catheters should be discontinued and replaced.

Management of the gastrointestinal system.   Maintenance of the gastrointestinal system involves gastric decompression and observation for complications. A nasogastric tube may be inserted to keep air and fluid from accumulating in the GI tract because paralytic ileus is a common transitory occurrence postoperatively. Gastric distention impairs diaphragmatic movement and interferes with effective ventilation. In addition, vomiting and the potential aspiration of gastric contents are avoided by insertion of a nasogastric tube.

Bowel sounds must be assessed frequently. Abdominal girths may be measured every 8 hours in the presence of abdominal distention. Ascites, which may be detected on abdominal examination, is secondary to the shifting of fluid into the extracellular fluid spaces. Evaluating the pH of gastric drainage for increased acidity is advisable. It is required if the drainage results in a positive Hematest. Antacid therapy may then be required in order to avoid the development of stress ulcers. Gastrointestinal bleeding is sometimes a serious problem in children who have had repair of coarctation. Special care must be taken to avoid this potentially serious complication.

The feeding of children who have had cardiovascular surgery is generally delayed for a minimum of 16 to 24 hours. Oral feedings can be resumed and advanced slowly when the stability of the gastrointestinal tract has been reestablished, as evidenced by clinical examination. No attempt to feed these children early is recommended.

Management of the central nervous system.   Cerebral functioning must be monitored thoroughly and frequently during the postoperative period. Neurological damage may result from an intraoperative embolism, hypoxia, or prolonged hypotension secondary to low CO states. Embolization may cause cerebral bleeding, hemiplegia, or paraplegia. Thus, it is essential to monitor the child's level of consciousness and neuromuscular ability. Neurological damage may manifest itself by either local (focal seizures) or diffuse signs (changes in behavior or orientation). Optimal cardiovascular support is of paramount importance in decreasing the incidence of neurological complications.

"Postoperative psychosis" or "post-pump psychosis" is occasionally observed in the pediatric patient. This so-called psychosis, a severe behavior change, is likely to be a secondary reaction to sensory overload or deprivation or to increased anxiety during the child's postoperative stay in the ICU. (*see* p. 8). Manifestations of the behavior change include the following signs: disorientation, inappropriate behavior for age, agitation, combativeness, insomnia, and hallucinations. Severe postoperative behavior change may be avoided by thoroughly evaluating the child's and parents' preoperative knowledge of the surgery and their mental and emotional response to the impending surgery, as well as by taking steps to ensure that adequate preparation is provided. Excessive preoperative anxiety may make it difficult for the child to adjust to the ICU setting. The child must be assured that parental support will not be denied and that medication will be given for control of pain.

Whenever a child manifests severe behavior change postoperatively, frequent reassurance and reorientation to time and place are required. Stimulation should be minimized whenever possible, and parents should be encouraged to remain with their child. Adequate opportunity to rest and sleep is extremely important. Whatever can be done to "normalize" the ICU environment should be attempted because, despite extensive physical needs, the child's emotional needs must not be forgotten (*see* p. 16).

Discharge from the ICU. The critical care management of the child after cardiovascular surgery is all-inclusive because optimal cardiovascular functioning affects all other organ systems. Once hemodynamic, respiratory, and renal stability is achieved, the child is prepared for discharge from the ICU. Progressive decannulation is planned, along with the removal of chest tubes, Foley catheter, and, eventually, peripheral IV lines. Diet and activity can be advanced simultaneously. The parents and child may need support in the transition from the ICU, with the security of monitors and one-to-one nursing, to nursing care in a ward. Successful critical care management of the child who has had cardiac surgery requires the cooperative and coordinated efforts of many clinicians in the ICU and is evidenced by the return of the child to normal functioning.

REFERENCES

1. Morgan.
2. Garson et al.
3. Guntheroth.
4. Silverman et al.
5. Allen et al.
6. Hastreiter and Van Der Horst.
7. King et al.
8. Perloff. 360.
9. Rudolph and Heymann.
10. Fontan and Baudet.
11. Rowe et al. 304.
12. Edmunds and Ebert. 372.
13. Ravitch et al. 598.
14. Ravitch et al. 602.
15. Padula. 186.

BIBLIOGRAPHY

Allen, H. D., L. W. Lange, D. J. Sahn, and S. J. Goldberg. 1978. Ultrasound cardiac diagnosis. *Pediatric Clinics of North America.* **25**:677–706.

Anderson, R. W. 1976. Shock and circulatory collapse. *In* D. C. Sabiston and F. C.

Spencer, editors. 1976. Gibbon's Surgery of the Chest. W. B. Saunders Co., Philadelphia. third edition.

Anthony, C., R. Arnon, C. Fitch. 1979. Pediatric Cardiology. Medical Outline Series, Medical Examination Publishing Co., Inc., Garden City, New York.

Behrendt, D. M., and W. H. Austen. 1980. Patient Care in Cardiac Surgery. Little, Brown Co., Boston. Third edition.

Buda, A. J., M. Pinsky, N. B. Ingels. G. T. Daughters, E. B. Stinson, and E. L. Alderman. 1979. Effect of intrathoracic pressure on left ventricular performance. *The New England Journal of Medicine*. **301**:453–459.

Carew, J., P. Reynolds. Nursing Care of the Post-Operative Cardiac Patient. Paper presented at the Pediatric Intensive Care Conference, Childrens' Memorial Hospital, Dallas, May, 1978.

Clowes, G. H. 1969. Bypass of the heart and lungs with an extracorporeal circulation. *In* J. H. Gibbon, F. C. Spencer, and D. C. Sabiston, editors. *Gibbon's Surgery of the Chest*. W. B. Saunders Co., Philadelphia. Second edition.

Edmunds, J. F., G. A. Barker, and A. Conn. 1980. Current concepts in cardiovascular monitoring in children. *Critical Care Medicine*. **8**:548–553.

Edmunds, L. H., and P. A. Ebert. 1977. The heart: congenital diseases. Part II. *In* J. Dunphy and L. Way, editors. Current Surgical Diagnosis and Treatment. Lange Medical Publications, Los Altos, California. Current Surgical Diagnosis and Treatment. Third edition.

Filipek, J. E. 1980. Postoperative care of the pediatric cardiac patient. *(CCQ) Critical Care Quarterly*. **3**:45–53.

Fink, B. W. 1975. Congenital Heart Disease: A Deductive Approach to Its Diagnosis. Year Book Medical Publishers, Inc., Chicago.

Fontan, F. and Baudet, E. 1971. Surgical repair of tricuspid atresia. *Thorax*. **26**:240–248.

Garson, A., R. S. Benson, L. Ivler, and L. Patton. 1978. Parental reactions to children with congenital heart disease. *Child Psychiatry and Human Development*. **9**:86–94.

Glancy, D. L. 1980. Medical management of adults and older children undergoing cardiac operations. *Heart Lung*. **9**:277–283.

Glenn, W., A. Liebow, and G. Lindskog. 1975. Thoracic and Cardiovascular Surgery with Related Pathology. Appleton-Century-Crofts, East Norwalk, Conn. Third edition.

Gorlin, R. 1977. Practical cardiac hemodynamics. *New England Journal of Medicine*. **296**:203–205.

Guntheroth, W. G. 1978. Initial evaluation of the child for heart disease. *Pediatric Clinics of North America*. **25**:657–676.

Hastreiter, A. R. and R. L. Van Der Horst. 1977. Hemodynamics of neonatal cyanotic heart disease. *Critical Care Medicine*. **5**:23–28.

Kawabori, I. 1978. Cyanotic congenital heart defects with decreased pulmonary blood flow. *Pediatric Clinics of North America*. **25**:759–776.

Kawabori, I. 1978. Cyanotic congenital heart defects with increased pulmonary blood flow. *Pediatric Clinics of North America*. **25**:777–796.

King, T. D., S. L. Thompson, and C. Steiner. 1976. Secundum ASD: nonoperative closure during cardiac catheterization. *(JAMA) Journal of the American Medical Association*. **235**:2506–2509.

King, O. M. 1975. *Care of the Cardiac Surgical Patient*. C. V. Mosby Co., St. Louis.

Lang, P., R. G. Williams, W. I. Norwood, and A. R. Castaneda. 1980. The hemodynamic effects of dopamine in infants after corrective cardiac surgery. *The Journal of Pediatrics*. **96**:630–634.

Midgley, F. M., L. P. Scott, L. W. Perry, S. R. Shapiro, and D. W. McClenathan. 1978. Subclavian flap aortoplasty for treatment of coarctation in early infancy. *Journal of Pediatric Surgery*. **13**:265–268.

Moore, G. C. Post-operative ventilation of the cardiac patient. Paper presented at the Pediatric Intensive Care Conference, Childrens' Memorial Hospital, Dallas, May 1978.

Morgan, B. C. 1978. Incidence, etiology, and classification of congenital heart disease. *Pediatric Clinics of North America*. **25**:721–724.

Morrow, A. G. 1978. Hypertrophic subaortic stenosis. *Journal of Thoracic and Cardiovascular Surgery.* **76**:423–430.

Nelson, R. M. 1977. Extracorporeal circulation. *In* D. C. Sabiston, editor. Davis-Christopher Textbook of Surgery — the Biological Basis of Modern Surgical Practice. W. B. Saunders, Co., Philadelphia. Eleventh edition.

Padula, R. T. 1976. Postoperative management. In D. C. Sabiston and F. C. Spencer, editors. *Gibbon's Surgery of the Chest.* W. B. Saunders Co., Philadelphia. Third edition.

Parenzan, L., G. Locatelli, O. Alfieri, V. Massimo, G. Invernizzi, and A. D. Pacifico. 1978. The Senning operation for transposition of the great arteries. *Journal of Thoracic and Cardiovascular Surgery.* **76**:305–311.

Perloff, J. K. 1978. Clinical Recognition of Congenital Heart Disease. W. B. Saunders Co., Philadelphia. Second edtion.

Ravitch, M. M., K. J. Welch, C. J. Benson, E. Aberdeen, and J. G. Randolph. 1979. Pediatric Surgery. Volume I. Year Book Medical Publishers, Inc., Chicago. Third edition.

Rowe, R. D., R. M. Freedom, A. Mehrizi, and K. R. Bloom. 1981. The Neonate with Congenital Heart Disease. W. B. Saunders Co., Philadelphia.

Rudolph, A. M. and M. A. Heymann. 1977. Medical treatment of the ductus arteriosus. *Hospital Practice.* **12**(2):57–65.

Sacksleder, S., J. H. Gildea, and C. Dassy. 1978. Common congenital cardiac defects. *American Journal of Nursing.* **78**(2):266–272.

Sade, R. M., D. M. Cosgrove, and A. R. Castaneda. 1977. Infant and Child Care in Heart Surgery. Year Book Medical Publishers, Inc., Chicago.

Silverman, N. H., A. B. Lewis, and M. A. Heymann. 1975. Echocardiographic assessment of ductus arteriosus in premature infants. *Circulation* **50**:821–826.

Stevenson, J. G. 1978. Acyanotic lesions with normal pulmonary blood flow. *Pediatric Clinics of North America.* **25**:725–742.

Thorpe, C. J. 1979. A nursing care plan—the adult cardiac surgery patient. *Heart & Lung.* **8**:690–698.

CHAPTER 4

NEUROLOGICAL DISORDERS

Donna H. Groh
Sherry Waples Benica
with Susan B. De Jong

SELECTED ASPECTS OF NEUROANATOMY AND PHYSIOLOGY

The human brain is an extremely complex, highly specialized system that coordinates and integrates the functioning of all other body systems. A basic overview of the organization, structure, and function of the brain will be presented in order to provide a basis for understanding the specific pathological conditions discussed. Aspects of structure and function related to the spinal cord and the peripheral nervous system are beyond the scope of this chapter.

Neural Tissue

There are two types of cells constituting neural tissue in the brain: neurons and neuroglia. These two types of cells are closely correlated and integrated so as to function as a single unit. Neurons are specialized, excitable cells that receive sensory (afferent) input from peripheral nerves or sensory receptor organs, and transmit motor (efferent) output to muscles and glands. Neurons that transmit signals to other neurons are called internuncial or association neurons.

Each neuron has a cell body and one or more processes extending from it. Processes that conduct information toward the cell body are called dendrites. An axon is a single long process that conducts information away from the cell body. Axons and dendrites, collectively, are called nerve fibers (Fig. 4-1).

Neurons conduct two types of neural signals throughout the body. Electrical signals are conducted along the length of a neuron, and chemical signals are transmitted between neurons. The area where neurons come in contact with other neurons or effector organs is called the synapse, which is the only location that an impulse can pass from one neuron to another or to an effector organ.

Neuroglia are the support cells, providing nutrition and protection for the neurons in the central nervous system (CNS). Schwann cells have this function in the peripheral nervous system. The neuroglia outnumber the neurons approximately 10 to 1, and comprise about 40 percent of the volume of the brain and

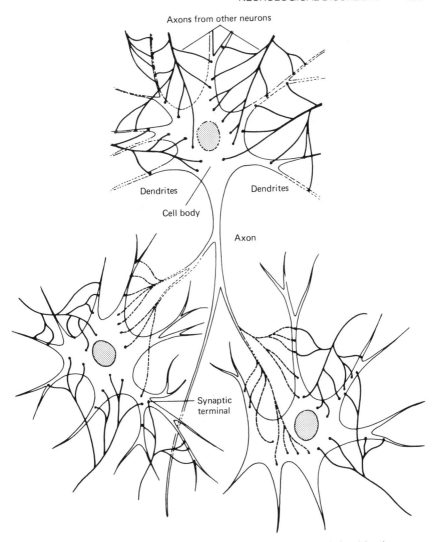

Figure 4-1. Diagrammatic representation of the components and relationship of neurons. (*See* text for discussion.)

spinal cord. There are four distinct types of neuroglial cells, each of which plays a specific role in the function of support and protection of the neurons (Fig. 4-2). Microglia are phagocytic cells that ingest and digest tissue debris. Ependyma are involved in cerebrospinal fluid (CSF) production. Astroglia (astrocytes) provide essential nutrients to neurons and assist in maintaining the right balance of bioelectrical potentials for impulse conduction. Oligodendroglia are responsible for myelin production in the CNS.

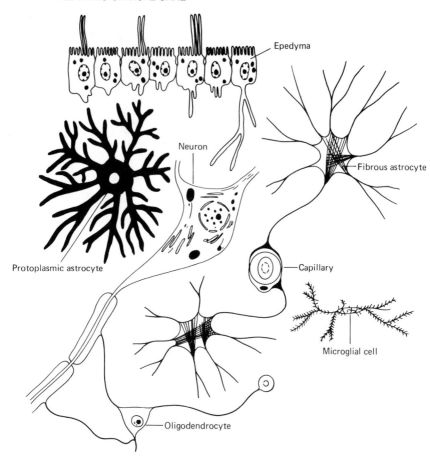

Neuron

Epedyma

Fibrous astrocyte

Protoplasmic astrocyte

Capillary

Microglial cell

Oligodendrocyte

Figure 4-2. Diagrammatic representation of the main types of neuroglial cells. (*See* text for discussion.)

Meninges and Skull

The tissue of the brain is protected by bone (the skull) and by three layers of connective tissue: the dura mater, the arachnoid, and the pia mater (Fig. 4-3). The dura mater has two layers and is tough, inelastic, and leatherlike. The outer endosteal layer forms the inner periosteum of the skull, while the inner meningeal dura is a thick membrane that covers the brain and dips in between brain tissues to provide support and protection. There are four major sheaths of the meningeal dura that extend into the cranial cavity: (1) the falx cerebelli separates the two cerebellar hemispheres, (2) the falx cerebri separates the two cerebral hemispheres along the longitudinal fissure, (3) the tentorium cerebelli separates the cerebrum from the cerebellum, and (4) the diaphragma sellae overlies the pituitary.

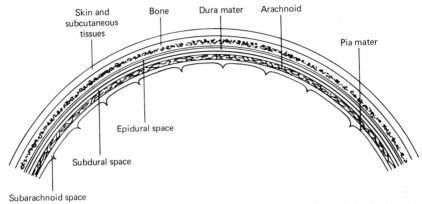

Figure 4-3. Diagrammatic representation of the protective coverings of the brain. (*See* text for discussion.)

The arachnoid is a thin, fibrous, avascular membrane lying over the brain. The subarachnoid space, between the arachnoid and the pia mater, contains cerebral arteries, veins, and the CSF that bathes the CNS. The pia mater is a vascular layer through which blood vessels pass to nourish the neural tissue of internal structures. This layer is directly continuous with the brain and follows every contour of the external structure.

Cranial Sutures

The principal sutures of the skull are the sagittal, coronal, and lambdoidal sutures (Fig. 4-4A). The junction of these sutures forms the anterior and posterior fontanels (Fig. 4-4B).

At birth, cranial sutures are separated by membranous material, and for the first few days after birth, the cranial bones may override one another. Growth of the cranial bones occurs perpendicular to the suture line, and closure of the sutures occurs in a definite and precise order.

There is variation in the ages at which closure of the sutures occurs, but all sutures and fontanels should ossify by the following ages: the posterior fontanel by age 3 months, union of the sutures by age 6 months, and closure of the anterior fontanel by age 20 months. Complete union does not occur until approximately 12 years of age. Thus, after this time, the sutures cannot be separated by increased intracranial pressure (ICP).

The Brain: Structure and Functional Organization

The brain is the most energy-consuming tissue in the body and is sustained primarily by the oxidative metabolism of glucose. The brain receives about 20 percent of the cardiac output, demands 20 percent of the body's oxygen consump-

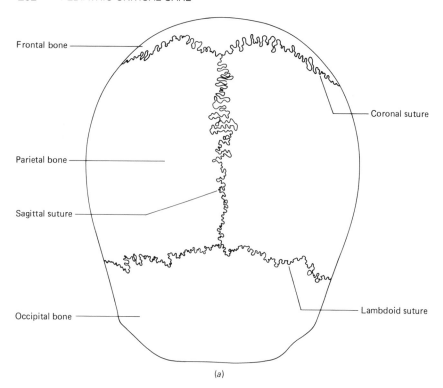

Frontal bone

Coronal suture

Parietal bone

Sagittal suture

Occipital bone

Lambdoid suture

(a)

Figure 4-4. Representation of (A) the principal sutures and (B) the anterior and posterior fontanels of the skull.

tion, and requires approximately 400 kilocalories of energy daily. The brain is unceasing in its activity, functioning to integrate and coordinate the sense organs and effector systems of the body, process incoming information and outgoing impulses, store experiences, and effect behavior. There are five major subdivisions of the brain, each of which serves as a specialized organizational center related to the above functions (Figs. 4-5 and 4-6).

Myelencephalon. The medulla oblongata is located in the myelencephalon, which is the caudal portion of the brainstem and is continuous with the pons and midbrain. The medulla oblongata is the reflex center for cardiac, respiratory, sneezing, coughing, swallowing, salivation, vomiting, and vasoconstrictor reflexes. On the posterior surface are two enlargements that are the dorsal columns' ascending tracts. These tracts are responsible for conscious muscle proprioception and two-point tactile discrimination. They also carry pressure and vibratory sensations. The nuclei of the 9th to the 12th cranial nerves are also contained in the medulla oblongata.

Metencephalon. The pons and cerebellum are located in the metencephalon. The pons is a bridge of fibers connecting the halves of the cerebellum and joining the midbrain above with the medulla oblongata below. The lower portion of the pons

Anterior fontanel

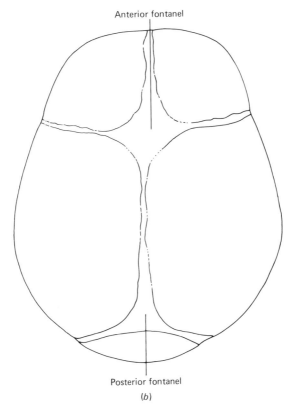

Posterior fontanel

(*b*)

Figure 4-4. (*Continued*)

has a role in respiratory regulation. The nuclei of the 5th to the 7th cranial nerves are also located in the pons.

The cerebellum consists of a middle portion (vermis) and two lateral hemispheres. The activities of the cerebellum are unconscious. The main function is that of a reflex center that controls the coordination and refinement of muscular movements related to posture and equilibrium.

Mesencephalon. This portion of the brain (known as the midbrain) is comprised of the corpus quadrigemina, the tegmentum, and the cerebral peduncles. The midbrain lies above the pons. The superior and inferior colliculi of the corpus quadrigemina mediate visual and auditory reflexes. The substantia nigra and red nucleus (in the tegmentum) are part of the extrapyramidal or involuntary motor pathways. The cerebral peduncles are composed of motor fiber bundles descending from the cerebrum.

Diencephalon. This portion of the brain consists of structures surrounding the third ventricle and forming the inner core of the cerebrum. The thalamus acts as a relay station in the brain for all the main sensory pathways which synapse with

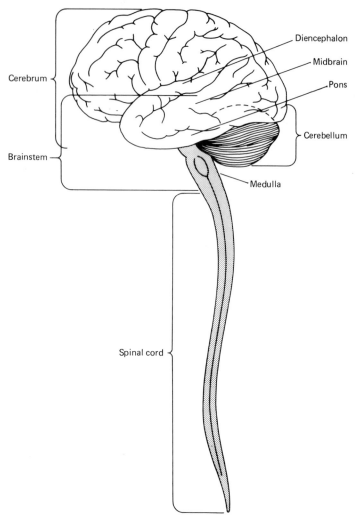

Figure 4-5. Lateral view of the brain and spinal cord (central nervous system), indicating major anatomical structures.

thalamic nuclei on the way to the cerebral cortex. Primitive sensations of pain, pressure, touch, and temperature are centered in the thalamus.

The hypothalamus, lying beneath the thalamus, regulates peripheral autonomic nervous system control of behavior and emotional expression. The hypothalamus also regulates hormonal secretion related to body water and electrolyte composition (via antidiuretic hormone), body temperature, endocrine functions of sexual and reproductive activity, hunger, and thirst.

Telencephalon.   The cerebral cortex, the limbic system, and the basal ganglia are all located in the telencephalon. The two cerebral hemispheres are joined by a

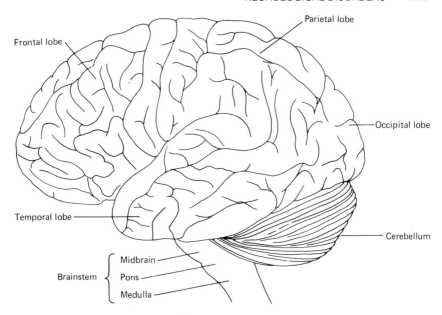

Figure 4-6. Lateral view of the brain, illustrating the lobes and brainstem.

band of fibers called the corpus callosum. The limbic system refers to a ring of structures around the corpus callosum. The primary function of the limbic system is related to experiences and expressions of mood and emotion, most especially fear, rage, and emotions of sexual behavior. This area is also believed to play a role in memory.

The basal ganglia are gray masses of nuclei located deep within the white matter of the cerebrum, and have multiple connections with other portions of the CNS. The basal ganglia are believed to play an important (but poorly understood) role in motor functions related to automatic movements of the body. Damage here can result in tremor, rigidity, and involuntary movements.

The cerebral cortex has a surface of gray matter. It is arranged in numerous convolutions called gyri. This intricate folding makes it possible for a large surface area to be contained within the narrow confines of the cranial cavity. The furrows between the folds are called sulci or (when deep) fissures.

Under the gray matter of the cerebrum lie the cerebral fiber tracts that comprise the white matter. These tracts serve to correlate the action of the two cerebral hemispheres in coordinated functions, such as using both arms to catch a ball.

The functional areas of the cerebral cortex are viewed as either primary or association. The primary areas are those in which a function actually occurs, but the association areas are necessary for integration and for the higher levels of intellect and behavior.

The frontal cortex contains the primary motor area, which is responsible for voluntary movements. The frontal eye field, in this area, is the center for voluntary movements of the eye, as well as conjugate deviation of the eyes and head. The motor function of articulating speech, is also located in the frontal cortex.

Aspects of personality, such as complex intellectual activities, some memory functions, sense of responsibility, creative thought, and judgment, are located in the prefrontal cortex.

Integration of sensory information and high-level processing are controlled by the parietal cortex. Conscious awareness and fine discrimination of general sensations such as pain, temperature, pressure, and proprioception are made possible in this area. Language is a function that is located throughout many areas of the parietal cortex.

The temporal lobe is the primary sensory receptive area for auditory information. This lobe also has a role in certain memory processes and the understanding of spoken language.

The primary visual cortex is located in the occipital lobe, where visual impulses are received and interpreted, and where sense of colors becomes conscious.

Centers for sensory and motor activities are duplicated in each hemisphere and are, for the most part, associated with the opposite side of the body. This concept is termed contralateral control.

Ventricles and CSF

The ventricles are a series of four interconnected cavities within the brain that contain CSF (Fig. 4-7). There is one lateral ventricle in each hemisphere, while the third is in the diencephalon, and the fourth ventricle is in the pons and medulla. The lateral ventricles connect with the third ventricle via the foramen of Monro. The fourth ventricle is then connected to the third via the aqueduct of Sylvius. The foramen of Luschka and the foramen of Magendie are openings extending from the fourth ventricle to the subarachnoid space of the brain and spinal cord.

CSF is formed in three different ways. Most of it is produced by the choroid plexuses in the cerebral ventricles. Smaller amounts are formed by the blood vessels of the meningeal and ependymal linings of the CSF chambers. Even smaller quantities are produced by the blood vessels of the brain and spinal cord.

CSF differs from other extracellular fluid: its sodium concentration is 7 percent greater, its glucose concentration is 30 percent less, and its potassium concentration is 40 percent less.

The major function of CSF is to provide cushioning for the brain, but it also provides nourishment for brain metabolism. CSF fills the cerebral ventricles and subarachnoid space, and it then flows from the choroid plexuses to the archnoid villi. Almost all of the CSF formed each day is reabsorbed into the blood through the arachnoid villi, which are extremely permeable, allowing for free flow of CSF as well as of protein molecules and other particulate matter.

Normal pressure in the CSF system of a person in a horizontal position averages 10 mm Hg, though it can be as low as 5 mm Hg or as high as 15 mm Hg. Regulation of CSF pressure is determined by the rate of CSF formation and by the degree of resistance to absorption through the arachnoid villi. If either of these parameters is increased, CSF pressure will rise; conversely, if either is decreased, the pressure will fall.

Autoregulation of Cerebral Blood Flow

Blood flows to the brain by way of the two carotid arteries and, to a lesser extent, via the two vertebral arteries, which unite to form the basilar artery of the hindbrain. The basilar artery then combines with the two internal carotid arteries,

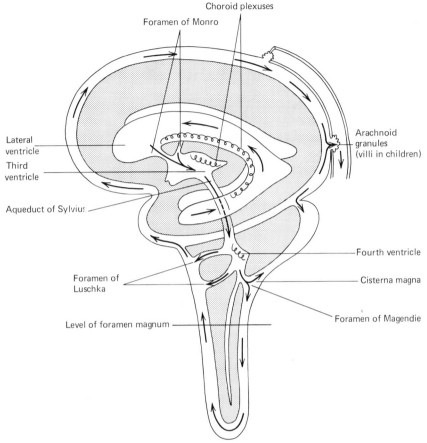

Figure 4-7. Diagrammatic representation of the ventricles and cerebrospinal fluid flow (indicated by arrows).

which also connect with each other by way of the circle of Willis (Fig. 4-8). The rate and volume of blood flow through the brain constantly adjusts itself to meet the metabolic demands of the brain. This is accomplished by a number of control systems.

Chemical regulation. Regulation of cerebral blood flow (CBF) is primarily determined by the carbon dioxide (CO_2) content of cerebral tissue. Increased levels of CO_2 cause vasodilation; decreased levels of CO_2 produce vasoconstriction. Therefore, when CBF is diminished, there is a buildup of CO_2 and other metabolites in the cerebral blood. Vasodilation then occurs, increasing CBF in order to carry off the excess CO_2 from cerebral tissue. The effect of CO_2 on CBF is the most important factor in autoregulation of CBF.

The utilization of oxygen (O_2) by the brain and the rate of metabolism remain in balance, even during sleep and periods of strenuous exercise. If CBF decreases

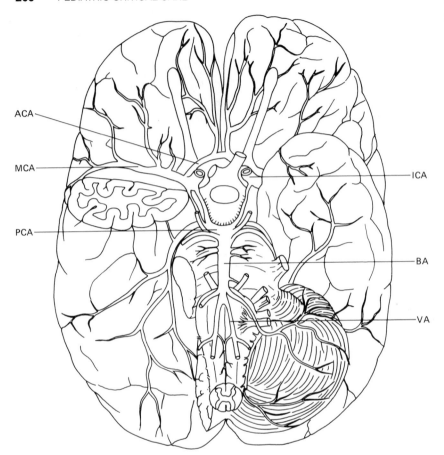

Figure 4-8. Cerebral blood flow. (*See* discussion on p. 206.) ACA, anterior cerebral artery; BA, basilar artery; ICA, internal carotid artery; MCA, middle cerebral artery; PCA, posterior cerebral artery; VA, vertebral artery.

significantly, there will be an insufficient supply of O_2 for metabolism. The O_2-deficiency autoregulatory mechanism, which is present in almost all tissues of the body, will then be activated. An O_2 deficit below a partial pressure of arterial O_2 (PaO_2) of 50 mm Hg will cause immediate vasodilation, thereby increasing CBF and the amount of O_2 available for metabolism.

Metabolic regulation. Metabolic factors are primarily responsible for distribution of blood flow within localized areas of the brain. If the metabolic demands of the brain increase and/or an O_2 deficit exists, metabolites will be released into the circulation, thereby causing vasodilation. The resulting increased CBF meets the increased metabolic needs and, at the same time, removes the metabolites from cerebral circulation, thus restoring homeostasis. The most common metabolite influencing CBF is the hydrogen ion. An excess of hydrogen ions will cause vasodilation, whereas a deficit will cause vasoconstriction. Other metabolites such as ADP (adenosine 5'-diphosphate) or adenine, or changes in potassium and osmolality levels, can also cause changes in local CBF.

Neurogenic regulation. Cerebral blood vessels are innervated by both sympathetic and parasympathetic nerves. Until recently, it was believed that these nerves had no influence on the regulation of CBF. It is now known that neurogenic influences normally have a minor effect. In a state of stress, however, neurogenic regulation can be important. During extreme stress, there is an increase in sympathetic tone, which leads to vasoconstriction of the arteries supplying the brain and, therefore, to a possible reduction in CBF.

Myogenic regulation. Vascular smooth muscle responds rapidly to changes in pressure gradients. Because of this intrinsic ability of the vasculature, compensatory adjustments to changes in cerebral perfusion pressure (CPP) can occur rapidly. Myogenic autoregulation is effective over the range of perfusion pressures from 50 to 150 mm Hg.

Temperature regulation. Changes in temperature, as regulators of CBF, are difficult to evaluate because of the variations in blood pressure, in the partial pressure of arterial CO_2 ($PaCO_2$), and in hemoconcentration that accompany body temperature change. It is, however, generally accepted that CBF and metabolism undergo changes of between 7 and 15 percent for each degree centigrade of temperature change. In going from 37 to 42°C (98.6 to 107.6°F), CBF and metabolism increase, whereas profound hypothermia will greatly reduce CBF and metabolism.

PRINCIPLES OF NURSING CARE

The nurse is the patient's first line of defense against neurological disaster.[1] By close and accurate observation, the nurse will be able to alert the critical care team to the often subtle changes in the patient's status that may require immediate intervention or an alteration in therapy.

The ultimate goal for any child with a neurological disorder is protection against residual neurological dysfunction. This goal is best achieved through application of two related principles of nursing care. The first is maximal preservation of cerebral tissue, which is best accomplished by ensuring that the child maintains optimal oxygenation, cardiac output, and glucose levels. The second principle is the prevention of additional cerebral injury caused by hypoxia, hypercapnia, and/or compromised CPP.

The cerebral autoregulatory mechanisms serve to maintain homeostasis: upon insult, the brain's autoregulation will initially work to accomplish the first principle (i.e., preservation of cerebral tissue). In severe neurological insult, however, the autoregulatory system attempts to promote maximal oxygenation and remove excessive CO_2 and other cellular metabolites. This is accomplished only by generalized vasodilation, but, at this point, the cerebral autoregulatory mechanisms are counterproductive. The vasodilation speeds up metabolism and further increases CBF, thereby intensifying the already existing state of hyperemia.

The objective of critical care management is to interrupt this counterproductive cycle (vasodilation, increased CBF, increased metabolism, and increased hyperemia) in order to prevent additional cerebral injury. Nursing measures that will assist in fulfilling the two principles of nursing care include the following actions: accurate monitoring and recording of respiratory status, including ventilatory settings, arterial blood gases, and breath sounds; monitoring of arterial, central venous, pulmonary artery, jugular venous, and intracranial pressures; and continuous calculation of CPP by subtracting the ICP from the mean arterial pressure (MAP):

$$CPP = MAP - ICP.$$

In addition, the neurological assessment by the nurse is of utmost importance, and the maintenance of fluid and electrolyte balance is crucial. Other measures used to help prevent increases in ICP involve maintaining good body alignment in the patient, providing comfort measures, and ensuring a quiet environment (*see* p. 225).

The nurse's role within the multidisciplinary critical care team is to provide a constant level of maximal surveillance and to maintain continual communication with all other members of the team, while at the same time delivering fundamental nursing care.

NEUROLOGICAL ASSESSMENT

It is crucial for nurses to have a clear understanding of neurological assessment and classification systems for evaluation of pediatric patients. It is primarily the nurse who is in the position to observe subtle changes in the patient's status that may indicate improvement or deterioration, thus requiring alterations in therapy. Most institutions use the Glasgow Coma or Responsiveness Scale[2,3] for neurological assessment.

The Glasgow Coma Scale

The Glasgow Coma Scale (Table 4-1) is divided into three sections: eye opening, best verbal response, and best motor response. Points are assigned for each section and are then totaled. A score of 3 would indicate deepest coma, whereas a patient with a score of 15 would have normal neurological functioning. Each section of the scale will be reviewed, with specific attention to age-appropriate examples.

The first section, which deals with eye opening, is perhaps the easiest to assess in a child. Spontaneous eye opening receives the highest score in this section, followed by eye opening in response to verbal stimulation. The third level of response is eye opening to painful or noxious stimuli, such as pinching the trapezius muscle or applying pressure with the knuckle over the sternal area. (It is not necessary to leave a thumbnail imprint on the earlobe or to do extensive pinpricking of all extremities. Pinpricking can be valuable when trying to ascertain the level of sensation if spinal cord injury is suspected, but, in this case, the aim is a gross assessment of the level of consciousness.) Finally, the lowest level is the absence of eye opening in response to any stimulus.

The second section of the scale attempts to assess a best verbal response. This section is particularly difficult to adapt to young children who have not yet developed meaningful speech and for whom crying is often the only verbal response

TABLE 4-1 The Glasgow Coma Scale

Criteria	Points
I. Eye opening	
Spontaneous	4
To speech	3
To pain	2
None	1
II. Best verbal response	
Oriented	5
Confused	4
Inappropriate	3
Incomprehensible	2
None	1
III. Best motor response	
Obeys command	6
Localizes pain	5
Withdraws from pain	4
Flexes to pain	3
Extends to pain	2
Flaccid	1

Adapted from Jennet, B., and G. Teasdale. 1977. Aspects of coma after severe head injury. *Lancet.* I:878–881.

that can be evaluated. Almost any painful or frightening experience, however, should elicit a cry from children in this age-group.

The infant who does not cry in response to any stimulus, who cries continuously and cannot be comforted, or who produces a high-pitched cry is considered to have given an inappropriate verbal response. It is important to remember that parents can be valuable resources when assessing an infant's cry.

In general, it is almost impossible to differentiate between a confused, an inappropriate, and an incomprehensible response in a small infant. For practical purposes, only oriented, inappropriate, or none are used to evaluate best verbal response.[4] Observing the infant's response to parents, toys, and the environment is an additional means of assessing the infant's orientation.

For children who have developed meaningful speech, a better assessment can be made. An oriented response would be one in which the child can correctly answer the question, "What is your name?" Children of 3 years or older should be able to indicate their age either by verbalization or by the use of fingers. A child of 6 years should be able to verbalize the following: home address, grade in school, name of teacher, and names of siblings.

It is important to consider the type of question to be asked. Inquiries such as "Where were you?" or "What were you doing before you came to the hospital?" may be threatening. The child may have been engaged in a forbidden activity (e.g., riding a bicycle in the street), and may not respond for fear of punishment. In fact, the child may perceive the hospitalization as the punishment. The child may also have no memory of the event or may be confused by the questions and, therefore, be unable to answer.

A child who gives an incorrect answer to the above questions (name, age, home address, etc.) can be considered confused. An inappropriate response is one that has no relationship to the question posed. For example, when asked "How old are you?" the child replies "There are bugs on my bed." A child who merely moans, grunts, or screams is classified as exhibiting an incomprehensible response. The category of "no verbal response," is self-explanatory.

Best motor response constitutes the third section of the Glasgow Coma Scale. Once again, this is difficult to judge in infants, but can be adapted more easily for older children. The infant who exhibits spontaneous movement and normal reflexes would be classified at the highest level; however, if there is movement only in response to pain or noxious stimuli, the behavior should be described as withdrawal, flexion, or extension.

When assessing an older child, the nurse must give commands that are reasonable for the developmental level. Most children between 12 and 18 months of age can follow commands such as "touch your nose," "hold my hand," or "kick your feet," but they may not understand "wiggle your toes."

When judging motor response to pain, the nurse must keep in mind that the difference between localizing to pain and withdrawing from pain is very pronounced. For example, if the child reaches for and grabs the catheter during suctioning, this would be an example of localizing to pain. If, however, there is turning of the head or pulling away in response to suctioning, this would be termed withdrawal from pain. Localizing to pain must involve an active attempt to remove the painful stimulus.

Flexion to pain occurs when the affected extremity is drawn up against the body; extension to pain occurs when the extremity is extended to its full length away from the body. A flaccid response is indicated by the absence of muscle tone. Often, these responses of flexion and extension are classified as either decorticate or decerebrate rigidity; however, this terminology is quite imprecise. There is one type of decorticate rigidity, but there are five types of decerebrate rigidity:[5]

Decorticate rigidity: triple flexion of the upper limbs (which are adducted), clenched fists, lower limbs hyperextended.

Full decerebrate rigidity: clenching of the jaw, extension of all four limbs (the upper more so than the lower), arms adducted and internally rotated, shoulders lifted, feet in plantar flexion.

Unilateral decerebrate rigidity: extensor motor activity of limbs on one side and spontaneous or evoked normal mobility on the opposite side.

Combined decerebrate rigidity: extensor rigidity on one side and decorticate on the other; painful stimuli increase the amount of posturing without modifying the pattern.

Mixed decerebrate rigidity: flexor rigidity of lower limbs and hyperextension of upper limbs; this pattern clearly emerges as a reaction to painful stimuli.

Alternating decerebrate rigidity: characterized by widely variable postural attitude; influenced by metabolic or respiratory disturbances; prolonged stimulus often evokes immediate extensor rigidity followed by flexion.

The application of these definitions in the clinical setting can be very confusing, whereas the documentation of responses as simply decorticate or decerebrate is inaccurate. It is far better to describe the exact motions that the patient exhibits.

It is obvious that there are problems with using the Glasgow Coma Scale to assess small children. However, with modification, the scale can be useful and effective as a neurological assessment tool.

Assessment of Cranial Nerves

In order to comprehensively complete the neurological examination, it is necessary to assess the cranial nerves. Assessment of the cranial nerves should be performed with a logical, systematic approach in order to determine the level to which neurological deterioration has progressed. It is also imperative to have some understanding of cranial nerve function and location. Used in conjunction, these two factors will provide a clear picture of the patient's neurological status and will facilitate anticipation of changes in the patient's condition.

Deterioration of neurological functioning can be indicative of increasing ICP, causing compression of the cranial nerves and leading to the possibility of transtentorial herniation. The tentorium cerebelli is a tentlike membrane that lies over the cerebellum, and the tentorial notch is the area through which the brainstem passes (Figs. 4-9 and 4-10). Transtentorial herniation (herniation of the cerebrum through the tentorial notch) which results in brainstem compression, may occur when ICP reaches a critical point.

Arising directly from the brain are the 12 pairs of cranial nerves, which supply structures in the head, neck, and trunk (Table 4-2 and Fig. 4-11). (The 1st, or

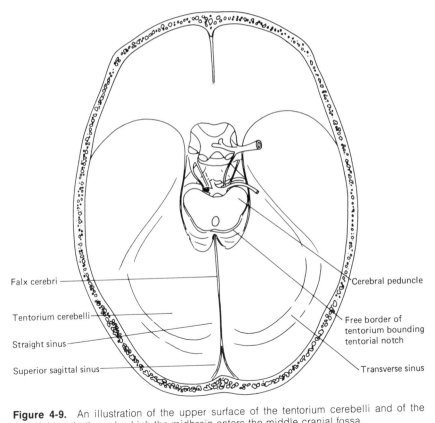

Figure 4-9. An illustration of the upper surface of the tentorium cerebelli and of the tentorial notch, through which the midbrain enters the middle cranial fossa.

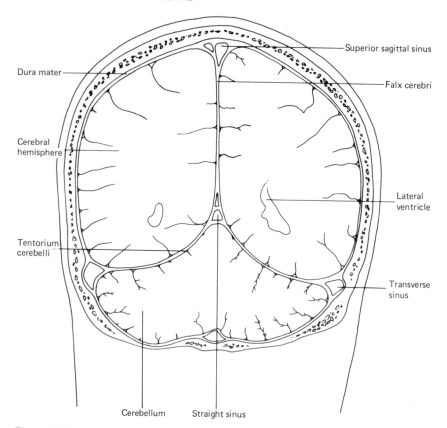

Figure 4-10. A coronal section of the head, illustrating the tentorium cerebelli and its relation to the cerebellum.

olfactory, cranial nerve transmits only sensory impulses associated with the sense of smell, and it is therefore not an essential element in the neurological examination of the critically ill child.)

Optic nerve (2). The optic nerve is responsible for vision and contains only sensory fibers. These fibers, however, transmit impulses from the optic nerve to the 3rd, 4th, and 6th cranial nerves in the midbrain. These three nerves are responsible for pupillary reactions; therefore, damage to the optic nerve will inhibit normal pupillary responses. The functioning of the optic nerve can also be assessed by testing the threat reflex, which is elicited by quickly bringing a hand close to the child's eyes. If the child's eyes close or blink, the optic nerve is intact. The absence of a response indicates damage to either the optic nerve or to the 5th nerve, which innervates the muscle of the eyelid.

Oculomotor nerve (3). The oculomotor nerve carries motor impulses and controls all the extrinsic muscles of the eye (with the exception of the lateral rectus and the superior oblique muscles, which control pupillary dilation and constriction). The

TABLE 4-2   The Cranial Nerves

Nerve	Function	Distribution
Olfactory (1)	Sensory	Olfactory mucosa
Optic (2)	Sensory	Visual neurons in retina of the eye
Oculomotor (3)	Motor	Extrinsic muscles of the eye, with the exception of the lateral rectus and superior oblique muscles
Trochlear (4)	Motor	Superior oblique muscles of the eye
Trigeminal (5)	Sensory and motor	Muscles of mastication and major sensory supply of the face and head
Abducens (6)	Motor	Lateral rectus muscle of the eye
Facial (7)	Sensory and motor	Facial muscles, tongue, and salivary and lacrimal glands
Vestibulocochlear (8)	Sensory	Organs of equilibrium and hearing; internal ear
Glossopharyngeal (9)	Sensory and motor	Tongue and pharynx
Vagus (10)	Sensory and motor	Larynx, pharynx, esophagus, bronchi, lungs, heart, stomach, and small intestines
Accessory (11)	Motor	Trapezius muscle and the neck
Hypoglossal (12)	Motor	Extrinsic and intrinsic muscles of the tongue

neural pathway for the pupillary light reflex is very intricate, involves several brain structures, and is not yet fully understood.[6] Because of this complexity, there can be many variations in pupillary reactions to light.

A change in the equality and reactivity of one or both pupils from one assessment to the next is one of the initial signs of increasing cerebral dysfunction. Compression or stretching of the 3rd nerve results in a dilated pupil ipsilateral to the pressure. Paralysis of the sympathetic fibers, indicating injury to the pons, results in small, nonreactive pupils bilaterally. Damage to the parasympathetic fibers in the midbrain causes dilation of the pupils. Fixed and dilated pupils, therefore, indicate prolonged O_2 deficit, possible midbrain dysfunction, or extensive brain damage.

"Hippus" is the term used to describe the balance between the sympathetic and parasympathetic functions that keeps the pupil in a constant state of motion. (Sympathetic response causes miosis, and parasympathetic response causes mydriasis, the two of them combining to maintain equilibrium.) With the introduction of a bright light, the presence of hippus may be more evident, but, when there is neurological impairment, this normal state is disrupted and hippus is decreased.[7]

Some individuals normally exhibit anisocoria (unequal pupils), or they may have normally dilated pupils. Argyll Robertson pupils, which do not react to light but which do react to accommodation, are also sometimes seen in the healthy individual, but most often in the diabetic. Because these variations are seen in the general population, it is important to obtain information regarding the normal status of the child's pupils.

In order to properly examine the pupils, the room should first be darkened. Size, shape, and equality should be assessed by means of a small ruler graduated in millimeters. Reactivity is determined by observing for constriction as a light is

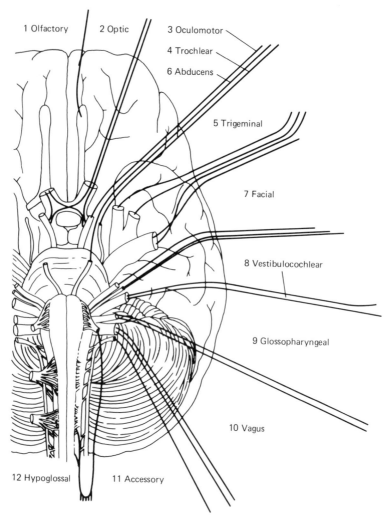

Figure 4-11. Sites of origin of the cranial nerves.

shone into the eye from the side. Shining the light in from the front of the eye will test accommodation rather than reaction to light. It should also be noted whether the response is brisk or sluggish, and if this response is consistent with previous examinations of the child. A once briskly reactive pupil that becomes sluggish can be a sign of impending danger.

Trochlear nerve (4) and abducens nerve (6). These two nerves also carry motor impulses: the trochlear innervates the superior oblique muscle of the eye and controls downward and outward movements; the abducens innervates the lateral rectus muscle and is responsible for horizontal movement of the eye to the ipsilateral lateral position. The integrity of these nerves can be tested in the unconscious patient by use of the doll's-eye maneuver (testing the oculocephalic reflex) and by caloric stimulation (testing the oculovestibular reflex).

The doll's-eye maneuver is performed by holding the child's eyelids open and briskly rotating the head from side to side. A positive response is called controversive conjugate eye deviation, which means that if the head is rotated to the left, the eyes deviate to the right, as would the eyes of a doll. The neck is then briskly flexed and extended. A positive response consists in deviation of the eyes upward when the neck is flexed and downward when the neck is extended. Pupils that remain fixed in the midline and do not deviate when the head is moved indicate an abnormal finding and midbrain involvement.

Caloric stimulation (testing of the oculovestibular reflex) is usually performed by the physician. A small catheter is placed in the external ear canal near the tympanic membrane, and iced water is slowly introduced until either nystagmus or ocular deviation occurs. In the unconscious patient with intact brainstem functioning, the eyes deviate toward the irrigated ear and remain there for as long as 2 to 3 minutes before returning to their original position. Vertical eye movement can be tested by instilling water into both auditory canals simultaneously. The use of iced water should produce downward eye movement, whereas the introduction of warm water should elicit an upward gaze.

Trigeminal nerve (5). The 5th cranial nerve is the largest of the cranial nerves. It has both motor and sensory fibers, and it controls mastication and the corneal reflex, which may be elicited by stroking the cornea lightly with a wisp of sterile cotton. The normal response is immediate closure of the eyelid. The absence of this reflex indicates dysfunction in the reflex pathway.

Facial nerve (7). The facial nerve also carries both motor and sensory fibers and can be easily tested in the clinical setting. In response to supraorbital pressure, an ipsilateral facial grimace should be elicited. The absence of this response indicates facial nerve dysfunction or deep coma.

Vestibulocochlear nerve (8). The 8th cranial nerve carries only sensory fibers and is generally not part of the nurse's clinical evaluation, but is always a part of a comprehensive neurological evaluation in a less acute setting. Functioning of this nerve can be tested, however, by a procedure involving auditory stimulation and electroencephalographic recording. There is some evidence that this test, called brainstem auditory-evoked response, can be a valuable tool in predicting outcome.[8]

Glossopharyngeal nerve (9). The 9th cranial nerve is composed of both motor and sensory tracts and controls the gag reflex, which is easily elicited by the use of a tongue blade or during suctioning. Loss of the gag reflex indicates pressure or damage at the level of the 9th cranial nerve.

Vagus nerve (10). It is at the level of the 10th nerve in the medulla that rising ICP will begin to impinge on the center of vital-sign control. Although it is certainly important to carefully observe and note any changes in vital signs, one must remember that these changes are indeed very late signs and are poorly correlated with increases in ICP. The "classic signs" of increased ICP (hypertension, widened pulse pressure, and bradycardia) can no longer be considered the heralding signs of neurological disaster.

Accessory nerve (11) and hypoglossal nerve (12). Both of these nerves are composed of motor fibers. The accessory nerve is responsible for shoulder movements, turning movements of the head, voice production, and movement of the viscera. The hypoglossal nerve controls tongue movements. These nerves are not key elements in the neurological examination of the critically ill child: because these nerves arise from the base of the brainstem, it is superfluous to test their functioning for indications of increasing ICP.

DIAGNOSTIC STUDIES FOR NEUROLOGICAL ASSESSMENT

Lumbar Puncture

Lumbar puncture (LP) is one of the most basic diagnostic tools for assessment of CNS disorders. It provides a means of measuring CSF pressure and of obtaining CSF for chemical analysis.

LPs are routinely performed on patients with suspected meningitis, on children with brain tumors, and on those with suspected Reye's syndrome (stages I or II) in order to provide a means of differential diagnosis. (LPs are rarely used in cases of head trauma, arteriovenous malformations, status epilepticus, or Reye's syndrome [stages III, IV, or V.])

It is important to remember that when increased ICP is suspected, an LP may carry the risk of precipitating transtentorial herniation, which can occur as the result of a sudden decompression effect when the CSF is drained.

Computerized Axial Tomography

Computerized axial tomography (CAT) is a sophisticated scanning technique that is used for the diagnosis of many neurological disorders. This technique provides visualization of the brain through a series of segmental pictures. Alterations in CBF, mass lesions, hemispheric shifting, size of the ventricles, and density of the brain tissue can all be determined by CAT scanning. Visualization can be further enhanced by radioisotope injection. Often, sequential CAT scans may be performed several days apart in order to document improvement or deterioration. Because CAT is a sophisticated diagnostic tool, it may not be available in all treatment centers. It may therefore be necessary to transfer the child to a facility that can provide this service.

Arteriogram

Cerebral angiography is a well-established and still valuable x-ray technique that utilizes radiopaque contrast material. It provides visualization of CBF and can demonstrate mass lesions, aneurysms, arteriovenous malformations, or lack of CBF. Arteriograms are most frequently used when the CAT scan provides insufficient data for definitive diagnosis or for documentation of cerebral death.

Electroencephalogram

The electroencephalogram (EEG) records the electrical activity of the brain, including many different electrical rhythms and discharges. These various patterns can be distinguished from one another based on location, frequency, amplitude, form, and functional properties. Interpretation involves identifying patterns by means of a combination of the above criteria.

In the clinical setting, the EEG can be used as an initial diagnostic tool and for the diagnosis of seizure type and response to therapy. It is also useful in predicting outcome after a neurological insult, in determining the effectiveness of barbiturate coma, and in documenting cerebral death.

HEAD TRAUMA

Head injury in children is a major health problem in the United States. Nearly 5,000,000 children per year sustain a head injury, most of them associated with automobile accidents.[9] Mortality rates vary markedly, depending on the treatment center, the severity of injuries seen, and the length of time elapsed between injury and the initiation of treatment. Rates as high as 70 percent and as low as 7 percent have been reported.

Clinical Presentation

There are two different types of injuries that may be sustained: acceleration/deceleration injuries and skull distortion/head rotation injuries. Acceleration/deceleration injuries occur when the head strikes, or is struck by, an object. These traumas generally result in contusions and lacerations; epidural, subdural, or intracerebral bleeds; or skull fractures. These manifestations of injury are classified as coup or contrecoup. Coup injuries affect cerebral tissue directly beneath the site of impact. Contrecoup injuries affect the side of the brain that is diametrically opposite to the site of impact.

The brain is suspended within the cranial vault and can glide freely within it. Skull distortion/head rotation injuries occur when the impact is such that the brain is wrenched within the vault, with resultant laceration and tearing of blood vessels. These injuries are exacerbated if accompanied by a skull fracture.

There is often no evidence of tissue damage initially. If there is, it will manifest itself as contusions, lacerations, or bleeds, with diagnostic studies indicating a severely swollen brain with obliteration of CSF spaces and congestion of blood vessels. These injuries produce immediate deep coma. Contusions, lacerations, and bleeds are not commonly seen in children. It is more likely that they will exhibit the pediatric concussion syndrome.[4] The child loses consciousness initially, then reawakens and remains lucid for several minutes or for as long as a few hours. The child then begins vomiting and becomes increasingly drowsy. Loss of consciousness ensues, the pupils dilate 1 to 2 millimeters, and abnormal posturing may be present. This state may resolve itself quickly, persist with eventual resolution, or lead to progressive coma.

Pathophysiology

Lesions sustained during head injury are classified in two ways: first, as either primary or secondary injuries and, second, as either brainstem or space-occupying lesions. Primary injuries are the direct and immediate result of the biomechanical forces applied to the brain. There is usually no visual evidence of primary injuries either on CAT scan or autopsy. Secondary injuries are those superimposed on the primary damage. Causes of secondary injuries may be hypoxia, hypercapnia, systemic hypotension, and/or increased ICP.

Lower brainstem injuries almost always lead to death because the brainstem

TABLE 4-3   Effects of Trauma on Cerebral Blood Flow

Body system	Effects ·
Autonomic nervous	Cellular injury causes a release of histamine, which dilates cerebral blood vessels, thereby increasing cerebral blood flow.
Chemical	Cellular injury results in an increased production of lactic acid and leads to metabolic acidosis, which requires increased cerebral blood flow. Hypoxia and hypercapnia of cerebral tissue also elicit increased cerebral blood flow by the production of lactic acid and excess hydrogen ions and by the resultant metabolic and respiratory acidosis.
Thermal and metabolic	Injury to the hypothalamus may damage the temperature-regulating system, which results in hyperthermia and increased blood flow requirements. Increased metabolic activity as a result of injury requires increased cerebral blood flow.

controls vital functions. All other lesions (hyperemia, contusions, lacerations, hemorrhage, and/or hematomas) are considered space-occupying—a term based on the Monro-Kellie hypothesis, which states that the sum of all volume compartments within the intracranial vault is constant. Brain and neuroglial tissue occupy 70 percent of the space; CSF, blood, and interstitial water occupy 10 percent each. The various volumes adjust accordingly to maintain the equilibrium.

When there is an increase in cerebral mass, CSF moves into the dural sac, thereby maintaining a balance, and ICP remains constant. Eventually this compensatory mechanism is exhausted, the ventricles collapse, and ICP rises. Because of the increased ICP, cerebral vessels dilate to maintain CBF despite the resulting decrease in CPP. Finally, the MAP becomes equal to the ICP: CBF ceases and neural death results.

In addition to the increase in CBF that results from increased ICP, the cerebral trauma itself directly influences CBF (Table 4-3). Cellular injury stimulates the release of histamine, which causes vasodilation. Thus, the cerebral vessels dilate, and CBF and ICP are increased. Also related to cellular injury is the increased production of lactic acid. Greater than normal quantities of lactic acid result in metabolic acidosis. By way of compensation, the cerebral vessels dilate in order to increase CBF so that excess hydrogen ions can be carried away, thus normalizing pH. Once again, the increased CBF results in increased ICP. Along these same lines, hypoxia and/or hypercapnia will cause an excess of lactic acid and/or hydrogen ions, resulting in metabolic acidosis. The same compensatory mechanism is activated in an attempt to normalize pH.

Injury near or around the hypothalamus may interfere with temperature regulation. Hyperthermia increases metabolic activity, which necessitates increased blood flow. Once again, the increased CBF results in elevated ICP. Seizures will also increase the metabolic demands of the body, thereby increasing CBF and, in turn, ICP.

Diffuse cerebral swelling (Fig. 4-12) will be evident on the CAT scan of a child with a severe head injury. This swelling is the direct result of the increased CBF, but secondary tissue edema also occurs. Diffuse cerebral swelling begins with

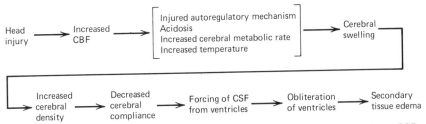

Figure 4-12. Mechanism of diffuse cerebral swelling. CBF, cerebral blood flow; CSF, cerebrospinal fluid.

cerebral congestion as a result of the increased CBF. Cerebral compliance is decreased, resulting in obliteration of the ventricles. The CSF is forced from these compartments into the brain tissue, causing secondary tissue edema.

Diagnosis

Determination of the severity of the head trauma and, therefore, of the treatment indicated is based on neurological and CAT scan findings (Fig. 4-13). A child with a Glasgow Coma Scale score of 5 or lower, or whose CAT scan shows diffuse cerebral swelling, requires immediate intervention. The hyperemic state of the brain will be seen as increased density on the initial CAT scan. A follow-up CAT scan 7 to 20 days after the injury will show a decreasing density toward a normal state. If an intracranial mass or lesion is evident on CAT scan, surgery is indicated.

Critical Care Management

Because of the limited understanding of initial injury and its traumatic effect on neural tissue, there is as yet no means of treating the mechanical effects produced by the primary injury. All therapy is centered around the secondary lesion and the ischemic damage that results from it. These secondary lesions can result from any or all of the following causes: hypoxia, hypercapnia, systemic hypotension, and/or increased ICP.

Increases in ICP are not generally seen in the first 24 hours after a head injury because the primary injury does not manifest itself early and secondary lesions have not yet developed. Elevations in ICP, if they are to occur, do so 24 hours to 5 days after the injury. The first 24 hours of care are thus devoted to stabilizing all body systems. Current modes of therapy are discussed in the section on increased ICP (*see* p. 225).

REYE'S SYNDROME

Reye's syndrome (RS) is a noncommunicable illness that strikes healthy children between the ages of 2 months and 19 years. It is no longer considered rare, but rather a poorly understood disease that is devastating and often fatal.

RS was first identified in 1963 by R. D. Reye, an Australian pathologist. He described 21 children who exhibited the same clinical symptoms and pathological

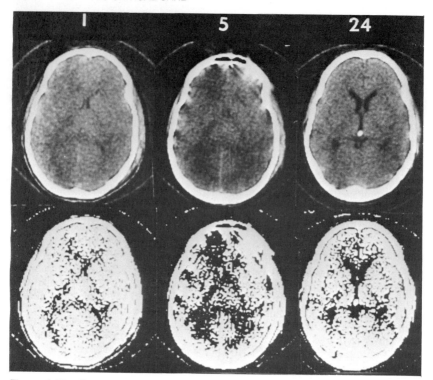

Figure 4-13. Computerized axial tomography (CAT) scan findings in a 16-year-old patient with a head injury. Day 1 (top): diffuse cerebral swelling with compression of the ventricles in the unconscious patient; Day 1 (bottom): changed density setting, revealing high density in white matter. Day 5 (top): diffuse cerebral edema with compressed ventricles as in Day 1, but decreased density in white matter; Day 5 (bottom): changed density setting, revealing decreased density in white matter that is consistent with edema. Day 24 (top): recovery scan, showing normal ventricles; Day 24 (bottom): changed density setting, showing normal density of white matter.

findings. The most prominent features were altered consciousness leading to convulsions, alteration in muscle tone and reflexes, vomiting, and fever. Of those 21 children, 17 died, their autopsies demonstrating cerebral edema, fatty infiltration and enlargement of the liver, and fatty changes in the kidneys, myocardium, and pancreas.

The etiology of this syndrome is still unclear. RS is now the second highest cause of death in children (after encephalitis) among the virus-related CNS diseases. It is ranked by the national Center for Disease Control (CDC) in Atlanta as one of the top 10 causes of death among all children's diseases.

The incidence of RS seems to be increasing, but this may be a result of better identification and reporting. Because RS mimics other disease states such as encephalitis, drug ingestion, and diabetic coma, it may have been diagnosed as such in the past.

RS most often strikes preschoolers and early school-age children. It affects males and females equally, and whites more often than blacks, although recent

NEUROLOGICAL DISORDERS**223**

data from the CDC show that black children under 1 year of age have a higher incidence of RS than whites in that age group.

RS almost always follows a viral illness such as influenza, varicella, the common cold, or a gastrointestinal virus. It occurs during all months of the year, but most frequently from November to March, when influenza is most prevalent.

Although RS has been linked to viral illnesses (most specifically varicella and influenza B), the ingestion of substances such as hypoglycin A, aflatoxin, antiemetics, and salicylates, and exposure to pesticides or chemical fertilizers have also been implicated.[10]

After conducting a collaborative study, the CDC has issued a warning. Their study suggests a relationship between the use of aspirin and/or antiemetics and the onset of RS. The study indicates that children who were administered aspirin or antiemetics for treatment of a viral illness were more likely to develop RS than those who received an aspirin substitute or no treatment at all.

Pathophysiology

There are several pathophysiological alterations with RS, including hyperammonemia, fatty infiltration of the liver, fatty changes in the kidneys and myocardium, and diffuse cerebral edema.

Early hyperammonemia occurs in most cases, and the degree of elevation seems to correlate well with the clinical presentation and prognosis. The increased ammonia level is believed to be the result of an error or deficiency in the urea cycle. An acquired and transient dysfunction of hepatic mitochondrial urea-cycle enzymes has been implicated, although the exact mechanism for this dysfunction has not been defined.[10] It has also been suggested that inherited or acquired urea-cycle abnormalities could remain undetected until stressed by a viral infection or a toxin.[10] The relative state of starvation, dehydration, and fever accompanying a viral infection or toxin reaction leads to increased protein catabolism with a resultant increased ammonia level.

The fatty infiltration and degeneration of the viscera, most notably the liver, are characterized by a panlobular, diffuse distribution of fatty droplets. Although the mechanisms responsible for these changes have not been identified, the mobilization of lipid from adipose tissue stores, reflected by increased serum levels of free fatty acids, may be involved.[11] Hepatocyte necrosis, inflammation, and bile duct changes are not usually seen.

It has been generally assumed that the encephalopathy of RS is a result of liver failure, with no specific direct injury to cerebral cells. The changes in brain tissue cells seen on microscopic examination are swollen or shrunken neurons, swollen astrocytes, and swollen oligodendrocytes. Myelin appears well preserved, and inflammation is not evident. Neuronal changes seen on occasion suggest a hypoxic or ischemic etiology.[12]

The mortality rate in the the initial group that Reye described was 81 percent. Today, nationwide, 30 to 50 percent of the children who contract RS will die, even with aggressive supportive therapy. Cases that are diagnosed early result in the highest survival rate. Most survivors recover completely; 10 to 25 percent suffer minor to severe disability due to brain damage.

Clinical Presentation

RS typically develops in a previously healthy child after a viral illness. (In rare instances, RS has occurred abruptly, without a preceding viral illness.) There is

TABLE 4-4   Clinical Staging of Reye's Syndrome

Stage*	Signs
I	Vomiting, lethargy, sleepiness, laboratory evidence of hepatic dysfunction, type 1 EEG
II	Disorientation, delirium, combativeness, hyperventilation, hyperactive reflexes, appropriate response to painful stimuli, evidence of hepatic dysfunction, type 2 EEG
III	Obtundation, coma, hyperventilation, decorticate rigidity, preserved light reflexes and oculovestibular reflexes, liver dysfunction, type 2 EEG
IV	Deepening coma, decerebrate rigidity, loss of oculocephalic reflexes (often asymetrical), large and fixed pupils, disconjugate eye movements in response to caloric stimulation, minimal liver dysfunction, type 3 or 4 EEG with evidence of brainstem dysfunction
V	Seizures, loss of deep tendon reflexes, respiratory arrest, flaccidity, type 4 EEG, liver-function tests often normal

Adapted from Lovejoy, F. H., A. L. Smith, M. J. Bresnan, J. N. Wood, D. d. Victor, and P. C. Adams, 1974. Clinical staging in Reye Syndrome. *American Journal of Diseases of Children.* **128**(7):36–41.

EEG, electroencephalogram.

*Progression of stages can occur rapidly, and duration of one stage before progression to the next is unpredictable. In general, rapid progression through the first three stages is an ominous prognostic sign.

generally a brief period of recovery from the preceding illness that may last from a few hours to several days. During this time the child is no longer exhibiting active symptoms of the viral illness, but has not yet returned to a complete state of health.

It is at this point that the child will exhibit prolonged and violent vomiting and varying degrees of personality change and unusual behavior. The child may complain of headache, and may be irritable, restless, or sleepy. Within 24 to 48 hours, varying degrees of coma become apparent, ranging from extreme sleepiness to disorientation, screaming, and hostility. This leads to complete coma and, possibly, seizures. The course of this disease is rapid: only 3 to 5 days usually elapse from the onset of vomiting to coma and (if it is to occur) death.

Children younger than 2 years of age are somewhat more difficult to assess because they can rarely describe how they feel. Vomiting is usually the first sign, and the child may be listless, with a normal or subnormal temperature.

Infants younger than 12 months of age may not exhibit the typical pattern of vomiting, but may have diarrhea instead. The infant may only exhibit crankiness, which may be difficult to interpret as a serious sign. But crankiness at a time when the infant seems to be recovering from the virus should serve as a warning sign of RS. Infants can progress from crankiness to coma very quickly, sometimes in a matter of minutes.

As a standard point of reference, a description of the clinical staging of RS has been developed.[13] It is currently used by many centers that routinely care for children with RS (Table 4-4).

Diagnosis

Because the etiology of RS is unclear and the causative agent unknown, diagnosis is made on the basis of the patient's history and laboratory studies. The diagnosis

TABLE 4-5 Laboratory Data in Reye's Syndrome

Test	Normal values	Values with RS
Serum glutamic ox-aloacetic transaminase	5–40 U/ml	Elevated to twice the normal values
Serum glutamic pyruvic transaminase	5–35 U/ml	Elevated to twice the normal values
Bilirubin	0.2–0.9 mg/dl	Normal
Serum ammonia	30–70 µg/dl	Elevated to twice the normal values
Serum glucose	70–110 mg/dl	Normal or low
Prothrombin time	11–16 seconds	Prolonged
Partial thromboplastin time	Control specimen used	Prolonged

RS, Reye's syndrome.

of RS should be considered for any child presenting with an altered level of consciousness and/or coma of unknown etiology. Every effort should be made to obtain a complete and accurate history from the parents.

Laboratory data are summarized in Table 4-5. Often, an LP and a toxicology screening are performed to rule out other illnesses. A liver biopsy may be performed to confirm the diagnosis. Although some investigators have suggested that this syndrome can be diagnosed by history and laboratory data alone, the value of the liver biopsy in distinguishing RS from other disease states has been demonstrated.[14–16] A cutaneous needle biopsy reveals the typical pattern of fatty droplets uniformly distributed throughout the hepatic cells.

A CAT scan is usually performed to document the extent of diffuse cerebral edema, which is a determining factor in planning the course of management.

Critical Care Management

Because the etiology of RS is still unknown, treatment is primarily supportive. In the past, various treatments have been attempted: exchange transfusions, peritoneal dialysis, "total body washout," and decompression craniectomy. With the exception of decompression craniectomy, these therapies have proved to be of little value. Craniectomy itself is considered to be little more than a last attempt to relieve increased ICP that is refractory to all current therapies.[10]

Most centers that routinely treat RS use a combination of controlled hyperventilation, osmotic diuretics, barbiturate coma, and hypothermia. Each of these modalities will be discussed in detail in the next section.

CRITICAL CARE MANAGEMENT OF THE CHILD WITH INCREASED ICP

Any child with a severe neurological problem runs the risk of developing the serious consequences of increased ICP. Children who have sustained a head injury or who have RS are at greatest risk. Critical care management of increased ICP is complex and generally proceeds in an ordered sequence, depending on the child's clinical presentation and course.

Initial Therapy

Initial therapy is primarily supportive for children with the potential for increased ICP. It is also the first line of action for those already exhibiting signs of deteriorating neurological functioning.

Fluid management. Because of their impaired neurological state, these children are given nothing by mouth (NPO). Intravenous (IV) fluids are initiated, but generally restricted to two-thirds of the child's maintenance level. Fluid restriction at this time is prophylactic: by decreasing the overall circulating blood volume, cerebral blood volume is also decreased, thus minimizing the amount of fluid available for diffuse cerebral swelling.

Steroid therapy. In addition to fluid restriction, the use of steroids is advocated in the early management of increased ICP. Dexamethasone is usually the drug of choice because of its minimal salt-retaining property as compared with other steroids. This is an important quality because salt retention can result in fluid retention, which has an adverse effect in those patients with the potential for, or who already have, increased ICP.

Direct measurement of ICP in patients with severe head injury has demonstrated that the desired effect of dexamethasone is dose dependent. Normal doses of 1 mg/kg/day result in no significant effect. Only higher than normal doses (1.5 mg/kg/day) have been shown to reduce posttraumatic brain edema.[4,17] Steroids are administered in four divided doses over 24 hours for 5 days, then gradually tapered during the next several days. Despite the lack of conclusive data regarding the effects of steroids on patients with RS, steroids are nevertheless frequently used as part of the initial therapy.

There are two dangers associated with the use of steroids that are of special concern in the care of the critically ill child. First, these drugs increase the risk of infection by inhibiting the immune system. (It is imperative that strict hand washing and aseptic techniques be enforced in the critical care setting.)

Second, steroids result in gastrointestinal hyperacidity and therefore predispose the patient to gastrointestinal bleeding. The child should have a nasogastric tube inserted in order to permit aspiration of stomach contents and routine measurement of gastric pH. If the pH falls below 5, an antacid should be administered, preferably one with a low sodium content. Often, an antihistamine specific to the gastric parietal cells is ordered. Cimetidine hydrochloride is the drug of choice, administered in a dose of 20 to 40 mg/kg/day in four divided doses. This medication generally lessens the amount of antacid required, thus reducing the fluid volume administered to the patient.

Initial therapy is primarily prophylactic. At the first sign of deteriorating neurological status or increasing ICP, advanced therapy is indicated.

Advanced Therapy

When advanced therapy is necessary, the child's condition is such that many treatment modalities are required simultaneously.

Controlled hyperventilation. Ventilation is controlled to maintain the $PaCO_2$ in the range of 20 to 25 mmHg and the PaO_2 in the range of 100 to 130 mmHg. The child is ventilated with a large tidal volume and a rapid respiratory rate for age. Promoting respiratory alkalosis partially or completely compensates for the acidosis of insulted brain tissue. In addition, hypocapnia results in constriction of cerebral blood vessels and, thus, in a limitation of CBF.

Tracheal intubation is necessary in order to provide controlled ventilation. Muscle paralysis is generally required to facilitate a state of controlled ventilation. Paralyzing agents permit ventilation of the child without pulmonary competition, and they prevent straining on the endotracheal tube or coughing, which may precipitate increases in ICP. Tubocurarine chloride was at one time the paralyzing agent used. It is now known that this drug causes the release of histamine. In addition, it has a vasodilating effect. Although there have been no studies on the effects of tubocurarine on ICP, it is obvious that the side effects of this drug have at least the potential for increasing ICP. Pancuronium bromide is now the most frequently used neuromuscular blockade agent. It can be administered by either intermittent bolus at 0.2 mg/kg or by way of continuous infusion at a dose of 0.1 mg/kg/hr.

Once mechanical ventilation has been established, small doses of morphine sulfate (0.1 to 0.2 mg/kg), diazepam (0.04 to 0.20 mg/kg), or sodium pentothal (3 to 5 mg/kg) are administered to provide sedation, especially before any procedures that may precipitate increases in ICP. (Pancuronium, a paralyzing agent, does not in any way sedate the child.) Almost any procedure or treatment can cause pain and/or anxiety for the child. Although the child does not physically respond, the body reacts by increasing metabolism, which results in increased blood flow (including CBF) and, thus, in increased ICP.

It is the nurse's responsibility to maintain a patent airway in the patient. Breath sounds should be assessed frequently, and routine suctioning of the endotracheal tube should be performed with extreme care. Suctioning must be performed quickly (with manual hyperinflation on 100 percent O_2 both before and after suctioning) in order to avoid dangerous increases in ICP. Frequent repositioning will help diminish the risk of pulmonary complications such as atelectasis or pneumonia.

If chest physiotherapy is indicated, the nurse must monitor the ICP at all times during treatment, as well as during suctioning and repositioning. These activities often cause increases in ICP. If elevations in ICP occur, the treatment should be stopped, manual hyperventilation started, and the physician notified.

The nurse must also take into consideration the use of paralyzing agents and their effects on the respiratory system. If the cough and gag reflexes are inhibited, the child will be unable to protect the airway from aspiration. Therefore, it is extremely important to assess breath sounds, maintain a patent airway, and insert a nasogastric tube (to keep the stomach free of gastric contents and to minimize the chances of vomiting).

Because of the effects of pancuronium, the child is no longer able to blink. Meticulous eye care is imperative in order to prevent corneal abrasions. The child's total lack of mobility necessitates good skin care and repositioning to prevent decubiti, a cushioned ring under the head to prevent alopecia, and passive range-of-motion exercises to prevent joint contractures.

It is necessary to insert an arterial line in order to accurately monitor the child in a state of controlled hyperventilation. An arterial cannula greatly facilitates collection of blood samples for arterial blood gas and chemistry analysis. Arterial blood gases should be monitored on a routine basis to ensure that the patient is being maintained in a state of hyperventilation as well as to ensure adequate O_2 perfusion.

Direct, continuous measurement of systemic blood pressure is another advantage to the use of an arterial line and is essential to the management of these patients. In addition, MAP must be known in order to calculate CPP.

ICP monitoring.   Direct monitoring of ICP is essential for guiding therapy and should be instituted as soon as the child's airway is intubated and ventilation is controlled. The ability to monitor ICP directly is the most significant element in the management of patients with increased ICP. Mild to moderate elevations of ICP can be detected before the appearance of clinical symptoms, and, in addition, patients are not subjected to unnecessary therapy.

Monitoring ICP involves the use of a sensor, a transducer, and a recording device. An intracranial sensor device is inserted, and changes in ICP are transmitted to a transducer, where the mechanical impulses are converted to electrical impulses. These electrical impulses are transmitted to the recorder (monitor) and converted into visible oscillations and digital display.

The sensor can be placed in the subarachnoid space or the lateral ventricle. A ventricular catheter can also be used to facilitate drainage of CSF in order to reduce ICP. The following are potential problems with the use of this system: possible ventricular infection; bleeding or increased edema; difficult insertion because of cerebral edema (with resultant compression of the ventricles, which makes them very small and difficult to distinguish); obstruction of the catheter with brain tissue because of cerebral edema; possible CSF leakage, resulting in false ICP readings; and increased risk of contamination and infection.

A subarachnoid screw is used most frequently to monitor ICP. This involves the insertion of a screw through a burr hole into the subarachnoid space or, occasionally, into the subdural space. The difficulties with this system, far fewer than those presented by the ventricular catheter, include possible meningitis resulting from contamination, and occlusion of the proximal end of the screw by cerebral tissue in cases of severely increased ICP, thereby resulting in false readings. Insertion of the subarachnoid screw by the neurosurgeon can be easily accomplished in the intensive care unit with the patient under local anesthesia.

It is best to keep the head of the child's bed elevated approximately 30 degrees to promote cerebral venous drainage. In addition, whenever the child is repositioned, the head must be maintained in the midline position in order to avoid compression of the jugular veins and compromising of venous drainage.

The transducer must be aligned either with the point of entry of the screw into the skull or at the level of the cerebral ventricles (approximately the level of the top of the ear,. The level of alignment is determined by the preference of the neurosurgeon. Once this has been established, the nurse should maintain the transducer at that level throughout the course of the treatment in order to ensure accurate readings.

Ongoing neurological assessment is also of utmost importance, but is limited to ICP readouts and evaluation of pupil size and reactivity because the use of pancuronium prevents further neurological examination.

Pupil size and reaction to light must be evaluated frequently, especially during any elevations in ICP or changes in vital signs. ICP readouts must be continually monitored. In addition, the nurse must continually calculate CPP. Monitoring of the ICP must include both the digital readout of pressure and the pressure wave form. Dampening of the wave form, with a concomitant decrease in the readout pressure, may indicate interference with, or obstruction of, the monitoring device.

Osmotherapy.   Limitation of fluid intake to two-thirds of the maintenance level, which was begun as prophylaxis, now becomes essential. A dehydrated state is necessary to control ICP. Therefore, fluid intake may be restricted to even one half of the child's maintenance level. Regulation of this dehydrated state is accomplished by maintaining serum osmolality at a level of greater than 290 milliosmoles/liter, preferably in the range of 310 to 320 milliosmoles/liter. Acute diuresis can be initiated with agents such as furosemide (0.5 to 1.0 mg/kg), but mannitol in doses of 0.25 to 1.00 g/kg is frequently recommended to treat subsequent rises in ICP.

Mannitol is the diuretic of choice because of its forceful and rapid effect, which is specific to edematous cerebral tissue. However, in children who have sustained severe head trauma, another diuretic may be administered in place of mannitol for the first 24 to 48 hours after injury because mannitol causes transient vasodilation, which could be detrimental to a freshly injured brain in a hyperemic state. When 48 to 72 hours have elapsed since the injury, diffuse cerebral swelling is thought to be a combination of hyperemia and secondary tissue edema, so that the vasodilating effect of mannitol is no longer as much of a threat to the patient, but it nevertheless remains a consideration.[18,19]

Dangers associated with the excessive use of mannitol are (1) the effects of severe hypovolemia on cerebral perfusion and systemic cardiovascular dynamics,[10] and (2) electrolyte imbalance.

Fluid status is an area of major concern for the nurse. The child's total fluid intake must be precisely regulated. Total fluid intake includes not only the routine IV fluid, but also fluid infused with medications, flushes, any fluids administered through the nasogastric tube, and fluids used to calculate cardiac output. The nurse must be careful to infuse no more than the ordered rate per hour through all possible sites.

Because of the severely restricted fluid intake, the child's renal status must be closely monitored. Urine output of 0.5 to 1.0 ml/kg/hr ensures that adequate fluid to metabolize waste products is provided. The urine should be routinely tested for pH, glucose, ketones, protein, and blood. For accurate measurement of urine output, a Foley catheter must be inserted. The indwelling catheter provides an additional portal of entry for bacteria, placing the child at risk for urinary tract infection. Scrupulous aseptic technique during insertion is a necessity, and routine catheter care with an iodine-based antiseptic may help to avoid this potentially serious complication. In addition, careful assessment of the child for the presence of urinary tract infection, including a routine urine culture, will facilitate early detection and treatment if an infection occurs.

Fluid balance is more difficult to maintain if the child requires osmotherapy to control ICP. Mannitol has a rapid effect, and it can cause sudden fluid loss from the vascular space, with an accompanying decrease in systemic arterial blood and venous filling pressures. Mannitol also increases serum osmolality and can lead to electrolyte imbalance. The nurse must therefore closely monitor vital signs and urine output while administering this drug and after the infusion is completed. Specific gravity of the urine should be routinely monitored, as well as urine osmolality and electrolyte levels. Serum osmolality and electrolyte levels should also be monitored. All of these measures can alert the nurse to problems before they become dangerous to the patient. If all therapy thus far described fails to control the ICP, extraordinary therapy is indicated.

Extraordinary Therapy

Hemodynamic monitoring. Before introducing either of the treatment modalities of extraordinary therapy, extensive hemodynamic monitoring must be established, in addition to systemic arterial pressure (SAP) and ICP monitoring. Left

TABLE 4-6   Possible Pulmonary and Cardiovascular Changes After Neurological Insult

Cause	Changes	Treatment	Effects of treatment
Fluid overload	Increased PAOP, PAP, and CVP; normal to increased CO; increased pulmonary shunting; increased ICP	Diuretics and fluid restriction	Decreased PAOP, PAP, and CVP; normal to decreased CO; decreased pulmonary shunting; decreased ICP
Hypovolemia	Decreased PAOP, PAP, CVP, CO, pulmonary perfusion, and PaO_2	Colloid	Increased PAOP, PAP, CVP, CO, pulmonary perfusion, and PaO_2

CO, cardiac output; CVP, central venous pressure; ICP, intracranial pressure; PaO_2, partial pressure of arterial oxygen; PAOP, pulmonary artery occluded pressure; PAP, pulmonary artery pressure.

heart filling pressures are monitored by means of the Swan-Ganz catheter, which enables accurate monitoring of the pulmonary artery pressure (PAP), the pulmonary artery occluded pressure (PAOP), and the central venous presure (CVP), as well as providing for measurement of cardiac output by the thermodilution technique.

The Swan-Ganz catheter is crucial in guiding therapy. With the information obtained from this catheter, two distinct pulmonary and cardiovascular changes can be identified (Table 4-6).[20] These changes are not unique to patients with a neurological insult, but can occur in any critically ill child.

The first change is evidenced by an increase in all filling pressures, a normal to high cardiac output, and increased pulmonary shunting as determined by arterial blood gas analysis, with the result of a possible increase in ICP. In general, the problem is fluid overload. Fluid restriction and diuretics will, most of the time, correct this situation. Filling pressures return to normal, arterial oxygenation is improved, and ICP usually decreases.

The second change is evidenced by low filling pressures, a decrease in pulmonary perfusion, and a possible increase in ICP. Usually, the cause is hypovolemia, and the addition of colloid will, most of`the time, correct the problem.

Children with either problem present in the same way (i.e., with a drop in PaO_2 and, sometimes, with an increase in ICP). Without information about left heart and pulmonary pressures obtained from the Swan-Ganz catheter, these problems are indistinguishable.

Another invasive pressure that assists in guiding therapy is the jugular venous line. A catheter placed in the jugular venous bulb facilitates measurement of CBF, jugular O_2 content, and cerebral metabolic rate.[4] Measurements from this line permit the lowering of the $PaCO_2$ to less than 20 mmHg in an effort to control ICP, as long as jugular venous PO_2 is maintained at 35 mmHg.

Barbiturate coma.   After the establishment of necessary hemodynamic monitoring lines, barbiturate coma is induced for control of ICP. The use of barbiturates in large doses may serve to protect the brain and effectively reduce ICP by the reduction of cerebral metabolism and the promotion of cerebral vasoconstriction. Sodium pentobarbital (Nembutal) is administered initially in a bolus dose of 3 to 5 mg/kg over 30 minutes and subsequently by continuous IV infusion at 2 mg/kg/hr to maintain serum barbiturate levels in the range of 2.5 to 3.5 mg/dl. Blood levels in excess of 4 mg/dl usually lead to systemic hypotension, and the use of vasopressors may be required to maintain SAP, thereby preserving a CPP of greater than 50 mmHg.[10]

It is the nurse's responsibility to accurately calculate, prepare, and administer the infusion. Barbiturates can cause severe hypotension; therefore, the nurse must closely monitor vital signs to ensure adequate SAP and CPP at all times. Barbiturate coma serves to sedate and calm the patient and may eliminate the child's responsiveness to environmental stimuli. (It is likely, however, that the child can still hear.) Because the level of coma induced by continuous barbiturate infusion prevents muscular movement, the infusion of pancuronium can be discontinued.

Surface hypothermia.   When other measures to control ICP are insufficient, surface hypothermia may be used to lower body temperature from 37°C (98.6°F) to 31°C (87.8°F). This serves to additionally reduce CBF and, therefore, ICP. Some authorities advocate using hypothermia immediately after initiating controlled hyperventilation,[10] whereas others believe that this method of controlling ICP should be reserved until other therapies, including barbiturate coma, have proved ineffective.[4] Hypothermia complicates the management of fluid and electrolyte status and, in theory, may interfere with immune and inflammatory responses.

Because there is a 40 percent decrease in O_2 consumption with body temperature at 31°C (87.8°F), all metabolic demands of the body are reduced and CBF is decreased.[4] The initial response of the body to hypothermia is a sympathetic one: shivering, vasoconstriction, increased O_2 consumption, bronchodilation, and an increase in body functions. Fortunately, this autonomic response is inhibited by barbiturate coma, and the patient suffers none of these effects if an adequate serum level of barbiturate is ensured. The ultimate and desired effects of hypothermia are a decreased heart rate and cardiac output, directly related to the decreased metabolic demands of the body.

When the decision to use surface hypothermia to control ICP is made, the child's body temperature must be monitored by either the thermistor on the Swan-Ganz catheter or by an esophageal temperature probe. These methods provide an accurate measurement of the child's core temperature at the level of the heart and great vessels. Rectal or skin temperature measurements do not correspond accurately to core temperature when surface hypothermia is used.

Hypothermia is evoked by cooling with hypothermia blankets. The child is cooled rapidly until the core temperature drops to 32 to 32.5°C (89.6 to 90.5°F) and then allowed to drift gradually to 31°C (87.8°F). Cooling to below 30°C (86°F) can result in devastating complications: spontaneous ventricular fibrillation and asystole occur at a body temperature of approximately 29°C (84.2°F).

Cooling to 31 to 32°C (87.8 to 89.6°F) is not without side effects, which must be evaluated carefully in order to prevent serious complications. As already mentioned, the immune responses may be inhibited by hypothermia. In addition, the child whose treatment necessitates hypothermia is critically ill and further at risk for infection because of the multiple portals of entry from hemodynamic monitoring and IV lines, urinary catheter, and endotracheal tube. Caregivers must maintain scrupulous aseptic technique and a high level of suspicion regarding infection.

Hypothermia also results in a shift of extracellular fluid from the intravascular to the interstitial spaces. Because this third spacing of fluid can result in hypovolemia and electrolyte imbalance, the child's fluid and electrolyte status must be monitored with increased vigilance. Hyperkalemia and hypernatremia are the most significant electrolyte imbalances seen in these children. In addition, as the result of unrelieved pressure, the child's skin may become edematous and more prone to breakdown. Meticulous skin care is a necessity, in conjunction with an alternating pressure mattress, a cushioned head-protector, and frequent position changes. Blood viscosity is also increased as the result of fluid shift from the plasma to the surrounding tissues. Serum osmolality and hematocrit are monitored closely. Should either parameter indicate danger to the patient, then IV fluid administration should be reevaluated.

In addition, cardiac conduction is altered by hypothermia. Conduction abnormalities that may be seen include a prolonged P-R interval, lengthened QRS complex, prolonged Q-T interval, and inversion of the ST segment, all of which place the child at risk for the development of serious arrhythmias. The electrocardiogram must be monitored closely in order to ensure detection of conduction aberrations before serious disturbances in rhythm occur. This is of special importance because barbiturates adversely affect myocardial contractility.

In those patients in whom barbiturate coma and hypothermia have been induced, two major pulmonary and cardiovascular changes have been identified (Table 4-7).[20] The first change is thought to be caused by a progressive loss of brainstem functioning. It is evidenced by a low SAP, decreased pulmonary vascular resistance (PVR), an initially high cardiac index (CI), a normal to low PAP and a low CVP. The administration of catecholamines has little effect on this condition; the administration of fluids only increases the SAP and the ICP. The child then develops a progressively falling cardiac output, and death almost always follows.

The second change is evidenced by a normal to increased SAP, a high PVR, a

TABLE 4-7 Possible Pulmonary and Cardiovascular Changes After Inducement of Barbiturate Coma and Hypothermia

Cause	Changes	Treatment	Effects of treatment
Loss of brainstem functioning	Decreased SAP and PVR; increased CI; normal to decreased PAP; decreased CVP	Catecholamines Administration of fluids	Minimal Increased SAP and ICP, leading almost always to death
Unknown	Normal to increased SAP; increased PVR; decreased CI; increased PAOP; normal PAP and CVP	Peripheral vasodilators Colloid	Decreased PVR and CVP Increased SAP and normal ICP, the latter of which then results in increased CI, decreased SAP and PVR, increased oxygenation, and decreased pulmonary shunting

CI, cardiac index; CVP, central venous pressure; ICP, intracranial pressure; PAOP, pulmonary artery occluded pressure; PAP, pulmonary artery pressure; PVR, pulmonary vascular resistance; SAP, systemic arterial pressure.

low CI, a high PAOP, and a normal PAP and CVP. In these children, the administration of neither fluids nor diuretics improves pulmonary perfusion, and, frequently, the addition of fluid causes a rise in the ICP; however, the use of vasodilators (usually sodium nitroprusside) has proved helpful (*see* Table 6-18, p. 384). As the PVR and CVP fall, adequate amounts of colloid can be administered to support circulation. This treatment avoids serious increases in ICP and results in an improved CI, a lowered SAP and PVR, improved arterial oxygenation, and a decrease in pulmonary shunting.

The nurse should be aware of these patterns and the appropriate treatment. In addition, the nurse must be knowledgeable about the drugs used. Nitroprusside can cause severe hypotension very quickly. Colloid should be available at the bedside, ready to be administered, if hypotension occurs. The child may be on dopamine for various reasons (for one of the above-mentioned changes or for the maintenance of adequate CPP or urine output). Dopamine can cause hypertension and is caustic to the veins. As with any drug infusion, the nurse must accurately calculate, prepare, and administer the infusion, as well as be prepared for any adverse effects.

Withdrawal of therapy.　　Full therapy is generally maintained for at least 72 hours. At this time, therapy is withdrawn, if the child has been free of increased ICP for 24 hours. Withdrawal of therapy progresses in an ordered sequence, beginning with the last therapy initiated.

Rewarming from hypothermia should proceed very gradually at a rate of no faster than 0.5°C (0.9°F) per hour until the temperature reaches 35°C (95°F). Active rewarming should be stopped at this point and the temperature allowed to rise gradually back to normothermia. Rapid rewarming causes the plasma fluid that has been extravasated into the body tissues to reenter the intravascular space at a rapid rate. This sudden expansion of the circulating blood volume may result in hypokalemia and congestive heart failure. Fluid and electrolyte status must be monitored carefully and left heart filling pressures monitored continuously in order to evaluate myocardial functioning and fluid balance.

During rewarming, if the child is not maintained in barbiturate coma, reinstitution of the IV administration of pancuronium may be necessary. This measure is indicated until the core temperature is at least 35°C (95°F) in order to avoid shivering and the concomitant increases in both general metabolic rate and ICP.

Barbiturate therapy is discontinued after normothermia is achieved, provided that no increases in ICP have occurred. The infusion is stopped and blood levels are closely monitored.

Continuous IV administration of barbiturates results in addiction of the child to these medications within 72 hours. In addition, the half-life of these medications is 18 to 24 hours and is prolonged by cooling, which slows the metabolism of this drug by the liver. When the medication infusion is discontinued, it may be longer than 24 hours before the child shows signs of responsiveness because the serum level of the drug remains elevated. Parents need to be prepared for this occurrence because they are understandably eager to see their child wakeful and responsive.

The child will demonstrate signs and symptoms of barbiturate withdrawal as the serum level of the drug decreases. These symptoms include tremors, crying, extreme irritability, and sleep disturbances, all of which can cause a great deal of parental anxiety. Parents will require a great deal of support during this period in order for them to help their child cope with this difficult period. Parents may be comforted to know that their child will not remember past events, but they must also realize that a great deal of reorientation is required because these children have no memory of where they are or how they came to be there.

Often, as therapy is withdrawn, increases in ICP may occur. If these rises in ICP return to baseline spontaneously within 5 to 10 minutes, they may be an indication of the child's response to the environment. If, however, the ICP elevation is sustained and/or requires therapy to lower it, the most recently discontinued therapy is reinstituted and maintained until there has been a period of 24 hours free of ICP elevation.

Once spontaneous respiration is reestablished, efforts to wean the child from mechanical ventilation can begin.

Emotional Support

Preservation of the critically ill child's life and the quality of the child's future is dependent on all the complex and technical aspects of the critical care management of increased ICP that have been described. In addition, however, it must be borne in mind that a child—a member of a family—occupies the intensive care bed. It is difficult to imagine a more stressful situation for the child's parents. Individuals working closely with the child and family should talk to the child, explaining procedures, unexpected noises, and the presence of others around the bed. It is also important to use touch to convey warmth and comfort to the child. Parents appreciate the concern that caregivers demonstrate by these simple measures and are thereby encouraged to do the same for their child. Parents may also read stories to their child or provide information about family members and friends, as well as participate in aspects of the child's physical care, such as bathing, skin care, or passive range-of-motion exercises.

It is especially important for the family to participate during the recovery phase. Parents should become active in the rehabilitation of their child because they best know the personality and special abilities of their child, as well as how their child can best be encouraged to relearn or remaster previously gained skills. A collaborative effort on the part of the family and the health care team ensures holistic, family-centered care.

BRAIN TUMORS

In infancy and childhood, intracranial tumors are among the most frequently occurring neoplasms, generally ranked third after leukemias and renal/adrenal tumors in the period between birth and 5 years of age. Between the ages of 5 and 15 years, however, brain tumors rank second only to leukemias among childhood neoplasms.

Intracranial tumors are not often diagnosed in infancy, but, from the age of 2 years on, the frequency of diagnosis according to age distribution is relatively proportionate. At 16 years of age, there is a sharp increase in frequency of diagnosis because the types of tumors typical of this age (pituitary adenomas, glioblastomas, meningiomas, and neurinomas) are more prevalent after puberty.[21]

Sexual predilection shows a preponderance of males over females, related to tumor type. This is especially pronounced in the first 6 years because of the high percentage of medulloblastomas, ependymomas, and sarcomas, all of which are more common in males. In a study of 700 children and adolescents with brain tumors, the male:female ratio was 4:3.[22]

Tumor site shows a distinctly different distribution in children as opposed to adults. The vast majority (two-thirds) of tumors occur infratentorially in children under 10 years of age, after which age the distribution is one third infratentorially and two-thirds supratentorially, which is more similar to the adult pattern.[23]

Clinical Presentation

Intracranial tumors are frequently difficult to diagnose in children for several reasons. Infants under the age of 12 months exhibit few signs of increased ICP because of the elasticity of their skulls. Eventual hydrocephalus may be the only sign. Young children (up to the age of 10 to 12 years) may remain asymptomatic even with a large tumor because the cranial sutures will still readily spread to accommodate increasing pressure. In addition, the immature brains of young children are prone to lesions that can become quite extensive in a relatively short period of time.

Often, the symptoms exhibited by a child with a brain tumor are the same as those of many other mild childhood diseases and, therefore, are not closely investigated. The most common signs and symptoms of intracranial tumors will be reviewed in the following sections.

Headache. Young children who are unable to express themselves verbally will not be able to voice complaints of headache. Headache, however, is one of the most important signs of increasing ICP and is present with almost all tumors of the posterior cranial cavity. It should be remembered that, because headache is more unusual in childhood maladies than in those of adults, it should be investigated very closely whenever it manifests itself in children.

In infants, headache will often be expressed as restlessness, increased irritability, and an aversion to being touched. Infants may cover their head protectively with their hands, shielding their eyes, forehead, or the back of their head. Children who are old enough to identify pain will complain of discomfort in a localized region, frequently in the frontal area. (The localization is not often diagnostic of tumor site.) The pain is usually dull and persistent.

Headache associated with vomiting generally occurs in the morning upon awakening. Cerebral blood volume increases during sleep because of hypoventilation (which raises the $PaCO_2$ level) and recumbent positioning. The sudden shift to an upright position precipitates changes in hemo- and CSF dynamics. Vomiting and the accompanying hyperventilation usually relieve or alleviate the headache. A key observation is that the child's appetite is unaffected.

Sudden "bursting" pain with vomiting is a particularly important sign because it may be indicative of an acute increase in ICP with CSF block. Transient blindness may also accompany this symptom. The particular danger is that, if the increase in ICP is sustained, CBF may be compromised.

In addition to headache, there may be irritation of cranial nerves, resulting in rigidity of the neck—a sign that is frequently mistaken for a sign of meningitis. This irritation may cause the child to tilt the head in a protective posture and to be unwilling to alter this position.

Vomiting. Vomiting is the second most common symptom of a brain tumor. It occurs in children of all ages, as the result of increased ICP, regardless of tumor type and location. It may be a transient symptom, relieved when the cranial sutures spread to accommodate the increased pressure.

The vomiting is usually not accompanied by nausea. It generally occurs in the morning, just after the child arises. Because of the transient nature of this symptom, the pattern of early-morning occurrence, and the fact that the child feels well after vomiting, it is frequently not viewed as a serious warning signal and may be attributed to other vague childhood illnesses or to a reluctance to attend school.

Visual disturbances. Visual disturbances are rarely noticed as an early symptom of brain tumors in infants and are difficult to assess in very young children. Papilledema and the resulting secondary optic atrophy are caused by increased ICP. The infant's malleable skull will accommodate the increasing pressure to such a degree that papilledema in this age group is rarely seen.

In school-age children, the teacher may be the first to notice a visual difficulty, but the children themselves rarely complain of decreased vision. Referral to an ophthalmologist may or may not result in early detection of a space-occupying lesion. Funduscopic examination will reveal the papilledema that is almost always present with tumors of the posterior cranial area, as well as the primary optic atrophy that results from direct pressure on the optic nerve. This pressure usually occurs with tumors such as craniopharyngiomas, located in the sellar-chiasmatic area.

Strabismus and diplopia are more frequently seen with infratentorial tumors and are a result of pressure on the cranial nerves, particularly the abducens nerve (6) and sometimes the oculomotor nerve (3). If the trochlear nerve (4) is affected unilaterally, the child is frequently able to correct for this by tilting the head to the opposite side, thus avoiding diplopia.

Bilateral scotomas (blind gaps in the visual field) and hemianopsia, which are rarer, are caused by pressure from hydrocephalus on the nerve fibers of the optic nerve (2). These visual field defects are usually present only at an advanced stage of disease.

Cerebellar and cranial nerve manifestations. Cerebellar signs and cranial nerve palsies will more frequently be noticed as indications of a serious problem. Ataxia is the most common early sign of cerebellar dysfunction. Initially, it may be ascribed to clumsiness, but falling, running into objects, and poor fine motor control become more obvious as cerebellar dysfunction increases.

Cranial nerve palsies resulting from pressure on the affected nerve are also easily noticed. The nerves most frequently affected are the facial (7), glossopharyngeal (9), vagus (10), trigeminal (5), and abducens (6)[24] (*see* p. 215).

Changes in vital signs. Respiratory changes such as disturbances in frequency, rhythm, and amplitude may be caused by increased ICP. Because of the compensatory capacity of regulating systems, however, these changes are not usually observed in the early stages of intracranial tumors. Nor do observable circulatory disturbances usually occur as initial signs. Increased ICP can cause widened pulse pressure and bradycardia (although, with chronically increased pressure, tachycardia may be seen instead of bradycardia). A disturbance in temperature regulation as a result of increased ICP is a very late and acute sign.

Changes in vital signs may also be caused by direct invasion of the brainstem by the tumor. In the case of invasion of the hypothalamus (as with a craniopharyngioma), severe hypo- or hyperthermia may result. In any event, the tumor is usually well advanced before any of these changes in vital signs is evident.

Seizures. Focal symptoms such as seizures may occur because of the local effects of tumor growth. Of all children with brain tumors, 38 percent present with seizures.[25] Seizures are generally produced by cerebral tumors, particularly if localized in the temporal region. These seizures may be generalized major motor, petit mal, focal, or Jacksonian. Focal and Jacksonian seizures are most indicative of a local cerebral lesion.

In some patients, the seizures may occur in conjunction with the symptoms of increased ICP. These seizures can often be traced back several years in the child's history, having been treated as symptoms of an idiopathic seizure disorder. Childhood seizures, especially in infants and toddlers, are often associated with transient metabolic and febrile diseases. If adequate diagnostic investigation is not performed, the presence of a tumor could be overlooked.

Pathophysiology and Associated Medical Management

Management of brain tumors is primarily dependent on the tumor type and location. Some of the more common tumor types are reviewed below. Although nursing intervention for postoperative care is presented, a lengthy discussion of chemotherapy and radiation techniques is beyond the scope of this text.

Infratentorial tumors. The majority of brain tumors that occur in childhood are located infratentorially. Tumors in this area will lead to functional disorders and impairment of vital structures earlier in their course than is the case with supratentorial tumors. The most important factor is tumor location with regard to the CSF passages. Even a small tumor can give rise to severe symptoms of increased ICP by producing obstructive hydrocephalus; however, it is also possible for tumors in this region (most particularly cerebellar tumors and, occasionally, tumors of the brainstem) to grow quite large without obstructing CSF flow.

Medulloblastoma: Medulloblastomas are neuroepithelial in origin and are the most malignant tumors of childhood and adolescence. They constitute about 20 percent of all intracranial tumors in children and are most frequent between the ages of 3 and 8 years.[26]

These tumors extend from the roof of the fourth cerebral ventricle, involve the vermis (the median connecting lobe of the cerebellum), and expand in every direction. Often, the tumor grows into the lumen of the fourth ventricle and may fill it completely. This tumor may become quite large before detection, and initial symptomatology is that of increased ICP secondary to hydrocephalus from fourth ventricular obstruction.

Because medulloblastomas characteristically seed tumor cells through the CSF pathways, ventriculoperitoneal (VP) shunt insertion is contraindicated. Treatment consists of surgical removal of as much tumor mass as possible, followed by radiation. There is some evidence that chemotherapy may affect recurrent medulloblastoma. Prognosis remains rather poor, with the best survival rate reported as 25 to 35 percent over a 5-year period.[25]

Cerebellar astrocytoma: These tumors are found almost exclusively in childhood and early adolescence, with a peak incidence between 7 and 9 years of age. They are the most benign tumors in childhood, constitute 16 percent of all childhood intracranial tumors, and show a female predilection.

Astrocytomas may localize in the midline, localize within a cerebellar hemisphere, or extend from the vermis into the cerebellar hemisphere. They are cystic in nature and do not seed into the CSF pathways.

Complete surgical removal is usually possible, but, with incomplete removal, postoperative radiation can increase long-term survival. With complete removal, 90 percent or more of all patients can survive for years or even decades.[26]

Brainstem glioma: Brainstem glioma is rare, but is seen almost exclusively in children and adolescents. Situated in the area of the pons, medulla, and midbrain, these tumors are highly malignant. They produce cranial nerve impairment instead of symptoms of generalized increased ICP.

Because of their location, surgical removal of gliomas is not possible, but biopsy may be performed to confirm the diagnosis and obtain tissue samples. Because approximately 20 percent of these tumors are cystic, drainage of the cyst may produce relief of symptoms.[25] Radiation may increase survival time to as long as 4 years, and steroids may be used to decrease edema in the surrounding tissue.[25] Chemotherapy has not proved to be beneficial.

Supratentorial tumors. The signs and symptoms produced by tumors of the cerebral hemispheres are the same for children as for adults. Recognition of these signs, however, is much more difficult in children. Infants and young children may be unable or unwilling to cooperate with the examiner. Motor functions, speech, and sensory processes that can provide information about localization of a tumor are not matured. The initial manifestations of these tumors are usually the signs and symptoms of generalized increased ICP or of focal seizures.

Cerebral astrocytoma: Cerebral astrocytomas occur in all age-groups, but there is an increased incidence after the age of 13 years. These tumors, considered semibenign, are neuroepithelial in origin. They may affect any portion of the cerebral hemisphere, but are frequently situated in the frontal lobe. They generally invade the white matter and frequently extend into the cerebral ventricles. These tumors, though firm and cartilaginous on the surface, may degenerate into many small, fluid-filled cysts at their depths.

Management consists of total surgical removal, if possible. If total removal cannot be achieved, radiation therapy (and possibly chemotherapy) should be considered. Astrocytomas do not metastasize, but may recur after incomplete removal; therefore, the long-term prognosis is poor.[27]

Ependymoma: Cerebral ependymomas are tumors that occur preferentially in childhood and adolescence. They are neuroepithelial in origin and generally arise from the ependymal lining of the lateral ventricles.[28] The tumors are firm, circumscribed, cauliflowerlike masses that may reach the size of a child's fist. They may occur in any lobe, but more frequently in the frontal and parietal lobes. With its main mass located in the white matter, the tumor may break through the ventricular wall and continue growing into the lumen of the ventricle.

Ependymomas frequently metastasize into surrounding tissue and are known to shed cells into the CSF and to seed further tumor growth along the CSF pathways. Treatment depends on the exact location and size of the tumor. Total surgical removal of the mass, if possible, can provide a good prognosis. Frequently, however, the tumor involves a complete hemisphere or extends over both hemispheres. In addition, involvement of the ventricles makes surgical intervention very hazardous.[29] High-dose radiation is generally used. If CSF seeding is suspected, systemic and intrathecal chemotherapy is effective. Prognosis varies with the deree of malignancy, but improves with the use of multimodal therapy.

Craniopharyngioma: Craniopharyngiomas are congenital in origin, arising from epithelial remnants of the craniopharyngeal duct. They are cystic in nature, filled with cloudy fluid, and, in the pediatric population, frequently calcified. They may cause blockage of CSF flow by pushing the floor of the third ventricle upward and by compressing the walls of the ventricle.

Children may present with hypothalamic disturbances, fatigue, sleepiness, obesity, or pituitary dysfunctions attributable to abnormal production of growth, adrenocorticotrophic, or gonadotrophic hormones. Visual field disturbances are also a frequent finding because of compression of the optic nerves, the chiasm, and the optic tracts. Depending on the exact location of the tumor, there may be bitemporal hemianopsia, homonymous hemianopsia, primary narrowing of the visual field, loss of visual acuity due to primary optic atrophy, or blindness. Although peak incidence is between the ages of 10 and 16 years, these tumors can occur in any age-group.

The treatment of choice is complete surgical removal without interfering with hypothalamic functioning. Endocrine replacement may be necessary. Subtotal removal necessitates the use of radiation postoperatively. Prognosis is generally good, but worsens if a second resection becomes necessary.

Tumors of the optic pathway: Optic nerve gliomas are characteristically slow-growing, nonmetastasizing tumors with long periods of dormancy. They are frequently associated with generalized neurofibromatosis and on the surface appear as an expansion of the optic nerve. In addition, they tend to expand anteriorly or posteriorly from the chiasm, and small cystic areas may be seen. The first sign of these tumors may be a unilateral, forward displacement of the eyeball or a mechanical limitation of ocular movement.

Treatment varies, with some groups advocating total surgical removal with or without radiation,[30] whereas others propose a more conservative approach with radiation only.[25] Treatment and prognosis depends on the degree of intracranial expansion, and recurrence is possible even many years later.

Pinealoma: Pinealomas, which are of neuroepithelial origin, are rare, but are more frequently seen in children and adolescents than in adults. These tumors show an overwhelming (80 percent) predilection for males.[31] Pinealomas grow by expansion, pushing the quadrigeminal plate (corpora quadrigemina) downward and the corpus callosum upward to penetrate the caudal portion of the third ventricle. They may even force themselves beneath the tentorium. These tumors are hard and tough, sometimes calcified, and may contain small cysts within the tumor tissue.

Surgical removal is difficult because of the firm attachment to deep cerebral veins and the brainstem. Shunting may be performed to relieve hydrocephalus, and radiation may result in survival for as long as 5 to 10 years.

Critical Care Management

Preoperative. The time from diagnosis of an intracranial tumor to surgical intervention is usually very short. The child and parents may have little time to adjust to the diagnosis and come to terms with the need to undergo a life-threatening procedure. The parents may experience guilt feelings for not having noticed early warning signs and symptoms. The nurse should make sure that both the parents and the child receive an introduction to the intensive care unit, nursing personnel, and postoperative equipment (*see* Chapter 1). Instruction for the child should be geared to the appropriate developmental stage and level of understanding.

Postoperative. Most surgical procedures for intracranial tumors are quite lengthy, and anesthesia effects may be prolonged postoperatively. Airway patency is of utmost importance, and ventilator support may be required initially. In addition, dressings over the operative site must be assessed frequently for drainage or bleeding.

Neurological assessment: A complete neurological assessment should be performed by the nurse immediately after surgery and hourly thereafter for at least 24 hours. Level of consciousness and pupillary reactions are the most important parameters. Children with infratentorial tumors may initially be more difficult to arouse postoperatively because the reticular activating system, which controls wakefulness and sleep, may have been disturbed. Once the child is awakened, however, any deterioration in level of consciousness should be regarded as a serious sign.

Children with craniopharyngiomas or tumors of the optic pathway should be assessed for visual field defects. If these defects persist postoperatively, it is important, in administering care, to approach the child from a midline position rather than from one side or the other, out of the field of vision.

Changes in motor strength may be subtle or sudden, but are important in localizing areas of damage. Findings should be compared with preoperative base line assessments to evaluate possible deficits. Increased ICP from brain swelling is a danger throughout the initial period of 72 hours postoperatively. (A more thorough discussion of neurological assessment is presented on p. 210.)

Hypo- or hyperthermia can occur after surgery in the areas of the hypothalamus and the brainstem; however, the possibility of infection should be considered if fever develops 48 to 72 hours postoperatively.

Fluid and electrolyte management: Postoperatively, the child will usually receive IV fluids at a rate of two-thirds to three-quarters of the maintenance level. This decreases the possibility of fluid overload, with a resultant increase in ICP.

The child should be NPO until fully recovered from anesthesia and until the cough and gag reflexes are intact. Once started on oral fluids, the child must be watched closely for vomiting because of both the danger of aspiration and the danger of increased ICP caused by vomiting.

Urine volume and specific gravity must be monitored closely to evaluate for diabetes insipidus (DI) or for syndrome of inappropriate antidiuretic hormone (ADH) secretion. DI is most common after excision of a craniopharyngioma, but syndrome of inappropriate ADH secretion may be seen after excision of any intracranial tumor (*see* p. 349).

Positioning and comfort measures: Postoperative positioning is extremely important. The child should be kept with the head of the bed elevated approximately 30 degrees. A side-lying position may prevent aspiration and the exertion of pressure on the incision site. The neck should not be flexed when the child turns, and the head and neck should always be kept in the midline position. If a large tumor has been excised, the child should not be placed on the operative side in order to prevent sudden shifting of the brain.

Headache is a rare postoperative complaint but incisional discomfort or neck stiffness with tumors of the posterior cranial fossa may require medication such as acetaminophen or aspirin. Narcotics, which are rarely required, may suppress the level of consciousness.

Ventriculostomies: Some children may have ventriculostomies in place postoperatively in order to facilitate drainage of CSF. These should be connected to a closed drainage system to minimize the chances of infection. The volume of drainage can be measured in a number of ways, depending on the drainage system used, but it should be measured carefully and calculated into the daily fluid balance. Drainage should be observed for any change in quality, such as increased bleeding or cloudiness.

The ventriculostomy can also be used to monitor ICP postoperatively (*see* p. 228). The system can be arranged for continuous monitoring with intermittent drainage of CSF, if desired. In addition, if required, the ventriculostomy can be converted at a later time to a permanent shunt.

ARTERIOVENOUS MALFORMATION

An arteriovenous malformation (AVM) of the brain is a rare congenital lesion that is asymptomatic in a large number of patients. If symptoms are to occur, they generally do so during the second to fourth decades of life. The most common initial symptom is hemorrhage or seizure.

Pathophysiology

AVMs arise early in fetal life, at approximately the third week of gestation.[32] At this point, the primitive arteries, veins, and capillaries divide into the mature vascular system. If this state of development is disrupted, a direct communication between an artery and vein without the usual capillary bed will result. This communication then develops into an AVM.

As the child's brain develops, the AVM evolves into a lesion characterized by many large, rudimentary vascular channels. The feeding arteries and draining veins are grossly dilated and are virtually indistinguishable as arteries or veins. The AVM generally extends from the cerebral cortex into the white matter of the brain substance. Any cerebral tissue within the AVM is considered nonfunctional.

Specific anatomic information about AVMs is scanty, but it is generally accepted that most AVMs receive their blood supply from at least two of the major cerebral arteries and, often, from all three. There is evidence of increased blood flow to the area of the AVM, which results in increased pressure and distended venous vessels.[32] The arteries may become hypertrophic, with a consequent degeneration of the arterial wall, thereby providing a possible explanation for the appearance of aneurysms on the arteries supplying the AVM.[32] Often, the brain tissue adjacent to AVMs shows atrophy on CAT scanning. This change is generally believed to be the direct result of ischemia produced by the "steal" syndrome. Because of the large, primitive vascular channels of an AVM, there is increased blood flow to the area. Blood is therefore diverted from surrounding brain tissue to the AVM. In other words, the AVM "steals" blood from regional brain tissue.

Both the AVM and the effects of the "steal" syndrome can produce symptoms at any time in the individual's life-span. It has been estimated that 0.14 percent of the population have AVMs, and it is generally accepted that the majority of patients will exhibit symptoms before the age of 40 years.[33] There does not seem to be any genetic predisposition to AVM, and the distribution between males and females is equal.

Approximately 70 to 93 percent of AVMs are supratentorial; the remainder are infratentorial.[33] AVMs occur equally in the right and left hemispheres, but the area of greatest occurrence seems to be the region of the middle cerebral artery. The parietal region is often involved, and these malformations (as well as frontal AVMs) are generally fed by branches of the middle and anterior cerebral arteries.

Clinical Presentation

The presenting signs and symptoms of greatest importance in an individual with an AVM are subarachnoid hemorrhage, convulsive seizures, headache, arterial bruit, syncope, hemispheric neurological deficit, and mental confusion. These symptoms most often appear in adolescence and early adulthood. Consequently, the diagnosis of AVM in the young child is rare.

Hemorrhage. Hemorrhage occurs in approximately 50 percent of patients with AVMs (85 percent in children).[32] Once hemorrhage has occurred, the probability of a second bleed increases; however, there appears to be no cause-and-effect relationship between activity level, blood pressure, or other external factors (such as stress) with either the first or succeeding bleeds. There is some controversy as to whether hemorrhage correlates with the size of the lesion or with its location, but it is generally agreed that the rupture occurs at the arteriovenous junction, where the vessel walls are most fragile.

Hemorrhage can occur intracerebrally, into the subarachnoid space, into the ventricles, or into a combination of any of these locations. Intracerebral hematomas frequently occur in combination with subarachnoid bleeds and will therefore produce focal neurological deficits. Younger patients have a greater incidence of intracerebral hematomas and will exhibit such deficits as hemiplegia, homonymous hemianopsia, a visual field defect, or aphasia.[34]

Special attention should be given to the child who presents with an intracranial bleed of unknown etiology because this may be an indication of a cryptic AVM.[34] These lesions are very small and are generally not visualized either on arteriogram or on CAT. Often, these AVMs are completely obliterated in the course of rupturing.

Seizures. Seizures are the second most common presenting symptom of an AVM and may be either focal or major motor. Focal seizures are generally of the motor variety (or they may be psychomotor), and they occur as frequently as major motor seizures. Lesions located in the frontal region are usually the cause of major motor seizures, whereas focal seizures are primarily associated with lesions involving the parietal lobe. In general, lesions of the temporal and frontal lobes produce seizures more often than do other supratentorial locations.[35]

Seizures are believed to be caused by cerebral ischemia in areas surrounding the AVM. This ischemia is most probably the result of the cerebral "steal" syndrome. Both seizures and hemorrhage can occur simultaneously, although one generally precedes the other.

Headaches. Headaches are also common presenting symptoms of AVMs, but, in isolation, they are difficult to evaluate because they are common occurrences in the general population. Severe, recurrent headaches that mimic the migraine (i.e., those that are consistently unilateral) are more frequently investigated in more depth. It has been suggested that headaches and their intensity may be caused by a mechanism involving the arterial supply to the dura mater or the venous drainage from the AVM.[32] Many patients have experienced these headaches for months to years before the diagnosis of the AVM and have become addicted to drugs—an additional consideration in determining their treatment.[33]

Other presenting symptoms such as hemiparesis, syncope, dysphasia, visual disturbance, or mental confusion are much less common, but will provoke the individual to seek medical attention. Arterial bruit is a rare symptom that is usually associated only with carotid-cavernous fistulas, extracranial malformation, and AVMs presenting in the neonatal period.[35]

Diagnosis

Definitive diagnosis of AVM can be made only after radiological evaluation. Cerebral angiography remains the primary investigative method, but CAT scanning provides additional valuable information.[36] More specifically, CAT scanning is helpful in identifying areas of calcification, ventricular dilation, alterations in the surrounding brain tissue, and intracranial hematomas from rupture of the AVM. After injection of the contrast medium, the tortuous channels of the AVM become much more apparent, and, if there is an associated hematoma, the adjacent vessels are also shown to be displaced.

Some investigators claim that CAT scanning is as accurate a screening technique as angiography in the detection of AVMs and that it is the superior modality for the diagnosis of intracranial hemorrhage.[37] In some cases, CAT scanning demonstrated AVMs that were not visualized by angiography.[36] Angiography, however, remains the definitive diagnostic tool for AVMs and is required for demonstrating the specific anatomy of the malformation.

Critical Care Management

Conservative treatment. AVMs can result in a catastrophic outcome if left to their natural course, but the dangers associated with more aggressive treatment are equally significant. Up to 50 percent of the untreated patients may experience serious consequences, including death, from rupture of the AVM.[38] Although an AVM most frequently becomes symptomatic in the second to fourth decades of life, this congenital malformation may manifest itself at any point in the individual's life-span. Therefore, the risk of serious consequences is proportionately greater the younger the individual is when symptoms begin.

Although there has been an increasing trend toward radical surgical excision of AVMs, conservative treatment is still used in some cases. This decision is generally based on one of two factors. First, depending on the site of the lesion, the consequences of the operation may be deemed to be more severe than the lesions's natural course. Second, the presence of relatively benign symptoms, such as infrequent seizures that are easily controlled, may be the basis for electing conservative treatment. In such cases, supportive therapy after a bleed and/or drug therapy to control seizures may be adequate.

A child who presents with seizures alone rarely requires critical care management. Most of the children who require intensive care will have sustained a bleed. Neurological assessment is of paramount importance. Often, the child is awake, in which case the focus of the examination should be evaluation for focal signs of the hemorrhage (i.e., hemiparesis, hemiplegia, dysphagia, visual disturbances, or headache). If the child is comatose, the examination should center on cranial nerve functioning, with close observation for subtle signs of improvement or deterioration.

Other nursing measures are primarily supportive. Unlike intracranial aneurysms, AVMs do not generally tend to rebleed in the period immediately after the first rupture. For this reason, it is unnecessary to restrict activity and maintain a quiet environment unless there is clinical evidence of an expanding mass lesion. It is important, however, to provide emotional support and age-appropriate diversional activities.

If the child's speech is impaired, an alternative method of communication must be devised to the satisfaction of the child, parents, and staff. If parents are encouraged to participate in the care of their child, some of their anxiety may be alleviated.

Parents can be involved in the care of the comatose child as well. They can be asked to make tape recordings of their voices (or of those of the child's siblings and classmates), which can then be played to the child during those times that the parents are unable to visit. Reading stories, assisting with the bath, stroking, and touching are other means by which parents can help to comfort their child.

Both the child and the parent should always be dealt with in an open and honest fashion. The nurse should provide information and education concerning the child's condition according to each individual's needs and level of understanding.

Some investigators have found that mortality among patients managed conservatively may be as high or higher than mortality from surgical treatment.[39-41] Whereas the initial course after diagnosis of an AVM may often be fairly benign, the long-term outlook is less benign. There is approximately a 10 percent mortality rate per decade because of recurrent hemorrhages. In addition, these patients may suffer psychologically from the knowledge that they harbor a potentially lethal malformation.[42] For these reasons, there has been an increasing trend toward more aggressive management of the child with an AVM.

Surgical intervention.   The first surgical excision of a cerebral AVM was performed in 1932. Other early attempts at surgical intervention included ligation of the carotid artery and clipping of the feeding arteries, as well as partial or total resection of the lesion. Ligation, clipping, and partial resection merely aimed at reducing the blood supply to the AVM and proved to be largely ineffective, and, in some instances, even more dangerous than the AVM itself. In those cases, the development of a collateral blood supply to the AVM resulted in an increased "steal" phenomenon, by which an increased blood flow from surrounding tissues was drawn to the lesion, causing additional ischemia in adjacent areas of the brain.

Current surgical treatment is therefore directed toward total excision of the malformation. This is particularly true for children, because the risk of rebleeding is already proportionately increased over their projected life-span and because the incidence of mortality associated with bleeds is increased in childhood.[34,43] The advent of microsurgical and electrocoagulation techniques has greatly facilitated the surgical management of AVMs. Lesions that were previously deemed inoperable are now accessible with the aid of the microscope. Success has been reported with surgical excision of AVMs in the speech and motor-sensory regions, which had long been considered inoperable because of the possibilities of severe postoperative deficit.[44] This success is attributed to the assumption that the brain tissue within the AVM space is hypoplastic because of the maldevelopment of the capillary system.

There are several well-documented potential hazards associated with surgical removal of an AVM: ischemia in surrounding brain structures and hyperemia in normal tissue proximal to the vascular occlusion. Ischemia generally presents as a problem when feeding arteries are ligated without removal of the abnormal mass, thereby precipitating the "steal" phenomenon. Hyperemia in proximal tissue is a much more significant problem.[45] It is believed that the normal brain tissue proximal to the AVM is subject to swelling as a result of the suddenly increased blood volume available to it when the AVM is removed.

In the initial postoperative phase, the key element is, once again, neurological assessment. The focus of the examination, however, is now primarily on cranial nerve functioning and on observation for signs of increased ICP, which would indicate impending transtentorial herniation. This could occur as a result of delayed hyperemia after surgical excision: it is extremely rare, very rapid, and almost always fatal. Direct ICP monitoring is therefore of questionable value and is rarely used. If there are no postoperative complications, nursing care primarily involves supportive measures.

Flow-directed embolization. A wide variety of flow-directed embolization techniques have received much attention and differing degrees of acceptance in recent years. The aim of this therapy is to occlude only the blood supply to the AVM, with arterial supply to normal tissues being preserved. Although all flow-directed embolization techniques are essentially the same, there are nevertheless several different methods employed and numerous types of embolic materials (including Silastic beads, adhesive polymers, and silicone fluid) that may be used.

So far, none of the flow-directed embolization techniques has proved to be successful at effecting a complete cure. Severe complications, such as profound cerebrovascular accident and gluing of catheters in place, have also been reported.

Combined treatment. Current therapy at some centers consists of a joint approach by the neuroradiologist and neurosurgeon.[38] The neuroradiologist obliterates portions of the AVM by flow-directed embolization and the neurosurgeon then excises the lesion. Postoperative care is the same as for surgical intervention, outlined above.

Radiation. Conventional and proton-beam radiotherapy have also been used in the treatment of these lesions. Radiation affects the AVM by causing endothelial hyperplasia and thickening of the vessel walls. In the past, the effect of radiotherapy on AVMs has been perceived as a very slow process, and reports on the long-term effects have been scanty. Recently, however, there has been some evidence to suggest that conventional and proton-beam radiation may be more effective than previously thought.[39] Long-term, follow-up studies are still being conducted.

STATUS EPILEPTICUS

Pathophysiology

Status epilepticus is a state of continual or recurrent seizure activity that is so prolonged or so frequent that consciousness is not regained without medical treatment. Status epilepticus can be classified as either idiopathic or symptomatic. Idiopathic status epilepticus is frequently precipitated in individuals with idiopathic seizure disorders by rapid weaning of their antiepileptic drugs or by a state of hyperpyrexia. Symptomatic status epilepticus may result from a number of acute or chronic underlying conditions (Table 4-8).

The seizures can be classified according to the clinical manifestations, the

TABLE 4-8 Causative Factors in Symptomatic Status Epilepticus

Type	Factor
Acute	Infection
	Purulent meningitis
	Encephalitis
	Aseptic meningitis
	Trauma/hypoxia
	Acute hypoxic injury
	Subdural hematoma
	Metabolic/toxic factors
	Dehydration or electrolyte imbalance
	Exogenous toxin
	Hypocalcemia
Chronic	Hypoxic or congenital injury
	Progressive encephalopathy
	Brain malformations
	Tumor
	Arteriovenous malformation
	Cerebral palsy

anatomic origin, and the EEG findings. Seizures can be either generalized or focal. Generalized status epilepticus is characterized by tonic-clonic, myoclonic, or absence seizures, and it involves both cerebral hemispheres. Focal status epilepticus is characterized by seizures that arise in a localized area of the brain. This type includes hemiconvulsion-hemiplegia epilepsy, focal seizures, epilepsia partialis continua, or complex partial seizures. The focus in this section will be on the more severe forms of status epilepticus, which require immediate management in order to prevent serious residual damage or death.

Generalized tonic-clonic epilepsy.   This is the most common form of status epilepticus in children and adults, and by far the most severe. It may occur in individuals with known seizure disorders or in those who have never had seizures. The incidence seems to be higher with symptomatic than with idiopathic etiology.[46]

Initially, the generalized tonic-clonic convulsions of status epilepticus are no different from those of a single major motor seizure. The duration of the attack is the basis for the differentiation. With continuation of the seizure, autonomic changes may occur, including tachycardia, hyperpyrexia, hypertension, and salivary hypersecretion. Neurological signs such as pupillary changes, Babinski's sign, and increased or decreased muscle tone may occur, either symmetrically or asymmetrically. Coma may persist after the convulsions for a variable period of time. Metabolic changes may include acidosis and increases in blood glucose, blood urea nitrogen, creatine phosphokinase, and white blood cell count. The EEG may exhibit a variety of changes, including focal or generalized slowing or bilateral spike-wave discharges.

Death or severe residual neurological deficit can occur as the result of uncontrolled generalized major motor seizures. Death is usually caused by the underlying disease, respiratory failure, cardiac arrhythmias, circulatory collapse, or injudicious use of medication.[46] Residual neurological deficit can include mental retardation, focal motor deficits, behavioral disorders, and chronic seizure disorder. Residual effects, which can occur even in children with no previous history of seizures, are likely to be more severe with younger children. The longer the duration of status epilepticus from the onset of the seizures until the time they are controlled, the more unfavorable the prognosis will be.

Hemiconvulsion-hemiplegia epilepsy. This form of status epilepticus manifests itself by continuous, repeated tonic-clonic movements that are localized to one side of the body. Consciousness may be altered, but may occasionally be maintained. This type of epilepsy represents a medical emergency and should be treated in the same fashion as generalized tonic-clonic status epilepticus.

Causative factors of hemiconvulsion-hemiplegia epilepsy involve a variety of disorders, including vascular occlusion. This disorder is seen most frequently in childhood, and it may be referred to as the convulsive form of infantile or childhood hemiplegia. The EEG demonstrates continuous focal slowing or focal discharge. Residual hemiparesis, chronic seizure disorder, and mental retardation may result.

Critical Care Management

Immediate aggressive treatment is required in order to prevent the severe consequences of generalized tonic-clonic or hemiconvulsion-hemiplegia status epilepticus. Specific aspects of management must be carried out in the following order.

General therapy. All efforts must be made to ensure cerebral oxygenation. The insertion of an oral airway and the suctioning of secretions may be adequate to maintain a patent airway. In the presence of cyanosis, O_2 should be administered, and endotracheal intubation may be necessary if adequate respiratory functioning is uncertain. It is unnecessary to place a hard object between the teeth during a seizure unless the patient's tongue and cheeks are being lacerated. The dangers associated with placing an object between the patient's teeth during a seizure are those of precipitating vomiting by the patient and of having one's fingers severely bitten. The patient should be protected from injury by padding the side rails and removing hard or sharp objects from reach. It is very important to measure and document blood pressure, heart rate, and respiratory rate, as well as to describe the convulsion, even in the first minutes of the seizure. Observation and recording of seizure activity should include the following information: the time at which the seizure began; the region of the body where the seizure began (if localized); a description of the type of muscle movement (i.e., twitching, jerking, or tonic-clonic); any occurrence of vomiting and/or incontinence; and the time at which seizure activity stopped.

Obtaining a brief history from the family is important in order to reveal a known seizure disorder, dosages of antiepileptic drugs, or events (such as trauma or infection) that may have precipitated the attack. During the physical examination, special attention should be given to any signs of infection or trauma, or to signs of an underlying neurological condition such as focal deficits, asymmetric pupil size, posturing, or signs of increased ICP.

Initial laboratory studies should include blood glucose, calcium, blood urea nitrogen, electrolytes, and complete blood count, as well as a toxicology screening, blood cultures, levels of antiepileptic drugs, and liver enzymes, if indicated by the patient's history. An IV infusion of 5 percent dextrose should be started for hydration, as well as for providing an access route for administration of medications. Some authorities advocate infusing a 50 percent dextrose solution at a dose of 2 ml/kg, followed by 1 to 2 ml/kg of 10 percent calcium gluconate if the dextrose infusion produces no change in the seizures.[46] Because of the possible cardiac effects of calcium, electrocardiogram monitoring is recommended.

Specific drug therapy. It is essential for nurses to be thoroughly familiar with the characteristics, dosages, and side effects of the more commonly used antiepileptic drugs. These drugs are administered by IV infusion because absorption of the medication from intramuscular injections varies significantly from one individual to another. It must be remembered that the high doses used to reach therapeutic levels may easily produce serious side effects in the cardiac and respiratory systems (Table 4-9).

The drugs most commonly used to control status epilepticus are diazepam, phenobarbital, and phenytoin sodium. If a single drug is ineffectual in arresting the seizures, a combination of these drugs may be necessary, but a maximum dosage of a single agent is better than small dosages of several different medications.

Diazepam: Diazepam, which has an effect on convulsive states of both cortical and centrencephalic origin, is often considered to be the initial drug of choice to combat status epilepticus. Its primary advantage is its rapid effect, which sometimes occurs within seconds. This drug is considered relatively safe for IV administration; however, if diazepam is used after phenobarbital or phenytoin has proved ineffective, the margin of safety for cardiac and respiratory side effects decreases. The major disadvantage of diazepam is its short-lived effect. Because it is rapidly metabolized, the seizures may begin again within an hour of the initial injection. Because of its relative insolubility in water, diazepam should not be diluted with water or saline solutions (to avoid its precipitating), and the IV site should be monitored closely for signs of thrombosis.

Phenobarbital: Phenobarbital is the safest of the barbiturates for IV administration, but it requires 20 to 60 minutes to reach peak concentration in the brain. Therefore, it is not likely to be as effective as diazepam for initial control of status epilepticus, but it is appropriate for sustaining control after the seizures have been initially stopped. Blood levels should be monitored frequently in the initial period of dosage regulation because, with the patient in a postictal or comatose state, it is difficult to rely on clinical appearance alone in assessing toxic states.

Phenytoin: Because of its lipid solubility, phenytoin rapidly enters the brain and reaches peak levels in half the time required for phenobarbital but less rapidly than that for diazepam. In addition, phenytoin levels fall rapidly unless sufficiently high doses are used initially to saturate other organs as well. Blood levels should be monitored closely to guard against toxicity. An advantage of phenytoin over both diazepam and phenobarbital is that it has much less of a sedative effect. Phenytoin, however, can cause hypotension and abnormalities in cardiac conduction.

Other agents: Other agents may be necessary if none of the above drugs proves successful in interrupting the seizures. Paraldehyde is frequently effective, particularly if a traumatic, vascular, toxic, or febrile etiology is suspected. A continuous infusion of 0.10 to 0.15 ml/kg is administered over 60 minutes. If the seizure is controlled, the infusion can be slowly decreased to the lowest dose that will sustain a state of seizure control. After maintenance levels of a long-acting anticonvulsant are attained, the infusion can be gradually discontinued.

In rare instances, when all other methods have proved ineffective in interrupting status epilepticus, it may be necessary to resort to a general anesthetic such as

TABLE 4-9 Antiepileptic Drugs

Drug	Loading dose	Rate of infusion	Therapeutic range	Side effects	Comments
Diazepam	100 µg/kg	Not to exceed 2 mg/min		Sedation, respiratory depression, hypotension, cardiorespiratory arrest, and laryngospasm	Should not be diluted or mixed with other drugs.
Phenobarbital	5 mg/kg	30 mg/min	10–40 µg/ml	Same as for diazepam	May act synergistically with diazepam
Phenytoin sodium	10–20 mg/kg	50 mg/min	10–40 µg/ml	Hypotension and cardiac conduction defects	Should not be diluted or mixed with other drugs. Precipitates in dextrose IV solutions; IV line should be flushed with NaCl. Concurrent administration with chloramphenicol sodium succinate may increase levels.
Paraldehyde	0.10–0.15 ml/kg	Over a period of 60 min		Pulmonary edema, pulmonary hemorrhage, hepatic and renal toxicity	Reacts with plastic; should be administered by means of a glass syringe. Should be protected from light.

IV, intravenous; NaCl, sodium chloride.

thiopental sodium or a curarizing agent in order to control the seizures. These agents should be administered only by an anesthesiologist.

Further diagnostic testing. After the seizures have been controlled, all efforts should be directed toward determining the etiology of the attack. If the patient has no known history of prior seizures, a CAT scan should be performed to rule out a mass lesion. An LP is indicated if meningitis is suspected.

Emotional Support

The family needs strong emotional support at this time to deal with their feelings. They may experience guilt, shame, or shock at the unpleasantness and suddenness of the seizures. They may be concerned about the possibility of social stigma for their child and themselves. It is important to help the family to identify these feelings and to discuss them in an honest and open way (*see* Chapter 1).

MENINGITIS

Meningitis is the most common infection of the CNS in infants and children. It is a serious, life-threatening infection with no preventive treatment. Early clinical assessment, recognition, and treatment determine the prognosis. Although meningitis can be caused by many organisms, bacterial or viral organisms are the most common causative agents.

Pathophysiology

The meninges are protective membranes that cover and support the brain and spinal cord. Meningitis occurs when bacterial or viral organisms enter the CNS and infect the meninges. These organisms frequently reach the meninges by way of the bloodstream, from another site of infection. This is why septicemia often accompanies meningitis. Meningitis may also be caused by direct invasion of organisms through the nose, ears, or sinuses, or the portal of entry may be provided by skull fracture or a surgical procedure. The meninges respond to this invasion by inflammation, an increase in the white blood cell (WBC) count, and the formation of exudate. The infection is spread downward into the spinal cord by CSF.

In addition to local inflammatory reactions, the meningeal infection causes an increased secretion of CSF, which contributes to the symptoms of increased ICP that are characteristic of meningitis. Because of the inflamed meninges, the brain becomes hyperemic and swollen, thereby further contributing to the increase in ICP.

The already increased ICP may be aggravated by an inappropriate release of ADH. Cerebral swelling is intensified by the fluid retention that results from syndrome of inappropriate ADH secretion, which frequently accompanies meningitis. This syndrome manifests itself in children with meningitis by hyponatremia and an increase in urine specific gravity and serum osmolality, all in the absence of dehydration (*see* p. 350).

Depending on the organism causing the infection, the brain can become covered with a thick exudate. If left untreated, the infection can extend to other areas of the brain, causing obstruction of the CSF passages, subdural effusions, brain abscess, and thrombosis of the meningeal veins. Meningitis caused by *Neisseria meningitidis* can cause disseminated intravascular coagulation, septicemia, and shock (*see* Chapter 7).

Etiology

Acute bacterial meningitis. The etiology of acute bacterial meningitis varies with the age and environment of the patient. Meningitis in newborns is frequently attributed to birth-related difficulties (e.g., prematurely ruptured membranes, prolonged labor, or excessive infant manipulation), and the causative organisms originate in maternal flora. The newborn's immature immune system, however, may also be a contributing factor. In the first 2 months of life, the organisms that most frequently cause meningitis are the gram-negative bacilli, especially group B streptococcus and *Escherichia coli*. (*E. coli* rarely causes meningitis after infancy.) Meningitis in the newborn is usually severe, and the outcome is poor.

The organisms that usually cause meningitis in children over the age of 2 years are *Hemophilus influenzae* type B, *Streptococcus pneumoniae*, and *N. meningitidis*. *H. influenzae* is the predominant organism in children between the ages of 2 months and 5 years. It is rare in children under the age of 2 months because they are passively protected by maternally acquired bactericidal substances, and it is uncommon in children over the age of 5 years because of acquired immunologic protection. *H. influenzae* appears to have a seasonal pattern, occurring primarily in the autumn and early winter. Although all other pathogens can occur at any time of the year, they seem related to sporadic epidemics.

N. meningitidis and *S. pneumoniae* occur more frequently in children over the age of 1 year. The risk of *N. meningitidis* and *S. pneumoniae* increases if children live in a crowded family environment. *S. pneumoniae* occurs more often and in a more severe form in children with immunoglobulin deficiencies, asplenia, or sickle cell disease.

During the neonatal period, meningitis occurs more frequently in males. After infancy, the incidence of meningitis is the same for males and females. Meningitis occurs most frequently between the ages of 6 and 12 months, and the mortality from meningitis is highest between birth and 4 years of age.

Aseptic meningitis. Aseptic (viral) meningitis is seen with relative frequency, and its course is usually self-limiting. The following enteroviruses are the most common agents: coxsackievirus, echovirus (enteric cytopathogenic human orphan virus), and mumps virus.

Enteroviruses, found in human feces and oropharyngeal secretions, are transmitted by direct contact. These viruses are more prevalent in the summer and autumn. Infants and young children are the most susceptible groups, with some children experiencing several separate episodes of viral meningitis from different causative viruses. Aseptic meningitis can occur at any age.

Clinical Presentation

Acute bacterial meningitis. The clinical presentation of acute bacterial meningitis depends on the age of the child and, to some extent, on the causative organism.

The classic symptoms associated with acute bacterial meningitis are often absent in infants and young children. Infants typically present with very subtle, nonspecific signs: poor sucking, difficulty with feeding, irritability, a high-pitched cry, and, sometimes, tense and bulging fontanel. Specific meningeal signs (fever, severe headache, and nuchal rigidity progressing to severe opisthotonus) are often absent, and thus it is difficult to diagnose the meningitis.

Older children present with the classic symptoms generally associated with meningitis (*see above*). These symptoms may be followed by changes in the child's level of consciousness. Seizures may often be the first indicators of this change in sensorium, followed by a deterioration of neurological status.

Meningitis caused by *N. meningitidis* is unique in that it frequently presents with a petechial or purpuric rash. This type of meningitis is usually accompanied by septic shock.

Aseptic meningitis. The onset of aseptic meningitis may be insidious or sudden. It will, however, usually exhibit an acute presentation. Infants and young children with aseptic meningitis generally do not look as ill as children who present with bacterial meningitis.

Infants and young children exhibit irritability when disturbed. Older children present with severe headache and a dulled sensorium. Both groups present with high fever, nausea, vomiting, nuchal rigidity, and general malaise. Children with aseptic meningitis rarely present with seizures.

Critical Care Management

Diagnosis. The definitive diagnosis of menigitis is made only after examination of the CSF. When meningitis is first suspected, an LP should be performed (to obtain CSF for analysis) before the administration of antibiotics. The LP permits measurement of CSF pressure, which is of no value in diagnosing meningitis, but which can indicate the degree of increased ICP.

The CSF is evaluated for appearance, Gram stain, culture, WBC count, protein, and glucose (Table 4-10). The culture analysis of CSF usually determines the type of organism causing the meningeal infection, with the exception of *N. meningitidis*, which frequently causes clinical symptomatology before the organisms actually invade the CSF. The appearance of the CSF should be colorless and clear. Although a traumatic LP can cause the CSF to be bloody, it should clear as successive samples are obtained. If the CSF remains bloody, it may be indicative of a CNS bleed.

Acute bacterial meningitis: Bacterial meningitis can cause the CSF to be cloudy or turbid in appearance because of the presence of microorganisms or a high WBC level. Normally, very few WBCs are present in CSF. A WBC count of greater than 500/mm^3 is indicative of an infection. (The WBCs usually seen with bacterial meningitis are polymorphonuclear cells.)

Meningitis causes the blood-brain barrier to become more permeable, thereby allowing large molecules to cross into the CSF. The increased permeability allows WBCs to enter the CSF, transporting protein molecules with them. This causes the CSF protein level to rise as the WBC count rises. The CSF protein level is further increased when WBCs disintegrate and release protein into the CSF.

In general, CSF glucose levels will vary with serum glucose levels. Bacterial meningitis causes CSF glucose levels to fall because of the glycolytic properties of the bacteria. In addition, "the large numbers of white blood cells that may be necessary to combat meningeal infection may, by their metabolic requirements, contribute to the decreased CSF glucose levels."[47]

Rapid identification of the organisms causing meningitis can be obtained by a

TABLE 4-10 Cerebrospinal Fluid Findings and Bacterial and Aseptic Meningitis

CSF analysis	Normal values		Meningitis values	
	Children <2 mo	Children >2 mo	Bacterial	Aseptic
WBC count	0–8/mm³	0–5/mm³	Greater than 500/mm³	50–500/mm³
WBC type	Mononuclear	Mononuclear	Polymorphonuclear	Mononuclear
Appearance	Clear	Clear	Cloudy or turbid	Clear to opalescent
Protein levels	15–150 mg/100 ml	15–45 mg/100 ml	Elevated	Normal to slightly elevated
Glucose levels	20–40 mg/100 ml	70–90 mg/100 ml	Decreased	Normal
CO_2 levels	25 mEq/liter	NA	NA	NA
pH	7.35–7.40	NA	NA	NA

CO_2, carbon dioxide; CSF, cerebrospinal fluid; NA, not applicable; WBC, white blood cell.

Gram stain. Although this will allow the administration of appropriate antibiotics early in the disease process, a CSF Gram stain should never be substituted for a complete CSF analysis.

Children with meningitis who receive antibiotic treatment before CSF is obtained for analysis will frequently have negative CSF cultures and Gram stains. Because it is necessary to determine the causative organism, however, a laboratory technique known as countercurrent immunoelectrophoresis (CIE) is used in these cases. CIE identifies the bacterial antigen in the child's blood, CSF, or urine, and does not require the presence of viable organisms. This technique, which takes only 30 minutes to perform, is an important diagnostic tool in the evaluation of children with pretreated meningitis.

Aseptic meningitis: The CSF in the child with aseptic meningitis is much closer to normal than the CSF in the child with bacterial meningitis. The appearance of the CSF can be clear to opalescent. It has very few WBCs, and they are usually mononuclear cells. The CSF protein and glucose levels in aseptic meningitis remain within normal parameters, and the Gram stain is negative.

The following diagnostic studies are also indicated with meningitis: blood cultures (to rule out septicemia); complete blood count; electrolyte evaluation; and nasopharyngeal and throat cultures (to help identify the causative organisms).

Clinical management
ACUTE BACTERIAL MENINGITIS

Acute bacterial meningitis requires prompt recognition and treatment in order to prevent long-term sequelae or death. After an LP is performed, large doses of antibiotics should be administered by IV infusion. The initial choice of antibiotics is dependent on the child's age and the probable causative organism. A delay in the delivery of treatment can drastically affect the outcome and increase the likelihood of sequelae. It is for these reasons that treatment is initiated before the specific organism is identified. Broad-spectrum antibiotics are used in order to provide the best possible coverage. Children under 2 months of age with a gram-negative infection are usually administered ampicillin and either gentamicin sulfate or kanamycin sulfate by IV infusion.

Children over 2 months of age are treated with ampicillin and chloramphenicol sodium succinate until the causative organism is positively identified. Although ampicillin provides broad-spectrum coverage, its widespread use has promoted the development of ampicillin-resistant strains of *H. influenzae.* It is for this reason that initial treatment must include chloramphenicol. Infants and children with suspected pneumococcal, streptococcal, or meningococcal meningitis are frequently started on penicillin. If not, when cultures confirm the diagnosis, antibiotic therapy is changed to include penicillin. Recommended dosages of these medications are listed in Table 4-11.

After bacterial meningitis is confirmed, infants under 2 months of age should receive IV antibiotics for at least 3 weeks. If therapy is discontinued before this time, these infants are at risk for relapse, which would require additional therapy. Children over 2 months of age should receive IV antibiotics for 1 to 2 weeks.

A repeat LP should be performed 24 to 36 hours after the institution of antibiotic therapy. Often, there is worsening in the CSF cell count and in the glucose and protein levels, but the CSF culture and Gram stain should be negative. Gram-negative organisms, frequently seen in infants, often require several days of antibiotic therapy before the CSF is sterilized. There is some controversy as to whether a third LP is necessary at the conclusion of IV antibiotic therapy. If the

TABLE 4-11   Recommended Dosages of Drugs Used in Treating Acute Bacterial Meningitis

Drug	Recommended Dosage*	
	Children <2 mo	Children >2 mo
Ampicillin	100 mg/kg/day, q 12 hours	150-400 mg/kg/day, q 4 hours
Penicillin	150,000 U/kg/day, q 8 hours	250,000–300,000 U/kg/day, q 4 hours (maximum: 20 million U/day)
Kanamycin sulfate	20 mg/kg/day, q 12 hours	30 mg/kg/day, q 8 hours
Gentamicin sulfate	5 mg/kg/day, q 12 hours	7.5 mg/kg/day, q 8 hours
Chloramphenicol sodium succinate	25 mg/kg/day, q 12 hours	50–100 mg/kg/day, q 6 hours

*Total daily dosages are provided, followed by the schedule of administration.

disease has had an uncomplicated course, a third LP may not be indicated. However, if the course has been complicated, it may be indicated. Results from the LP must be evaluated very carefully so as not to prolong therapy unnecessarily.

Infants and children with suspected or confirmed meningitis should remain in respiratory isolation for 24 hours after the initial dose of appropriate antibiotics is administered. Isolation must be enforced until the organism is identified. After this identification has occurred, the need for isolation is reevaluated because *N. meningitidis* is the only organism that requires isolation.

Neurological evaluations and the measurement of vital signs should be performed frequently, depending on the child's clinical condition. The neurological evaluation should include pupillary responses, level of consciousness, movement of extremities, degree of nuchal rigidity, and evaluation of the fontanel and the head circumference. A tense, bulging fontanel or an increasing head circumference can signal increased ICP, secondary to hydrocephalus or subdural effusion.

IV fluids should be monitored closely to correct any existing fluid deficit, but they should be calculated and administered at two-thirds of the maintenance level to limit cerebral edema. Weights, intake, and output must be measured accurately. The child should be assessed for signs of syndrome of inappropriate ADH secretion (*see* p. 350).

The infant or child with meningitis must be continually assessed for potential complications. During the early phase of meningitis, it is not uncommon for the infant or child to develop respiratory insufficiency or seizure activity. Supplemental O_2, intubation, and assisted ventilation are often necessary to ensure adequate oxygenation. Anticonvulsants are administered to control seizure activity (*see* p. 249). Signs of increasing ICP and impending septic shock should be continually monitored.

Comfort measures should be used to decrease general stimulation of the irritable infant or child. By lowering the bright lights in the hospital room and by speaking quietly and softly to the child, the nurse can decrease the external stimuli that can be irritating to the child with meningitis. The nurse should also find a comfortable position for the child. Often, a side-lying position is most comfortable because it does not aggravate the child's nuchal rigidity.

Parents should be instructed to observe the ill child's siblings and friends for signs and symptoms of concurrent cases of meningitis. Proper evaluation and treatment should be provided if the sibling or friend develops symptoms suggestive of meningitis. Prophylactic treatment for children intimately exposed to a positive case of *N. meningitidis* is recommended. The drug of choice is rifampin, 20 mg/kg/day, administered orally in divided doses every 12 to 24 hours. Recently, prophylactic treatment for children exposed to *H. influenzae* has gained popularity, with rifampin again being the drug of choice.[48]

Often, despite quick recognition of meningitis and the administration of IV antibiotics, children develop long-range sequelae. *H. influenzae* appears to be associated with more residual problems than other forms of bacterial meningitis: significant hearing loss, seizures requiring long-term therapy, paralysis, and partial blindness. Other residual problems that are seen less frequently are speech loss, behavioral problems, and mental retardation. The complications that are seen from other causative organisms are not as significant. Perhaps this is because, with other meningeal infections, the child either lives (normally) or dies.

Aseptic meningitis: Supportive care is the accepted mode of treatment for the child with aseptic meningitis. Often, the withdrawal of CSF during the LP alleviates the child's meningeal signs.

As with bacterial meningitis, vital signs and neurological status should be evaluated closely. If the child is febrile, measures to relieve or reduce the fever should be provided. These measures include the administration of antipyretic agents (aspirin 65 mg/kg/day or acetaminophen [Tylenol] 10 mg/kg, repeated every 4 to 6 hours) and sponging the child with tepid water if the temperature remains elevated despite medication. Care must be taken to avoid chilling the child because shivering increases the metabolic rate.

Before *N. meningitidis* is definitely ruled out, the child should be placed in respiratory isolation, and antibiotic therapy should be instituted.

Complications from aseptic meningitis are rare because this disease is usually self-limiting and is resolved within a week.

Emotional support. The anxiety of parents often heightens when they are told that their child has meningitis. Most parents still associate meningitis with death because of a lingering memory of preantibiotic times. The critical care team should provide the family with information on the plan of treatment and the child's prognosis. Precipitating events should be discussed immediately, with appropriate attention given to their severity. The family should be encouraged to verbalize any feelings or doubts they may have about their child's illness, especially with regard to the initial problems of this disease. Reinforcement of their ability to be good parents is often necessary.

BRAIN DEATH

Brain death (cerebral death) is generally accepted as one of the criteria of death by the medical and legal professions as well as by public opinion. Cerebral death involves permanent and irreversible death of the brainstem. Once this has occurred, further life support measures are futile and should be discontinued. It is now considered appropriate medical practice to identify brain death and withdraw support, thus sparing the family prolonged emotional trauma.

The need for a definition of cerebral death became apparent under two conditions. First, improvements in resuscitative measures sometimes led to only partial success, as in the case of an individual whose brain is irreversibly damaged but whose heart continues to beat as long as adequate respiration is supported. A situation such as this places a burden on the family, the hospital, and on those people awaiting a hospital bed. Second, with advances in organ transplantation, it became obvious that patients in irreversible coma could serve as organ donors.

Cerebral death is not only a medical issue, but also a religious, ethical, and legal one. For these reasons, brain death has been carefully studied, and several sets of criteria have been established.

Criteria for Brain Death

The Harvard Criteria.   In 1968, the Ad Hoc Committee of the Harvard Medical School published its four criteria of brain death.[49] The first criterion is unreceptiveness and unresponsiveness. The patient must exhibit complete unawareness of stimuli. Even the most intense stimulus must evoke no response whatsoever.

Second, there must be no movement or breathing. There must be observation of the patient by a physician for a minimum of 1 hour, during which time there is no sign of muscle movement, spontaneous ventilation, or response to stimuli. In order to assess for spontaneous respiratory effort, the mechanical ventilator should be discontinued for 3 minutes. The patient's CO_2 tension should be within normal limits and the patient should have been breathing room air for at least 10 minutes before discontinuation of the respirator. In order to meet this criterion, there must be total absence of ventilation during the 3-minute interval as well as no sign of respiratory effort.

The third criterion is absence of reflexes. The pupils must be fixed and dilated, and there must be no ocular movement (to either the doll's-eye maneuver or caloric stimulation), no corneal reflex, no cough or gag reflex, no evidence of postural activity, and no deep tendon reflexes.

Fourth, the patient must have an isoelectric EEG. A minimum of 10 minutes of recording time is preferred, and there must be no change in the EEG in response to noise or painful stimulation.

The committee also specified that neurological testing must be repeated within 24 hours of the first examination and that the results must be the same. To be valid, these neurological tests must be performed under two conditions: the absence of hypothermia in the patient below 32.2°C (90°F) and the absence of CNS depressants such as barbiturates.

The committee advocated that the family and all health care professionals involved in the patient's care should be informed of the determination of brain death and that the family should in no way be forced to make a decision regarding the determination. It also recommended that the patient be declared dead before discontinuation of any ventilatory support in order to avoid the legal implications of discontinuing support on a ventilator-dependent patient who is not dead.

A collaborative study.   A second set of criteria for brain death was devised in 1977 by a nationwide collaborative study conducted by the National Institute of Neurological Diseases and Stroke.[50] This study emphasized four prerequisites that must be met before the institution of brain death protocol: (1) the absence of sedative-drug intoxication, (2) normothermia, (3) the absence of cardiovascular shock, and (4) the absence of a repairable lesion.

According to this study, the criteria of cerebral unresponsiveness, apnea, and cerebroelectrical silence proved to be 99 percent accurate in diagnosing brain death. To improve this degree of accuracy, the study suggested the following additional standards, which have varying sensitivities as indicators of brainstem dysfunction: the absence of pupillary, corneal, oculoauditory (blinking to a clap), oculocephalic, oculovestibular, cough, gag, and swallowing reflexes. Although the addition of any or all of these factors to the basic criteria did not improve the accuracy of the final diagnosis, the study nevertheless advocated that the absence of these cephalic reflexes be made a component of the criteria.

The collaborative study indicated that spinal reflexes do not differentiate a dead brain from a dormant one and, therefore, should not be included in the criteria. The study did, however, suggest a safeguard: a confirmatory test with regard to CBF should be performed in all cases in which an early decision is desirable, especially if base-line criteria are subject to doubt.

Conference of Royal Colleges and Faculties of the United Kingdom.   In 1974, the Royal Colleges were asked to consider the diagnosis of death and developed diagnostic criteria for determining when death has occurred in those patients whose vital functions are being mechanically maintained.[51]

In general, the Royal Colleges of the United Kingdom concur with the Harvard Committee with regard to the definition of cerebral death. They have refined the Harvard Criteria, however, and believe their own criteria to be capable of distinguishing between those patients who have some chance for recovery and those for whom no such possibility exists.

The first item defined by the Royal Colleges committee concerned the circumstances under which the diagnosis of brain death should be considered. The patient should be in a deep coma, with no suspicion of its being drug related. The committee recommended an extensive study of the patient's drug history and the allowance of enough time for any drug effects to be excluded. Profound hypothermia should also be ruled out as a causative factor of deep coma, as should abnormalities in serum electrolytes, blood glucose, and acid-base balance.

Lack of spontaneous ventilation, immobility, and unresponsiveness must not be the result of neuromuscular blockade. The effects of these blocking agents can be ruled out by eliciting spinal reflexes or by demonstrating normal neuromuscular conduction with the use of a nerve stimulator. Hypnotic and narcotic effects should also be excluded as possible causes of respiratory failure.

In addition, there should be no doubt that the patient's condition is due to irreversible brain damage. A diagnosis of a disorder that has the potential of leading to brain death should be firmly established; however, if the patient has suffered from hypoxia or circulatory insufficiency (with an indefinable period of cerebral anoxia), it may take much longer to confirm the diagnosis of brain death.

Diagnostic testing to confirm cerebral death must include the absence of all brainstem reflexes on neurological examination. The examination should be repeated to ensure that no error has been made. The interval between examinations depends on the progress of the patient, but it should not exceed 24 hours. (Body temperature should not be less than 35°C (95°F) during the neurological examination.)

The committee has established that spinal cord functioning can persist even when brainstem functioning is destroyed; that EEGs, angiography, or CBF measurements are not necessary for the diagnosis of brain death; and that only in doubtful cases should a neurologist or neurosurgeon be consulted.

Summary. The goal of all these criteria is to demonstrate that the brain is unable to return to a functioning state, but the methods that are used vary widely. Some consider it enough to demonstrate a state in which return of bodily functioning has not occurred. Others believe in additional testing, such as EEGs or angiograms, to confirm the diagnosis. Still others advocate a set of criteria that would indicate, beyond doubt, widespread brain necrosis, which could only be shown on postmortem examination.

All criteria for brain death, however, agree on three basic predictors: coma with unresponsiveness, apnea, and absence of brainstem reflexes. Time intervals recommended for repetition of the neurological examination vary, as do recommendations for the use of further diagnostic testing. It is generally accepted that contrast angiography will definitely demonstrate obstruction of CBF, whereas the EEG could be falsely interpreted as isoelectric in some overdose states as well as in hypothermic states.

Other methods for testing CBF are being studied (e.g., nitrous oxide clearance, ultrasound, and Doppler signals). These techniques are still in an experimental stage and are not widely used as criteria for brain death.

There are three areas in which the issue of brain death has important implications: organ transplantation, withdrawal of life support therapy, and the law. It is generally agreed that organs removed from patients who are brain dead have a greater chance of providing successful functioning than organs that are removed after circulatory arrest. The majority of institutions have recourse to a safeguard on this issue: the declaration of death should be made by the physician whose primary concern is the donor patient and who is independent of the organ transplantation team. Although this is generally accepted practice, there is still controversy over whether the attending physician should be involved in asking the family for organ donations.

The timing for withdrawal of life support systems has been well defined and is crucial for legal reasons: death should be declared before the withdrawal of any therapy. There have been enough court cases to establish the precedent of cerebral death warranting withdrawal of support.

Family Support

This is a most difficult time for families. The early diagnosis of cerebral death and the subsequent withdrawal of support may protect the family from prolonged agony and false hope. It is firmly recommended that the burden of the decision to withdraw support not be placed on family members.

The nurse is usually present when parents are informed of the diagnosis of brain death and can provide some emotional support (*see* Chapter 1). The nurse should also remain with the family while they visit their child for the last time, but should give them time alone with their child if they so desire. Some parents feel more comfortable saying their good-byes before the withdrawal of support and then going home. In these cases, the nurse should assure them that their child will not be left alone during the withdrawal of support and for the subsequent period in which the heart is still functioning. Families often ask the nurse whether they should go home or stay with the child. Nurses can best help parents by not imposing their own values on them and by assuring them there is no correct answer. Each family must act according to what is best for them.

Implications for the Nursing Staff

This is also a time of emotional turmoil for the nursing staff, which has invested much time and energy into the care of the child. The nurse is always present when support is withdrawn. It is the nurse who is left alone with the child while the heart slowly dies. If the family is there, the nurse remains with them to provide emotional support. In addition to supporting the child and the family, the nurse must perform postmortem care, which can be a painful experience.

It is sometimes difficult for nurses to accept a family's decision to stay with their child or to leave. Nurses must suppress those feelings that arise from their own value systems (if different from those of the family) and support the family's decision. At times, a nurse may not be ready to accept the diagnosis of cerebral death. This denial only causes more stress in an already stressed nurse.

Depending on the relationship between the nurse and the family, it may be comforting to share the grief with the family. Often, the nurse receives emotional support from other nurses. Nurses should offer assistance to their co-worker in the delivery of postmortem care, which should not be performed solely by the nurse who has provided care to the child. The staff members usually talk about the death among themselves. This offers the primary nurse the opportunity to cry and/or ventilate feelings. Brain death is perhaps the most difficult of deaths with which to deal, and it is therefore imperative that emotional support systems be readily available (*see* Chapter 9).

REFERENCES

1. Rudy.
2. Jennet and Teasdale.
3. Obrist et al.
4. Raphaely et al.
5. Bricolo et al.
6. Plum and Posner. 43–44.
7. Plum and Posner. 42.
8. Starr.
9. Bruce et al. (1978)
10. Boutros et al.
11. Chaves-Carballo et al.
12. Partin et al.
13. Lovejoy et al.
14. Glasgow et al.
15. Samaha et al.
16. Gall et al.
17. Gobiet.
18. Bruce et al. (1979) (*Child's Brain*)
19. Bruce et al. (1981) 137.
20. Bruce et al. (1979) (Grant proposal)
21. Koos and Miller. 17.
22. Koos and Miller. 18.
23. Hausman. 8–12.
24. Damon and Taylor.
25. Schut and Rosenstock.
26. Koos and Miller. 305.
27. Koos and Miller. 103.
28. Koos and Miller. 89.
29. Koos and Miller. 93.
30. Koos and Miller. 175.
31. Koos and Miller. 227.
32. Stein and Wolpert. Part I.
33. Michelsen.
34. Mori et al.
35. Perret and Nishioka.
36. LeBlanc et al.
37. Terbrugge et al.
38. Stein and Wolpert. Part II.
39. Drake.
40. Olivecrona and Riives.
41. Troupp et al.
42. Trumpy and Eldevik.
43. Sing Cho So.
44. Kunc.
45. Mullen et al.
46. Rothner and Erenberg.
47. Blount et al.
48. Daum et al.
49. Report of the Ad Hoc Commitee of the Harvard Medical School.
50. Collaborative study.
51. Report of the Conference of Royal Colleges.

BIBLIOGRAPHY

Apuzzo, M. L. J., K. M. A. Sheikh, J. S. Heiden, M. W. Weiss, and T. Kurze. 1979. Definition of cellular immune responses to brain antigens in human head trauma. *Journal of Neurosurgery.* **51:**317–322.

Baliga, R., L. E. Fleishmann, C. Chang, A. P. Sarnaik, A. K. Bidani, and E. L. Arcinue. 1979. Acute renal failure in Reye's syndrome. *American Journal of Diseases of Children.* **133:**1009–1013.

Belkengren, R. P. and S. Sapola. 1981. Reye's syndrome: clinical guidelines for practitioners in ambulatory care. *Pediatric Nursing.* **7:**26–28.

Berenstein, A. 1980. Flow-controlled silicone fluid embolization. *American Journal of Roentgenology.* **134:**1213–1218.

Berman, W., F. Pizzi, L. Schut, R. Raphaely, and P. Holtzapple. 1975. The effects of exchange transfusion on intracranial pressure in patients with Reye's syndrome. *Journal of Pediatrics.* **87:**887–891.

Black, P. M. 1978. Brain death. Part I. *New England Journal of Medicine.* **299:**338–344.

Black, P. M. 1978. Brain death. Part II. *New England Journal of Medicine.* **299:**393–401.

Blount, M., A. Kinney, and K. Donohue. 1974. Obtaining and analyzing cerebrospinal fluid. *The Nursing Clinics of North America.* **9:**593–610.

Bobo, R. C., W. K. Schubert, J. C. Partin, and J. S. Partin. 1975. Reye syndrome: treatment by exchange transfusion with special reference to the 1974 epidemic in Cincinatti, Ohio. *Journal of Pediatrics.* **87:**881–886.

Boutros, A. R., S. Esfandiari, J. P. Orlowski, and J. S. Smith. 1980. Reye syndrome: a predictably curable disease. *Pediatric Clinics of North America.* **27:**539–551.

Bricolo, A., S. Turazzi, A. Alexandre, and N. Rizzato. 1977. Decerebrate rigidity in acute head injury. *Journal of Neurosurgery.* **47:**680–698.

Bruce, D. A., R. C. Raphaely, A. I. Goldberg, R. A. Zimmerman, L. T. Bilaniuk, L. Schut, and D. E. Kuhl. 1979. The pathophysiology, treatment, and outcome following severe head injury in children. *Child's Brain.* **5:**174–191.

Bruce, D. A., L. Schut, L. A. Bruno, J. H. Wood and L. N. Sutton. 1978. Outcome following severe head injuries in children. *Journal of Neurosurgery.* **48:**679–688.

Bruce, D. A., L. N. Sutton, and L. Schut. 1981. Acute brain swelling and cerebral edema in children. *In* de Vlieger, M., S. A. deLange, and J. W. Beks, editors. Brain Edema. 1981. John Wiley & Sons, Inc., New York.

Bruce, D. A., D. Swedlow, R. Raphaely, W. Obrist, and T. Atkins. 1979. The pathophysiology and consequences of acute head injury in children. From a grant proposal. Section IV. 205–242.

Chaves-Carballo, E., G. A. Carter, and D. A. Wiebe. 1979. Triglyceride and cholesterol concentrations in whole serum and in serum lipoproteins in Reye syndrome. *Pediatrics.* **64:**592–597.

Collaborative Study. 1977. An appraisal of the criteria of cerebral death: a summary statement. *(JAMA) Journal of the American Medical Association.* **237:**982–986.

Cooper, P. R., S. Moody, W. K. Clark, J. Kirkpatrick, K. Maravilla, A. L. Gould, and W. Drane. 1979. Dexamethasone and severe head injury. *Journal of Neurosurgery.* **52:**705–708.

Cromwell, L. D., and A. B. Harris. 1980. Treatment of cerebral arteriovenous malformations: a combined neurosurgical and neuroradiological approach. *Journal of Neurosurgery.* **52:**705–708.

Damon, J. and L. F. Taylor. 1980. Brain tumors in children. *Nursing Clinics of North America.* **15:**99–113.

Daum, R., M. Glode, D. Goldmann et al. 1981. Rifampin chemoprophylaxis for household contacts of patients with invasive infection due to h. influenzae type B. *Journal of Pediatrics.* **98:**485–491.

DeVivo, D. C., J. P. Keating, and M. W. Haymond. 1975. Reye syndrome: results of intensive supportive care. *Journal of Pediatrics.* **87:**875–880.

Drake, C. G. 1979. Cerebral arteriovenous malformations: considerations for and experience with surgical treatment in 166 cases. *Clinical Neurosurgery.* **26:**145–208.

Ellis, G. H., L. D. Mirkin, and M. C. Mills. 1979. Pancreatitis and Reye's syndrome. *American Journal of Diseases of Children*. **133**:1014–1016.

Enevoldsen, E. M., and F. T. Jensen. 1978. Autoregulation and CO_2 responses of cerebral blood flow in patients with severe head injury. *Journal of Neurosurgery*. **48**:689–703.

Feign, R., and P. Dodge. 1976. Bacterial meningitis: newer concepts of pathophysiology and neurological sequelae. *Pediatric Clinics of North America*. **23**:541–556.

Friedman, P., J. L. Salazar, and O. Sugar. 1978. Embolization and surgical excision of giant arteriovenous malformation. *Surgical Neurology*. **9**:149–152.

Gaddy, D. 1981. Meningitis in the pediatric population. *The Nursing Clinics of North America*. **15**:83–97.

Gall, D. G., E. Cutz, H. J. McClung, and M. L. Greenberg. 1975. Acute liver disease and encephalopathy mimicking Reye Syndrome. *Journal of Pediatrics*. **87**:869–874.

Gilder, S. S. B. 1968. Twenty-second World Medical Assembly: death and the W.M.A. *British Medical Journal*. **3**:493–494.

Glasgow, A. M., R. B. Cotton, and K. Dhiensire. 1972. Reye's syndrome: Blood ammonia and consideration of the nonhistologic diagnosis. *American Journal of Diseases of Children*. **124**:827.

Gobiet, W. The influence of various doses of dexamethasone on intracranial pressure in patients with severe head injury. *Stadium Anaesthetist*. **26**:187–195. (Abstract).

Gudeman, S. K., J. D. Miller and D. P. Becker. 1979. Failure of high-dose steroid therapy to influence intracranial pressure in patients with severe head injury. *Journal of Neurosurgery*. **51**:301–306.

Guyton, A. C. 1981. Textbook of Medical Physiology. W. B. Saunders Co., Philadelphia. Sixth edition.

Hahn, J. F. 1980. Cerebral edema and neurointensive care. *Pediatric Clinics of North America*. **27**:587–592.

Hausman, K. A. 1978. Brain tumors in children. *Journal of Neurosurgical Nursing*. **10**:8–12.

Hooshmand, H. 1974. Toxic effects of anticonvulsants: general principles. *Pediatrics*. **53**:551–556.

Jennet, B. and G. Teasdale. 1977. Aspects of coma after severe head injury. *Lancet*. **1**:878–881.

Kerber, C. W., W. O. Bank, and L. D. Cromwell. 1979. Calibrated leak balloon microcatheter: a device for arterial exploration and occlusive therapy. *American Journal of Roentgenology*. **132**:207–212.

Kooi, K. A. 1978. Fundamentals of Electroencephalography. Harper & Row, Publishers, Inc., New York. Second edition.

Koos, W. T. and M. H. Miller. 1971. Intracranial Tumors of Infants and Children. C. V. Mosby Co., St. Louis.

Krugman, S., R. Ward, and S. Katz. 1977. Infectious Diseases of Children; C. V. Mosby Co. St. Louis Sixth edition.

Kunc, Z. 1974. Surgery of arteriovenous malformations in the speech and motor-sensory regions. *Journal of Neurosurgery*. **40**:293–303.

Kutt, H. 1974. The use of blood levels of antiepileptic drugs in clinical practice. *Pediatrics*. **53**:557–560.

Lalli, S. 1978. The complete Swan-Ganz. *RN*. **41**(*9*):3–15.

Lamas, E., R. D. Lobato, J. Espanza, and L. Escudero. 1977. Dural posterior fossa AVM producing raised sagittal sinus pressure. *Journal of Neurosurgery*. **46**:804–810.

Langfitt, T. W. 1978. Measuring the outcome from head injuries. *Journal of Neurosurgery*. **48**:673–677.

LeBlanc, R., R. Ethier, and J. R. Little. 1979. Computerized tomography findings in arteriovenous malformations of the brain. *Journal of Neurosurgery*. **51**:765–772.

Levin, D. L, F. C. Morriss, and G. C. Moore, editors. 1979. A Practical Guide to Pediatric Intensive Care. C. V. Mosby Co., St. Louis.

Linnemann, C. C., C. A. Kauffman, L. Shea, G. M. Schiff, J. C. Partin, and W. K. Schubert. 1974. Association of Reye's syndrome with viral infection. *Lancet*. **2**:179–182.

Lombroso, C. T. The treatment of status epilepticus. *Pediatrics.* **53**:536–540.

Long, D. M., E. L. Seljeskog, S. N. Chou, and L. A. French. 1974. Giant arteriovenous malformations of infancy and childhood. *Journal of Neurosurgery.* **40**:304–312.

Lovejoy, F. H., A. L. Smith, M. J. Bresnan, J. N. Wood, D. I. Victor, and P. C. Adams. 1974. Clinical staging in Reye syndrome. *American Journal of Diseases of Children.* **128**(7):36–41.

Menkes, J. H. 1980. Management of status epilepticus. *Pediatrics in Review.* **1**:219–220.

Michelsen, W. J. 1979. Natural history and pathophysiology of arteriovenous malformations. *Clinical Neurosurgery.* **26**:307–313.

Mills, G. C. 1980. Preparing children and parents for cerebral computerized tomography. *Maternal Child Nursing.* **5**:403–407.

Mitchell, P. H. and N. Mauss. 1976. Intracranial pressure: fact and fancy. *Nursing 76.* **6**:53–57.

Mori, K., T. Murata, N. Hashimoto, and H. Handa. 1980. Clinical analysis of arteriovenous malformations in children. *Child's Brain.* **6**:13–25.

Mullen, S., F. D. Brown, and N. J. Patronas. 1979. Hyperemic and ischemic problems of surgical treatment of arteriovenous malformations. *Journal of Neurosurgery.* **51**:757–764.

Murray, J., P. Fleming, J. Weber, J. Hsuen, R. Bonnatyne, and C. Anglen. 1974. The continuing problem of purulent meningitis in infants and children. *Pediatric Clinics of North America.* **21**:967–980.

Obrist, W. D., T. A. Gennarelli, H. Segawa, C. A. Dolinskas, and T. W. Langfitt. 1979. Relation of cerebral blood flow to neurological status and outcome in head-injured patients. *Journal of Neurosurgery.* **51**:292–300.

Olivecrona, H. and J. Riives. 1948. Arteriovenous aneurysms of the brain: their diagnosis and treatment. *Archives of Neurology and Psychiatry.* **59**:567–602.

Partin, J. C., W. K. Schubert, and J. S. Partin. 1971. Mitochondrial ultrastructure in Reye's syndrome (encephalopathy and fatty degeneration of the viscera). *New England Journal of Medicine* **285**:1330–1343.

Patterson, R. H. and R. M. Voorhies. 1978. Surgical approaches to intracranial and intraspinal arteriovenous malformations. *Clinical Neurosurgery.* **25**:412–424.

Perret, G. and H. Nishioka. 1979. Report on the cooperative study of intracranial aneurysms and subarachnoid hemorrhage. Section VI. Arteriovenous malformations. *Journal of Neurosurgery.* **51**:467–489.

Plum, F., and J. B. Posner. 1980. The Diagnosis of Stupor and Coma. F. A. Davis Co., Philadelphia. Third edition.

Pool, J. L. and D. G. Potts. 1965. Aneurysms and Arteriovenous Anomalies of the Brain: Diagnosis and Treatment. Harper & Row, Publishers, Inc., New York.

Price, S. A. and L. M. Wilson. 1982. Pathophysiology Clinical Concepts of Disease Processes. McGraw-Hill Book Co., New York. Second edition.

Quesenbury, J. H. and P. Lembright. 1969. Observations and care for patients with head injuries. *Nursing Clinics of North America.* **4**:237–247.

Raphaely, R. C., D. B. Swedlow, J. J. Downs, and D. A. Bruce. 1980. Management of severe pediatric head trauma. *Pediatric Clinics of North America.* **27**:715–727.

Report of the Ad Hoc Committee of the Harvard Medical School. 1968. A definition of irreversible coma. *(JAMA) Journal of the American Medical Association.* **205**:85–88.

Report of the Conference of Royal Colleges and Faculties of the United Kingdom. 1976. Diagnosis of brain death. *Lancet.* **2**:1069–1070.

Reye, R. D. K. 1963. Encephalopathy and fatty degeneration of the viscera: A disease entity in childhood. *Lancet.* **2**:749–752.

Rosman, N. P. 1974. Increased intracranial pressure in children. *Pediatric Clinics of North America.* **21**:483–499.

Rothner, A. D. and G. Erenberg. 1980. Status epilepticus. *Pediatric Clinics of North America.* **27**:593–602.

Rudy, E. 1977. Early omen of cerebral disaster. *Nursing 77.* **7**:59–62.

Samaha, E. F., E. Glau, and J. L. Beradinelli. 1974. Reye's syndrome: clinical diagnosis and treatment with peritoneal dialysis. *Pediatrics.* **53**:336.

Schmidt, R. P. and B. J. Wilder. 1968. Epilepsy. F. A. Davis Co., Philadelphia.

Schut, L. and J. G. Rosenstock. 1974. Treatment of intracranial neoplasms in children. *Seminars in Oncology.* **1**:9–14.

Sibley, W. A. 1974. Diagnosis and treatment of epilepsy: overview and general principles. *Pediatrics.* **53**:531–535.

Shapiro, H. M. 1977. Physiologic and pharmacologic regulation of cerebral blood volume. *American Society of Anesthesiologists Refresher Course in Anesthesiology.* **5**:161–177.

Silverman, D., M. G. Saunders, R. S. Schwab, and R. L. Masland. 1969. Cerebral death and the electroencephologram. *(JAMA) Journal of the American Medical Association.* **209**:1505–1509.

Sing Cho So. 1978. Cerebral arteriovenous malformations in children. *Child's Brain.* **4**:242–250.

Starr, A. 1976. Auditory brain-stem responses in brain death. *Brain.* **99**:543–554.

Stein, B. M. and S. M. Wolpert. 1980. Arteriovenous malformations of the brain: current concepts and treatment. Part I. *Archives of Neurology.* **37**:1–5.

Stein, B. M. and S. M. Wolpert. 1980. Arteriovenous malformations of the brain: current concepts and treatment. Part II. *Archives of Neurology.* **37**:69–75.

Terbrugge, K., G. Scotti, R. Ethier, D. Melancon, S. Tchang, and C. Milner. 1977. Computed tomography in intracranial arteriovenous malformations. *Radiology.* **122**:703–705.

Troupp, H., I. Marttala, and V. Halonen. 1970. Arteriovenous malformations of the brain: prognosis without operation. *Acta Neurochirurgica.* **22**:125–128.

Trumpy, J. H. and P. Eldevik. 1977. Intracranial arteriovenous malformations: conservative or surgical treatment? *Surgical Neurology.* **8**:171–175.

Vaughan, V. C., and R. J. McKay, editors. 1979. Nelson Textbook of Pediatrics. W. B. Saunders Co., Philadelphia. Eleventh edition.

Venes, J. L., B. A. Shaywitz, and D. D. Spencer. 1978. Management of severe cerebral edema in the metabolic encephalopathy of Reye-Johnson syndrome. *Journal of Neurosurgery.* **48**:903–915.

Ventureyra, E. C. G., L. P. Ivan, and N. Nabavi. 1978. Deep seated giant arteriovenous malformations in infancy. *Surgical Neurology.* **10**:365–370.

Walter, A. E. 1977. An appraisal of the criteria of cerebral death: A summary statement. Report of a collaborative study. *(JAMA) Journal of the American Medical Association.* **237**:982–986.

Warwick, R. and P. L. Williams, Editors. 1973. The Gray's Anatomy. W. B. Saunders Co., Philadelphia. 35th edition.

Whaley, L. F. and D. L. Wong. 1979. Nursing Care of Infants and Children. C. V. Mosby Co., St. Louis.

CHAPTER 5

NEUROMUSCULAR DISEASES

Janet A. Koehler
with Susan B. De Jong

Neuromuscular disease is the collective term used to describe disorders that involve a disruption of any segment of the neuromuscular pathway — from the anterior horn cell, through the peripheral motor and/or peripheral sensory nerves and the neuromuscular junction, to the innervated muscle fibers. In general, these disorders are progressive and chronic in nature, but they may present acutely, thus requiring intensive care.

This chapter will focus on the pediatric age group (infancy to adolescence) in acute crisis from neuromuscular dysfunction. Acute crisis in neuromuscular disease may be described as any acute condition in which the child is in danger of respiratory failure secondary to muscle weakness or paralysis.

Two disorders of the neuromuscular junction (myasthenia gravis and infant botulism) and one disorder of the peripheral nervous system (Guillain-Barré syndrome) will be discussed. The emphasis will be on the acute presentation, pathophysiology, diagnostic criteria, and critical care management of these disorders.

SELECTED ASPECTS OF NEUROMUSCULAR PHYSIOLOGY

The Motor Pathway

The structure of the neuromuscular system involves both upper and lower motor units (Fig. 5-1). The upper motor unit extends from the cerebral cortex to the anterior horn cell in the spinal cord. The upper motor unit consists of nerves and their axons originating in the cerebral cortex. The nerves conduct impulses from the motor cortex to the pyramidal tract (also known as the corticospinal tract). The pyramidal tract is an anteriorly descending tract originating from the motor cortex and extending through the brainstem to the gray matter of the spinal cord. The function of the pyramidal tract is to carry impulses for voluntary movements. The extrapyramidal tract, which includes the basal ganglia and the cerebellum, is also part of the upper motor unit. The functions of the extrapyramidal tract include control of repetitive motor acts and coordination of movement.

In general, disorders of the upper motor unit (pyramidal and extrapyramidal

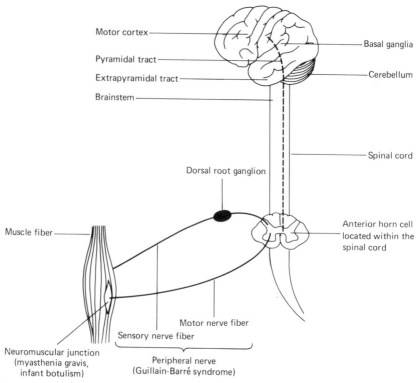

Figure 5-1. Schematic diagram of the upper and lower motor pathways.

tracts) disrupt voluntary and reflex motor functions. Frequently, upper motor lesions enhance involuntary and reflex activity as a result of the loss of ability by the central nervous system (CNS) to inhibit these actions.

The lower motor unit functionally consists of the anterior horn cell (also called the lower motor neuron), its axons, peripheral nerves, the neuromuscular junction, and the innervated muscle fiber itself. Each lower motor neuron and its group of innervated muscle fibers is known as a motor unit. Lesions of the lower motor neuron lead to disruption or loss of both voluntary and involuntary motor activities.

The Neuron and Peripheral Nerve Structure

A neuron consists of the nerve cell body and its processes, the axons and dendrites (Fig. 5-2). The nerve cell body is a diamond-shaped structure that maintains the viability of the axons. The processes are cytoplasmic extensions of the nerve cell body. Axons transmit impulses from the cell body to other nerve cells or to motor muscle fibers. Dendrites conduct impulses to the cell body.

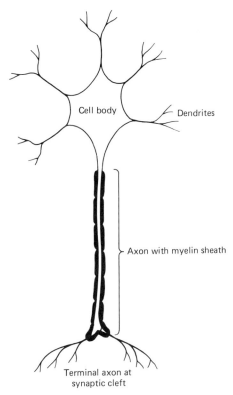

Figure 5-2. Schematic diagram of a neuron and its processes.

A myelinated axon consists of a central core or axis cylinder, a myelin sheath, and a neurilemma containing Schwann cells. (Fig. 5-3). The average length of an axon is 10 millimeters.[1] Myelin encompasses the entire axon and is divided into segments, at 1-millimeter intervals, by the nodes of Ranvier. When present, myelin (a fatty, insulating substance) determines the velocity of nerve impulse conduction. The neurilemma is a thin membrane that forms the outermost covering of the axon and myelin sheath. All peripheral nerves have a neurilemma, which is

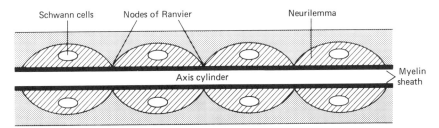

Figure 5-3. Schematic diagram of a myelinated axon.

necessary for peripheral nerve regeneration. Schwann cells, located within the neurilemma, produce myelin.

Nerve fibers, consisting of the axon and its sheath, are either myelinated or nonmyelinated. Most peripheral nerves are myelinated, whereas nerve fibers of the gray matter of the CNS are mostly nonmyelinated. The loss of myelin (demyelination) results in the loss of nerve impulse transmission.

The primary function of neurons is to conduct impulses along the nerve pathways. Sensory (afferent) neurons conduct impulses from the skin surface to the spinal cord and the CNS. Motor (efferent) neurons conduct impulses from the CNS and the spinal cord to the muscles and glands. Internuncial neurons conduct impulses between afferent and efferent neurons within the CNS.

Peripheral Nerve Pathways

A peripheral nerve is formed of axons originating in (1) cell bodies within the CNS (anterior horn cell gray matter), or (2) sensory ganglia (dorsal root ganglia), or (3) autonomic ganglia outside the CNS. Three types of fibers function within each peripheral nerve: (1) sensory fibers from the dorsal root ganglia, (2) motor fibers from the anterior horn cells, and (3) autonomic fibers from cell bodies within the CNS and the autonomic ganglia (Fig. 5-4).[2]

The motor and autonomic fibers form the anterior (ventral) root and the sensory fibers form the posterior (dorsal) root. The anterior and posterior roots join to form the peripheral nerve, which contains axons with sensory, motor, and autonomic functions.

Nerve Impulse Transmission

The integrity of the neuromuscular system depends on nerve impulse transmission to the muscles. Incomplete or disrupted transmission leads to muscle paralysis or weakness.

Nerve impulses are propagated disturbances (action potentials) that are transmitted along the axon to its termination in muscle, effector organ, or other nerve cell body. The stimulus for nerve impulse transmission may be electrical (from adjacent nodes of Ranvier), chemical (from one neuron to another across a synaptic cleft), or mechanical (from electrodes placed on the nerve). The conduction of

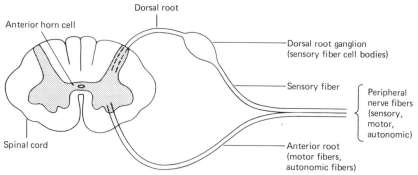

Figure 5-4. Schematic diagram of the peripheral nerve pathway.

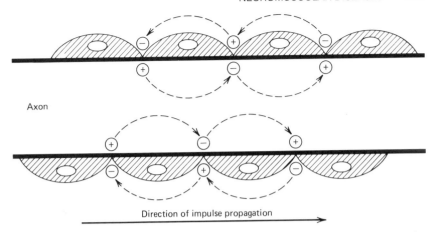

Axon

Direction of impulse propagation

Figure 5-5. Saltatory conduction in a myelinated axon. The broken line represents the local current (the movement of positive charge). The current causes a change in the cell membrane permeability resulting in depolarization. The depolarization at one node of Ranvier generates another impulse to the adjacent node.

nerve impulses is a self-propagating process, occurring at a constant velocity, and requiring the expenditure of energy by the nerve. Conduction velocity is faster in myelinated fibers than in nonmyelinated fibers. Conduction along myelinated axons is achieved through saltatory conduction in which the nerve impulse jumps from one node of Ranvier to another. The mechanism for this transmission is the presence of a local electrical current that circulates from the node that the impulse has reached and returns to the original node in the extracellular fluid. This current causes a change in membrane permeability, resulting in depolarization, which then generates another impulse to the adjacent node (Fig. 5-5).[1]

Electrical disturbances (called nerve impulses or action potentials) travel along the axons to a muscle, effector organ, or other nerve cell bodies. When an impulse moves along a myelinated fiber, it "jumps" from one node of Ranvier to another. This type of transmission is electrical in nature (saltatory conduction). The cause of this transmission is a local current that circulates from the point that the impulse has reached through the next node, causing a change in membrane permeability, which generates another impulse (Fig. 5-5).[1]

The nerve cell membrane is polarized at rest (resting membrane potential) because of the exterior and interior concentrations of ions. The exterior of the cell membrane is positively charged, whereas the interior net charge is negative. The net charges along the membrane are dependent on the efflux and influx of sodium (Na^+) and potassium (K^+) ions. The movement of these ions depends on the sodium and potassium pump.

Stimulation of the cell membrane will cause an increased permeability to sodium, causing extracellular sodium to move into the cell, thereby reversing the resting cell membrane potential. This change (depolarization) results in a negatively charged extracellular space and a positively charged intracellular space. This situation permits an action potential (or flow of electrically charged ions) to pass down the axon (Fig. 5-6). When the inside of the nerve fiber has attained a high level of positive charge, the membrane again becomes impermeable to

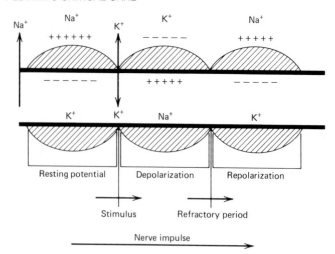

Figure 5-6. Nerve impulse transmission. The nerve cell membrane is polarized with the interior net charge negative and the exterior net charge positive (resting membrane potential). Following stimulation, depolarization takes place with the reversal of net charges, the influx of sodium ions (Na^+) and the efflux of potassium ions (K^+). The impulse travels down the axon. A refractory period precedes repolarization in which electronegativity is reestablished interiorly.

sodium, and potassium diffuses back into the cell. This process (repolarization) reestablishes intracellular electronegativity.

The nerve fiber must repolarize before the next impulse transmission. The duration of the refractory period, or the time between depolarization and repolarization, varies according to the size of the nerve fiber. In addition, the refractory period may be absolute or relative. During the absolute refractory period, no response by the nerve can be elicited, even in the presence of a strong stimulus. In the relative refractory period, a nerve response may be stimulated, but the stimulus must be greater than that needed to stimulate a resting nerve.

The diameter of the nerve fiber and the thickness of the myelin sheath determine the velocity of nerve impulse conduction. As the diameter of the nerve fiber increases, the rate of conduction may increase to a velocity of up to 120 m/sec or more.[1]

The Neuromuscular Junction

Nerve impulse transmission to muscle fiber takes place at the neuromuscular junction by means of a chemical mechanism. The impulse, traveling along the axon by an electrical process, must be transmitted across a synaptic cleft to the motor end plate of the muscle fiber.

The neuromuscular junction is a complex structure that consists of the motor nerve axon and axon terminals, the motor end plate (the flat area on the muscle fiber where the motor nerve innervates), the synaptic cleft (the area of chemical tranmission between the axon terminals and the motor end plate), synaptic vesicles, which store acetylcholine (ACH), and ACH receptor sites on the motor end plate (Fig. 5-7).

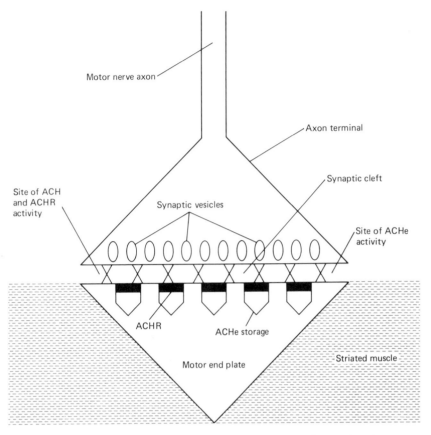

Figure 5-7. Schematic diagram of the neuromuscular junction. A nerve impulse causes the synaptic vesicles to release acetylcholine (ACH), which binds to the ACH receptor (ACHR) sites in the motor end plate. Acetylcholinesterase (ACHe) destroys ACH at the neuromuscular junction, causing termination of the nerve impulse.

When the nerve impulse reaches the axon terminals, ACH is released by the rupturing of the synaptic vesicles. ACH is a chemical neurotransmitter that alters the permeability of the muscle cell membrane by making it permeable to sodium. ACH diffuses through the synaptic cleft to the ACH receptors at the motor end plate of the muscle.

As ACH combines with its receptor site, there is a transient increase in muscle cell permeability to sodium. This creates an electrical action potential as the net charge of the cell becomes positive. The muscle cell membrane depolarizes, followed by depolarization of the entire muscle fiber. The end result is muscular contraction.[1] The chemical transmission ceases (1) as ACH diffuses away from the junction and (2) through the action of acetylcholinesterase, an enzyme produced at the motor end plate. It hydrolyzes ACH and allows the muscle cell membrane to return to its resting potential.

Any disruption along the transmission pathway at the neuromuscular junction results in neuromuscular fatigue (the inability to sustain muscular contraction).

NURSING ASSESSMENT OF THE NEUROMUSCULAR SYSTEM

The primary indicator of neuromuscular disease is weakness. The origin and progression of weakness can be ascertained through a detailed history obtained from the parents of the infant or child. The physical examination of the child will accurately outline the extent of weakness, further deterioration, or regression of symptoms. The infant and older child need to be evaluated in different ways because of the differences in normal growth and development.

Weakness

Weakness, or diminished strength in a specific muscle or group of muscles, is the result of dysfunction in either the upper or lower motor units. The neuromuscular examination should determine if the weakness is upper or lower motor unit in origin, and a general physical examination will aid in determining if a systemic illness, with associated weakness, is present.

Upper motor unit disease is characterized by increased deep tendon reflexes, Babinski's sign, ankle or patellar clonus, persistent infantile reflexes, and spasticity. There is no muscular atrophy or fasciculation. Hypotonia is the most common sign of upper motor unit disease in infants. The weakness is usually mild and involves muscles of the affected area (e.g., trapezius or deltoid).[3]

Lower motor unit disease is characterized by absent or decreased deep tendon reflexes, profound weakness, hypotonia, and muscular atrophy and fasciculation.[3] (Fasciculations are rarely seen in infants because of overlying subcutaneous fat.) Table 5-1 summarizes the characteristics of upper and lower motor unit disease.

Whether weakness is acute or chronic can be determined by obtaining a detailed history from either the parents or from the older child or adolescent. In the newborn, weakness is characterized by a weak cry, poor sucking reflex, difficulty with breathing, decreased body movement, and hypotonia ("floppy infant"). After the neonatal period, delayed development of motor skills is the most common manifestation of weakness.

Whether the onset of weakness is acute or progressive gives insight into the origin of the weakness. Weakness presenting acutely indicates vascular or traumatic origins. Weakness presenting insidiously over a day to several days indicates an exogenous or endogenous toxic process, an electrolyte imbalance, or an infectious process. Questioning should focus on (1) exposure to infectious processes such as mumps, measles, or recent infection, (2) exposure to specific toxins, and (3) possible circumstances leading to electrolyte imbalance. Weakness associated with a progression over several weeks to months is associated with diseases of a neoplastic, degenerative, or metabolic nature. Factors that may aggravate the weakness should also be explored (e.g., time of day, physical exertion, muscle cramps or twitching after exercise). These factors will aid in the determination of whether the weakness is of acute or chronic origin.

Weakness is further defined as static, progressive, or episodic. For the infant, a review of baby pictures and records is helpful in determining if the process is

TABLE 5-1 Characteristics of Upper and Lower Motor Unit Disease

Upper motor unit disease	Lower motor unit disease
Hypotonia (decreased resistance to passive movement) or spasticity (increased muscle tone in response to passive stretching)	Hypotonia; no spasticity
Mild weakness (usually involving the anti-gravity muscles)	Profound weakness
Increased deep tendon reflexes	Decreased or absent deep tendon reflexes
Persistence of infantile reflexes; Babinski's sign; and ankle or patellar clonus	No Babinski's sign or clonus
No muscular atrophy	Muscular atrophy (difficult to detect in infants)
No muscle fasciculations (rapid, visible contractions)	Muscle fasciculations (easily detected in older children; tongue fasciculations seen in infants)

progressive. In the older child, progressive symptomatology is characterized by a period of normal development followed by a loss of previously acquired skills.[4] A thorough developmental history, consisting of achievement of motor, language, and social behavior milestones, will help in determining progression.

Static clinical symptomatology implicates congenital abnormalities, traumatic processes, acute toxicity, or resolved infection.[4] Episodic weakness may be related only to a specific activity.

The neurological history and examination will further determine if the weakness deficit is focal or diffuse. If the deficit could be produced by a single, discrete anatomic lesion (e.g., single peripheral nerve paralysis), the disease is focal. If the deficit implicates two or more discrete anatomic lesions, the process is multifocal or diffuse. Most neuromuscular diseases are diffuse rather than focal, even if the weakness has a specific distribution.[5] Diffuse involvement may be due to toxic, degenerative, infectious, or dystrophic processes. Focal involvement is usually secondary to a vascular, neoplastic, or traumatic process.

In conjunction with the history of weakness, the physical motor examination entails the assessment of muscle size, tone, strength, and abnormal movements. The examinations of the infant and older child will be presented separately.

Motor Examination of the Infant

The predominant indicator of an infant with neuromuscular disease is the presence of hypotonia, which can be determined through observation of the infant's activity and evaluation of muscle tone and reflexes.

Muscle tone. The examination of the infant's neuromuscular status begins with thorough, planned observation. The infant's resting posture and spontaneous movements yield information about extremity weakness, distribution, and muscle group involvement. The "frog position" (hips held in abduction almost flat against a surface while they are in external rotation) is a sign of a hypotonic, floppy infant.

Muscle tone is further evaluated by assessing resistance to passive movement of an extremity. In the first 2 months of life, an infant's muscle tone is of the flexor type; after 2 months, extension becomes more pronounced, developing in a cephalocaudal direction. (In addition, after 2 months, spasticity will occur if an upper motor unit disease, such as cerebral palsy, is present.) Placement of the foot to the chin or head and adduction of the elbow past the midline toward the opposite side of the body are maneuvers possible only in the hypotonic infant.[3]

If the normal infant is held in ventral suspension, the head will be held at a 45-degree angle to the horizontal line, the back will be straight or only slightly flexed, the arms will be flexed at the elbows and partially extended at the shoulders, and the knees will be partially flexed. The hypotonic infant will exhibit head lag, a limp trunk, and dangling arms and legs.

Another method of detecting hypotonia is to pull the infant by the wrists from a supine to a sitting position. The normal infant will keep the head in the same plane as the body until sitting, when the head will balance momentarily and then bounce forward. The hypotonic infant's head will lag noticeably as the infant is raised, and there will be no momentary balancing of the head in the sitting position.

Muscle strength. Muscle strength in the infant can be judged by the strength of the sucking reflex, the level of general motor activity, and the speed with which motor skills have developed.[6]

Reflex activity. Tendon reflexes reveal the intactness of the reflex arc, which includes the sensory nerve endings in the tendons, sensory nerve fibers, spinal cord, motor neuron, and muscle. The reflexes are elicited by a light tap of a reflex hammer over a stretched tendon, thereby causing a muscle jerk. A positive response (jerk) reveals the intactness of the arc at the spinal level tested: e.g., biceps reflex, cervical level 5 and 6; and knee jerk, lumbar level 3 and 4.

The tendon reflexes of the infant may vary regionally. In the ill child, if all the reflexes are brisk, upper motor unit involvement should be suspected.[7] The common deep tendon reflexes tested are the biceps, triceps, brachioradial, patellar, and Achilles.

Babinski's sign is tested by stroking the lateral aspect of the sole, across the great toe. In normal infants, bilateral plantar flexion is elicited. An extensor response is abnormal and may be indicative of injury to the brainstem or spinal cord.[8] The symmetry of the response must also be evaluated: a unilateral extensor response or ankle clonus in an infant older than 2 months may indicate upper motor unit disease.[9]

Testing other reflexes found in infancy is useful in detecting asymmetry of movement. The following are some of the common reflexes: Moro's (startle), palmar grasp, plantar grasp, adductor spread of the knee, tonic neck, and Landau's.

A normal Moro's reflex consists of a sudden symmetrical extension and abduction of the arms laterally away from the body, accompanied by extension of the fingers and followed by a gradual adduction of the arms over the body with slight shaking movements.[10] Moro's reflex may be elicited by a sudden loud noise above the infant or by a sudden change in the infant's position.

The normal palmar grasp response is a grasping of the examiner's finger when it is placed in the infant's palm. The plantar grasp response consists of plantar flexion when the infant's toes are stroked. The adductor spread of the knee reflex is a visible contraction of the adductor muscles of the leg after a patellar reflex has been elicited on the opposite side.[10]

TABLE 5-2   Infant Reflexes of Position and Movement

Reflex	Age at appearance	Age at disappearance (after birth)
Moro's	Complete by 34th wk of gestation	1–3 mo
Tonic neck	Reliably present at 31st wk of gestation	5–6 mo
Palmar grasp	Strong enough to support infant's weight at 38th wk of gestation	4 mo
Plantar grasp	26th wk of gestation	8–15 mo
Babinski's	26th to 28th wk of gestation	Before 2 yr
Landau's	3 mo after birth	24 mo
Adductor spread of the knees	Birth	7 mo

The tonic neck reflex is present if the infant extends the arm and leg on the side to which the head is turned. The opposite arm is raised and flexed at the elbow. (The position assumed is commonly known as the fencing position.) The absence of the tonic neck reflex is abnormal; however, if the reflex persists past 6 months of age, the child will not be able to develop normal eye-hand coordination.

Landau's reflex is used to assess the maturity of the motor system. This reflex is elicited by flexion of the infant's head by the examiner, and it is characterized by an accompanying flexion of the legs onto the trunk. The absence of this response is indicative of cerebral palsy.[10]

These reflexes are all normally present in the newborn and disappear in a predictable order as voluntary actions by the infant take precedence. Persistence of the reflexes beyond the normal age of disappearance is often associated with CNS lesions and general developmental delay. Absence of the infantile reflexes indicate CNS or peripheral motor function depression. Asymmetrical responses indicate either a CNS or peripheral focal lesion. An asymmetrical Moro's reflex indicates neuromuscular dysfunction of the brachial plexus or of a single nerve. Any asymmetry of the palmar grasp reflex indicates weakness of the flexor muscles of the hands, possibly as a result of a lower brachial plexus palsy.[11] Depression of all these reflexes indicates CNS involvement due to trauma, toxin, or hypoxia. Table 5-2 presents the ages of onset and disappearance of the infant reflexes.

Motor Examination of the Older Child

The neuromuscular examination of the older child includes the evaluation of muscle tone and strength, gait, reflex activity, and muscle size. The older child will often be able to participate in the motor examination.

As with the infant, neuromuscular assessment of the older child is begun by astute observation. The child's facial expression and standing or sitting posture will yield information regarding motor status. Extraocular muscle functioning can be evaluated as the child follows an object, with the eyes only, through all visual fields. In the younger child, crying that results in asymmetrical facial expression may reveal facial nerve dysfunction. When the child is asked to stick out the tongue, weakness will be revealed if the tongue deviates to one side or if atrophy is present.

Muscle tone. Muscle tone may be assessed through passive range of motion of the extremities. During these movements, any involuntary resistance, spasticity, flaccidity, or rigidity of the extremities should be noted. Any decrease or increase in the expected range of motion of an extremity should also be assessed. Diminished muscle tone suggests lower motor unit disease, whereas rigidity or spasticity is indicative of upper motor unit disease.

Muscle strength. The strength of individual muscles in the extremities can be tested and graded by means of the following scale:[12]

0 — no movement
1 — movement with gravity eliminated
2 — full range against gravity
3 — movement against slight resistance
4 — movement against moderate resistance
5 — normal strength

In general, upper motor unit diseases produce weakness in the extensor muscles of the arms and in flexor muscles of the legs. Diseases of the peripheral nerves result in distal weakness, whereas most muscle disorders affect proximal muscles.[12]

The hip, back, and proximal leg muscles can be evaluated by having the child first sit up, and then stand up, from a supine position. The child should be observed for any unequal use of muscles (i.e., favoring one muscle group over another in changing position). Intercostal muscle functioning can be evaluated by watching the child's breathing pattern, by instructing the child to blow at a feather, or by instructing the child to take a deep breath. Shoulder muscle strength is evaluated by lifting the child from under the axillae. If shoulder weakness is present, the child will not be able to be supported after being lifted.

Muscle percussion. Muscle percussion is accomplished by means of a reflex hammer. When percussed, a muscle normally contracts, indicating muscle excitability. A brisk contraction is visible as a rippling of the skin. Myotonia (tonic spasm of a muscle) is present if percussion elicits a muscular contraction with rigidity preceding relaxation. Percussion may also elicit fasciculations (coarse, irregular twitches due to simultaneous contraction of the entire motor unit). Fasciculations are seen in anterior horn cell disease.

Muscle fatigue. Muscle fatigue is assessed by observing the effects of repetitive muscle contraction. The child is instructed to rapidly open and close the eyelids or hand. The child should normally be able to perform these simple tasks without tiring.

Gait. An abnormal gait is a common symptom of neuromuscular disease. If the child is unable to participate in walking exercises (as would often be true in an intensive care setting), the examiner should ask the parent to describe the child's walking pattern or, preferably, to imitate the child's walk. A normal gait depends on the proper functioning of the motor and sensory cortices, basal ganglia, cerebellum, spinal cord and tracts, peripheral nerves, neuromuscular junctions, and muscles.[13]

Specific gait abnormalities found in neuromuscular disorders include sensory ataxia, high steppage gait, and hip weakness gait. Sensory ataxia is the result of a disruption of input to the cerebellum from the peripheral nerves, posterior roots, or posterior columns of the spinal cord.[14] The child will have a positive Romberg's sign, a loss of position sense in the toes, and a loss of vibration sense. Pain, touch, and temperature sensation are not affected, except in the presence of a peripheral neuropathy. The child will have a wide-based gait and will experience difficulty with standing. Sensory ataxia is seen in polyneuritis (Guillain-Barré syndrome) and any other demyelinating disease.

High steppage gait is associated with weakness of dorsiflexion. The child walks by lifting the leg high, flexing it at the hip and knee, and advancing the foot by flinging it forward. The toe hits the ground before the heel or ball of the foot.[14] High steppage gait occurs in Guillain-Barré syndrome, poliomyelitis, and progressive muscular atrophy.

Hip weakness is characterized by a waddling gait and marked lordosis (anterior convexity of the spine). In hip weakness, which can be associated with any neuromuscular disease, the abductor and extensor muscles are affected.

Reflex activity.   The tendon reflexes may all be elicited in the older infant and child.[15] They are normally less active in the upper than in the lower extremities, and they are generally depressed or absent in lower motor unit disease (e.g., peripheral neuropathies or diseases that affect the spinal cord at the level of the reflex arc). Hyperactivity of tendon reflexes is indicative of upper motor unit disease, especially when associated with clonus.

Muscle size.   Muscle size should be assessed by inspection, palpation, and comparison of symmetry. Both upper and lower motor unit dysfunction affect the growth of muscle mass.

Significant muscular atrophy occurs in lower motor diseases, and it is characterized by muscle weakness and a rubbery texture of the muscle mass. In infants, muscular atrophy is generally not visible because of the large amount of subcutaneous fat, but it may be detected by palpation of the muscle. In older children, atrophy can be visualized by comparing the bilateral symmetry of muscle masses. Muscular hypertrophy (excessive muscle bulk) may also be evidenced by asymmetry. Unusually large muscle growth, primarily of the deltoid and gastrocnemius, may indicate pseudohypertrophy as a result of fat infiltration of the muscle.

Abnormal Muscle Movement

Abnormal muscle movements are involuntary in nature and generally reflect extrapyramidal syndromes or dysfunction on the cerebellar level or at that of the basal ganglia. These movements are absent during sleep, but are elicited during attempts to maintain a posture or perform a specific motor skill.

Tremor, the most common involuntary movement, is a series of rapid, rhythmic, alternate contractions of opposing muscle groups. Choreiform movements are spontaneous, irregular, purposeless, and asymmetric. They are abrupt in onset, rapid, and of brief duration. Athetoid movements are slower and more sustained than choreiform movements, and they primarily affect the distal portions of extremities. These movements are characterized by continuous, slow, snakelike motions of flexion, extension, adduction, and abduction.[16]

Dystonia, a tendency toward hyperextension of the joints, is especially prominent when the patient tries to walk.[17] Dystonic movements usually involve large portions of the body, and they have an undulant, sinuous quality.[18]

Spasms — involuntary, sudden, strong muscular contractions — can reflect disturbances in the muscle fiber itself, in the peripheral nerve, or at almost any level of the CNS, from the spinal cord to the cerebral cortex. Spasms often result in movement that affects one or more muscles. Clonic spasms are repetitive, rapid in onset, and brief in duration; tonic spasms are continuous and more prolonged.[18]

Cramps are painful spasms that may or may not produce movement. They are the result of a disturbance within the peripheral neuromuscular system,[19] and they tend to occur in response to a strong contraction of an already shortened muscle. Cramps are relieved by stretching the affected muscle.[20]

The Sensory Examination

After completion of the motor examination in the pediatric patient, a sensory examination should be conducted. The sensations of pain, touch, and position sense are dependent on the intactness of the peripheral nerves and the pain pathways to the thalamus and cerebrum. The thalamus, the sensory nucleus, is the area in which the synapsing of nerve impulses to the cerebral cortex takes place. The role of the cortex is discriminatory in that it makes fine sensory distinctions. Superficial sensation includes light touch, pain, and temperature. Deep sensation includes vibration sense, as well as pain from joints, muscles, ligaments, tendons, and bones.

Sensory testing is limited in infants and toddlers, and its results tend to be unreliable in this age-group because of the young child's inability to cooperate with the examiner. Only gross response to pain or touch can be elicited. With older children, the sensory examination can be more detailed because the children can actively participate in the examination.

Primary sensations (superficial sensation, deep sensation, and motion and position sense) can be tested in all parts of the body. Symmetry of response should be compared. Sensitivity to light touch can be assessed by moving a feather or a wisp of cotton along the skin. Sensitivity to superficial pain can be tested by alternating the sharp and blunt ends of a safety pin on the skin. Temperature sensation can be assessed through the use of test tubes filled with hot or cold water.

Vibration sense can be tested with a tuning fork. The child should indicate when the vibrations stop as the tuning fork is placed near the sternum, toes, knees, elbows, and iliac crest. Motion and position sense can be evaluated through passive range-of-motion exercises. Deep pain can be tested by applying pressure over the eyeballs, Achilles tendon, calf, and forearm muscles.

Cortical and discriminatory sensation can be assessed by the two-point or the one-point discrimination tests. Two-point discrimination is the ability to feel whether there are one or two pressure points on the skin. The arms, legs, chest, and abdomen can be tested. One-point discrimination, or point localization, makes use of only a single pressure point. The child, keeping the eyes closed to prevent visual detection of the applied stimulus, should be able to point to the area where the pressure is applied.

Sensory testing should be carried out in an unpredictable order so as to prevent

TABLE 5-3   Ongoing Neuromuscular Assessments in the Intensive Care Unit

Infants	Older children
Resting posture	Facial movements
Spontaneous activity	Passive movement of extremities
Passive movement of extremities	Muscle fatigue
Head lag	Abnormal muscle movements
Sucking reflex	Sensory levels of all body parts
Reflex activity	Primary sensations
	Superficial sensations of light touch, pain, temperature
	Deep pain and position sense
	One- and two-point discrimination

the anticipation of a particular stimulus, which would nullify the examination. By making the examination a game, the examiner can help the child feel less stressed, and thus the results obtained will be more conclusive.

(Table 5-3 summarizes the ongoing neuromuscular assessments in the intensive care unit.)

Diagnostic Studies

The diagnosis of neuromuscular disease is determined on the basis of diagnostic studies, as well as through neuromuscular physical assessment. The common adjuncts to diagnosis of neuromuscular disease are muscle biopsy and electrodiagnostic studies. The electrodiagnostic studies include electromyography (EMG), nerve conduction measurements, and repetitive nerve stimulation testing. Serum enzyme studies are used to distinguish between myopathies and neuropathies. Nerve biopsy may also be performed, but is rarely required.

EMG and muscle biopsy yield information about the motor unit, whereas nerve conduction studies are used to determine the structure and functioning of the motor and sensory nerves. Diseases of the neuromuscular junction are diagnosed by repetitive nerve stimulation studies.

Muscle biopsy.   Muscle biopsy is a diagnostic procedure that subjects a sample of muscle tissue to microscopic evaluation. By means of different staining techniques, knowledge is gained about the muscle's morphology, histology, and enzymatic activity. Common sites for biopsy are the biceps, quadriceps, gastrocnemius, and deltoid muscles.

The proper selection of the muscle site to be biopsied is dependent on the acute or chronic presentation of the neuromuscular disease as well as the integrity of the various muscle groups. Severely wasted muscle primarily contains fat and an increased amount of connective tissue, thus yielding limited, nonspecific information. In an acute, rapidly progressing disease that causes muscle weakness, the greatest number of diagnostic findings are discovered in the affected muscle. In chronic disease with associated muscle wasting, moderately weak muscles are biopsied.

Electrodiagnostic studies.   EMG and nerve conduction measurements are the most important facets of electrodiagnosis. These techniques may confirm the diagnosis or provide diagnostic information by identifying the site of dysfunction within the lower motor unit.

EMG provides information on the electrical activity or action potential of the motor unit. At rest, a normal muscle has no electrical activity, but, during contraction, the motor units acquire action potentials. In the presence of a diseased motor unit, electrical activity of various types may appear in the resting muscle, and the action potentials of motor units may evince abnormal forms and patterns of activity.[21]

There are several clinical uses of EMG. It can be used to (1) identify the site of lower motor unit disease, (2) distinguish the cause of muscle wasting from pain or disuse, or (3) determine the cause of muscle paralysis. The analysis of the recorded electrical activity (action potentials) is strikingly different in these two types of disorders with regard to insertion potentials, spontaneous action potentials, and muscle contraction potentials. (However, if the cause of weakness is primary muscle disease, EMG testing cannot identify the specific muscle disease.) EMG will identify a defect in nerve transmission at the neuromuscular junction, and it will aid in the detection of lower motor unit disease, as well as provide information on the distribution and relative number of the affected neurons.

Nerve conduction studies provide information primarily about the myelination of the fastest-conducting myelinated fibers.[22] Peripheral neuropathies that cause damage to the myelin sheath or Schwann cells result in a decreased velocity of nerve conduction. The conduction velocity of motor or sensory nerves varies with the patient's age because of changes in the fiber diameter, degree of myelination, and internodal distance.[23]

Repetitive nerve stimulation studies are used in the diagnosis of neuromuscular junction disorders. These studies produce maximal stress on neuromuscular junction transmission through repetitive stimulation. If a neuromuscular junction disorder such as myasthenia gravis is present, a progressive fall in the amplitude of the action potentials during repeated stimulation is the expected response.

Serum enzyme studies. Serum enzyme studies, particulary those of serum creatine phosphokinase (CPK) activity, are useful in differentiating myopathies from neuropathies. Elevated CPK levels, which may rise to three times the normal value in patients with neuromuscular disorders, almost always correlate with myopathic disease. In neuropathies, the serum CPK level is usually normal.

The use of creatine and creatinine determinations to evaluate muscle disease is based on the relatively constant ratio between muscle mass and urinary creatinine excretion. Total muscle mass is estimated from urinary creatinine levels. Any disease process that reduces muscle mass also decreases the rate of urinary excretion of creatinine.

(Table 5-4 summarizes the various components of the neuromuscular examination.)

PRINCIPLES OF NURSING CARE

The nursing principles in caring for the child with neuromuscular disease focus on two main areas: (1) the identification of potential problems and (2) the preservation of muscle integrity.

TABLE 5-4   Components of the Neuromuscular Examination

History of weakness: acute or chronic; static, progressive, episodic
Muscle tone: face, limbs, and trunk (resistance to passive movement, resting posture)
Muscle strength: graded on a scale of 0 to 5
Reflex testing: infant reflexes or deep tendon reflexes
Muscle percussion and palpation
Muscle size
Gait evaluation (older child)
Abnormal muscle movements: tremors, cramps, spasms, dystonia, and athetoid or
    choreiform movements
Sensory evaluation: pain, touch, vibration, position sense, and temperature
Electrodiagnostic studies
Muscle biopsy
Serum enzyme studies

Identification of Potential Problems

The most critical problem facing the child with neuromuscular disease is the crisis of respiratory failure, which may be secondary to increased neuromuscular fatigue, weakness, or paralysis. The nurse must be able to identify subtle changes in the child's status that may lead to respiratory problems. Some of these changes are weakening of the protective reflexes (cough, gag, swallow), decreasing chest excursion, progressive decreases in tidal volume, and fatigue in vocalization. The nurse must also recognize the signs and symptoms of acute respiratory failure. Consistency in assessment and documentation of respiratory evaluation is crucial for detecting the subtle changes that may precede respiratory failure. In addition to the crisis of acute respiratory failure, the potential problems of atelectasis and pneumonia must be anticipated and prevented with supportive care.

The child with neuromuscular disease may face long periods of immobility. The nurse must be aware of the complications of immobility: skin breakdown, muscle wasting, contractures, decalcification of bone, urinary retention, and bowel dysfunction. The immobile child will also be susceptible to autonomic instability, and thus the nurse must assess the child for orthostatic hypotension, transient hypertension, flushing, diaphoretic episodes, and transient tachycardia.

Another potential problem is sensory impairment, which occurs primarily in peripheral neuropathies. The child with sensory impairment will be susceptible to hypo- or hyperthermia burns. The child may also be frightened if touch sensation and position sense are lost. This situation becomes stressful for the child because of the fear of losing body integrity. The child will need to know, through visual examination, that all the limbs remain intact, especially after periods of sleep.

An ongoing potential problem is the lack of stress control. Children normally cope with stress through active play. The child with neuromuscular disease lacks this outlet and may react to stress by withdrawing emotionally as well as physically, thus masking regression or improvement of physical symptoms. Another reaction to stress is hostility or uncooperativeness. This outlet of expressing hostility verbally or through misconduct is limited by the child's functional capabilities during the hospitalization. The underlying problems for these children are their loss of control over their normal environment and their fear of the strange, new environment. Increased stress may lead to the development of gastrointestinal ulcers as well as to an exacerbation of muscle weakness.

The nurse caring for the child with neuromuscular disease needs to be aware of the stresses placed on the child. Stress can be minimized through the establishment of communication systems with the child and family early in the hospitalization. Sound communication will lead to the development of a trusting therapeutic relationship. Through knowledge of normal growth and development, the nurse can work with the family in developing age-appropriate schedules of care. The development of routines will aid in establishing a sense of control and security within the environment. Approaching the child in a consistent manner (praising the child when appropriate but being firm when indicated) will aid in developing trust and will thus help prevent emotional and physical regression.

Preservation of Muscle Integrity

The preservation of muscle integrity includes the maintenance of muscle tone and functioning, as well as joint mobility. In order to ensure muscle integrity, the nurse must plan for short periods of passive range-of-motion exercises, while avoiding overexerting the child, which leads to increased weakness. Consultations with the physical therapist, the occupational therapist, and the nutritionist will be helpful in planning for muscle preservation. The nutritionist will aid in assessing the caloric needs of the child so as to prevent muscle wasting and promote muscle growth (*see* p. 469). The physical and occupational therapists will aid in developing specific exercise routines, as well as constructing splints to maintain correct limb alignment. The child's base-line growth and development will suggest appropriate play activities that will provide diversion and exercise. The games also aid in assessing muscle strength, joint mobility, and gross motor movement.

An important nursing principle in neuromuscular disease is that of making consistent, age-appropriate assessments. In working with the pediatric population, the nurse will need to know what constitutes normal growth and development so as to be capable of establishing a sound base line for assessment. Each age-group has specific developmental milestones, socialization behaviors, and physical capabilities. Only through a sound knowledge of the pediatric population can the nurse detect the subtle changes of neuromuscular disease and be instrumental in preventing complications and in promoting the return of normal functioning.

GUILLAIN-BARRÉ SYNDROME

Guillain-Barré syndrome is an acute polyneuropathy that is characterized by a symmetrical ascending paralysis that may lead to respiratory failure. The syndrome is also referred to as acute infective polyneuritis, polyradiculoneuritis, or Landry's ascending paralysis.

All ages, all races, and both sexes are affected. The average incidence of the syndrome is 1.7 per 100,000 population.[24] Geographic location, season, and climate may affect the incidence of Guillain-Barré syndrome. In 1979, on the national level, there were an increased number of cases between January and March, with a peak incidence in February and early March.[25]

Etiology

Although the etiology of Guillain-Barré syndrome is idiopathic, the syndrome has recently been considered an immune reaction in which the primary target is the peripheral nervous system. The immune process may be triggered by exposure to an exogenous agent, recent infection, or vaccination. An antigen-antibody reaction occurs, causing lymphocytes to become sensitized to peripheral nerve antigen and to attack the myelin of peripheral nerve tissue. The following is a list of the possible precipitating factors of Guillain-Barré syndrome:

Tetanus antitoxin injection
Antirabies vaccination
Smallpox vaccination
Typhoid vaccination
Mumps-rubella vaccination
Varicella
Influenza
Infectious mononucleosis
Swine influenza vaccine
Enteric viruses

Pathophysiology

The pathophysiology of Guillain-Barré syndrome is primarily one of segmental demyelination (loss of the fatty myelin sheath) of the peripheral nerves (Fig. 5-8). This degenerative change affects spinal and cranial nerve roots in ascending order. Concomitant changes are inflammation, edema, and compression of the nerve roots. Although the myelin is affected, the structure of the axon is usually spared. The result of these degenerative changes is the slowing or total blocking of nerve conduction, causing total or partial ascending paralysis.

The anterior spinal roots (motor neurons) are primarily affected, causing disturbance in movement. The posterior spinal roots (sensory neurons) are also affected, resulting in sensation disturbance. The cranial nerves may also be involved. Autonomic functioning may be disturbed because the anterior and posterior roots join to form peripheral nerves, which relay sensory, motor, and

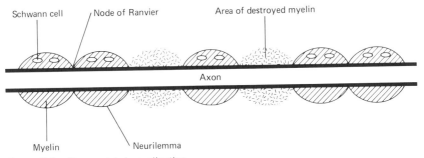

Figure 5-8. Segmental demyelination.

autonomic impulses. In Guillain-Barré syndrome, motor disturbance is more prominent than sensory disturbance.

The most distal axons, those in the legs, are affected first, due to the distance from the nerve cell body outside the spinal cord. Thus, the first usual symptom of Guillain-Barré syndrome is leg muscle weakness.

Clinical Presentation

The primary presenting feature of Guillain-Barré syndrome is symmetrical, distal, peripheral muscle weakness. Leg weakness is pronounced, but arm weakness may also be present. Paresthesia (numbness or tingling) of fingers and toes is present in a "glove-and-stocking" fashion. Muscle tenderness may also be present.

Diagnosis

The first exact criteria for the diagnosis of Guillan-Barré syndrome were formulated in 1960.[26] (Currently, there is no specific test to confirm the diagnosis of Guillain-Barré syndrome: the diagnosis is based on the collective information gained from the patient history, clinical symptomatology, progression, and laboratory results.) Since 1960, further diagnostic criteria for Guillain-Barré syndrome have been established in response to the increased incidence of the syndrome in association with the swine influenza vaccine. The criteria were divided into several categories: features required for the diagnosis of Guillain-Barré syndrome, features that strongly support the diagnosis, and features that rule out or cast doubt on the diagnosis. Preceding events (e.g., viral illness or vaccination) are not essential for diagnosis. The following are the required criteria for diagnosis of Guillain-Barré syndrome:[27]

1. Motor weakness of more than one extremity, the degree of weakness variable (with or without ataxia) up to total paralysis.
2. Loss of deep tendon reflexes (areflexia).

The following is a partial summary of the criteria that strongly support the diagnosis of Guillain-Barré syndrome but that are not individually diagnostic:[27]

1. The progression of paralysis reaches its peak within 3 to 4 weeks.
2. Relative symmetry of weakness/paralysis.
3. Mild sensory loss (possibly transient).
4. Cranial nerve involvement, primarily the facial nerve (7) although any cranial nerve may be involved.
5. Recovery begins 2 to 4 weeks after progression stops. Most patients have full functional recovery.
6. Variable degrees of autonomic dysfunction.
7. Patient is afebrile at time of first neuritic symptoms.
8. Electrodiagnostic studies show evidence of slowing or blocking of nerve conduction.
9. Sphincter functioning is usually not affected.
10. Albuminocytologic dissociation. Elevation of cerebrospinal fluid protein (50

to 250 mg/100 ml) at any stage of illness without a rise in cell count (less than 10 mononuclear cells/mm³) or in cerebrospinal fluid pressure.

Clinical Course

The initial weakness, beginning in the legs and/or arms, may progress to full, flaccid paralysis. Decreased muscle tone and strength are present in symmetrical distribution. Facial muscle weakness is present in most cases. Intercostal weakness may necessitate the need for ventilatory assistance. The height of paralysis is usually reached within a few days after onset, although the progression of paralysis may persist for up to 3 weeks.

Guillain-Barré syndrome occurs in all degrees of severity, but all affected patients will require hospitalization. Some children may never progress to full paralysis and may only require observation, whereas others will require acute care. Patients may recover within 2 weeks of onset, but recovery usually tends to take 4 to 8 weeks. The mortality rate is 3 to 4 percent.[28]

Sensory involvement is variable, but often minimal. Position sense as well as touch, pain, and temperature sensation may be impaired. Paresthesia tends to be intermittent during the initial stages of illness.

Cranial nerve involvement is present to some degree in the majority of patients. The facial nerve (7) is most frequently affected. Dysphagia and laryngeal paralysis have been reported, implicating the glossopharyngeal nerve (9) and the vagus nerve (10). Although any of the cranial nerves may be affected, the vestibulocochlear nerve (8) is rarely implicated.

Autonomic dysfunction manifests itself primarily by orthostatic hypotension and/or transient hypertension. Excessive sympathetic activity is evidenced by hypertension, persistent sinus tachycardia, episodes of delirious behavior, sudden profuse diaphoresis, and peripheral vasoconstriction.[29] Insufficient sympathetic activity results in orthostatic hypotension and poor venous tone, causing pooling in dependent areas.[29] Excessive parasympathetic activity results in bradycardia, facial flushing, and generalized extreme warmth. Insufficient parasympathetic activity results in sphincter disturbances.[29]

Other clinical features documented in relation to Guillain-Barré syndrome are papilledema, increased intracranial pressure, and acute glomerulonephritis. The increased intracranial pressure and papilledema may be the result of a cerebrospinal fluid absorptive defect secondary to the high cerebrospinal fluid protein.[30] (This explanation is not universally accepted and is being subjected to further research.) The presence of acute glomerulonephritis is poorly understood, but it has been identified in patients with microscopic hematuria or systemic hypertension after serial examinations.[31]

Recovery is dependent on the extent of demyelination. Remyelination occurs from the CNS outward at a rate of 1 mm/day.[32] The longest peripheral nerves are the last to recover. Intercostal functioning returns before phrenic nerve functioning. Chest wall movement can be identified, but without adequate alveolar ventilation because diaphragmatic function will not yet have returned.

Critical Care Management

The management of Guillain-Barré syndrome is symptomatic and depends on the stage of the illness and the extent of muscular involvement. (Table 5-5 summarizes the neuromuscular assessment for Guillain-Barré syndrome.) The general man-

TABLE 5-5   Neuromuscular Assessment for Guillain-Barré Syndrome

Parameter	Components of assessment
Muscle strength	Bilateral proximal and distal muscle strength
Bilateral sensory functioning of extremities	Pain, one- and two-point discrimination
	Touch
	Temperature
	Position
Cranial nerve involvement (intactness, absence, or weakening of functioning)	Cough and gag reflexes
	Swallow reflex
	Speech dysfunction
	Diaphragmatic movement
	Ability to manage secretions
	Facial muscle movement
	Eyelid and ocular muscle movement
Bilateral gross motor movement	Flexion and extension of arms and legs
	Raising of arms and legs
	Grip strength
Autonomic dysfunction	Absence/presence of diaphoresis
	Flushing/mottling of skin
	Pupillary size
	Fluctuating blood pressure
	Fluctuating heart rate
	Sphincter control
Altered level of consciousness	

agement is one of highly supportive care. Corticosteroid therapy has been used without conclusive results. Plasmapheresis has been investigated, based on the premise that the etiology is immunologic. By removal of the circulating antibody specific for peripheral nerves, clinical improvement should follow.

Respiratory care.   Respiratory failure is the most frequent complication of Guillain-Barré syndrome, secondary to phrenic nerve and intercostal muscle paralysis. Intercostal and diaphragmatic paralysis will produce alveolar hypoventilation.

Indications for artificial ventilation are the same as for other children with respiratory failure: a vital capacity of less than 15 ml/kg, a partial pressure of arterial oxygen (PaO_2) of less than 50 mmHg on 100 percent oxygen, a partial pressure of arterial carbon dioxide of greater than 50 mmHg, and clinical signs of progressive cyanosis, diminishing rate and depth of respirations, inability to speak or monosyllabic speech, inability to manage secretions, and altered level of consciousness. Endotracheal intubation is performed, and the child is placed on an appropriate ventilator. A tracheostomy is usually performed if the child shows no signs of recovery within 7 to 14 days. An arterial line may be inserted initially in order to provide for frequent arterial blood sampling during stabilization of ventilation. Transcutaneous partial pressure of oxygen ($TCPO_2$) and end-tidal carbon dioxide monitoring may also be instituted. Chest x-rays will be taken intermittently to assess the level of the diaphragm as well as the integrity of the pulmonary fields.

After intubation, nursing care focuses on airway maintenance and the prevention of pulmonary complications. Physiotherapy should be performed every 2 to 4 hours accompanied by hyperinflation and suctioning. Tracheal secretions should be evaluated for changes, and aspirates should be sent to the laboratory weekly for culture and Gram stain. Modified postural drainage may be instituted. Extreme position changes may produce the autonomic changes of hypotension and bradycardia. If the child has a tracheostomy, routine tracheostomy care must be provided.

As the child slowly regains strength, weaning from the ventilator begins with the goal of avoiding fatigue. The child will be switched from controlled ventilation to an intermittent mandatory ventilation (IMV) circuit in order to allow for spontaneous ventilation. Periods of continuous positive airway pressure (CPAP) may be instituted for short intervals daily to test inspiratory force and vital capacity. Arterial blood gases or $TCPO_2$ and end-tidal carbon dioxide may be monitored continuously in order to assess the weaning process. The intervals of CPAP will be increased as the IMV rate is decreased.

The final step in respiratory management is decannulation or extubation. Before this step, however, certain assessments need to be made: (1) the protective reflexes (cough and gag) must be present in order to prevent aspiration; (2) diaphragmatic strength and movement must be adequate in order to prevent hypoventilation and carbon dioxide retention; and (3) the child must be able to manage airway secretions. If these criteria are met, the child can be decannulated or extubated.

Neuromuscular examination. The neuromuscular examination will help determine the progression and extent of paralysis or weakness caused by Guillain-Barré syndrome. The neuromuscular assessments should be conducted every 2 hours until the child's condition has stabilized. The examination should include cranial nerve, gross motor movement, sensory, and autonomic assessments (*see* Table 5-5).

Fluid and electrolyte management. Serum calcium testing is conducted at least weekly during the course of illness. Hypercalcemia may result as calcium is mobilized from bone during prolonged immobility. If present, hypercalcemia may be treated with fluid increase (1.5 times the maintenance level). Serum electrolytes may be checked weekly. Lumbar puncture for cerebrospinal fluid evaluation may be repeated during the course of illness.

Nutrition. Nutrition is maintained by means of high-caloric enteral feedings to help prevent muscle mass loss (*see* p. 480). Care should be taken to prevent aspiration. Gastrointestinal problems include increased gastric acidity, abdominal distention, ileus, and diarrhea or constipation.

Gastric pH testing will detect increased acidity. Antacids may be administered to relieve this problem. Bowel sounds should be assessed in order to detect the development of an ileus, which may cause abdominal distention and poor absorption of feedings. Stool softeners such as dioctyl sodium sulfosuccinate (Colace) are commonly used to prevent constipation. Diarrhea is treated by changing the child's diet and by replacement intravenous (IV) fluid therapy.

Bladder care. Bladder functioning is not normally affected, but urinary retention may develop. Bladder size should be palpated. Credé of the bladder or intermittent catheterizations may be necessary, as may urine pH and dipstick determinations. Strict intake and output must be documented for fluid balance evaluation. Weight should be monitored twice weekly.

Autonomic dysfunction. Autonomic dysfunction is treated in the presence of a decreased cardiac output. Hypotension is corrected with volume or colloid administration, bradycardia with atropine sulfate, and hypertension, if life threatening, with hydralazine hydrochloride, 0.75 mg/kg/day (*see* p. 382).

Autonomic problems are usually transitory and do not require aggressive therapy. Temperature instability may be treated with hypo- or hyperthermia blankets and antipyretics. The child may become poikilothermic because of the loss of the ability to sweat. If a persistent fever develops (greater than 38.5°C [101.3°F]), blood and urine cultures and chest x-ray should be performed to rule out sepsis, urinary tract infection. pneumonia, or increased atelectasis.

Immobility. The problems of immobility will obviously be encountered with the paralyzed child. With supportive care, however, these problems can be minimized. If the child has hypercalcemia, the nurse should observe for cardiac arrhythmias. Meticulous skin care is necessary in order to avoid pressure areas and skin breakdown. The child's position should be changed every 2 hours. The use of an alternating-pressure mattress is helpful. Passive range-of-motion exercises should be instituted early to prevent contractures. Collaboration with the physical and occupational therapists will aid in developing a daily routine for the child and in fitting the child for splints to maintain limb positioning. Eye care is necessary if the ocular muscles are involved. Lacri-Lube or Tearisol should be applied to prevent exposure keratitis.

Communication. The recognition of the child's fears and feelings of loss of bodily control is a primary element in providing care during the acute phase of Guillain-Barré syndrome. In some instances, children may find themselves totally paralyzed, intubated, and helpless within 24 hours after admission to the pediatric

TABLE 5-6   Critical Care Management of Guillain-Barré Syndrome

Neuromuscular evaluation for progression of disease
Respiratory management
   Intubation/tracheostomy
   Mechanical ventilation
   Chest physiotherapy with hyperinflation
   Postural drainage
   Tracheal aspirates
   Weekly chest x-ray
   Tracheostomy care
$TCPO_2$, $ETCO_2$, and/or arterial blood gas monitoring
Serial tidal volume measurements
Laboratory studies:
   Calcium levels
   Serum electrolyte levels
   CSF evaluation
Symptomatic treatment for autonomic dysfunction
Corticosteroid therapy
Plasmapheresis
Electrodiagnostic studies
Maintenance fluids
High-caloric enteral feedings
Immobility care
Evaluation of GI and renal functioning
Emotional and psychological support

CSF, cerebrospinal fluid; $ETCO_2$, end-tidal carbon dioxide; GI, gastrointestinal; $TCPO_2$, transcutaneous partial pressure of oxygen.

TABLE 5-7 Possible Complications of Guillain-Barré Syndrome

Respiratory failure
Atelectasis/pneumonia
Gastric ulcer
Abdominal distention or ileus
Aspiration of enteral feedings
Complications of immobility
   Hypercalcemia
   Contractures
   Decubitus ulcers
   Joint fusion
Autonomic dysfunction (severe)
Increased ICP and papilledema secondary to high levels of CSF protein
Urinary retention
Exposure keratitis

CSF, cerebrospinal fluid; ICP, intracranial pressure.

intensive care unit. The parents will also find themselves fearful and helpless, initially. It is of the utmost importance that communication systems be established. The child and family gradually need to feel a sense of security in the intensive care environment.

If the child still has facial muscle control, it is possible to communicate by means of eye signals, head nodding, and silent speech. The use of picture boards and language charts is also helpful.

At the bedside, the nurse should always speak to the child, tell the child what will happen, talk about topics familiar to the child, and report news from home. The parents can become involved by reading stories and assisting in the child's daily care.

Establishing daily schedules is helpful in allowing the child to gain some control over the environment and in assisting the child to become familiar with the personnel who are active in the hospitalization.

The recovery period for Guillain-Barré syndrome may be as long as several months; thus, open communication and the establishment of trust are extremely important.

(Tables 5-6 and 5-7 summarize the critical care management and the possible complications of Guillain-Barré syndrome.)

MYASTHENIA GRAVIS

Myasthenia gravis is a chronic disease that may precipitate an acute crisis of respiratory distress or failure. The crisis may occur in undiagnosed myasthenia gravis and may be the precipitating factor for hospitalization and subsequent diagnosis. In diagnosed myasthenia gravis, the acute crisis is secondary to the over- or underdosage of anticholinesterase therapy.

The site of dysfunction in myasthenia gravis is the neuromuscular junction between the axon terminals and the motor end plates of striated muscles. The result is a lack of nerve transmission and subsequent muscle contraction. Primary symptomatology involves muscle fatigue and weakness of the voluntary muscles. The mechanism of dysfunction involves the nerve transmitter substance ACH and the ACH receptor (ACHR) sites.

Myasthenia gravis may affect any age-group: it may be the transitory type seen in neonates or the acquired type that affects individuals from young childhood through adulthood. Females are affected more frequently than males until the fourth or fifth decade of life, when males begin to predominate. The onset of the disease may be insidious or rapid. Respiratory compromise will afflict 40 percent of all patients, whereas approximately 20 percent will experience complete and permanent spontaneous remission of symptoms.[33] This section will deal with the pediatric age-group in acute crisis.

Etiology

Myasthenia gravis prevents sustained muscular activity secondary to the lack of nerve impulse transmission at the neuromuscular junction. Research initially revealed that the defect in myasthenia gravis is the lack of ACH activity due to increased acetylcholinesterase activity. Further research has shown, however, that the basic defect is a reduction of the number of available ACHRs at the neuromuscular junction, brought about by an autoimmune process. Patients with myasthenia gravis have only about 20 percent of the normal number of ACHRs at the neuromuscular junction.[34]

Pathophysiology

Autoimmunity is immunologic reactivity against self-antigens. It reflects a loss of tolerance (unresponsiveness) in that it results in the activation of immune cells that, under normal circumstances, are unresponsive.[35] The autoimmune response in myasthenia gravis results in the production of an autoantibody directed at the ACHR sites, causing either (1) a reduction in the number of functional sites or (2) structural changes leading to disruption in neuromuscular transmission. The origin of the autoimmune response in myasthenia gravis is still under investigation; however, there is some evidence that it may originate within the thymus gland, although the exact relationship between the thymus and myasthenia gravis is not fully understood.

Myoid (musclelike) cells are present in the thymus and have surface ACHRs. It is possible that the juxtaposition of myoid, ACHR-bearing cells with immunocompetent cells in the thymus may initiate the autoimmune response.[34] An immune reaction may be triggered if either the myoid cells or the thymus-dependent lymphocytes (T cells) are abnormal, and the ACHRs may thus be perceived as being "non-self."[34]

Part of the evidence that implicates the thymus in myasthenia gravis is that it is responsible for cell-mediated immunity through the maturation of T cells through the action of thymic hormones. Lymphocytes are involved in the production of anti-ACHR antibody.[34] Subtle changes have been found in the immunocompetent cells of the thymus in myasthenic patients, including the number of T cells and changes in their antigenic properties.[36]

In addition, 75 percent of myasthenia gravis patients have thymic abnormalities: 85 percent of these have thymic hyperplasia, whereas the remainder have thymomas.[34] The beneficial results of thymectomy in myasthenic individuals, ranging from complete remission to minimal improvement of symptoms, support the theory that the thymus is involved in the formation of antibodies against ACHRs.

Approximately 70 to 95 percent of patients with myasthenia gravis have detectable anti-ACHR antibodies.[34] These antibodies are present in the serum of most myasthenia gravis patients and are specific to myasthenia gravis.[37]

Anti-ACHR antibodies may produce a reduction of available ACHRs by several different actions: (1) increased degradation of ACHRs, (2) decreased synthesis of ACHRs, (3) blocking of ACHRs, and (4) destruction of ACHRs by complement and/or a cell-mediated mechanism.[34]

In summary, the following are the underlying defects found in myasthenia gravis:

1. An autoimmune process that causes a decrease in the number of ACHR sites.
2. An alteration in thymic functioning secondary to hyperplasia or thymomas.
3. The production of antibodies to ACHRs.

Clinical Presentation

The clinical presentation of myasthenia gravis is characterized by weakness of the voluntary muscles, worsening with activity and improving with rest. In milder forms, only the ocular muscles are involved, resulting in uni- or bilateral ptosis and diplopia. In the generalized form of myasthenia, symptoms may progress rapidly from ocular weakness to marked bulbar weakness (weakness originating at the level of the medulla oblongata and evidenced by dyspnea), resulting in respiratory failure.

The progression of symptoms in myasthenia gravis is as follows: ptosis, diplopia, jaw weakness, speech dysfunction (slurred speech and high-pitched, nasal voice), dysphagia, symmetrical or asymmetric limb weakness, and increasing respiratory difficulty. The complications resulting from this progression of symptoms include (1) aspiration secondary to the inability to manage secretions and protect the airway and (2) respiratory failure due to bulbar muscle weakness or paralysis. Myasthenic crisis may be recognized by the child's increasing weakness, ventilatory distress, and inability to swallow.

The diagnosis of myasthenia gravis is made on the basis of the presenting symptomatology and diagnostic testing. The diagnosis of myasthenic crisis is made on the basis of an edrophonium chloride (Tensilon) test, performed in the controlled setting of an intensive care unit.

Diagnosis of Myasthenia Gravis

The characteristic feature of myasthenia gravis is neuromuscular fatigue — the inability to sustain or repeat muscular contractions. Thus, myasthenia gravis may be diagnosed by means of repetitive nerve-stimulation testing. Stimulating electrodes, as well as recording electrodes, are placed on the muscle to be tested. Through repetitive nerve stimulation, a decreasing amplitude of the action potential is recorded, reflecting fatigue and posttetanic exhaustion of the involved muscle.

Normally, during repeated stimulation of motor nerves, the amount of ACH released per impulse declines after the first few impulses because the nerve terminal cannot maintain the original release rate.[38] However, the number of ACH to ACHR interactions in response to stimuli is more than sufficient to maintain neuromuscular transmission despite the decline of ACH release. The myasthenic patients lacks this margin of safety during neuromuscular transmission: because of the reduced number of ACHRs at the neuromuscular junction, fewer muscle fibers are activated by successive nerve impulses. Any change that reduces the probability of ACH and ACHR interaction results in the failure of neuromuscular transmission.[36]

In addition to nerve-stimulation studies, two different assay methods have been used recently in the diagnosis of myasthenia gravis, based on the antibody-to-ACHR theory. Radioimmunoassay measures the amount of antibody bound to solubilized ACHRs. Low antibody titers are found in mild myasthenia gravis, whereas high levels are found in patients severely afflicted by myasthenia gravis. ACHR-blocking assays measure the interference of antibodies on ACHR active sites.[38]

If myasthenia gravis is suspected on the basis of clinical symptoms, a Tensilon test is often performed to confirm the tentative diagnosis. (Atropine is generally administered before the test in order to counteract the muscarinic side effects of edrophonium, which is a short-acting anticholinesterase agent that prolongs the action of ACH.) The IV administration of edrophonium will cause a transient improvement in muscle weakness if the patient has myasthenia gravis. The peak action of the drug occurs after approximately 1 minute, and the patient may experience elation as well as increased muscle strength.

Diagnosis of Myasthenic Crisis

Myasthenic crisis is a period of acute weakness that may lead to respiratory failure. The weakness may be myasthenic in origin or cholinergic. The crisis may be brought on by an inadequate dosage of anticholinesterase agents or by influenza, emotional stress, or the menstrual cycle. Various categories of drugs may precipitate a crisis: procainamide hydrochloride (Pronestyl), propranolol hydrochloride (Inderal), quinidine sulfate, gentamicin sulfate, kanamycin sulfate, polymyxin B sulfate, neomycin sulfate, diuretics that promote hypokalemia, and sedatives with respiratory-depressant side effects. The anesthetics diethyl ether and halothane may also precipitate a crisis.[39]

When a child with diagnosed myasthenia presents with symptoms of increased weakness and respiratory difficulty, the Tensilon test is often performed to differentiate between myasthenic and cholinergic crisis (Table 5-8). The purpose of this diagnostic study is to determine whether the child is receiving an underdosage (myasthenic crisis) or overdosage (cholinergic crisis) of anticholinesterase drugs.

A small dose of edrophonium chloride (200 μg/kg IV) is administered under controlled conditions in an intensive care unit, where respiratory support measures are within easy access. (The child may be electively intubated before administration of the drug.) If the child is in myasthenic crisis, the child will become stronger as acetylcholinesterase is inactivated, permitting increased ACH action; if the child is in cholinergic crisis, the child will become weaker from excessive ACH accumulation, resulting in muscarinic and nicotinic side effects as well as in CNS depression. (If the child is in cholinergic crisis, atropine is administered as an antidote to diminish the severity of the side effects.)

Critical Care Management

The critical care management of the child in myasthenic crisis revolves primarily around the establishment of a suitable regimen of drug therapy that will counteract the debilitating weakness. During the period of crisis, maintenance of a patent

TABLE 5-8 Differentiation of Myasthenic from Cholinergic Crisis Following Tensilon Administration*

Myasthenic crisis	Cholinergic crisis
Decreased muscle weakness	Increased muscle weakness
Improved respiratory functioning	Muscarinic side effects
Improved voluntary muscle functioning	Abdominal cramping
	Nausea
	Vomiting
	Diarrhea
	Bradycardia
	Hypotension
	Bronchoconstriction
	Profuse sweating
	Excessive lacrimation
	Nicotinic side effects
	Skeletal muscle twitching
	Increased fatigue
	Paralysis of striated muscles, including the diaphragm and the intercostal muscles
	Respiratory failure

*The Tensilon test is used to differentiate myasthenic from cholinergic crisis. (A diagnosis of myasthenic crisis indicates that the patient has been receiving an underdosage of anticholinesterase drugs; a diagnosis of cholinergic crisis indicates that the patient has been receiving an overdosage of anticholinesterase drugs.) The patient receives 200 µg/kg of edrophonium chloride (Tensilon) by intravenous infusion. A differential diagnosis may be made, depending on the effects of the Tensilon. If a diagnosis of cholinergic crisis is made, an atropine antidote is administered to counteract the muscarinic effects of the Tensilon. Atropine may be given prophylactically before the administration of Tensilon.

airway and prevention of the complications of weakness and immobility are essential.

Anticholinesterase therapy.   Anticholinesterase therapy has been the primary drug therapy in myasthenia gravis for many years. Anticholinesterase medications provide symptomatic relief of weakness in the child with myasthenia gravis by inhibiting or inactivating acetylcholinesterase at the neuromuscular junction. This action permits an adequate accumulation of ACH for nerve impulse transmission.

At muscarinic sites, the resulting rise in ACH leads to increased parasympathomimetic activity of smooth and cardiac muscle and gland cells. At nicotinic sites, the accumulation of ACH causes stimulation of skeletal muscle and autonomic ganglia. Excessive accumulation of ACH leads to depression of skeletal muscle tone and ganglion nerve cell impulse transmission.[40]

Edrophonium chloride is useful for diagnostic evaluation in the early stages of crisis because of its short, reversible duration of action. Longer-acting cholinesterase inhibitors are used in the general managment of myasthenia gravis.

Pyridostigmine bromide (Mestinon) is the agent most widely used via the oral route. The onset of action occurs within 10 to 30 minutes, with a duration of action of from 3 to 8 hours. Oral ambenonium chloride (Mytelase) is indicated for bromide-sensitive patients. Mytelase has an onset of action of from 20 to 30 minutes, with a duration of action of 3 to 6 hours. Neostigmine methylsulfate

(Prostigmin), administered by IV infusion or intramuscularly, is often used during hospitalization.

The frequency of administration and the dosage of all these medications must be determined on an individual basis. The timing of doses of any of the anticholinesterase drugs depends on the clinical symptomatology of the patient between each dose. The majority of patients require frequent doses, ranging from 2-to-6 hour intervals, in order to avoid fluctuations in muscle strength. Atropine (0.5 mg orally) is often used as an adjunct to therapy to counteract the muscarinic side effects of overdosage.

The toxic side effects (muscarinic and nicotinic) of cholinesterase inhibitors are outlined in Table 5-8. The CNS may be affected by overdosage, resulting in confusion, slurred speech, convulsions, and coma. Underdosage may be detected by declining muscle strength and early respiratory depression. The child must be observed for these side effects while different anticholinesterase drug doses are being tested.

Steroid therapy.   Steroid therapy is an adjuvant treatment for myasthenia gravis in patients whose weakness cannot be controlled by anticholinesterase agents or by thymectomy. Although the precise mechanism of action of the corticosteroids has not yet been determined, their use is directed at the autoimmune mechanism of myasthenia gravis. They have been shown to decrease the size of the thymus, reduce the lymphocyte population, and diminish the antireceptor reactivity of peripheral lymphocytes.[38]

Steroid therapy may be initiated with high doses (50 to 100 milligrams) of prednisone, although a temporary increase in muscle weakness may develop, leading to respiratory insufficiency and requiring artificial ventilation. To avoid this problem, treatment with prednisone may be initiated at a lower dose (25 milligrams) and the dosage gradually increased by 5 to 10 mg/week until the optimal level is reached, when there is no fluctuation in muscle weakness. When the optimal dosage is attained, an alternate-day regimen may be started so that the same total maintenance dose is administered every other day. Alternate-day prednisone therapy will help to minimize the side effects of steroid therapy. The maintenance level, determined on an individual basis, may be decreased gradually over the course of a year to minimal yet effective doses.

Anticholinesterase therapy is not discontinued during steroid therapy because abrupt withdrawal could lead to an exacerbation of myasthenic weakness. The dosage of anticholinesterase drugs is regulated as required and eventually decreased to minimal maintenance dosages.

Steroid therapy is continued indefinitely and results in the development of adverse side effects, including fluid retention, gastrointestinal bleeding, decreased resistance to infection, hyperglycemia, and cataract formation. Strict intake and output determinations, daily weights, strict aseptic technique during all procedures, daily blood glucose tests or Dextrostix, and eye examinations will aid in the detection and prevention of these problems. Gastric pH testing will detect increasing gastric acidity, which, if untreated, may lead to gastrointestinal bleeding. Antacid therapy is a preventive course of action.

Adrenocorticotrophic hormone (ACTH) is sometimes administered by IV infusion or intramuscularly for a 10-day regimen. Approximately 2 to 3 days into therapy, the patient may begin to get weaker. The height of weakness is reached by the sixth to seventh day, and ventilatory support may need to be instituted. Recovery will begin at approximately the 10th day of therapy. The disadvantages of this therapy are (1) the necessity for repeated hospitalization for treatment every 60 to 90 days and (2) wide fluctuations in muscle strength.

Whether steroid or anticholinesterase drug therapy is indicated, base-line information regarding the patient's general status must be obtained in order to aid in determining the effectiveness of the therapy. This base-line information regarding vital signs, grip strength, degree of ptosis, and degree of respiratory effort must be compared to the same data obtained at the peak onset of action of therapy and at a minimum of every 4 hours.

Thymectomy.   A thymectomy may be performed to induce the remission of myasthenic symptoms in those patients whose symptoms are difficult to control with anticholinesterase therapy.

A thymectomy is performed in the presence of a thymoma or thymic hyperplasia. Irradiation of the thymus may precede surgery. The surgery itself entails either a transcervical approach or a sternum-splitting procedure that requires the postoperative use of chest tubes or a hemovac. Anticholinesterase drugs may be discontinued preoperatively and reinstituted postoperatively. Steroid therapy may also be initiated postoperatively. With the introduction of drug therapy, the symptoms of myasthenic or cholinergic crisis must be observed for.

Plasmapheresis.   Plasmapheresis, or plasma exchange, is a recent treatment for myasthenia gravis. The use of plasmapheresis is based on the belief that the mechanical removal of the circulating autoantibodies from the plasma should result in the clinical improvement of the myasthenic child.[41] The removal of circulating antibodies may affect neuromuscular transmission by altering the equilibrium between circulating antibodies and antibodies bound to the ACHRs and by allowing a proportion of newly formed ACHRs to function free of antibodies.[42] In myasthenia, plasmapheresis may be used to stabilize a rapidly deteriorating patient in crisis, to improve respiratory functioning before a thymectomy, to hasten the remission of postthymectomy patients, and to stabilize patients after the initiation of steroid therapy.[43]

Plasmapheresis is the process of removing plasma from the blood and replacing it with saline solution or albumin. The number of required plasma exchanges is based on the patient's response to the procedure. Large-vein access routes are used for the exchange, and the amount of plasma removed is determined by the patient's hematocrit level.[41]

Before the exchange, base-line information is needed concerning muscle strength, ptosis, respiratory functioning, protective reflex ability, and vital signs. A consent form is required. During the procedure, the child should be placed on a cardiorespiratory monitor. Vital signs must be monitored every 30 to 60 minutes. The exchange site should be observed for hematoma formation.

The complications of hypokalemia and hypocalcemia may occur during the exchange secondary to the changing plasma volumes. Signs of hypocalcemia are muscle pain and/or contractions, tetany, and lengthening of the Q-T interval on the electrocardiogram. Symptoms of hypokalemia are nausea, vomiting, weakness, shallow respirations, and T wave depression. Calcium gluconate and potassium chloride must be within easy access.

The child will continue to receive anticholinesterase therapy during the exchange and should be observed closely for signs of under- or overdosage. With the removal of the patient's plasma, there is a loss of plasma-bound medications (e.g., prednisone). Therefore, when possible, these medications should be administered after the exchange.

Nutritional support.   The nutritional needs of the child in myasthenic crisis can be met through enteral feedings. Precautions must be taken to prevent aspiration secondary to weakened protective reflexes. Slow, continuous nasogastric feedings or small, frequent feedings and careful positioning of the child will help to minimize the possibility of aspiration. Commercially prepared fluid diets are commonly administered via the nasogastric route (*see* p. 480).

If constipation develops, enemas should be avoided because they tend to precipitate a crisis. Mild laxatives may be administered prophylactically.

If the child's caloric needs are not being met by the enteral route, total parenteral nutrition is recommended by either peripheral or central routes. Strict monitoring of intake and output is necessary, as well as serum electrolyte monitoring (*see* p. 494).

Respiratory management.   For the child in myasthenic crisis, respiratory management is of paramount importance. Respiratory failure in myasthenia gravis is classified as restrictive in nature because its primary component is the loss of control of ventilation due to muscular paralysis or weakness. As the paralysis is reversed, ventilation resumes.

The child will be placed in a pediatric intensive care setting for intensive ventilatory support. The child will be intubated nasally and placed on a time-, volume-, or pressure-cycled ventilator. For long-term ventilation, a tracheostomy may be considered.

Initially, the child will be placed on controlled ventilation, and then weaned to an IMV circuit as muscle weakness decreases and spontaneous ventilation becomes possible. Rapid weaning in the myasthenic child may result in myasthenic crisis because of the increased work of breathing and the alteration in anticholinesterase consumption. During the weaning process, the child's duration and degree of respiratory effort without fatigue must be evaluated, as well as the return and strength of the cough and gag reflexes.

Positive end-expiratory pressure (PEEP) is used to increase the child's functional residual capacity and to improve oxygenation. Low pressures are preferred to prevent barotrauma to the trachea. Required oxygen concentrations are dependent on the child's arterial blood gases.

The duration of artificial ventilation is individually determined, based on the child's response to drug therapy, thymectomy, plasmapheresis, or any combination of therapies. During the period of ventilation, it is important to prevent complications: atelectasis, infection, artificial airway obstruction, and pneumonia. The child's fear and anxiety will also need to be minimized because these reactions may prolong a myasthenic crisis and the duration of artificial ventilation.

The following list is a summary of respiratory care in myasthenia gravis:

Endotracheal suctioning every two hours

Hyperinflation with 100% oxygen

End-tidal carbon dioxide monitoring

Transcutaneous PaO_2 monitoring

Arterial blood gases every shift until stable

Weekly tracheal aspirate culture

Chest physiotherapy with postural drainage every four hours

Repositioning every two hours

Tracheostomy care every shift if indicated

Weekly changes of tracheostomy tube
Chest x-ray weekly and as needed

The following list is a summary of the ongoing respiratory assessments associated with the treatment of the child with myasthenia gravis:

Breath sounds
Return of protective reflexes
Ability to manage secretions
Strength of spontaneous respirations
Duration of spontaneous respirations without fatigue
Signs and symptoms of respiratory insufficiency as ventilatory support is weaned
Signs of anticholinesterase over- or underdosage

Immobility.   The problems of immobility need to be considered for the child in crisis with extreme muscle weakness or paralysis. Repositioning every 2 hours, the use of an alternating pressure mattress, and meticulous skin care will aid in the prevention of decubitus ulcers. Passive range-of-motion exercises are conducted to maintain joint mobility. Care must be taken to avoid fatigue during these procedures because fatigue will prolong myasthenic crisis.

Stress control.   High levels of anxiety may contribute to the prolongation of myasthenic crisis. The child faced with acute hospitalization of unknown duration will be anxious and frightened. A primary concern in the critical care management of a child in crisis is the alleviation of stress.

The hospitalized child has specific needs with regard to controlling stress: (1) age-appropriate explanations for all treatments and procedures; (2) the knowledge that family members are nearby; and (3) age-appropriate diversional/play activities. These basic needs can be met through the early establishment of communication pathways.

The child may either not be strong enough to talk or be unable to talk because of intubation. The use of picture boards (with pictures of common objects and pictures that indicate feelings and normal patterns of daily living) may prove helpful. If the child is old enough and strong enough to write, pencil and paper should be provided. Parental visiting is strongly recommended. Familiar objects or toys from home will help provide the young child with a sense of security.

The adolescent in the pediatric intensive care unit requires special consideration with regard to privacy and to the need of controlling the environment to the greatest possible extent. Daily schedules may be adapted to these needs and may make use of appropriate input from the patient. Because the adolescent patient needs to maintain peer contact, visits from friends should be encouraged.

The parents of the child in the pediatric intensive care unit will also be under stress. Their stress can be alleviated through consistent communication from physicians and nurses and through involvement in their child's care as feasible. The child's emotional response to crisis reflects parental response to stress.

INFANT BOTULISM

Since infant botulism was first identified in 1976, over 188 cases have been reported to the Center for Disease Control (CDC) in Atlanta, Georgia. There are three kinds of botulism: adult, infant, and wound botulism. In adult botulism, the preformed toxin, released by the *Clostridium botulinum* spore, is ingested via a contaminated food source. Adult botulism results in rapid deterioration, total muscle paralysis, and, often, death.

In infant botulism, the spores of *C. botulinum* are ingested directly. Once ingested, these spores germinate, multiply, and colonize the gastrointestinal tract, where they manufacture botulin. As the toxin is absorbed from the gastrointestinal tract, it binds irreversibly with nerve terminals. Because the spores are ingested (rather than the toxin), the onset of symptoms and clinical course of infant botulism will vary from infant to infant.

Wound botulism occurs when there is a penetrating injury to the skin. Most commonly, *C. botulinum* will enter the wound when dirt or soil makes contact with it. Failure to cleanse the wound completely, followed by the placement of an occlusive dressing will create an anaerobic environment that allows proliferation of *C. botulinum*. The clinical course is similar to that of adult botulism.

Etiology

Infant botulism is an acute neuromuscular disease produced by the spores of *C. botulinum*. The exact source of these spores is unknown, although they are ubiquitous in nature. Studies have identified these spores in honey, topsoil, household dust, breast milk, and fresh fruits and vegetables.[44–46]

Because botulism occurs sporadically, it is presumed that some infants have an increased susceptibility to it. When a susceptible infant is exposed to environmental factors that contain *C. botulinum* spores, the infant is at risk for developing infant botulism.

Most infants who develop infant botulism are the products of a normal gestation and delivery, and are normal in their growth and development. Infant botulism appears to affect equal percentages of male and female infants. The age of the infant, however, appears to be a significant factor in the development of infant botulism: infants are at greatest risk between 3 weeks and 6 months of age. After 6 months of age, the risk of infant botulism is minimal. This decreased incidence may be due to colonization in the infant's gastrointestinal tract.

Some studies suggest that the infant's diet may contribute to the development of infant botulism. The colonization of the gastrointestinal tract with bacterial flora differs markedly in formula-fed and breast-fed infants. Formula-fed infants colonize their gastrointestinal tract with *Bacteroides fragilis* by the first week of life, whereas *B. fragilis* is not commonly found in the gastrointestinal tract of breast-fed infants until they are weaned from breast milk.[47] These differences may encourage the germination and growth of the *C. botulinum* spores.

Pathophysiology

Two theories are currently being investigated with regard to the muscle paralysis associated with infant botulism. The so-called presynaptic theory posits that the botulinal toxin inhibits the release of ACH from the synaptic vesicles: the postsynaptic theory assumes that the botulinal toxin interferes with the ACHRs at the motor end plate of the muscle. Whichever theory is accepted, the result is the same: the failure of ACH to bind to the ACHR sites, or to be released in sufficient amounts, interrupts normal nerve transmission and thereby inhibits muscle contraction.

Because the botulinal toxin is irreversibly bound to the neuromuscular junction, recovery from infant botulism occurs when there is growth of new nerve terminals. The return of muscle control begins with the regaining of functions that were the last to be lost.

Clinical Presentation

Although constipation is often the first sign of infant botulism, it is frequently missed or ignored. The most frequently recognized sign is the infant's loss of appetite and difficulty with feeding. This is apparent in the breast-fed infant when the mother continues to experience engorgement and discomfort after feedings, and in the bottle-fed infant when the infant no longer empties the bottle at feedings.

The gradual blockade of the neuromuscular junction in infant botulism correponds to the slow deterioration of the child's muscular and cranial nerve functioning. The slow blockade of ACHR sites causes the sympathetic system of the child to become overloaded, and this can contribute to the tachycardia that some infants present with.

Early in the disease, activities that require repetitive neuromuscular functioning are lost (e.g., crying, feeding, ocular and facial movements). The infant's inability to suck and swallow, and the loss of the cough and gag reflexes, indicate muscular paresis of the 9th cranial nerve. The infant gradually loses all facial expression (7th cranial nerve), eyelids begin to droop until the infant can no longer keep them open, and pupillary responses become sluggish (3rd cranial nerve).

The infant becomes progressively weaker and "floppier," with loss of peripheral movement and the characteristic loss of head control. When paralysis is almost complete, the infant will lose control of the diaphragm, and this loss will place the infant in danger of respiratory arrest.

The timetable for the progression of these clinical signs varies from 4 hours to 2 weeks, and the extent of clinical involvement varies from infant to infant.

Diagnosis

When the infant with severe neuromuscular depression is admitted to the intensive care unit, a wide spectrum of diseases must be ruled out; however, the most likely diagnosis for the acutely ill, floppy infant is meningitis. Therefore, a lumbar puncture (LP) should be performed. Meningitis is ruled out when the analysis of cerebrospinal fluid reveals a negative culture and sensitivity, a negative Gram stain, few white blood cells, a normal glucose level, and a clear appearance. Frequently, infant botulism will cause a transient elevation in the protein level of cerebrospinal fluid.

Routine laboratory tests should be performed on admission. These tests should include a complete blood count, blood urea nitrogen, electrolytes, and serum calcium and magnesium. In infant botulism, the results of these tests are usually within normal limits.

Although other tests that are less invasive are usually performed, a muscle biopsy and muscle enzymes can be obtained. In infant botulism, the results of these tests are generally negative, implying that the abnormality exists at the neuromuscular junction; however, a transient elevation in the level of muscle enzymes is not uncommon.

EMG is often helpful in the clinical diagnosis of infant botulism. The EMG pattern that is typical of infant botulism (and other primary muscle diseases) consists of brief, small-amplitude, abundant motor reaction potential (BSAP).[48]

The definitive diagnosis of infant botulism is made when C. botulinum is isolated from the infant's stool. Because the infant with botulism is usually constipated, obtaining a stool sample is often difficult. The infant can be stimulated to stool by means of glycerin suppositories. Once bowel movements have resumed, the infant's stool should be collected until 25 grams are obtained. This collection of stool should be kept on ice or frozen, and sent on dry ice to the CDC for analysis. Infant botulism is a disease that is reportable to the CDC.[45]

Critical Care Management

Infants with infant botulism should be admitted to an intensive care unit for close respiratory monitoring. Progressive neuromuscular blockade can deprive the infant of the cough and gag reflexes, resulting in an airway that is unprotected and vulnerable to aspiration. A nasogastric tube should be inserted to empty the stomach, thereby preventing vomiting and possible aspiration.

The infant's ability to breathe should be continually evaluated because respiratory arrest can occur suddenly and proceed rapidly. Respiratory function studies, including maximal inspiratory force (MIF) and vital capacity (VC), are performed daily. These tests provide an ongoing assessment of the child's respiratory progress.

Infants with infant botulism will have a decreased VC and MIF. VC is the maximal expired volume, expressed in milliliters and measured when the infant exhales completely into a spirometer. An adequate VC in the infant is 60 ml/kg. (Often, the infant must be stimulated to obtain a correct value.)

The MIF, measured with a hand-held manometer, can only be obtained when the infant is breathing spontaneously and when the manometer is placed over the infant's nose and mouth, creating a tight seal. An infant should have an MIF of greater than -20 to -30 cm/water. Values of less than -20 cm/water are indicative of poor respiratory musculature functioning. The VC and MIF, together with clinical assessment, can determine when elective intubation is necessary to ensure a safe airway and adequate gas exchange.

If the infant requires long-term respiratory management, a tracheostomy may be necessary. A tracheostomy avoids many of the hazards associated with long-term endotracheal intubation and also allows the infant more freedom of movement.

Meticulous nursing care is essential in order to prevent pneumonia and/or atelectasis. The infant should receive chest physiotherapy (postural drainage, percussion, and vibration) every 3 to 4 hours, and should be suctioned every 1 to 2 hours. These procedures will maintain a patent airway and promote removal of any tracheal secretions.

It is extremely important to realize that infants with infant botulism are vulnerable to events that impair or stress the neuromuscular junctions. For example, when the infant is positioned for an LP, the infant's pliable airway may be easily obstructed. Because the infant with botulism is incapable of exerting the degree of muscle activity that is needed to relieve this obstruction, the infant can sustain a respiratory arrest. When returned to a normal position, however, the infant will initiate spontaneous respirations.

Muscle paralysis renders infants with infant botulism totally dependent on excellent supportive care. It is essential that these infants be turned every 2 to 3 hours, and they should be placed on alternating pressure mattresses, if these are available. These measures preserve the skin and facilitate good respiratory care.

A program for physical therapy should be instituted as soon as the infant's airway is stabilized. Passive range-of-motion exercises should be performed several times a day in order to prevent muscle loss and wasting. These exercises, which can be taught to the parents, are an excellent way of involving the parents in the care of their infant.

The infant should be assessed for fluid and caloric requirements. Often, the infant with infant botulism will not tolerate nasogastric feedings (possibly because of the changes that have occurred in the infant's gastrointestinal tract and because of the lack of neuromuscular innervation). Therefore, the provision of fluids and calories via an intravenous infusion is often necessary. Peripheral hyperalimentation can be initiated in order to supply calories and to decrease muscle wasting. If long-term support is indicated, the infant may need a central venous line inserted for continued hyperalimentation and for intralipid administration. As neuromuscular control is regained, the infant can be restarted on nasogastric or oral feedings.

Adequate ventilation and the presence of a gag reflex are not sufficient indicators of returned muscle functioning to warrant the withdrawal of ventilatory support. When infants are started on nasogastric feedings and extubated/decannulated before the return of head control, they are at a higher risk for aspiration, which would require reintubation and the reinstitution of ventilation.

Although appearing very still and unresponsive, the infant with infant botulism continues to be quite aware of the noises and sounds in the environment. Parents should be encouraged to talk to and touch their infant. The nurse should work with the parents in developing a program of infant stimulation, which will provide the infant with stimuli that are familiar and soothing. When possible, the parents should be encouraged to hold and rock the infant. These actions are therapeutic for both the infant and the parents.

It is difficult to assess the return of neuromuscular control in the infant with infant botulism because there is no easy formula for assessing the complete return of functioning at the neuromuscular junction. The return of head control, however, is often used as the hallmark sign for the return of adequate and nearly complete muscle functioning.

Special Considerations

Antibiotic administration is not recommended for the following reasons: (1) antibiotic therapy may selectively suppress the bacterial flora in the gastrointestinal tract, which could lead to the increased proliferation of *C. botulinum;* (2) the administration of aminoglycoside antibiotics (e.g., tobramycin sulfate, gentamicin, or neomycin) can further decrease the amount of ACH released at the neuromuscular junction. This decrease in ACH seems to affect the innervation of the diaphragm, causing increased weakness and subsequent respiratory failure.[49]

The administration of an antitoxin has also been considered.[49] This has not been found effective, however, because the antitoxin does not release the toxin that is already bound to the nerve terminal and thus does not inhibit or interrupt the progressing paralysis.

REFERENCES

1. Meakin.
2. Swaiman and Wright. 79.
3. Swaiman and Wright. 6.
4. Swaiman and Wright. 4.
5. Swaiman and Wright. 5.
6. Alexander and Brown. 239.
7. Swaiman and Wright. 18.
8. Swaiman and Wright. 7.
9. Swaiman and Wright. 20.
10. Swaiman and Wright. 8.
11. Swaiman and Wright. 10.
12. Vaughn et al. 1733.
13. Swaiman and Wright. 13.
14. Swaiman and Wright. 14.

15. Swaiman and Wright. 11.
16. Mayo Clinic. 113.
17. Vaughn et al. 1734.
18. Mayo Clinic. 114.
19. Mayo Clinic. 115.
20. Mayo Clinic. 116.
21. Mayo Clinic. 229.
22. Ross et al.
23. Swaiman and Wright. 39.
24. Kennedy et al.
25. Nelson et al.
26. Osler and Sidell.
27. National Institute of Neurological and Communicative Disorders and Stroke.
28. Swaiman and Wright. 84.
29. Litchenfeld.
30. Bell and McCormick. 425.
31. Bell and McCormick. 426.
32. Samonds.
33. Fenichel.
34. Drachman. (1979)
35. Rana and Luskin.
36. Drachman. (1978) Part I.
37. Lindstrom et al.
38. Drachman. (1978) Part II.
39. Dahl.
40. Rodman and Smith. 268.
41. Blount et al.
42. Pinching et al.
43. Dau et al.
44. Chin et al.
45. Dowell.
46. Arnon et al.
47. Long and Swenson.
48. Clay et al.
49. Marks.

BIBLIOGRAPHY

Alexander, M. M., and M. S. Brown. 1974. Pediatric Physical Diagnosis for Nurses. McGraw-Hill Book Co., Inc., New York.

American Association of Critical Care Nurses. 1975. Core Curriculum for Critical Care Nursing. American Association of Critical Care Nurses.

Arnon, S. S., and J. Chin. 1979. The clinical spectrum of infant botulism. *Reviews of Infectious Diseases*. 1:614–621.

Arnon, S. S., T. F. Midura, K. Damus, B. Thompson, R. M. Wood, and J. Chin. 1979. Honey and other environmental risk factors for infant botulism. *Journal of Pediatrics*. **94**:331–336.

Arnon, S. S., T. F. Midura, K. Damus, R. M. Wood, and J. Chin. 1978. Intestinal infection and toxin production by Clostridium botulinum as one cause of sudden infant death syndrome. Lancet. **I**:1273–1276.

Bell, W. E., and W. F. McCormick. 1975. Neurologic Infections in Children. W. B. Saunders Co., Philadelphia.

Berg, B. 1977. Syndrome of infant botulism. *Pediatrics*. **59**:321–322.

Blount, M., A. Kenney, and M. Stone. 1979. Plasma exchange in the management of myasthenia gravis. *Nursing Clinics of North America*. **14**:173–190.

Bushnell, S. 1973. Respiratory Intensive Care: From Beth Israel Hospital, Boston, Little, Brown & Co., Boston.

Chin, J, S. S. Arnon, and T. F. Midura. 1979. Food and environmental aspects of infant botulism in California. *Reviews of Infectious Diseases*. 1:693–696.

Clay, S. A., C. Ramseyer, L. S. Fishman, and R. P. Sedgwick. 1977. Acute infantile motor unit disorder. *Archives of Neurology*. **34**:236–243.

Crowley, C., and A. Morrow. 1980. A comprehensive approach to the child in respiratory failure. *(CCQ) Critical Care Quarterly*. 3:27–43.

Dahl, D. 1976. The management of myasthenia gravis. *Drug Therapy*. 1:21–29.

Dau, P., J. Lindstrom, C. Cassel, E. Denys, E. Shev, and L. Spitler. 1977. Plasmapheresis and immunosuppressive drug therapy in myasthenia gravis. *New England Journal of Medicine*. 297:1134–1140.

Donohoe, K. N. 1079. An overview of neuromuscular disease. *Nursing Clinics of North America*. 14:95–106.

Dowell, V. R. 1978. Infant botulism: new guise for an old disease. *Hospital Practice*. 67–72.

Drachman, D. 1979. Immunopathology of myasthenia gravis. *Federation Proceedings*. **38**:2613–2615.

Drachman, D. 1978. Myasthenia gravis. Part I. *New England Journal of Medicine*. **298**:186–193.

Drachman, D. 1978. Myasthenia gravis. Part II. *New England Journal of Medicine.* **298:**186–193.

Farber, H. L. Wynn, H. Farr, J. Schacter, P. Lerke, and J. Chin. 1979. Infant botulism in 1931. *American Journal of Diseases of Children.* **133:**580–582.

Fenichel, G. 1978. Clinical syndromes of myasthenia in infancy and childhood. *Archives of Neurology.* **35:**97–103.

Foldes, F., Graser, G. 1971. Diagnostic tests in myasthenia gravis: overview. *Annals of the New York Academy of Sciences.* **183:**275–286.

Frohlich, E. D. 1976. Pathophysiology. J. B. Lippincott Co., Philadelphia. Second edition.

Ganong, W. F. 1981. Review of Medical Physiology. Lange Medical Publications, Los Altos, Calif. Tenth edition.

Genkins, G., P. Kornfeld, and K. Osserman. 1971. The use of ACTH and corticosteroids in myasthenia gravis. *Annals of the New York Academy of Sciences.* **183:**369–374.

Groenwald, S. 1980. Physiology of the immune system. *Heart & Lung.* **9:**645–650.

Grover, W., G. J. Peckham, and P. H. Berman. 1974. Recovery following cranial nerve dysfunction and muscle weakness in infancy. *Developmental Medicine and Child Neurology.* **16:**163–171.

Hedley-Whyte, J. 1965. Respiratory management of peripheral neurologic disease. *In* Bendixen, H., editor. 1965. Respiratory Care. C. V. Mosby Co., St. Louis.

Jones, J. 1980. Plasmapheresis: current research and success. *Heart & Lung.* **9:**671–674.

Kealy, S. 1977. Respiratory care in guillain barré syndrome. *American Journal of Nursing.* **77:**58–60.

Kennedy, R., M. Danielson, D. Mulder, and L. Kurland. 1978. Guillain barré syndrome — a 42 year epidemiologic and clinical study. *Mayo Clinic Proceedings.* **53:**93–99.

Lavigne, J. 1979. Respiratory care of patients with neuromuscular disease. *Nursing Clinics of North America.* **14:**133–143.

Levin, D., F. C. Morriss, and G. C. Moore. 1979. A Practical Guide to Pediatric Intensive Care. C. V. Mosby Co. St. Louis.

Lichtenfeld, P. 1971. Autonomic dysfunction in guillain barré syndrome. *American Journal of Medicine.* **50:**772–780.

Lindstrom, J., M. Seybold, V. Lennon, S. Whittingham, and D. Duane. 1976. Antibody to acetylcholine receptor in myasthenia gravis. *Neurology.* **26:**1054–1059.

Long, S. S., and R. M. Swenson. Development of anaerobic fecal flora in healthy newborn infants. *Journal of Pediatrics.* **91:**2:298–301, 1977.

Marks, R. G. 1978. Infant botulism, a newly recognized infectious disease. *Current Prescribing.* 67–75.

Mayo Clinic and Mayo Foundation for Medical Education and Research. 1976. Clinical Examinations in Neurology. W. B. Saunders Co., Philadelphia. Fourth edition.

McBride, M., and W. Sack. 1980. Emotional management of children with acute respiratory failure in the intensive care unit: a case study. *Heart & Lung.* **9:**98–102.

Meakin, A. 1977. The nerve impulse and disordered transmission. Related physiology. Part I. *Nursing Mirror.* **145:**17–18.

Meakin, A. 1977. The nerve impulse and disordered transmission. Part II. Myasthenia gravis. *Nursing Mirror.* **145:**34–35.

Midura, T. F. 1979. Laboratory aspects of infant botulism in California. *Infectious Disease Reviews.* **1:**652–654.

Mills, N., and H. Plasterer. 1980. guillain barré syndrome: a framework for nursing care. *Nursing Clinics of North America.* **15:**257–264.

Nastuk, W. 1971. Mechanism of neuromuscular blockade. *Annals of the New York Academy of Sciences.* **183:**171–182.

National Institute of Neurological and Communicative Disorders and Stroke. 1978. Criteria for Diagnosis of Guillain Barré Syndrome. *Annals of Neurology* **3:**565–566.

Nelson, D., R. Holman, E. Hurwitz, L. Schonberger, D. Bregman, and R. Kaslow. 1979. Results of the national surveillance for guillain barré syndrome. *Neurology.* **29:**1029–1033.

Osler, L., and A. Sidell. 1960. The guillain barré syndrome — the need for exact diagnostic criteria. *New England Journal of Medicine.* **262:**964–969.

Perlo, V., B. Arnason, D. Paskanzer, B. Castleman, R. Schwab, K. Osserman, A. Papatestis, L. Alpert, and A. Kark, 1971. The role of thytmectomy in the treatment of myasthenia gravis. *Annals of the New York Academy of Sciences.* **183**:308–315.

Pickett, J., B. Berg, E. Chaplin, and M. A. Brunstetter-Shafer. 1976. Syndrome of botulism in infancy: clinical and electrophysiologic study. *New England Journal of Medicine.* **295**:770–772.

Pinching, A., D. Peters, and J. Davis. 1976. Remission of myasthenia gravis following plasma exchange. *Lancet.* **II**:1373–1376.

Pinching, A. 1978. Myasthenia gravis — a frustrating disability. *Nursing Mirror.* **148**:16–18.

Polk, B. 1976. Cardiopulmonary complications of guillain barre syndrome. *Heart & Lung.* **5**:967–970.

Rana, A., and A. Luskin. 1980. Immunosuppression, autoimmunity, and hypersensitivity. *Heart & Lung.* **9**:651–657.

Rodman, M. J., D. W. Smith. 1974. Clinical Pharmacology in Nursing. J. B. Lippincott Co., Philadelphia.

Ross, A. J., B. E. Herr, M. L. Norwood, K. M. Donohoe, and R. T. Moxley. 1979. Neuromuscular diagnostic procedures. *Nursing Clinics of North America.* **14**:107–121.

Rowland, L. 1971. Immunosuppressive drugs in treatment of myasthenia gravis. *Annals of the New York Academy of Sciences.* **183**:351–357.

Samonds, R. 1980. Guillain barre syndrome. helping the patient in the acute stage. *Nursing '80.* **10**(8):35–41.

Sibley, W. 1972. Polyneuritis. *Medical Clinics of North America.* **56**:1299–1319.

Stackhouse, J. 1973. Myasthenia gravis. *American Journal of Nursing.* **73**:1544–1547.

Swaiman, K. F., and F. S. Wright. 1979. Pediatric Neuromuscular Diseases. C. V. Mosby, Co., St. Louis.

Turner, H. D., E. M. Brett, R. J. Gilbert, A. C. Ghosh, and H. J. Liebeschuetz. 1978. Infant botulism in England. Lancet. **I**:1277–1278.

Vaughn, V. C. and R. J. McKay, editors. 1979. *Nelson's Textbook of Pediatrics.* W. B. Saunders, Co., Philadelphia. Eleventh edition.

CHAPTER **6**

THE RENAL SYSTEM

Margaret D. Rielly

The kidneys are regulatory organs that function to maintain internal homeostasis of body fluids and electrolytes. The series of complex physiological mechanisms performed by the kidneys to ensure this balance effects many organ systems throughout the body. Fluid and electrolyte balance is accomplished through interdependent functions that primarily involve the renal and respiratory systems.

Nursing care planning for the child with renal dysfunction requires that the nurse possess a solid knowledge base regarding normal renal functioning. Therefore, this chapter begins with a discussion of the body's fluid composition, its electrolytes, and how the kidneys regulate these factors. Acid-base balance is then reviewed in detail, and metabolic disturbances of acid-base balance are covered briefly.

Principles of nursing care for the child with renal dysfunction are necessarily broad because there is such a wide spectrum of renal disorders. Each child's clinical presentation and course will dictate how these principles of nursing care are individualized and applied.

The section devoted to the nursing assessment of a child with renal dysfunction reviews the type of information the nurse would gather to assess renal functioning and the overall clinical presentation of the child.

The remainder of the chapter is devoted to discussions of renal disorders that are frequently encountered in the pediatric intensive care unit patient, including hypertension, acute renal failure, the hemolytic uremic syndrome, disorders of fluid balance, and disorders of antidiuretic hormone.

Nurses employed in pediatric ICUs need to be cognizant of the fact that nursing care of patients with renal disease primarily involves monitoring the clinical parameters of various organ systems other than the renal system. This includes primarily the cardiac and respiratory systems. In addition, it cannot be overemphasized that the nurse must be aware of the importance of reviewing the functioning of organ systems other than the renal system when assessing a patient for potential renal dysfunctioning.

SELECTED ASPECTS OF RENAL PHYSIOLOGY

Composition of Body Fluid Compartments

Water. The percentage of an individual's body weight that is composed of water varies with age and the amount of fatty tissue present. The water content of fat

TABLE 6-1 Total Body Water*

Age	Children	Males	Females
	%	%	%
0–1 mo	75.7		
1–12 mo	64.5		
1–10 yr	61.7		
10–16 yr		58.9	57.3
Young adult		60.6	50.2
Middle age		54.7	46.7
Elderly		51.5	45.5

Reprinted with permission from Brenner, B. M., and F. C. Rector, Jr., editors. 1976. The Kidney. Vol. I. W. B. Saunders Co., Philadelphia. 77. Original data from Edelman, I. S., and J. Leibman. 1959. Anatomy of body water and electrolytes. *American Journal of Medicine.* **27:**256–276.

*Values are given as a percentage of body weight.

cells is approximately 10 percent as compared with 75 to 80 percent for other body cells. Thus, the more adipose tissue an individual has, the smaller the percentage of total body weight that is water.

Total body water is divided into two main compartments: the intracellular fluid (ICF) and the extracellular fluid (ECF). The ECF can be subdivided into the intravascular and interstitial fluids. The intravascular fluid — **plasma** — is composed of 94 percent water. The interstitial fluid bathes all cells throughout the body. A minor portion of the interstitial fluid is located in transcellular compartments (e.g., the pleural, pericardial, and peritoneal) and as inaccessible bone water. The size of the ICF and ECF compartments, and the percentage of body weight that is water, change as a person ages. As a child grows, the formation of new cells increases the size of the ICF compartment. At the same time, the percentage of total body weight that is water steadily decreases (Table 6-1). Once a person reaches adulthood, the size of the various body fluid compartments remains relatively constant (Fig. 6-1).

Electrolytes. Electrolytes are substances that produce positively (cation) and negatively (anion) charged particles when placed in water. Each body fluid compartment contains different concentrations of electrolytes (Fig. 6-2). At present, the concentration of intracellular electrolytes cannot be accurately measured, and therefore, they are not included in Table 6-2. For electroneutrality to exist within any one fluid compartment, the number of cations must equal the number of anions. The main cation of the ECF is sodium (Na^+), whereas the main cation of the ICF is potassium (K^+). Chloride (Cl^-) and bicarbonate (HCO_3^-) are the most plentiful extracellular anions. The intracellular anions are composed largely of organic phosphate and cellular proteins with only a small amount of bicarbonate present. Interstitial and plasma fluids are similar in composition except for a difference in the amount of protein they contain. The protein concentration of plasma fluid is higher because proteins (due to their size) are confined by capillary membranes to the plasma. The high protein concentration of plasma results in equilibrium between plasma and interstitial fluid, which conforms to the Gibbs-Donnan principle which states that because proteins carry a negative charge, when equilibrium exists between the plasma and the interstitial fluid, the plasma will contain a larger number of diffusible cations and fewer diffusible anions than

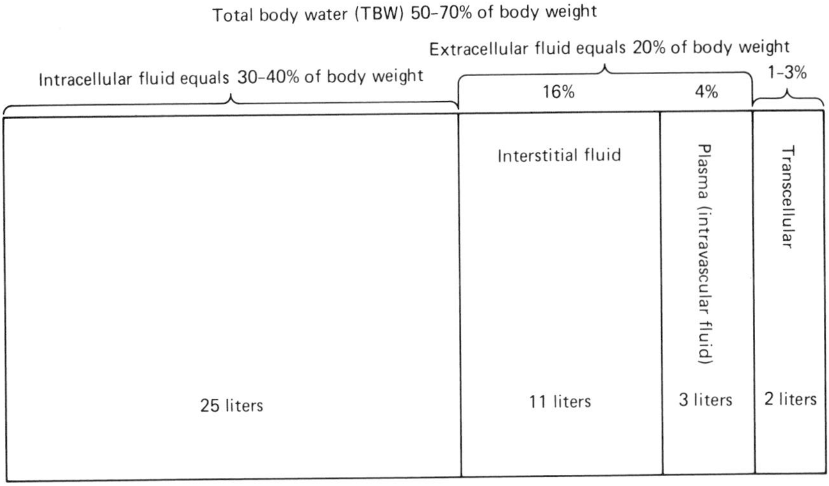

Total body water (TBW) 50-70% of body weight

Extracellular fluid equals 20% of body weight

Intracellular fluid equals 30-40% of body weight

				1-3%
		16%	4%	

	Interstitial fluid	Plasma (intravascular fluid)	Transcellular
25 liters	11 liters	3 liters	2 liters

Figure 6-1. Approximate size of the major body fluid compartments, expressed as a percentage of body weight and in mean absolute values for an adult human being who weighs 70 kg (154 lb). The ranges of normal among individuals are considerable. Thus, no single value should be interpreted too rigidly. *Reprinted with permission from* Valtin, H. 1973. Renal Function: Mechanisms Preserving Fluid and Solute Balance in Health. Little, Brown & Co., Boston. 16.

the interstitial fluid (Fig. 6-3).[1] The result is that the osmotic pressure of the plasma is greater than that of the interstitial fluid. An appreciation of the Gibbs-Donnan principle is fundamental to an understanding of how fluid shifts occur in the body.

Measurement of Solute

A knowledge of the vocabulary used to describe fluid and electrolyte homeostasis is essential to an understanding of fundamental concepts to be discussed in the remainder of this chapter. These terms pertain to the measurement of solutes in body fluids, and are defined as follows:

1. *Solute:* A substance dissolved in a solvent. 1 mole of a solute equals the molecular weight in grams or milligrams. A mole of an element is equal to the gram atomic weight of that element (e.g., one mole of sodium is equal to 23 grams). One millimole of sodium is equal to 23 mg.
2. *Milliequivalent:* Electrolyte concentrations in diluted body fluids are expressed as milliequivalents (mEq) per liter of fluid rather than as equivalents (1/1,000 equivalent = 1 mEq). The following formulas may be used to calculate the milliequivalents of a particular electrolyte:
   a. *univalent ions (e.g., sodium ion):* Divide the number of milligrams of the electrolyte by its atomic or molecular weight. To determine the number of milliequivalents of a particular substance of a univalent ion, use the following formula:

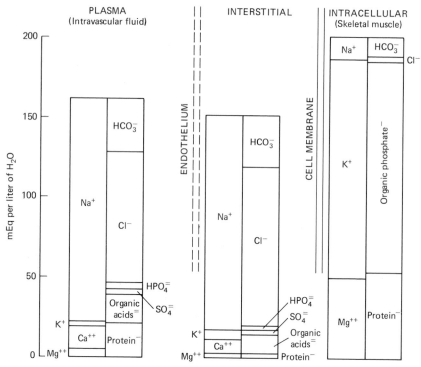

Figure 6-2. The main solute and electrolyte constituents of the major body fluid compartments. The concentrations are expressed as chemical equivalents to emphasize that the compartments are made up mainly of electrolytes, and that within any one space, the total number of negative charges equals the number of positive charges. The values given for intracellular fluid are approximations. Despite limitations, the diagram serves to emphasize important and typical differences between intracellular and extracellular fluid. *Reprinted with permission from* Valtin, H. 1973. Renal Function: Mechanisms Preserving Fluid and Solute Balance in Health. Little, Brown & Co., Boston. 20.

$$\text{mEq of a substance} = \frac{\text{number of milligrams of substance x the valence}}{\text{molecular or atomic weight}}.$$

For example, to determine how many milliequivalents of sodium there are in 46 mg, the following equation would be used:

$$\text{x mEq of sodium} = \frac{46 \text{ mg of sodium} \times 1}{23 \text{ mg of sodium}}.$$

$$\text{x mEq of sodium} = 2.$$

This means that there are 2 mEq of sodium in 46 mg of sodium.

TABLE 6-2 Average Concentration of Human Extracellular Fluid

Ions	Plasma (Intravascular fluid)	Interstitial fluid
Cations	mEq/kg H$_2$O	mEq/kg H$_2$O
Na$^+$	150	144
K$^+$	4–5	4–5
Ca^{++}	5	3
Mg^{++}	2	1.5
H$^+$	4×10^{-5}	4×10^{-5}
Total cation	**161**	**153**
Anions		
Cl$^-$	110	114
HCO$_3^-$	27	28
HPO$_4^-$ and H$_2$PO$_4^-$	2	2
SO$_4^-$	1	1
Proteinate	17	4
Organic acids	4	4
Total anion	**161**	**153**
Water	1,000 ml/kg H$_2$O 289 mOsm/kg H$_2$O	288 mOsm/kg H$_2$O

Reprinted with permission from Brenner, B. M., and F. C. Rector, Jr., editors. 1976. The Kidney. Vol. I. W. B. Saunders Co., Philadelphia. 82.

b. *multivalent ions (e.g., calcium ion):* The number of milligrams of substance is multiplied by the valence and then divided by the atomic or molecular weight:

$$\text{mEq of a substance} = \frac{\text{number of milligrams of substance} \times \text{valence}}{\text{atomic or molecular weight}}.$$

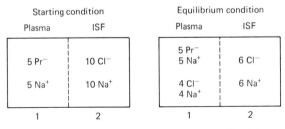

Figure 6-3. The Gibbs-Donnan principle. The effect of nondiffusable protein (Pr) anions on the distribution of diffusable cations and anions under closed-system conditions. Pr carries a negative charge and does not readily diffuse across vascular membrances. ISF, interstitial fluid. *Reprinted with permission from Pitts, R. F. 1974. Physiology of the Kidney and Body Fluids. Year Book Publishers, Inc., Chicago. Third edition. 20.*

For example, to determine the number of milliequivalents of calcium in 80 mg, the following equation would be used:

$$\text{x mEq of calcium} = \frac{80 \text{ mg of calcium} \times 2}{40 \text{ mg}}.$$

$$\text{x mEq} = \frac{160 \text{ mg}}{40 \text{ mg}}.$$

$$\text{x mEq of calcium} = 4.$$

3. *Osmole:* A measure of osmotic force. Osmotic force is a function of the number of discrete particles dissolved in solution. 1 mole of a substance is equivalent to 1 osmole if this substance does not dissociate into smaller parts. For example, 1 mole or 1 osmole of sodium is equal to 23 grams. The osmotic force of a substance is independent of valence, electric charge, and mass.

4. *Milliosmole (mOsm, equal to 0.001 osmole):* A measure of solute concentration, independent of valence, electric charge, or mass. A milliosmole equals millimoles multiplied by *n*, where *n* equals the number of electrolytic particles produced by dissociation of a millimole of a given substance. It is a measure of the number of discrete particles in a solution. For example:

$$\text{Univalent ions: 1 mM Na}^+ = 1 \text{ mOsm Na}^+.$$

$$\text{Multivalent ions: 1 mM Mg}^{++} = 1 \text{ mOsm Mg}^{++}.$$

The osmotic pressure is the same for uni- and multivalent ions. Multivalent ions exert no more osmotic pressure than univalent ions despite their higher chemical equivalents.

5. *Molarity (M, osmolarity):* Moles of solute per liter of solvent (same as millimoles per milliliter).

6. *Molality (m, osmolality):* Moles of solute per 1,000 grams of solvent (same as millimoles per milligram).

7. *Osmolality:* The tonicity (*see below*) of a fluid as compared with a second fluid (usually plasma). For example, a 3 percent saline solution is hypertonic because plasma is a 0.9 percent saline solution, which is isotonic. Osmolality can be expressed as milliosmoles per kilogram of solvent.

8. *Osmolarity:* Expressed as milliosmoles per liter of solvent.

9. *Isotonic:* A solution is isotonic if, when separated from a second solution by a semipermeable membrane, no transfer of water occurs. Both solutions have the same osmolality (Fig. 6-4).

10. *Hypertonic:* A solution is hypertonic if, when separated from a second solution by a semipermeable membrane, there is a net transfer of water from a solution of low solute concentration to one of a higher solute concentration (Fig. 6-4).

11. *Hypotonic:* A solution is hypotonic if, when separated from a second solution by a semipermeable membrane, there is a net transfer of water from a solution with a higher solute concentration to one with a lower solute concentration (Fig. 6-4).

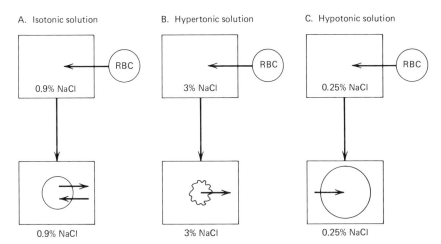

A. Isotonic solution   B. Hypertonic solution   C. Hypotonic solution

Figure 6-4. This figure depicts the effect of different concentrations of NaCl solution on a red blood cell (RBC). In A, no fluid movement occurs between the RBC and the isotonic solution because these two solutions both contain the same concentration of NaCl. In B, fluid moves out of the RBC into the hypertonic solution in an attempt to establish equilibrium. The RBC undergoes a process known as crenation. In C, when a RBC enters a hypotonic solution, fluid moves into the RBC and the cell swells and eventually bursts.

Thus, the osmolality of body fluids is determined by the concentration of osmotically active particles. Although the plasma protein concentration is approximately 15 mEq/liter, their contribution to the plasma osmolality is less than 1 mOsm/kg of water because they are large molecules.

Forces Responsible for Fluid Movement

There are specific forces regulated by the circulatory and renal systems that are responsible for the movement of the fluid between the interstitial fluid and the plasma. These forces were first described by Starling in 1896. The predominant force, which favors the filtration of fluid out of capillaries, is the intracapillary hydrostatic pressure. The forces opposing filtration include the plasma oncotic pressure and the tissue turgor pressure (*see* Fig. 6-12). The intracapillary hydrostatic pressure is provided by the mechanical pressure of the heart (e.g., blood pressure). The total difference in osmotic pressure that results from the Gibbs-Donnan principle is known as the oncotic pressure. In the case of the interstitial fluid and plasma, this pressure serves as a force that opposes filtration. The combination of all these forces results in a net filtration of fluid out of the arteriolar end of the capillary system into the interstitium and in a net reabsorption of fluid into the capillary as it approaches the venous system. Precapillary sphincters have the ability to alter the rate of fluid movement across capillary membranes through dilation and constriction. Fluids and proteins that are not returned to the capillary at the venular end are eventually returned to the venous system via the lymph channels.

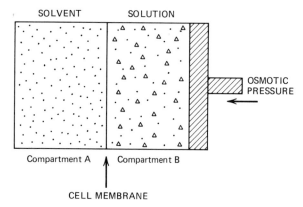

Figure 6-5. A representation of a kinetic formulation based on the diffusion of solvent but not of solute across a membrane. *Reprinted with permission from* Pitts, R. F. 1974. Physiology of the Kidney and Body Fluids. Year Book Medical Publishers, Inc., Chicago. Third edition. 25. (Courtesy of Charles C Thomas, Publisher, Springfield, Ill.)

There are various forces and transport mechanisms that describe the movement of water and solutes between the ICF and ECF compartments:

1. *Osmotic pressure:* The hydrostatic pressure that must be applied to a solution to prevent water solvent from crossing a cell membrane and entering the solution compartment (Fig. 6-5). Osmotic pressure helps maintain the tonicity of solutions.

2. *Passive transport:* The diffusion of solute from an area of high concentration to an area of lower concentration.

3. *Active transport:* Transport of solute that requires energy and results in the movement of solute against an electrochemical or concentration gradient.

4. *Facilitated diffusion:* The passive movement of solute from an area of high concentration to an area of lower concentration that involves preferential binding of solute to cell membrane proteins. This transport system can become saturated.

5. *Solvent drag:* The coupling of water and solute for transport. Movement is accelerated in the presence of an osmotic water flow and produces movement of solute in a "downstream" direction.

Anatomy of the Kidney

The kidneys are retroperitoneally positioned organs that lie on either side of the vertebral column and extend approximately from the 11th thoracic to the 2nd lumbar vertebrae. The right kidney lies at a lower level in the abdominal cavity than the left. The kidneys of a full-term infant at birth weigh approximately 24 grams and are 4.8 centimeters long. The growth of the kidneys parallels growth in the child, reaching adult weight and dimensions (196 to 282 grams and 11 to 12 centimeters in length) during adolescence.

Each kidney is sectioned into different anatomic compartments (Fig. 6-6). The two main areas are designated as the cortex and medulla. The cortex extends from

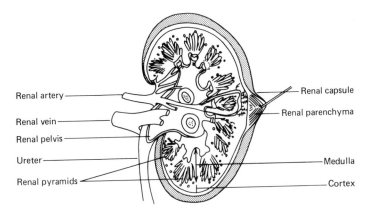

Renal artery

Renal vein

Renal pelvis

Ureter

Renal pyramids

Renal capsule

Renal parenchyma

Medulla

Cortex

Figure 6-6. A longitudinal section of the kidney showing gross anatomic features. *Adapted from* Langley, L. J., I. R. Telford, and J. B. Christensen. 1980. Dynamic Anatomy and Physiology. McGraw-Hill Book Co., New York. Fifth edition. 670.

the renal capsule to the bases of the pyramids. The medulla is subdivided into the outer and inner medulla and extends from the cortex to the renal pelvis.

The nephron is the functional unit of the kidney (Fig. 6-7). Each kidney contains approximately one million nephrons. Each nephron is composed of a glomerulus, Bowman's capsule, proximal convoluted tubule, descending and ascending limbs of the loop of Henle, distal convoluted tubule, and the collecting duct. The glomerulus is a spherical tuft of capillaries formed by the division of the afferent arterioles (Fig. 6-7). The epithelial cells that line the various portions of the tubules differ in their structure. It is believed that these structural differences are directly related to the functional differences between the tubule segments. The juxtaglomerular apparatus (JGA) is composed of specialized epithelial (macula densa) and vascular cells (granular cells) located in the early distal tubule and afferent arterioles of the glomerulus, respectively (Fig. 6-8). These two groups of cells of the same nephron come in close contact with each other and form part of the renin-angiotensin-aldosterone system. This feedback system regulates the size of the ECF compartments via its effect on sodium and water excretion.

As can be seen from Figure 6-9, there are two types of nephrons. The superficial cortical nephrons constitute seven-eighths of the total number of nephrons, and the juxtamedullary nephrons account for the other one eighth. The two types of nephrons differ in their location in the kidney, the length of their loop of Henle, and in the components of the vascular supply distal to the efferent arterioles. The cortical nephron has a short loop of Henle and a peritubular capillary network that surrounds its own tubules as well as those of other nephrons. The large glomeruli of the juxtamedullary nephrons lie in the deep cortical region. Their long loop of Henle extends into the inner medulla and is surrounded by a series of vascular loops called vasa recta, which are branches of the peritubular capillaries.

Renal vasculature.   The renal artery branches off the aorta and enters the kidney hilus alongside the renal vein and ureter (Fig. 6-10, p. 316). The renal artery soon branches into interlobar arteries, which extend through the renal parenchyma and branch to form the arcuate arteries at the corticomedullary junction. The arcuate arteries branch into interlobular arteries, which radiate through the cortex. At the

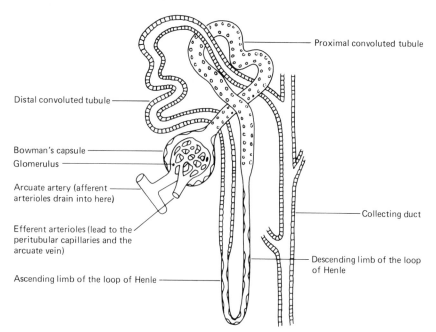

Figure 6-7. Component parts of a nephron. *Adapted from* Pitts, R. F. 1974. Physiology of the Kidney and Body Fluids. Year Book Medical Publishers, Inc., Chicago. Third edition. 4. (Adapted from Smith, H. W. 1935. The Kidney. Oxford University Press, New York.)

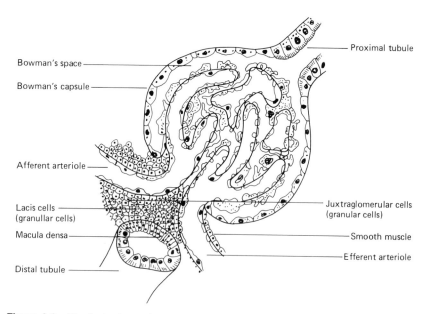

Figure 6-8. The juxtaglomerular apparatus. *Adapted from* Price, S. A., and L. M. Wilson. 1978. Pathophysiology. McGraw-Hill Book Co., New York.

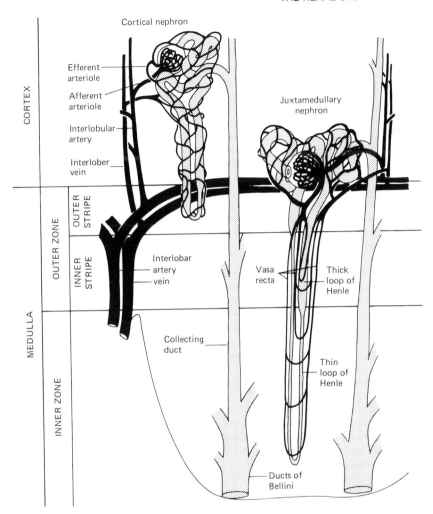

Figure 6-9. Comparison of the blood supplies of cortical and juxtamedullary nephrons. *Reprinted with permission from* Pitts, R. F. 1974. Physiology of the Kidney and Body Fluids. Year Book Medical Publishers, Inc., Chicago. Third edition. 8.

level of the cortex they form the afferent arterioles of the glomeruli. Each afferent arteriole has six to eight branches, which further divide to form the capillaries of the glomerulus. The venous system, which terminates with the renal vein, parallels the arterial vessels as they course through the kidney.

Physiology of the Kidney

Renal hemodynamics are an integral component of renal functioning. The kidneys of an adult weigh about 300 grams combined. Although this constitutes only 0.5

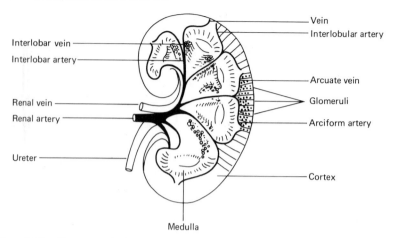

Figure 6-10. Gross morphology of the renal circulation. *Reprinted with permission from* Pitts, R. F. 1974. Physiology of the Kidney and Body Fluids. Year Book Medical Publishers, Inc., Chicago. Third edition. 3.

percent of the total body weight, the kidneys receive 20 to 25 percent of the cardiac output because of the low intrarenal arterial vascular resistance. Vascular resistance increases progressively as blood courses through the kidney. The fact that the cortex receives 90 percent of the total renal blood flow seems related to the kidney's role as a filtering organ and not its oxygen requirements. Extrinsic nervous, hormonal, and intrinsic autonomous factors interact to regulate resistance to blood flow throughout the kidney. The factors that are believed to play a role in the regulation of renal blood flow (RBF) are discussed below.

Autoregulation of RBF. Autoregulation as a theory of RBF regulation was first described in 1911 and has been confirmed experimentally several times since.[2] Autoregulation is described by the observation that the rate of RBF and the glomerular filtration rate (GFR) are held constant in the adult when the mean arterial pressure is varied between 80 and 180 mmHg. Autoregulation is lost at mean arterial pressures of less than 70 to 80 mmHg. In children, autoregulation is lost at mean arterial pressures lower than this. Autoregulation of RBF is considered to be an intrarenal control mechanism that functions independently of nervous control mechanisms. The autoregulation of GFR and control of RBF is mediated through changes in intrarenal vascular resistances.[3] Within the autoregulated range, afferent arteriolar resistance varies in direct proportion to arterial pressure to maintain a constant pressure within the capillaries in the glomerulus. This results in the maintenance of a relatively constant GFR. In contrast, low arterial pressures (less than 70 to 80 mmHg) are associated with a low GFR and are not subject to autoregulation.

Although the mechanism of autoregulation has not been fully identified, several theories have been advanced to explain the autoregulation of RBF.[4] One theory, the juxtaglomerular feedback theory, defines the autoregulation of RBF as an intrarenal control mechanism. The basic premise of this theory is that the RBF and the JGA of the kidney interact with the renin-angiotensin system to maintain a constant GFR.[4] Arteriolar resistance may be indirectly controlled via the renin-angiotensin system by the changes in the osmolality (sodium ion content) of the fluid delivered to the distal tubule,[5] or by the rate of sodium ion delivery to the macula densa.[6,7] Angiotensin II is thought to have a direct vasoconstrictive effect on afferent arterioles. Evidence at this point in time seems to favor the existence of an intrarenal mechanism for the control of RBF and GFR.

Formation of urine. The kidneys function as an excretory organ to maintain a constant internal balance of water and solutes. The amount of water and solutes excreted by the kidneys depends on the difference between the total amount taken into the body and the amount eliminated by nonrenal routes. The excretion of water and solutes by the kidneys also depends on feedback from extrarenal control mechanisms (neural, hormonal, etc.), which function to detect fluid and electrolyte disturbances.

The concentration of solutes excreted in the urine is a result of how the solutes are processed by the kidneys at the glomerular and tubular levels. The processes involved are filtration, reabsorption, and secretion (Fig. 6-11). Filtration is the diffusion of substances from the capillary into Bowman's space. Filtration occurs under hydrostatic pressure to separate plasma water and its nonprotein constituents from blood cells and protein molecules. Reabsorption and secretion of solutes can be active or passive. Reabsorption refers to the direction of transport of water and/or solute from the Bowman's space or tubular lumen into the peritubular capillary. Secretion is the addition of substances to the tubular fluid from tubular epithelial cells or peritubular blood.

As blood flows through the glomerular capillaries, water and solutes are removed and transported into Bowman's space. This fluid is referred to as glomerular filtrate or an ultrafiltrate of plasma. In children this fluid is normally formed at a rate of 80 to 120 ml/min/1.73 m². The glomerular capillary membrane restricts the passage of protein molecules into Bowman's space, making glomerular filtrate free of these substances.

As can be seen from Figure 6-12, glomerular filtration is the result of the Starling forces — primarily the glomerular capillary hydrostatic pressure and the hydrostatic pressure in Bowman's space.[8] Net ultrafiltration occurs at the afferent end of the capillary, where the mean hydrostatic capillary pressure is greatest.

Modification of glomerular filtrate. Once the process of ultrafiltration is complete, the glomerular filtrate flows from Bowman's space through the tubules. The final composition of glomerular filtrate depends on the processes of filtration, reabsorp-

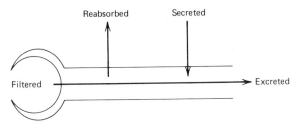

Figure 6-11. Fluid is filtered at the glomerulus. The amount filtered relative to its concentration in plasma depends on the size of the molecule and any protein binding. The net amount excreted is reduced by absorption and increased by secretion. These processes may be active or passive. *Reprinted with permission from* Hamburger, J. C., J. Crosnier, and J. P. Grunfeld. 1979. Nephrology. John Wiley & Sons, Inc., New York. 62.

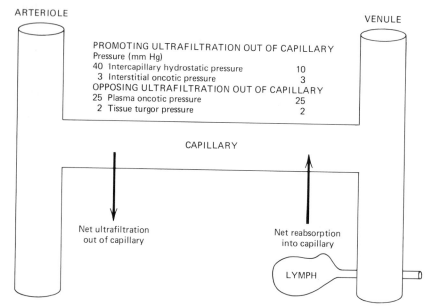

ARTERIOLE

VENULE

PROMOTING ULTRAFILTRATION OUT OF CAPILLARY
Pressure (mm Hg)
40 Intercapillary hydrostatic pressure   10
3 Interstitial oncotic pressure   3
OPPOSING ULTRAFILTRATION OUT OF CAPILLARY
25 Plasma oncotic pressure   25
2 Tissue turgor pressure   2

CAPILLARY

Net ultrafiltration
out of capillary

Net reabsorption
into capillary

LYMPH

Figure 6-12. The Starling hypothesis of fluid exchange between plasma and interstitium. The four factors that determine this exchange are known as "Starling forces." *Reprinted with permission from* Valtin, H. 1973. Renal Function: Mechanisms Preserving Fluid and Solute Balance in Health. Little, Brown & Co., Boston. 26.

tion, and secretion. These transport processes are coordinated in a manner that permits movement of one solute without disturbing the pattern of excretion of another. The energy required for transport processes in the kidney is produced by aerobic (cortex and medulla) and anaerobic (medulla) metabolism. Most of the energy generated is used in the active transport of sodium ions during reabsorption (1 calorie is required for each milliequivalent transported). Table 6-3 lists the quantities of major electrolytes that are filtered, reabsorbed, and excreted.

Under normal conditions, the proximal tubule is responsible for the reabsorption of 60 to 80 percent of the glomerular filtrate. Sodium ions are reabsorbed along with chloride ions and water in isosmotic proportions. The transport of chloride ions out of the tubular lumen is influenced by the amount of other anions present in tubular fluid. A high concentration of sulfate or bicarbonate ions in the tubular fluid decreases the reabsorption of chloride ions. Bicarbonate ion reabsorption in the proximal tubule accompanies the reabsorption of sodium ions and promotes the secretion of hydrogen ions into the tubular lumen.

Glomerular filtrate is isosmotic when it reaches the loop of Henle. The reabsorption of sodium chloride and water in this segment of the nephron provides the mechanism for the concentration and dilution of urine. In general, sodium ions and water diffuse into the interstitium from the descending limb of the loop of Henle, whereas in the ascending limb, sodium ions are reabsorbed secondary to the active transport of chloride ions.[9] The relative impermeability of the thick ascending limb to water accounts for the tubular fluid being hyposmotic as it enters the distal tubule.

TABLE 6-3 Filtration, Reabsorption, and Excretion of Ions and Water

Substance	Plasma concentration	Rate of glomerular filtration	Gibbs-Donnan factor	Quantity filtered	Quantity excreted	Quantity reabsorbed	Percent reabsorbed
	mEq/L	L/24 hr		mEq/24 hr	mEq/24 hr	mEq/24 hr	
Sodium	140	180	0.95	23,940	103	23,837	99.6
Chloride	105	180	1.05	19,845	103	19,742	99.5
Bicarbonate	27	180	1.05	5,103	2	5,101	99.9+
Potassium	4	180	0.95	684	51	633	92.6
Water	0.94 liter/liter	180 liter/24 hr	—	169.2 liter/24 hr	1.5 liter/24 hr	167.7 liter/24 hr	99.1%

Reprinted with permission from Pitts, R. F. 1974. Physiology of the Kidney and Body Fluids. Yearbook Medical Publishers, Inc., Chicago. Third edition. 101.

Although less than 10 percent of the filtered load of water and electrolytes is reabsorbed in the distal tubule, the late segment of the distal tubule serves as the primary site of potassium ion secretion. Through the action of aldosterone, the distal tubule (macula densa) plays a role in enhancing the rate of sodium ion reabsorption when fluid and electrolyte disturbances occur (e.g., decreased effective circulating volume of blood, as occurs with hemorrhage or burns).

The collecting duct is highly permeable to water in the presence of antidiuretic hormone (ADH),[10] and therefore, in conjunction with the loop of Henle, it plays a major role in determining the final concentration of urine.

Regulation of sodium and control of ECF volume. The regulation of sodium balance and the size of the ECF compartment are intimately related. A positive sodium ion balance usually results in expansion of the ECF volume. This functions as a feedback control over the rate of renal sodium ion excretion. ECF volume is maintained within a narrow range even though dietary intake of sodium may vary considerably on a day-to-day basis. In general, the urinary excretion of sodium ions is equal to the dietary intake. This balance is maintained through glomerular filtration and tubular reabsorption (glomerular tubular balance).[11]

ECF volume homeostasis appears to be controlled by a negative feedback system, which controls the size of ECF compartments and the osmolality of these fluids. It has been reported that progressive increments in dietary sodium intake result in a temporary increase in sodium ion reabsorption and weight gain with a new steady state near base line being reached in a few days.[12] A subsequent increase in excretion of sodium and water occurs, resulting in the reestablishment of zero base line at a higher level of salt intake. Whereas volume expansion is associated with a decreased tubular fractional reabsorption of sodium ions, contraction of the ECF compartment results in an increase in the fractional reabsorption of sodium ions in the proximal tubule. Volume control mechanisms are more closely related to tubular reabsorption of sodium ions than to glomerular filtration.[13]

The renin-angiotensin system is believed to play a role in the regulation of ECF volume and sodium ion excretion. The JGA of the kidney, which is composed of the macula densa and granular cells of afferent arterioles, is the structural unit through which the renin-angiotensin system operates (*see* Fig. 6-8). During periods registered as volume deficiencies (low systemic arterial pressure) the renin-angiotensin system stimulates release of aldosterone, which by increasing sodium ion reabsorption, attempts to maintain the circulating blood volume relatively constant. Under low-volume conditions, the JGA is stimulated to secrete renin, an enzyme that acts on angiotensinogen to ultimately produce angiotensin II (Fig. 6-13). Angiotensin II exhibits two main effects on the systemic arterial blood pressure. First, it causes vasoconstriction of peripheral arterioles, resulting in increased peripheral resistance. Second, it stimulates the adrenal cortex to secrete aldosterone. This results in an increased reabsorption of sodium ions, an increase in the ECF volume, and an improved cardiac output, thus maintaining circulating blood volume relatively constant.

Under normal circumstances, aldosterone has two important regulatory activities: regulation of ECF volume and regulation of potassium metabolism. Aldosterone has been shown to decrease the renal excretion of sodium ions and increase the excretion of potassium and hydrogen ions. Potassium ions can regulate the secretion of aldosterone independently of the renin-angiotensin system. A high dietary intake of potassium will increase the plasma concentration of potassium

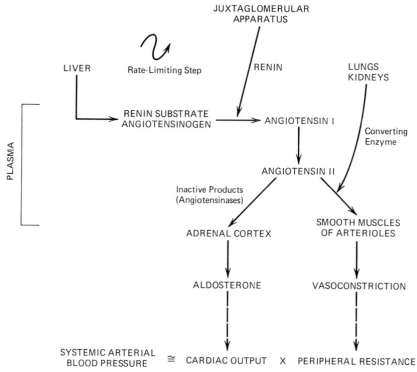

Figure 6-13. Dynamics of the renin-angiotensin system and its possible relation to the systemic arterial blood pressure. *Reprinted with permission from* Valtin, H. 1979. Renal Dysfunction: Mechanisms Involved in Fluid and Solute Imbalance. Little, Brown & Co., Boston. 396.

ions and stimulate aldosterone secretion. This leads to increased reabsorption of sodium ions and an increased urinary potassium ion excretion. The mechanism for this is unknown.

The release of renin is controlled indirectly by angiotensin II in the following ways:

1. Baroreceptors in the afferent arterioles sense changes in perfusion pressure and effective circulating blood volume. An increase in perfusion pressure (ECF volume expansion) will decrease the release of renin and vice versa.

2. Changes in the amount of sodium chloride flowing by the macula densa may influence the release of renin. Although the mechanism is not well understood, it has been proposed that kidney cells that secrete renin somehow sense an increase or decrease in the sodium chloride concentration at the macula densa. These cells respond by altering the secretion of renin in inverse proportion to the amount detected.

3. The sympathetic nervous system, through the action of catecholamines on afferent arterioles of the JGA, controls the release of renin. Stimulation of

alpha- and beta- (primarily beta) adrenergic receptors increases the release of renin. The renal sympathetic nerves most likely play the most important role in controlling the rate of renin secretion.

Other substances, such as potassium ions, ADH, and prostaglandins, have been associated with alterations in the release of renin.

Physical factors, such as hydrostatic and oncotic pressures, may play a role in sodium ion reabsorption and secretion. It appears that the oncotic pressure in the peritubular capillaries perfusing the proximal tubule, rather than the hydrostatic pressure,[14] has a direct effect on the proximal tubular reabsorption of sodium ions.[15,16] For example, an increase in plasma oncotic pressure would facilitate movement of sodium ions from the interstitial fluid into peritubular capillaries.

A "third factor," or natriuretic hormone, has been proposed as having a role in sodium ion excretion.[17,18] No definitive information on the molecular nature of the hormone or its mechanism of action has been elucidated.

Regulation of potassium. The kidney is the primary end organ in the regulation of potassium. This regulation must be precise because ECF levels must be maintained within narrow limits to avoid catastrophic effects on various organ systems (e.g., cardiac). The net excretion of potassium ions is affected by several factors including sodium ion concentration, urine flow rate, and acid-base balance. The link between potassium ion secretion and sodium ion reabsorption appears to be indirect, with the ratio between the two processes being 10:1.[19] The mechanisms whereby sodium ions influence the rate of potassium ion excretion have not been fully identified, although distal tubular reabsorption and secretion of potassium ions appear to be the mechanisms involved. During sodium ion depletion, increased potassium ion reabsorption in the collecting duct results in a low rate of urinary potassium ion excretion. A high urinary flow rate (as caused, for example, by diuretics such as furosemide, ethacrynic acid, and chlorothiazide) increases the rate of delivery of sodium ions, water, and potassium ions to the distal tubule. This results in increased distal tubular secretion and, ultimately, in excretion of potassium ions.

In acute acidosis, potassium ions shift out of cells into the ECF as hydrogen ions move into cells. In alkalosis, hydrogen ions move out of cells and potassium ions move into cells. The rate of potassium ion excretion by the kidneys depends on the intracellular concentration of potassium ions.[20] Therefore, in acidosis, when intracellular potassium ion concentration is low, the kidney conserves potassium ions by decreasing the rate of distal tubular potassium ion secretion. In alkalosis, the renal excretion of potassium ions is increased because the distal tubular cells contain higher concentrations of potassium ions. The mechanisms for the changes in distal potassium ion secretion probably involve reciprocal movement of hydrogen and potassium ions at the peritubular membrane of distal tubular cells.

Regulation of calcium. Calcium exists in the body in two forms: (1) bound to protein or complexed with other anions and (2) ionized. Ionized calcium and a portion of the calcium bound to protein are filtered at the glomerulus, but only the ionized (active) form can be reabsorbed. Parathyroid hormone (PTH) is the main determinant of calcium ion excretion. PTH causes an increase in calcium ion reabsorption primarily by its action on the distal tubule.[21] Metabolic acidosis causes calcium ion excretion to increase, whereas metabolic alkalosis decreases calcium ion excretion. The mechanisms of these effects are unknown. Severe hypercalcemia is associated with decreased reabsorption of calcium and sodium ions, whereas administration of magnesium and/or an osmotic diuretic increases the rate of calcium ion excretion.

Regulation of phosphorus. PTH is the main factor that influences renal excretion of phosphate. PTH decreases the proximal and distal reabsorption of phosphorus ions. Thiazide diuretics and furosemide are known to induce phosphaturia. Acidification of the urine increases the reabsorption of phosphorus ions, and alkalinization decreases reabsorption.

Regulation of magnesium. Reabsorption of magnesium is inhibited by volume expansion, loop diuretics, thiazides, PTH, acute metabolic acidosis, and hypercalcemia. Acidification of the urine increases the reabsorption of magnesium and alkalinization decreases reabsorption.

Concentration and dilution of urine. The human kidney is able to vary urine osmolality between 50 and 1,200 mOsm/kg H_2O. The concentration or dilution of urine depends on the body's need to excrete or retain water. Countercurrent multiplication and countercurrent exchange are the mechanisms that control urinary dilution and concentration. A countercurrent system is one in which the inflow and outflow paths lie adjacent to each other and material or energy is transferred between the two paths.

Countercurrent multiplication: The ascending and descending limbs of the loop of Henle serve as the countercurrent multipliers. The fluid within the limbs flows in opposite directions and is separated by a membrane that is relatively impermeable to water. The limbs function to increase the concentration gradient between the top of the limb(s) and the bend in the loop of Henle. The steps in countercurrent multiplication are depicted schematically in Figure 6-14. The active transport of chloride ions out of the ascending limb into the descending limb, via the interstitium, is believed to initiate the process.[9,22] Sodium ions are passively transported with chloride ions. This transfer of sodium and chloride is not accompanied by water because the ascending limb is relatively impermeable to water. A maximum osmotic gradient of 200 mOsm/kg H_2O at any horizontal level is established by the transfer of solute. This is known as the single effect (*see* Step 1, Fig. 6-14). As osmotic fluid continues to enter the descending limb of the proximal tubule, hyposmotic fluid flows from the ascending limb into the distal tubule. The single effect occurs again to create a 200 mOsm/kg H_2O gradient between the two limbs of the loop of Henle. By the time the fluid reaches the bend in the loop of Henle, its concentration can be 400 mOsm/kg greater than at the top of the descending limb. Countercurrent multiplication, therefore, increases the magnitude of the single effect along the length of the loop of Henle, from the cortex down into the papilla. The longer the loop of Henle in an individual nephron, the more concentrated the tubular fluid is at the bend of the loop. Juxtamedullary nephrons are, therefore, well-suited to the process of countercurrent multiplication. The increasing concentration of tubular fluid as the descending limb extends down into the outer medulla and papilla is probably the result of two factors: (1) passive diffusion of sodium and chloride ions from the interstitium into the descending limb, and (2) passive diffusion of water in the opposite direction. The relative contribution of these two factors remains unknown. As the tubular fluid moves up the ascending limb, the movement of sodium and chloride ions into the medullary interstitium creates a significant concentration gradient between the interstitium and the hyposmotic tubular fluid. This provides the major osmotic force that

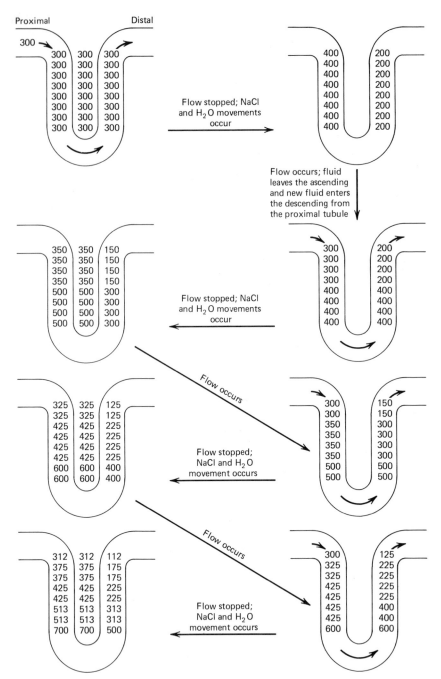

Figure 6-14. Countercurrent multiplier system in the loop of Henle. *Reprinted with permission from* Vander, A. J., J. H. Sherman, and D. S. Luciano. Human Physiology. The Mechanisms of Body Function. McGraw-Hill Book Co., New York. Second edition. 341.

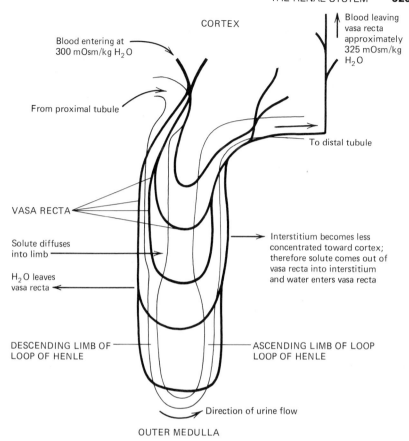

CORTEX

Blood entering at
300 mOsm/kg H$_2$O

Blood leaving
vasa recta
approximately
325 mOsm/kg
H$_2$O

From proximal tubule

To distal tubule

VASA RECTA

Interstitium becomes less
concentrated toward cortex;
therefore solute comes out of
vasa recta into interstitium
and water enters vasa recta

Solute diffuses
into limb

H$_2$O leaves
vasa recta

DESCENDING LIMB OF
LOOP OF HENLE

ASCENDING LIMB OF LOOP
LOOP OF HENLE

Direction of urine flow

OUTER MEDULLA

Figure 6-15. Illustration of countercurrent exchange. (*See* text for discussion.)

allows the subsequent removal of water from collecting ducts in the process of urinary concentration.[23]

Countercurrent exchange: The vessels involved in countercurrent exchange are the vasa recta. The ascending and descending limbs of these capillary loops encircle juxtamedullary nephrons. (Vasa recta are highly permeable to water and surrounded by a hyperosmotic interstitium.)

The purpose of the countercurrent exchange mechanism is twofold: (1) It prevents excessive concentration of the plasma as it leaves the kidneys, and (2) it maintains the osmotic gradient between the medullary interstitium and the tubular fluid in the loops of Henle. The countercurrent exchange system is illustrated in Figure 6-15. Blood entering the vasa recta has an osmolality of approximately 300 mOsm/kg H$_2$O. As the blood flows down the descending limb of the vasa recta through the hyperosmotic interstitium of the medulla, solute diffuses into the descending limb and water diffuses out into the interstitium. As the blood moves up through the ascending limb (toward the cortex), the interstitium becomes less concentrated. As a result, solute diffuses from the ascending limb of the vasa recta back into the interstitium and water diffuses back into the vasa recta. The osmolality of the blood leaving the vasa recta is only slightly higher (325 mOsm/kg H_2O) than that which entered the descending limb, indicating minimal net removal of solute from the interstitium. The blood carried by the vasa recta provides medullary and papillary tissues with needed oxygen and nutrients. At the same time that nutrients are being supplied to tissues in this area, the water that is reabsorbed from the collecting ducts in the final stage of urine formation is being removed from the inner tissue regions of the kidney by the vasa recta.

The fluid entering the distal tubule from the loop of Henle is hyposmotic. The reabsorption of water can be regulated independently of sodium through the concentration of plasma ADH. In the presence of high plasma levels of ADH, the permeability of the distal tubule and collecting duct increases. This allows for the passive reabsorption of water from the tubule into the concentrated medullary interstitium. Water is reabsorbed until osmotic equilibrium is reached between the fluid of the distal tubule and the interstitial fluid. As a result, the urine formed is hyperosmotic to plasma and no free water is excreted. In the absence of ADH, the collecting duct is relatively impermeable to water. Because no water is reabsorbed into the interstitium from the tubule, the urine will be hypotonic and free water is therefore excreted in the urine.

Development of renal functioning. Growth and development of the kidney is a dynamic and continuous process that progresses rapidly during the first 6 to 12 months of life. Immediately after birth the kidneys assume excretory and regulatory functions. As a result of high intrarenal vascular resistance in the newborn period, RBF is approximately 20 times lower than in the adult. The high vascular resistance is thought to result from several factors, including a high sensitivity of the vasculature to circulating catecholamines and to indirect effects of the renin-angiotensin system. During this first year of renal maturation, RBF increases because a greater fraction of the cardiac output is diverted to the kidneys.

GFR increases after birth until 1 to 2 years of age, at which time adult values are attained. The increase in GFR parallels the increase in RBF as well as the functional development of juxtamedullary and superficial nephrons.

Although the kidneys of infants have a limited capacity to excrete excess sodium ions under a condition of salt loading, they can efficiently conserve sodium ions when necessary. Sodium is an important element for growth, and its conservation is therefore significant during the first year of life. Excessive retention of water in the ECF and hypernatremia are two conditions that may develop secondary to the kidneys' inability to excrete sodium ions under certain conditions.

Young infants cannot concentrate their urine much beyond 600 to 700 mOsm/liter. These values are approximately 50 percent of the levels commonly observed in older children and adults (600 to 1,200 mOsm/liter). This failure to maximally concentrate urine is attributed to an inability to generate a sufficient concentration gradient in the inner medulla of the kidney. The subsequent low solute content prevents the formation of hypotonic fluid in the medulla and a maximally concentrated urine. A short loop of Henle, a low rate of solute excretion, problems with the release of ADH have all been identified as potential contributory factors in an infant's inability to maximally concentrate urine.

Infants have a somewhat lower serum concentration of bicarbonate ions. The etiology of this low serum concentration is not well understood. Although the kidneys maintain acid-base homeostasis under normal conditions, they are unable to excrete an acid load. This is due almost exclusively to a lack of sufficient amounts of urinary buffers. This may result from a limited capacity to reabsorb filtered bicarbonate ions and a limited capacity of the renal tubular cells to produce enough ammonium ion (NH_4^+). The net result is that net acid excretion is less than in the older child or adult. The production of ammonium ion reaches adult levels by the age of 2 years. A low serum bicarbonate ion concentration, a low to normal serum pH level, and an inability to secrete an acid load are all important factors that contribute to a tendency toward the development of acidemia in the infant.

The limited functional capacity of the kidneys predisposes the infant to the potential development of a variety of imbalances, including dehydration and acidosis.

ACID-BASE REGULATION

General Concepts

Acid-base regulation is accomplished by the interaction of physiochemical and physiological reactions. Balance is reflected by the value of the serum pH. This value is normally maintained within a narrow range of 7.35 to 7.45. The Henderson-Hasselbalch equation describes the relationship between pH, bicarbonate ion concentration (HCO_3^-), and the carbonic acid concentration (H_2CO_3). Carbonic acid is in equilibrium with dissolved carbon dioxide (CO_2) in the plasma. Since there are normally approximately 500 molecules of dissolved CO_2 for every molecule of H_2CO_3, the potential supply of H_2CO_3 for buffering far exceeds the actual supply. A meaningful form of the Henderson-Hasselbalch equation in terms of physiology and clinical practice is as follows:

$$pH = pK^1 + \log \frac{[HCO_3^-]}{[\text{dissolved } CO_2 + H_2CO_3]},$$

where pK^1 is a dissociation constant equal to a value of 6.1.

The ratio of bicarbonate ions to carbon dioxide content in the body determines the value of pH. The normal ratio is 20:1. Therefore, the concept of pH can also be expressed as a proportion:

$$pH \propto \frac{HCO_3^-}{CO_2}.$$

The bicarbonate ion concentration is regulated by the kidneys, and the carbon dioxide concentration is regulated by the lungs.

Buffers are substances that eliminate or minimize changes in the pH of a solution when hydrogen (H^+) or hydroxide (OH^-) ions are added. Buffers are composed of acid-base pairs that consist of a weak acid and its conjugate base (e.g., bicarbonate and sodium bicarbonate [$NaHCO_3$]). The addition of an acid or a base to a solution that contains buffers yields a weaker acid or a base and a salt.

1. Addition of an acid:

$$HCl + NaHCO_3 \rightarrow H_2CO_3 + NaCl \ (H^+ \text{ buffered}).$$
$$\text{strong acid} + \text{buffer} \rightarrow \text{weak acid} + \text{salt}.$$

2. Addition of a base:

$$NaOH + H_2CO_3 \rightarrow NaHCO_3 + H_2O \ (OH^- \text{ buffered}).$$
$$\text{strong base} + \text{buffer} \rightarrow \text{weak base} + \text{water}.$$

The body has physiological defense mechanisms that operate to minimize changes in the acid-base composition of the body. The major defense mechanisms are the chemical buffer systems, the lungs, and the kidneys.

First Line of Defense

The body's first line of defense is bicarbonate and nonbicarbonate buffer systems that exist in the plasma, interstitial fluid, erythrocytes, and ICF. Bicarbonate is the principal buffer system of plasma and interstitial fluid, whereas the protein and phosphate buffer systems predominate in the ICF. Hemoglobin is the main buffer contained in erythrocytes, although oxyhemoglobin is also present. Approximately 15 percent of hydrogen ions are buffered by plasma, 30 percent by the interstitial fluid and 55 percent by buffers in the ICF.

Bicarbonate buffer system. The bicarbonate buffer system exists in the plasma and interstitial fluid. The general equation that describes the system's function is as follows:

1. Dissolved CO_2 in lungs $= PaCO_2 \rightarrow CO_2 + H_2O \overset{*}{\rightleftarrows} H_2CO_3 \rightleftarrows H^+ + HCO_3^-$.
   (*, carbonic anhydrase)
2. The addition of a fixed acid to the system results in:

$$H^+Cl^- + Na^+HCO_3^- \rightarrow H_2CO_3 + NaCl \rightarrow H_2O + CO_2 \text{ (eliminated by}$$
$$\text{(acid)} \qquad\qquad\qquad\qquad\qquad\qquad\qquad\qquad \text{the lungs).}$$

3. The addition of a base to the system results in:

$$Na^+OH^- + H_2CO_3 \rightarrow H_2O + Na^+HCO_3^- \rightarrow \text{flows into the ECF.}$$
$$\text{(base)}$$

To maintain a fixed ratio, the concentrations of carbon dioxide and bicarbonate ions in the body can be varied independently by physiological responses. Normally, the main reaction above (No. 1) favors the formation of carbon dioxide over bicarbonate ions by a ratio of 800:1. Hydrogen ion balance in the body has a direct effect on the bicarbonate ion concentration of plasma. Endogenous acid production (volatile acids) and catabolism (fixed acids) result in the addition of hydrogen ions to the body fluids. The daily production of acid in children is normally 2 to 3 mEq/kg/day. This acid is buffered by bicarbonate ions, generating carbon dioxide (eliminated by the lungs) and sodium sulfate and sodium phosphate, which are excreted by the kidneys as ammonium and phosphate ions. Sodium and bicarbonate ions are returned to the ECF by the kidney. This normally prevents depletion of bicarbonate ion stores, although depletion can occur if there is a large amount of acid to be buffered.

Nonbicarbonate buffer systems. These systems involve primarily the action of hemoglobin and oxyhemoglobin in erythrocytes. The term "Buf$^-$" will be used to represent the anion component of nonbicarbonate buffer systems in the body.

1. Addition of an acid to the system results in:

$$HCl + NaBuf \rightarrow NaCl + HBuf.$$
Acid

2. Addition of a base to the system results in:

$$NaOH + HBuf \rightarrow NaBuf + H_2O.$$
base

The bicarbonate and nonbicarbonate buffer systems affect each other by alternating the concentration of buffers between erythrocytes and plasma.

Blood buffer base and base excess. Whole blood buffer base (BB) is equal to the sum of all the conjugate bases in 1 liter of blood (which consists primarily of bicarbonate). This is expressed as $BB = Buf^- + HCO_3^-$. The normal value is 48 mEq/liter.[24]

Base excess (BE) represents any change in the conjugate base concentration from the normal value (BB). This is expressed as BE = observed BB − normal BB. The normal value for BE in adults is 0, and for infants is −3.3 mEq/liter. If the value is negative, base has been lost or acid has been added. For example:

A BE of −10 mEq/liter = a BB of 38 mEq/liter.
A BE of 0 mEq/liter = a BB of 48 mEq/liter.
A BE of +10 mEq/liter = a BB of 58 mEq/liter.

Second Line of Defense

The second line of defense is the regulation of the partial pressure of arterial carbon dioxide ($PaCO_2$) by the respiratory system. The respiratory system responds quickly and makes the necessary adjustments in acid-base balance (minutes to hours). This is accomplished through the formation of H_2O and CO_2 from H_2CO_3. The respiratory system is the primary regulator of $PaCO_2$. This relationship is described by the following relationship:

$$PaCO_2 \propto \frac{CO_2 \text{ production}}{\text{alveolar ventilation}}.$$

Carbon dioxide production is directly proportional to $PaCO_2$, whereas alveolar ventilation is indirectly proportional (e.g., as $PaCO_2$ increases, pH decreases and alveolar ventilation must increase to decrease $PaCO_2$ and maintain balance).

Carbon dioxide production and homeostasis affects hydrogen ion metabolism through its action on the carbonic acid (H_2CO_3) concentration. Carbon dioxide produced in tissues diffuses into erythrocytes in the plasma. Within erythrocytes the hydration of carbon dioxide ($H_2O + CO_2 \rightarrow HCO_3^- + H^+$) proceeds quickly. The bicarbonate formed diffuses into the plasma in exchange for chloride ions. The majority of carbon dioxide added to capillary blood is carried to the lungs as bicarbonate ions, although a small amount is carried as dissolved carbon dioxide in erythrocytes and carbamino hemoglobin in the plasma. The hydrogen ions formed during the hydration of carbon dioxide are buffered by hemoglobin. As alveolar oxygen tension rises in the lungs, carbon dioxide diffuses out of the pulmonary capillaries into the alveoli and is eliminated.

Bicarbonate ion concentration is estimated from the total carbon dioxide (TCO_2) concentration of plasma. Carbon dioxide concentration tension influences both bicarbonate ion reabsorption and hydrogen ion excretion by the kidney. An increase in the formation of intracellular carbon dioxide (as in acidosis) results in the formation of hydrogen and bicarbonate ions that are quickly distributed in the ECF. This causes an increase in $PaCO_2$ and an increase in the excretion of hydrogen ions in the urine. Hyperventilation results in an increased hydrogen ion excretion and an elevated plasma bicarbonate ion level.

Third Line of Defense

The kidney is the definitive organ of regulation in the maintenance of acid-base balance. Renal acid-base regulation occurs slowly (hours to days). The principal mechanism of action is the regulation of the plasma bicarbonate ion concentration. Regulation is accomplished through the excretion of acid (hydrogen ions) and reabsorption of bicarbonate ions.

Acid excretion. Hydrogen ions that are excreted into the urine are buffered by the following two mechanisms:

$$1.\ H^+ + HPO_4^= \text{ (urine)} \rightarrow H_2PO_4^- \text{ (Fig. 6-16).}$$

Phosphate accounts for the majority of titratable acid (the amount of hydrogen ions present in combination with the base components of all filtered buffer substances that are excreted in the urine). The rate of titratable acid excretion depends on the availability of urinary phosphate, buffers, bicarbonate ions, and the severity of the acidosis. Acidification of the urine allows the kidneys to excrete

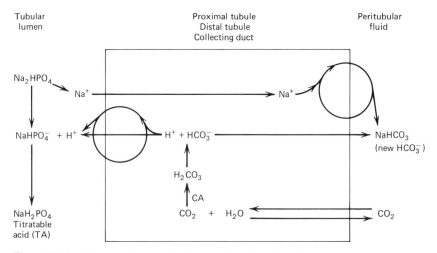

Figure 6-16. The formation of titratable acid in the urine. CA, coenzyme of carbonic anhydrase. *Reprinted with permission from* Valtin, H. 1973. Renal Function: Mechanisms Preserving Fluid and Solute Balance in Health. Little, Brown & Co., Boston. 184.

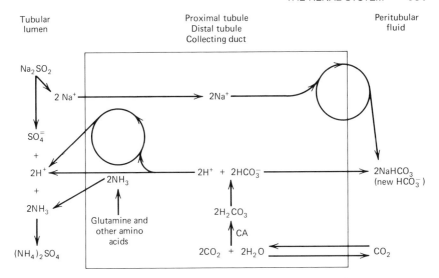

Figure 6-17. Mechanism for the renal excretion of ammonium ion (NH_4^+). CA, coenzyme of carbonic anhydrase. *Reprinted with permission from* Valtin, H. 1973. Renal Function: Mechanisms Preserving Fluid and Solute Balance in Health. Little, Brown & Co., Boston. 188.

hydrogen ions into the urine and convert $HPO_4^=$ to $H_2PO_4^-$. At maximal acidity of the urine (pH = 4.0), urinary phosphate is almost all in the form of $H_2PO_4^-$.

The only way to increase the net excretion of hydrogen ions is to increase the excretion rate of buffers. The rate of ammonia production by tubular epithelial cells represents the key mechanism that regulates acid-base balance in health and disease (Fig. 6-17). Control of renal ammonia (NH_3) production and excretion is influenced by the urinary pH and the severity of the acidosis. A low pH promotes ammonia diffusion into the tubular lumen, and a state of acidosis will increase production and excretion of ammonia into the renal tubule.

$$\textbf{2. } NH_3 + H^+ \rightarrow NH_4^+ \text{ (ammonium).}$$
(diffuses freely)(trapped in the urine)

The action of ammonia and phosphate buffers results in the removal of hydrogen ions from tubular fluid. This permits the entry of more hydrogen ions into the lumen to be buffered and results in the return of bicarbonate ions to the ECF.[23]

The kidney plays an important role in the maintenance of acid-base homeostasis. The regulation of plasma bicarbonate ion concentration depends on renal mechanisms. Bicarbonate ions that are consumed in buffering acids are regenerated by the kidney and reabsorbed to maintain a normal bicarbonate ion concentration in the ECF. Figure 6-18 describes the two processes of bicarbonate ion regeneration and reabsorption by the kidney. For every filtered bicarbonate ion that combines with a hydrogen ion in the renal tubule, a filtered sodium ion is reabsorbed along with a bicarbonate ion. Bicarbonate ions are formed when carbon dioxide combines with water in the tubular cell. The net result of these

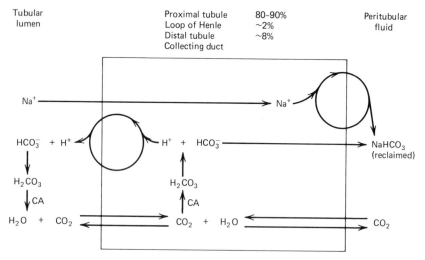

Figure 6-18. Mechanism for the reabsorption and regeneration of bicarbonate (HCO_3^-). CA, coenzyme of carbonic anhydrase. *Reprinted with permission from* Valtin, H. 1973. Renal Function: Mechanisms Preserving Fluid and Solute Balance in Health. Little, Brown & Co., Boston. 176.

reactions is the excretion of hydrogen ions and the return of sodium bicarbonate to the peritubular fluid. The bicarbonate ion that is filtered is not necessarily the same ion that is reabsorbed. The initiating event in the reabsorption of bicarbonate ion is sodium ion reabsorption. Sodium ion-hydrogen ion exchange occurs in the process of bicarbonate ion reabsorption. Sodium ions diffuse passively from tubular fluid into cells, and hydrogen ion secretion is active.[25]

Bicarbonate ion reabsorption. The general characteristics of bicarbonate handling have been described.[26,27] Under normal circumstances nearly all of the filtered bicarbonate ion is reabsorbed in the proximal tubule and the thick ascending limb of the loop of Henle. Several factors are known to affect the rate of bicarbonate ion excretion. Plasma potassium ion concentration is inversely related to the rate of proximal tubular reabsorption of bicarbonate ion.[28] Volume expansion decreases bicarbonate ion reabsorption. An inverse correlation also exists between plasma chloride ion concentration and bicarbonate ion reabsorption. The mechanism for this is not fully understood. PTH and ECF volume expansion are two factors that are known to inhibit bicarbonate ion reabsorption, whereas adrenal corticosteroids have the opposite effect.

Acid-Base Disturbances

This section will be concerned primarily with metabolic disorders.

Metabolic acidosis. The development of metabolic acidosis is initiated by a decrease in the plasma bicarbonate ion concentration. This is caused either by a disproportionate loss of bicarbonate ions from the ECF or by the addition of a strong acid (other than carbonic acid) to the ECF. The conditions that result in metabolic acidosis are listed in Table 6-4.

TABLE 6-4   Causes of Metabolic Acidosis

General mechanisms	Specific mechanisms	Example
Gain of strong acid by ECF	Gain of exogenous acid (HCl)	NH₄Cl acidosis
	Incomplete oxidation of fat (ketone body acidosis)	Diabetic or starvation ketoacidosis
	Incomplete oxidation of carbohydrate (lactic acid)	Lactic acidosis
	Gain of H_2SO_4, H_3PO_4, and (?) organic acids	Uremic acidosis
Loss of HCO_3^- from ECF	Via the kidney	Renal tubular acidosis
	Via the GI tract	Diarrheal acidosis

Reprinted with permission from Winters, R. W. 1973. The Body Fluids in Pediatrics: Medical, Surgical and Neonatal Disorders of Acid-Base Status, Hydration and Oxygenation. Little, Brown & Co., Boston. 51.
ECF, extracellular fluid; GI, gastrointestinal.

Conditions associated with an elevated anion gap* include uremia, diabetic ketoacidosis, salicylism, and lactic acidosis. Conditions associated with a normal anion gap include those conditions associated with a loss of bicarbonate (dilutional acidosis, gastrointestinal tract losses, or diarrheal dehydration) and excessive addition of chloride to the body (drugs such as ammonium chloride).

Buffer reactions include the following:

1. If bicarbonate is lost it must be regenerated:

$$H_2CO_3 + Buf^- \rightarrow HBuf + HCO_3^-.$$

2. If acid is gained:

$$HX + HCO_3^- \rightarrow H_2CO_3 + X^-.$$

This leads to a decreased BB, a negative BE, a decreased pH, and a decrease in plasma bicarbonate ion concentration.

Partial compensation in metabolic acidosis is accomplished by the respiratory system and is usually rapid. There is an increase in alveolar ventilation (rate and depth), leading to a decrease in $PaCO_2$ and an increase in serum pH. The initial stimulation for increased ventilation comes from serum pH and is registered by peripheral chemoreceptors. The stimulation is sustained by central medullary chemoreceptors, and therefore, the stimulation for hyperventilation arises from the cerebrospinal fluid (CSF), not the blood. Although blood pH may return to normal, hyperventilation may continue for 12 to 24 hours because of the slow

*Anion gap (also known as "R" fraction) = $Na^+ - (Cl^- + HCO_3^-)$ and is expressed in milliequivalents per liter. The normal value for adults is 8 to 12 mEq/liter. There are no published data available for children.

diffusion of bicarbonate ions across the blood-brain barrier from the CSF to plasma. The kidneys will act slowly to conserve bicarbonate ions and excrete excess hydrogen ions.

Correction of severe metabolic acidosis involves the administration of alkali (e.g., sodium bicarbonate). Usually, one half of the bicarbonate ion deficit is replaced over the first 12 hours, and serum electrolytes and arterial blood gases are monitored to assess the need for additional therapy.

Clinical signs and symptoms of metabolic acidosis include hyperventilation, peripheral vasodilation, hypotension, hyperkalemia, anorexia, nausea, vomiting, stupor, and altered tissue perfusion resulting from decreased cardiac contractility.

Metabolic alkalosis.   Metabolic alkalosis is initiated by an increase in the plasma bicarbonate ion concentration. It occurs as the result of the administration or increased production of alkali (bicarbonate, acetate, or lactate), the loss of hydrogen ions from the ECF (e.g., hydrochloric acid lost during vomiting, as in pyloric stenosis), or a disproportionate loss of chloride (e.g., diuretics in combination with a low-sodium diet). Table 6-5 lists those conditions that can result in metabolic alkalosis. Metabolic alkalosis results in an increased plasma bicarbonate ion concentration, increased serum pH, increased BB, and a positive BE.

Respiratory compensation in metabolic alkalosis is irregular and unpredictable. It generally involves a decrease in alveolar ventilation, which in turn, increases $PaCO_2$. The kidney reacts slowly to increased bicarbonate ion excretion along with sodium or potassium ions. If the total body supply of sodium and/or potassium ions becomes threatened, the body will preserve cation stores — rather than excrete them with bicarbonate ions — in order to correct the acid-base disturbance.

Correction of metabolic alkalosis involves urinary excretion of excess bicarbonate ion. This may be accomplished by the administration of chloride. Some types of metabolic alkalosis are responsive to chloride therapy (e.g., vomiting, diuretics, and gastric suction losses). In these conditions, less than 10 mEq/liter of chloride ion is usually lost in the urine. There are some types of metabolic alkalosis that are resistant to chloride therapy (e.g., Bartter's syndrome). Children

TABLE 6-5   Causes of Metabolic Alkalosis

General mechanisms	Specific mechanisms	Example
Gain of HCO_3^- by ECF	Gain of exogenous HCO_3^-	Ingestion or infusion of HCO_3^-
	Oxidation of salts of organic acids	Ingestion or infusion of lactate, citrate, or acetate
	Loss of HCl	Vomiting of gastric juice
	Loss of H^+ via the kidney	Diuretic therapy; K^+ depletion
	(?) Extrarenal transfer of H^+ to ICF	(?) K^+ depletion

Reprinted with permission from Winters, R. W. 1973. The Body Fluids in Pediatrics: Medical, Surgical and Neonatal Disorders of Acid-Base Status, Hydration and Oxygenation. Little, Brown & Co., Boston. 58.
ECF, extracellular fluid; ICF, intracellular fluid.

with these conditions tend to excrete more than 20 mEq/liter of chloride in their urine, and they may require additional forms of therapy.

NURSING ASSESSMENT OF THE CHILD WITH RENAL DYSFUNCTION

Assessment of the child with potential renal dysfunction requires that the nurse analyze and synthesize data obtained from the simultaneous monitoring of several parameters. Although a child's primary reason for admission to the intensive care unit (ICU) may not be directly related to a kidney dysfunction, many children who require the care of an ICU have the potential to manifest abnormalities of renal functioning. The pediatric ICU nurse, therefore, must be astutely aware of signs and symptoms that signal the onset of renal dysfunction. A knowledge and understanding of the basic physiological concepts presented in the preceding sections will assist the nurse in the recognition of fluid, electrolyte, and acid-base disturbances. Understanding basic laboratory studies and clinical conditions that predispose patients to developing disturbances of fluid and electrolyte balance enables the nurse to make a thorough assessment. Assessment of a child's renal status is a difficult task because, unlike the neurological or cardiovascular system, assessment of the renal system is indirect and primarily depends on observation of secondary signs and symptoms (e.g., changes in cardiac or respiratory status).

This section will describe the components of fluid balance in a pediatric ICU patient as well as review specific laboratory tests that are used to assess renal functioning.

Assessment of Fluid Balance

Accurate assessment of fluid balance in acutely ill pediatric patients requires that the nurse working in an ICU setting have knowledge of the components of fluid intake and output as well as an understanding of the physiological mechanisms that funtion to define a patient's fluid status.

Components of fluid balance. Nurses routinely measure and record patients' fluid intake and output. The ability to accurately assess the meaning of a patient's fluid balance depends on a thorough knowledge and understanding of the various components of fluid balance.

The total intake of water includes all fluids taken into the body (orally, nasogastrically, intravenously, etc.) plus the "hidden" intake — the water produced by the oxidation of protein, carbohydrate, and fatty acids. The amount of water produced by oxidation is dependent on the metabolic rate and the type of substances available for oxidation. The total output of water includes losses in perspiration (increased with fever), urine, stool, and insensible losses. The fluid intake normally approximates the output.

Maintenance fluid requirements in children are based on estimates of caloric expenditure and are calculated by using the child's body weight in kilograms (Fig. 6-19). The amount of fluid a child requires as intake during a 24-hour period is determined by the amount lost from the body during the same time period. Normal maintenance requirements of fluid define what the individual needs to take into the body. The day-to-day maintenance fluid requirement is generally deter-

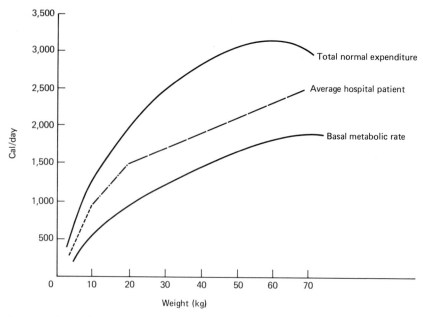

Figure 6-19.   Estimated caloric expenditure under basal conditions (bottom curve), under conditions of bed rest (middle curve), and under conditions of full activity (top curve). The middle curve can be divided into three segments according to slope: from 3 to 10 kg = 100 cal/kg (----); from 10 to 20 kg = 50 cal/kg (.—.—); and over 20 kg = 20 cal/kg (———). These slopes can be used to formulate reasonable estimates of caloric expenditure for maintenance fluid therapy without the use of the graph. *Adapted with permission from* Winters, R. W. 1973. The Body Fluids in Pediatrics: Medical, Surgical and Neonatal Disorders of Acid-Base Status, Hydration and Oxygenation. Little, Brown & Co., Boston. 117.

mined by the output. The relative contribution of the kidneys, lungs, etc., to the total fluid output depends on the specific pathological condition present. Maintenance fluid requirements are calculated by using the figures presented in Table 6-6. The components of normal maintenance requirements and their relative contribution to fluid homeostasis are listed below in Table 6-7. The usual requirements in the absence of sweating equal 100 ml fluid/100 cal expended. For example, a 17-kg child would require the following amount of maintenance fluids:

$$1,000 + 7 \times 50.$$

$$1,000 + 350 = 1,350 \text{ ml/24 hr.}$$

Under normal circumstances the amount of "hidden" water intake produced per 100 calories expended is equal to 12 milliliters. In patients who develop pathologic states, such as acute renal failure, the two sources of "hidden" water intake become more important. The water of oxidation is one source. The oxidation of fat produces more energy and water than carbohydrate or protein. Preformed water is another component of "hidden" water intake. This is defined as water

TABLE 6-6   Maintenance Fluid Requirements

Weight	Fluid requirement*
kg	
3–10	100 cal/kg
11–20	1,000 + 50 cal/kg
>20	1,500 + 20 cal/kg

*ml/kg = cal/kg.

gained by the ECF when cells are catabolized. The total amount of "hidden" intake may become significant if oliguria persists over several days or if catabolic stress is high.

Maintenance requirements for electrolytes are also based on estimates of caloric expenditures. These requirements are listed in Table 6-8. The maintenance fluid and electrolyte requirements do not apply to newborn infants or when the body is in an unbalanced state. Fluid requirements will increase in the presence of fever. Caloric expenditure will increase by 12 percent for each degree centigrade rise in body temperature above normal. Sweating will increase fluid requirements by 30 milliliters for each degree centigrade increase in the ambient temperature above 30.5°C (87°F).

Assessment of Hydration Status

There are several parameters that the nurse can use to assess hydration status in pediatric patients. These parameters as well as clinical symptoms related to fluid imbalances are described in Table 6-9. Several of these important clinical parameters the nurse may assess are described below.

Weight.   Determination of serial body weights is an important indirect measurement of total body water and, consequently, the status of internal fluid homeostasis. Rapid changes in body weight from one day to the next represent a change in the amount of total body water, not an increase or decrease in lean body mass. A loss or gain of 1 kilogram (2.2 pounds) corresponds to a loss or gain of approximately 1 liter of fluid. It should be fairly easy to distinguish fluid gain from a gain in lean body mass if the nurse recalls the normal rate at which children grow. Infants lose up to 10 percent of their birth weight in the first few days of life. This weight is

TABLE 6-7   Components of Normal Maintenance Requirements

Component	Fluid requirement
Output	ml/100 cal
Insensible water loss	45*
Sweat	0–25
Urine	50–75
Stool	5–10
"Hidden" intake	12

*15 via lungs, 30 via skin.

TABLE 6-8 Maintenance Electrolyte Requirements

Electrolyte	Requirement
Na$^+$	2.5 mEq/100 cal
K$^+$	2.5 mEq/100 cal
Cl$^-$	5.0 mEq/100 cal
Glucose	5.0 g/100 cal

gained back in the first 10 days of life. From this point on, there is a steady increase in weight gain as the infant's weight is doubled in 4 months and tripled by the end of the first year of life. After 1 year of age, there is a gain of approximately 3 kg/yr (6.6 lb/yr). The school-age child gains 1 to 3 kg/yr (2.2 to 6.6 lb/yr). Rapid changes in body weight usually indicate the sudden loss or gain of body fluid. The calculation of fluid intake and output on a 24-hour basis provides the nurse with information needed on a daily basis to assess the significance of a loss or gain of body weight.

Vital signs. The pulse rate, respiratory rate, and blood pressure are important parameters in the assessment of the renal system. The rate and quality of the pulse is a reflection of the effective circulating blood volume, which is affected by sodium ion balance and fluid shifts. Changes in blood pressure and pulse rate are associated with conditions in which the vascular compartment is compromised. It is important to determine both the blood pressure and the pulse rate because, together, they provide information that ensures a more complete assessment of fluid balance. Children who retain excess fluid may have respiratory changes characterized by an increase in the rate and a change in the quality of breath sounds (moist rales may be present). Difficulty in breathing is often identified by the presence of substernal or intercostal retractions and nasal flaring. Children who have severe depletion of body fluids will have an increased respiratory rate, but breath sounds may be normal. Physical assessment of the cardiovascular system (*see* p. 98) and the respiratory system (*see* p. 33) provides indirect, but nevertheless valuable, information regarding a child's fluid balance.

Urine output. The quality and quantity of urine produced by a child is often extremely helpful in assessing hydration status. Any change in the urine output of children who are critically ill is evaluated carefully. Retention of excess fluid, as in acute renal failure, results in oliguria, whereas conditions like diabetes insipidus produce an excess volume of urine. It is important for nurses to recognize changes in the quantity and characteristics of urine that may indicate the early onset of renal dysfunction. The laboratory assessment of renal functioning is described in detail below.

Assessment of Renal Functioning

An assessment of renal functioning can be made by examining the results of some laboratory tests and by assessing the child's clinical status. The extent of renal impairment is primarily determined by the analysis of the creatinine clearance, plasma creatinine levels, and blood urea nitrogen (BUN).

Creatinine clearance. Creatinine is a substance that is derived from muscle creatine and creatine phosphate. Under normal conditions in any individual, the

Table 6-9 Clinical Symptoms of Volume Expansion and Contraction

Assess/observe	Volume expansion	Volume contraction
Skin turgor	Moist, good turgor, pitting edema may be present, circulation depends on severity of edema.	Dry, poor turgor, pale. Extremities may be cool if peripheral circulation is impaired.
Eyes	Periorbital edema.	May look sunken. Absence of tears.
Fontanel, anterior	Bulging or full.	Normal or sunken.
Mucous membranes	Moist.	Dry, cracked, coated tongue. Absence of salivation.
Pulse	Bounding, increased rate.	Increased rate, weak, thready.
Respirations	Increased rate, may have retractions, use of accessory muscles.	Increased rate.
Breath sounds	Moist rales.	Normal.
Blood pressure	Normal or high.	May be normal or high initially, but then may decrease. Narrow pulse pressure.
Weight	Increased.	Decreased. Compare vs. preillness weight.
Thirst	Not present.	Usually present.
Urine Specific gravity Osmolality Volume	Depend on renal functioning.	Specific gravity and osmolality increased with dehydration. May exhibit less frequent voidings of smaller volumes.
Neurological status/behavior	Depending on cause of condition, may see subtle or significant changes in child's behavior. Family's assessment of child's behavior and affect important.	May include irritability, high-pitched cry, or lethargy.

daily production and excretion of creatinine is constant (Fig. 6-20). Therefore, plasma creatinine levels and creatinine excretion reflect muscle mass and renal functioning. The creatinine clearance test is used in children as an estimate of GFR. Because creatinine is excreted solely by the kidney, if the GFR decreases, the filtered load of creatinine decreases and a positive balance within the body develops. The positive balance is reflected as an increased plasma creatinine level. When steady state is reestablished, the excretion of creatinine once again equals the production (which may, in fact, be the same at an impaired level of renal functioning as it was when renal functioning was normal). The only difference is that in steady state renal failure, the serum creatinine is reset at a higher level. In a person with impaired renal functioning, excess creatinine will not necessarily be excreted and may accumulate slowly in the body. Creatinine clearance can be calculated with the following formula:

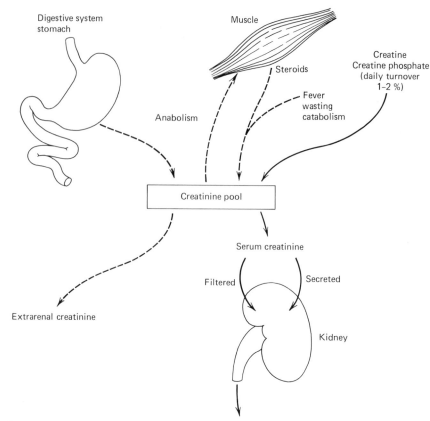

Figure 6-20. Representation of creatinine metabolism. *Reprinted with permission from* Lieberman, E. 1976. Workup of a child with azotemia. *In* Lieberman, E. editor. 1976. Clinical Pediatric Nephrology. J. B. Lippincott Co., Philadelphia. 47.

$$C_{cr} = \frac{U_{cr} \times V}{P_{cr}},$$

where U_{cr} is the concentration of creatinine in the urine (mg/100 ml), P_{cr} is the creatinine concentration in the plasma, and V is the urine flow rate (ml/min). Normal adult female and male values are 87 to 147 ml/min/1.73 m^2 and 88 to 174 ml/min/1.73 m^2, respectively. Mean normal values for children (age 3 to 13 years) are 113 ml/min/1.73 m^2, with a range of 94 to 142 ml/min/1.73 m^2.[29]

The calculation of a child's creatinine clearance requires that a 24-hour urine be collected. At the midpoint of the 24-hour period, a blood sample is taken for determination of creatinine concentration. Estimation of GFR using endogenous creatinine clearance is not always an accurate measurement of renal functioning in children because of the difficulty encountered in the collection of a 24-hour urine specimen. Children in steady state should have a urinary excretion of creatinine of at least 10 to 15 mg/kg/24 hr. If the quantitative creatinine excretion is less than this, the nurse should suspect that the collection is incomplete. The following formula is frequently used in the pediatric age group to quickly assess GFR:

$$\text{GFR (ml/min/1.73 m}^2) = 0.55 \times \text{L/P}_{cr}(\text{mg/dl}),$$

where, L is the child's length (in centimeters) and P_{cr} is the plasma creatinine value. This formula is clinically useful for all children over 6 months of age.[30]

Plasma creatinine. Plasma creatinine levels (Table 6-10) are used as an indirect estimate of renal functioning in children. The use of serial plasma creatinine levels in an individual serves as a useful indicator of the existence of intrinsic renal disease and its progress. Nonrenal factors that may affect the plasma creatinine level include catabolic states (e.g., excessive exercise or muscle wasting). It should also be noted that the measurement of plasma creatinine varies depending on the measurement technique used.

BUN. As can be seen from Figure 6-21, urea is the end product of protein metabolism. Urea is excreted almost exclusively by the kidneys through a combination of filtration and reabsorption. The final concentration of BUN is affected by several factors. The major factor affecting BUN is the availability of amino acids. Normal protein sources for the formation of urea include dietary intake (especially proteins) and tissue sources. If there is inadequate dietary protein to meet the body's needs, body tissue is broken down. This can result in a decreased muscle mass and hypoalbuminemia. An increase in the availability of amino acids results from such factors as the degradation of blood after gastrointestinal (GI) hemorrhage and dietary consumption of large amounts of meat. If a child with decreased renal functioning consumes a large amount of protein in his diet, the BUN will initially increase because the kidneys are unable to excrete the urea load.

The normal range of BUN is 9 to 18 mg/dl. Azotemia is an elevated BUN level that exceeds the normal range established for a laboratory. Azotemia may occur secondary to nonrenal causes or secondary to renal disease. Prerenal azotemia refers to situations in which the kidneys respond appropriately to a nonrenal pathological process. The result is an elevated BUN. Common causes in pediatrics include dehydration (secondary to GI losses or burns) and hypotension (secondary to hemorrhage). Prerenal azotemia is often reversed with replacement of

TABLE 6-10 True Plasma Creatinine Concentration in Children

Age	Surface area	Height	Plasma creatinine mg/100 ml ± 1 SD
yr	m^2	cm	
0	0.21	50	0.50 ± 0.08
0.5–3	0.36–0.60	67–96	0.32 ± 0.07
3–5	0.60–0.75	96–110	0.38 ± 0.07
5–7	0.75–0.87	110–122	0.42 ± 0.08
7–9	0.87–1.00	122–133	0.50 ± 0.10
9–11	1.00–1.17	133–142	0.52 ± 0.09
Adult male	1.76	174	0.97 ± 0.12
Adult female	1.56	163	0.77 ± 0.12

Reprinted with permission from Lieberman, E. 1976. Workup of a child with azotemia. *In* Lieberman, E., editor. 1976. Clinical Pediatric Nephrology. J. B. Lippincott Co., Philadelphia. 516.

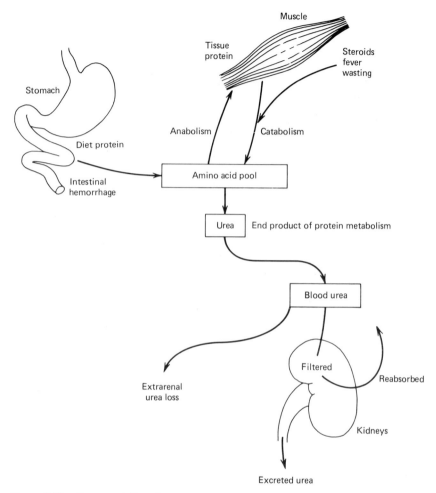

Figure 6-21. Representation of urea metabolism. *Reprinted with permission from* Lieberman, E. 1976. Workup of a child with azotemia. *In* Lieberman, E. editor. 1976. Clinical Pediatric Nephrology. J. B. Lippincott Co., Philadelphia. 46.

fluid losses and correction of their cause. If a child has a prerenal form of azotemia, the BUN often decreases to 50 percent of the initial value within 24 hours after rehydration. Renal disorders will not elevate the BUN out of the normal range until there is approximately a 40 to 50 percent reduction in the GFR.

Although the BUN is a useful screening test for renal disease, it is not an accurate indicator of renal functioning. BUN is affected by many nonrenal factors (e.g., dehydration and GI hemorrhage). Plasma creatinine and BUN levels are used together to assess renal functioning. The plasma BUN:creatinine ratio, normally 10:1, may provide the clinician with additional important information. An increase in the ratio may result from increased reabsorption of urea (dehydration), increased production of urea (increased dietary protein intake, GI bleeding, hemolytic anemia or fever), or a decreased production of creatinine. Decreased ratios are not common, but some causes include decreased urea production (low dietary protein intake or liver failure), decreased reabsorption of urea (overhydration), and an increased production of creatinine (rhabdomyolysis).

The tests described below provide indirect information on various aspects of renal functioning.

Osmolality.   Urine osmolality is a more accurate measurement of the kidney's ability to concentrate the urine than the specific gravity. Osmolality is dependent only on the discrete number of particles of solute in solution — not on the size, molecular weight, or electrical charge of the molecule. Urine osmolality can range from 50 to 1,200 mOsm/kg H_2O.

Plasma osmolality may be a useful measurement. It can be calculated with the following equation:

$$\text{Osmolality} = Na^+ \times 2 + \frac{\text{glucose}}{18} + \frac{\text{BUN}}{3}.$$

The normal plasma osmolality is 285 to 295 mOsm/kg H_2O. The urine:plasma ratio of osmolality may provide important information about specific disorders. For example, a urine:plasma ratio of less than 1:1 generally indicates the presence of a vasomotor nephropathy, whereas a ratio of greater than 2:1 suggests that oliguria may be due to hypovolemia.

Electrolytes

The measurement of plasma electrolytes provides general information about fluid, electrolyte, and acid-base balance. The normal values are provided in Table 6-2.

Under steady-state conditions, the electrolyte composition of urine is independent of renal functioning and depends on the quality and quantity of the dietary intake. For example, if one considers the daily urine output to be 1.5 liters, the following estimates of electrolyte concentration can be used as guidelines: sodium ions, 50 to 130 mEq/liter; chloride ions, 50 to 130 mEq/liter; potassium ions, 20 to 70 mEq/liter. If the body composition is not stable, the concentration of individual electrolytes is most meaningful when determined by calculating the fractional excretion of a particular electrolyte. The following formula is used to calculate this measurement:

$$FE_x = \frac{U_x/P_x}{U_{cr}/P_{cr}} \times 100,$$

where x is an undetermined electrolyte, FE is the fractional excretion, U_x is the urine concentration of the electrolyte, P_x is the plasma concentration of the electrolyte, U_{cr} is the urine concentration of creatinine, and P_{cr} is the plasma concentration of creatinine.

Characteristics of Urine

Specific gravity.   The specific gravity of urine is a measurement of urine concentration, which is dependent on the number, size, and weight of the particles in the urine. Specific gravity is not the best indicator of the kidney's ability to concentrate or dilute the urine because a falsely high value can be obtained when high-molecular-weight substances (e.g., protein, mannitol) are present in the urine. The normal range for specific gravity is 1.001 to 1.025.

pH.   Urine pH ranges from 4.7 to 8.0. An early morning specimen will usually reveal a pH of less than 5.3. Inability to maximally acidify the urine may be due to a tubular defect in the kidney (RTA).

Formed elements.   On microscopic examination of the urine, it is not unusual to see some formed elements. In general, the upper limits of normal in children are as follows: red blood cells (RBCs), less than 1 cell per high-power field (freshly spun urine); white blood cells (WBCs), 0 to 4 cells per high-power field (freshly spun urine).[30]

The presence of RBC casts in the urine indicates that the RBCs originate in the kidney. WBC, hyaline, and granular casts may also be found in the urine, and their presence is usually benign, although WBC casts may indicate infection. The presence of protein (most often measured by dipstick, which estimates the concentration in the urine), may be significant. A more accurate estimate of the concentration of protein in the urine can be calculated from a 24-hour urine collection. There is normally less than 150 mg of protein/100 ml of urine excreted per 24 hours. Abnormal amounts may be found in the urine of a patient with abnormal kidney functioning or with urinary tract infections. No ketones or glucose should be found in the urine.

A positive result may be obtained on a dipstick if more than 1 to 2 RBC/mm^3 are present in the urine. Hemoglobinuria will result in a similar reading. A false-positive dipstick for hematuria may be produced by myoglobin.

PRINCIPLES OF NURSING CARE FOR THE CHILD WITH RENAL DYSFUNCTION

Nursing care of the critically ill child with a kidney disorder can be separated into several phases. The combination of these phases results in the nurse implementing a specific plan of care for this child. The nurse must first gather information from several sources.

Information important to the care of the child with potential renal dysfunction includes the intake and output of fluids and electrolytes, body weight, body temperature, pulse rate, respiratory rate, and blood pressure. Although the clinical presentation of the child is very important, subjective information obtained from the child and the nurse's observations regarding the child's behavior are often valuable.

The nurse is in a unique position because of the amount of time spent directly caring for and observing the child. Formulation of an appropriate assessment of the child requires that nurses not only be able to accurately measure and record information but that they also have a firm knowledge base of renal physiology and pediatric nursing. Knowledge of what types of children have the potential to develop fluid and electrolyte imbalances or renal dysfunction places nurses in a position where they must be able to anticipate what signs and symptoms may develop and when in the course of the child's illness he or she may be more susceptible or vulnerable (or how the disorder may present).

After an assessment is formulated, a plan of nursing care can be developed. The nursing care plan is based on principles of nursing care related to the child with renal dysfunction: (1) maintenance of fluid and electrolyte balance, and (2) maintenance of optimal nutrition. Implementation of the plan is only effective and adequate if the nurse understands the rationale for the plan. This thorough understanding will allow the nurse freedom to clarify various aspects of the treatment plan for the child and the family.

Principle 1: Maintenance of Fluid and Electrolyte Balance

Critically ill children are susceptible to the development of fluid and solute imbalances. Any conditions that promote excessive fluid loss or prevent the intake of adequate amounts of fluid will predispose the child to volume depletion. Volume expansion is prompted by an excessive accumulation of water and solute in the body. The dynamics of volume expansion and contraction are referred to in the section on disorders of fluid balance (*see* p. 346). One of the nurse's primary responsibilities in caring for a child with renal dysfunction involves monitoring fluid intake and output.

The amount of allowed daily fluid intake depends on an assessment of several parameters. Intake is usually restricted to an amount equal to the insensible water loss plus the urinary output. The child's ideal body weight (dry weight) is used as a reference for the calculation of this amount. The fluid intake may be changed daily, depending on changes in body weight or the presence of clinical symptoms that may indicate ECF volume expansion or contraction.

Restriction of dietary intake of sodium and/or potassium may be necessary in children with renal dysfunction. Limiting sodium intake may help prevent accumulation of fluid in the ECF. Limiting potassium intake will help prevent the development of hyperkalemia. The amount and types of fluids and electrolytes that can be provided safely to these children may vary, depending on the severity of the renal condition.

Principle 2: Maintenance of Optimal Nutrition

An understanding of the basic principles of nutritional management of children with renal dysfunction will allow the nurse to interpret and clarify dietary plans and fluid restriction to the child and family. Dietary management consists primarily of controlling the intake of fluids, calories, protein, sodium, and oftentimes, potassium. A nutritional assessment is an important component of the overall assessment of the child with real or potential renal dysfunction. (*see* p. 467 for a description of the assessment of nutritional status in critically ill children.)

Adequate amounts of protein are needed to build, maintain, and repair body cells and tissues. The intake of excessive amounts of protein (especially of low biological value) leads to the production and retention of urea nitrogen. The recommended intake of protein in children with acute renal failure is at least 0.50 to 0.75 g/kg/day, two-thirds of which should be of high biological value. In children who do not have acute renal failure, it is recommended that the protein intake be liberalized to 1 to 2 g/kg/day.

Enough calories must be provided daily to prevent the breakdown of body protein for energy use. When tissue protein is broken down to be used for energy, potassium ions and water are released from cells and the production of hydrogen ions increases. Whereas metabolism of fats and carbohydrates does not increase the work load of the kidney, protein metabolism does. Concentrated sources of calories from both carbohydrates and fats are encouraged.

DISORDERS OF FLUID BALANCE

There are two categories of fluid disorders that occur in critically ill children. Some clinical conditions result in expansion of body fluids, and others result in the contraction of body fluid compartments from fluid depletion. A description of the pathogenesis of these conditions and the effect they have on body fluid compartments can be found in Table 6-11. The signs and symptoms of volume contraction and expansion described in Table 6-9 can be used by the nurse as guidelines for assessment. The symptoms will vary depending on the severity of each child's illness and his or her individual response.

Three specific conditions that often develop in children who are in the ICU will be described in this section. These conditions are acute dehydration, the syndrome of inappropriate ADH (SIADH), and diabetes insipidus (DI).

ACUTE DEHYDRATION

The development of acute dehydration in infants and children is often secondary to abnormal GI losses from diarrhea. If losses are not continuously replaced with the proper amount and type of fluid and electrolytes, severe imbalances can occur. Diarrhea may be accompanied by dehydration, shock, and acid-base disturbances (acidosis). In this section we will discuss hypertonic (hypernatremic), hypotonic (hyponatremic), and isotonic (isonatremic) dehydration. Dehydration may therefore be categorized according to the compositional changes in plasma.

Pathophysiology and Clinical Manifestations

Isotonic dehydration. In isotonic dehydration, the net loss of fluid and electrolytes is isotonic, leaving the remaining body fluids isotonic also. This means that the net loss of fluid and electrolytes was in isotonic proportions. As can be seen from Table 6-11, the entire isosmotic loss is sustained by the ECF, and no redistribution of water occurs as a result of the loss. Plasma volume and the circulating blood volume are reduced. Symptoms associated with a reduced blood volume and reduced blood flow to the skin, muscle, and kidney may be present in addition to signs and symptoms of circulatory shock.

Hypertonic dehydration. The net fluid loss in hypertonic dehydration is accompanied by a proportionately smaller net loss of electrolytes than water. The net loss is hypotonic and the remaining body fluids are hypertonic. This type of dehydration is seen commonly in infants who have diarrhea and are given fluids to drink that contain a large amount of solute, or in infants in which the intake of water has been severely reduced. The combination of a proportionately larger output of water and larger intake of electrolytes results in a hypertonic ECF. Water moves from the ICF spaces into the ECF. The ECF therefore is better defended than in isotonic dehydration and suffers a smaller loss. Thus, for the

TABLE 6-11 Pathogenesis and Fluid Effects of Volume Expansion and Contraction

Disorder	Example	Changes in volume		Changes in ECF concentration			
		ECF	ICF	Na⁺	Protein	Osm	Hct
1. *Isosmotic contraction:* Loss of isosmotic fluid from plasma. ISF moves into plasma. Result is contraction of entire ECF volume. No shift of fluid from intravascular spaces occurs. Plasma circulatory compromise sets in early.	Diarrhea with concurrent loss of electrolytes in urine	↓	—*	—	↑	—	↑
2. *Hyperosmotic contraction:* Water is lost in excess of solute. Water lost first from plasma. ISF flows in to replace water lost from plasma, and intracellular water flows into the interstitium. The volume of all major compartments is reduced. Symptoms of contraction less severe than with isotonic contraction because ECF volume protected by ICF shift into ECF.	Dehydration, insensible water loss, or fever	↓	↓	↑	↑	↑	—
3. *Hyposmotic contraction:* Loss of solute in excess of water relative to normal plasma. NaCl lost from ECF, so osmolality decreases. Fluid shifts from ECF into cells.	Dehydration	↓	↑	↓	↑	↓	↑
4. *Isosmotic expansion:* A positive balance of an isosmotic solution (NaCl). Selective expansion of ECF due to solute retention here (edema).	Edema	↑	—	—	↓	—	↓
5. *Hyperosmotic expansion:* A positive balance of ECF solute in excess of water. Causes a shift of water from the ICF into the ECF space until osmotic equilibrium is reached.	NaCl poisoning	↑	↓	↑	↓	↑	↓
6. *Hyposmotic expansion:* A positive balance of water. Both ECF and ICF spaces expand.	SIADH	↑	↑	↓	↓	↓	—

ECF, extracellular fluid; Hct, hematocrit; ICF, intracellular fluid; ISF, interstitial fluid; SIADH, syndrome of inappropriate antidiuretic hormone same degree of water loss, an infant who develops hypernatremic dehydration will exhibit fewer symptoms of ECF volume deficit than the infant who develops isonatremic dehydration, although there is also more nervous system disturbance. This is marked by lethargy, hyperirritability upon stimulation, muscle rigidity, and convulsions. Hypernatremic dehydration can result from a variety of conditions, including those that increase the insensible water losses (fever) and diseases that produce excess water loss in the urine (DI).

Hypotonic dehydration. In hypotonic dehydration the net loss of fluid is hypertonic, leaving behind a hypotonic ECF. As a result of the discrepancy between the osmolality of the ECF and the ICF, water moves from the ECF into the ICF, reducing the ECF volume even further. Infants with hypotonic dehydration may commonly exhibit symptoms of severe ECF contraction, including shock. Hypotonic dehydration may result from a continued intake of solute-poor fluids (e.g., tea) in the treatment of diarrhea. It may also occur secondary to the intravenous infusion of large amounts of dextrose and water that contains no salt. Severe neurological complications may occur as a direct result of brain tissue swelling. The signs of dehydration tend to be more severe with smaller fluid losses in children with hypotonic dehydration, whereas hypertonic dehydration is associated with proportionately larger degrees of water loss for the same intensity of clinical signs.

In children with dehydration, assessment includes a review of both the clinical and the biochemical information available. Clinical parameters include body weight, circulatory status, urine output, and the presence of signs and symptoms of dehydration. Biochemical information includes plasma concentrations of sodium, potassium, chloride, BUN, blood acid-base status, hemoglobin, urine pH, and urine specific gravity. The three types of dehydration can be rather easily classified according to the plasma sodium concentration (expressed in milliequivalents per liter): isotonic (130 to 150), hypertonic (greater than 150), and hypotonic (less than 130).

The clinical severity of dehydration is determined from the loss of body weight. Upon admission to the hospital the child is weighed. The pre-illness weight is then compared with the admission weight, and the body weight loss is estimated. Body weight changes when considered over a short period of time (24 hours) can be equated with a change in fluid status, either a gain or loss. Mild dehydration corresponds to a fluid deficit of 50 ml/kg (5 percent) in infants and 30 ml/kg (3 percent) in older children and adults. The first clinical signs of dehydration usually appear when approximately 5 percent of the body weight has been lost. These signs and symptoms include pale, cool skin, slight oliguria, a slightly increased pulse rate, and thirst. Although infants may be thirsty, they may, at times, fail to adequately communicate their need for fluids. Moderate dehydration corresponds to a fluid loss of 100 ml/kg (10 percent) in infants and 60 ml/kg (6 percent) in older children and adults. Symptoms become more severe at this state and include a decreased blood pressure, increased pulse rate, signs of early shock, oliguria, grayish skin color, and skin that is cool and has a loss of elasticity. Severe dehydration occurs when fluid loss reaches 150 ml/kg (15 percent) in infants and 90 ml/kg (9 percent) in older children and adults. Symptoms of circulatory shock prevail in severe dehydration. These include a low blood pressure, tachycardia, poor peripheral circulation resulting in cool, pale, mottled skin with poor capillary refill, and prerenal azotemia. The mucous membranes are very dry and cracked, and the anterior fontanel in young infants is sunken.

Critical Care Management

The goals of treatment in severe dehydration involve restoration of circulating blood volume, correction of ECF volume deficits, correction of acid-base imbalances, normalization of plasma electrolyte concentrations, and normalization of body weight to the pre-illness level.

Replacement of both normal ongoing losses and abnormal fluid losses must be considered when calculating fluid therapy. In nearly all situations, normal ongoing water losses can be estimated by multiplying the basal energy expenditure (which is derived from weight and age) by 1.5. Abnormal ongoing water losses are replaced in exact proportions to those lost. Replacement of fluid to restore blood volume usually takes 2 hours. The result is an improvement in the peripheral circulation, an increase in blood pressure, a decrease in the pulse rate, an increase in the GFR, and a secondary increase in urine flow rate. Replacement of ECF deficits is indicated by a decrease in the BUN, resolution of most signs and symptoms of dehydration, and a partial correction of the sodium deficit. The amount of sodium replaced is equal to the isotonic concentration of the calculated deficit volume. For example, in hypernatremic dehydration, in which the estimated fluid loss is 100 ml/kg, the sodium concentration in the fluid lost may be approximately 130 mEq/liter. The sodium deficit would be replaced with 13 mEq/100 ml, along with the accompanying anion (chloride).

Intracellular stores of potassium may become reduced with diarrheal dehydration and need to be replaced via the ECF during the recovery phase. This is usually accomplished through the intravenous route. Hypocalcemia may be present in children with hypernatremic dehydration and/or hypokalemia, although it is rarely severe enough to cause tetany or to warrant vigorous replacement therapy. Restoration of ECF volume deficits usually takes only 18 to 24 hours, whereas normalization of the plasma potassium concentration may take several days. A steady increase in body weight indicates a gain in body fat and protein stores to replace those lost during the acute phase of the illness.

DISORDERS OF ADH

Through the interaction of ADH, aldosterone, and other, as yet unexplained, mechanisms, the regulation of body fluid volume and osmolality is accomplished. ADH, also called arginine vasopressin, is produced by the cells of the supraoptic and paraventricular nuclei of the hypothalamus. After production in the hypothalamus, ADH is stored in the posterior pituitary gland. The supraoptic-neurohypophyseal tract connects the nuclei to the gland.

The secretion of ADH is stimulated by three different conditions: (1) an increase in plasma osmolality, (2) a decrease in ECF and/or intravascular volume, and (3) a direct neuronal stimulation of the supraoptic and paraventricular nuclei (fear, pain, trauma, stress reactions). Under the first condition, osmoreceptors in the brain respond to a 2 percent increase in osmolality in blood perfusing the supraoptic nuclei by stimulating the release of ADH, prompting an antidiuresis. In contrast, a 2 percent decrease in osmolality will inhibit ADH release, prompting a diuresis. Nonosmotic control of ADH is the responsibility of volume receptors and baroreceptors. Volume receptors located in the left atrium respond to a decrease in the intravascular and/or ECF volume by stimulating the release of ADH and the retention of water by the kidneys. On the other hand, left atrial distention causes the inhibition of ADH release. Baroreceptors located in the carotid sinus, left atrium, and pulmonary vein affect ADH secretion through afferent impulses. A decrease in afferent impulses will increase ADH secretion. For example, a person standing quietly in the upright position probably experiences constant ADH release.

The primary site of ADH action is the distal tubule and collecting duct of the kidney. ADH release increases the permeability of these tubules to water and increases the reabsorption of urea. Water is passively reabsorbed from the tubule into the ECF by osmosis. With inhibition of ADH release, the tubules become resistant to the movement of water from the tubules into the renal interstitium.

The close proximity of the supraoptic and paraventricular nuclei of the hypothalamus to other centers in the brain that control basic physiological processes is important to remember. The importance will become more apparent in the discussion of the etiology and pathophysiology of the clinical disorders associated with ADH release.

SYNDROME OF INAPPROPRIATE ADH

SIADH secretion occurs frequently in pediatric ICU patients. In patients with SIADH, ADH is present under conditions that are inappropriate to the current volume and osmolality of body fluids. In the face of serum hypoosmolality and expanded ECF volume, ADH secretion persists and is, therefore, inappropriate. There are a number of different conditions that are associated with the development of SIADH (Table 6-12). Of paramount importance in pediatric ICU patients is the development of SIADH in association with pathological conditions of the central nervous system (CNS). These conditions include those associated with inflammation and infection, for example, meningitis (*see* p. 250), encephalitis, and brain abscesses; injury, for example head trauma (*see* p. 219), subarachnoid hemorrhage; brain tumors (*see* p. 234), and Guillain-Barré syndrome (*see* p. 282). The stimulation of the neurohypophyseal system in these CNS conditions, which results in the release of ADH, is believed to be independent of the normal physiological stimuli. In some of the malignant neoplasms, it is thought that the tumor cells produce an ADH-like substance. The release of this substance is independent of hypothalamic control.

Pathophysiology and Clinical Manifestations

SIADH develops when a normal or high plasma concentration of ADH is accompanied by a normal or high exogenous fluid intake. The dilution and expansion of body fluids that result are indicative of the failure of the kidneys to excrete sufficient free water to establish and maintain fluid balance in the child. In addition to the dilutional hyponatremia that occurs secondary to total body water expansion, it is believed that this ECF expansion inhibits the reabsorption of sodium ions, thus aggravating the hyponatremia. The mechanism for this is not completely understood. If SIADH is allowed to continue, eventually a new steady state is reached in which the plasma sodium concentration levels off at hyponatremic values. The cardinal features of SIADH have been defined to include (1) hyponatremia with corresponding hypoosmolality of plasma and ECF; (2) renal

TABLE 6-12   Disorders Associated with the Syndrome of Inappropriate Antidiuretic Hormone Secretion

Lungs	CNS	Other tumors	Drugs
Tuberculosis	Meningitis	Duodenal carcinoma	Chlorpropamide
Pneumonia	Abscess	Pancreatic carcinoma	Vincristine sulfate or cyclophosphamide
Carcinoma	Tumors	Thymoma	Clofibrate
Others	Acute intermittent porphyria	Others	Others
	Head injuries		
	Encephalitis		
	Subarachnoid hemorrhage		
	Psychogenic illness		
	Others		

Reprinted with permission from Valtin, H. 1979. Renal Dysfunction: Mechanisms Involved in Fluid and Solute Imbalance. Little, Brown & Co., Boston. 42.
CNS, central nervous system.

excretion of sodium that increases with the development of SIADH, then when a new steady state is attained, excretion levels off; (3) the absence of clinical evidence of fluid volume depletion (e.g., normal blood pressure, normal skin turgor); (4) osmolality of urine that is greater than that appropriate for the concomitant tonicity of plasma [Urine is not necessarily hyperosmotic to plasma, but is relatively hyperosmotic with respect to the water balance and the hypoosmolality of the plasma. Under these conditions a more diluted urine would normally be expected.]; (5) normal renal functioning; and (6) normal adrenal functioning.[31]

Clinical features of SIADH include those signs of the underlying disease and those associated with hyponatremia and ECF expansion. The symptoms of SIADH become more severe as the plasma sodium concentration decreases. At concentrations of 120 to 125 mEq/liter, nonspecific symptoms (including nausea, vomiting, and anorexia) appear. As the plasma sodium concentration levels drop to 110 to 115 mEq/liter, the child becomes lethargic, restless, uncooperative, and may exhibit a positive Babinski's sign. In addition, the child may show signs of decreased or sluggish deep tendon reflexes. Although no increase in intracranial pressure occurs with SIADH, the child may experience headache, muscle weakness, and lethargy, which may progress to coma. Due to the fact that SIADH is frequently associated with CNS disease, it may become difficult to distinguish symptoms of SIADH from those caused by the CNS disorder. In SIADH there are no clinical signs or symptoms of dehydration, blood pressure and skin turgor are normal, the serum BUN level is normal to low, and the fluid retention that occurs with SIADH is usually not severe enough to cause detectable edema.

Critical Care Management

The goal of therapy in SIADH is to create a negative water balance. The treatment of SIADH is directed toward the underlying disease process, when possible, and toward the hyponatremic state. Resolution of hyponatremia is achieved initially by restricting the daily fluid intake to an amount less than or equal to the insensible water loss. As the amount of free water excretion increases, fluid intake is liberalized to an amount equal to the insensible water loss plus the urine output over 24 hours. In children, this amounts to approximately 60 to 75 ml/100 calories expended. In accordance with maintenance requirements, sodium and potassium intake should each equal 2 to 3 mEq/100 calories expended. The requirement for glucose would remain at 5 g/100 calories expended. Gradually, excess water is excreted and the plasma sodium concentration returns to a normal level. Infrequently, hyponatremia is so severe that an intravenous infusion of hypertonic saline solution is required. Although this measure may be necessary to prevent swelling and compression of brain cells, it is important to point out that fluid restriction, not sodium administration, is the mainstay of treatment for SIADH. Successful treatment of the primary underlying disease in patients with SIADH results in prompt resolution of the SIADH.

Children susceptible to the development of SIADH are those in whom the associated disorders listed in Table 6-12 exist. The most common predisposing condition in the pediatric ICU patient is one involving the CNS. Once the SIADH-prone patient can be identified, nurses can take measures to carefully monitor the child for the development of this condition. Assessment and monitoring of the neurological and hydration status of a child are the two primary responsibilities of the nurse caring for patients with SIADH. Assessment of the neurological status (*see* p. 210) involves observing the patient for changes in behavior and level of consciousness, assessing the quality of deep tendon reflexes (*see* p. 277), and testing muscle strength (*see* p. 276). Assessment of hydration status (*see* p. 337) involves accurately measuring and recording all components of fluid intake and output as well as monitoring the development of clinical signs that may accompany volume expansion (*see* Table 6-11).

Although the nurse may not observe clinical signs of dehydration or fluid retention in the child, monitoring the intake and output of fluids, as well as the laboratory tests performed on plasma and urine, often enables the nurse to detect changes that accompany the development of SIADH. Of paramount importance are the sodium concentration of plasma and urine and the osmolality. As mentioned previously, there may be only slight edema in patients with SIADH. There is rarely more than a 5 percent increase in body weight over the normal "dry" weight.

Many times, patients in the ICU have restricted activity or may be comatose. In these patients, blood tends to pool in the peripheral vascular beds, resulting in a decreased left atrial filling pressure. The volume receptors located in the left atrium respond by signaling the release of ADH. Since procedures that tend to alter left atrial filling pressure affect ADH release in a rather predictable manner, procedures that encourage blood return to the capacitance vessels of the thorax should act to decrease the plasma concentration of ADH. It has been found that tilting the head of the patient's bed down 5 to 10 degrees will significantly decrease the peripheral venous concentration of ADH when compared with ADH levels obtained when the head of the patient's bed was raised 15 to 20 degrees.[32] When caring for patients with SIADH, the nurse should remember that the position of the head of the bed may have an important influence on plasma ADH levels. Although tilting the head of the bed down 5 to 10 degrees may be contraindicated in some pediatric ICU patients (CNS disturbances associated with an increased intracranial pressure), the nurse should be aware of the effects produced if the head is raised to an angle greater than or equal to 15 to 20 degrees. Other procedures designed to promote blood return to the chest would be beneficial under these conditions.

The effectiveness of the treatment plan for SIADH can be determined by following serial measurements of urine volume, serum and plasma sodium concentration and osmolality, and body weight.

DIABETES INSIPIDUS

There are three different types of DI that are described in the literature: (1) psychogenic DI or primary polydipsic DI, (2) pituitary, central, or hypothalamic DI, and (3) nephrogenic DI (Table 6-13). The differential diagnosis, pathophysiology and clinical manifestations, and the critical care management of these disorders are described below. Pituitary DI is the type most often seen in pediatric ICU patients.

Differential Diagnosis

Several tests are available to distinguish pituitary DI from psychogenic polydipsia and from nephrogenic DI. The water deprivation test (WDT) is simple to perform but is generally not practical or useful in pediatric ICU patients. However, the

TABLE 6-13 Causes and Treatment of Diabetes Insipidus

Types	Causes	Treatment
Primary polydipsic DI (compulsive water drinker; psychogenic polydipsia).	Acquired: (1) emotional; (2) nonpsychogenic(?), e.g., tumors or other lesions causing chronic stimulation of the thirst center(?).	Psychiatric.
	Hereditary(?): Described in species other than man, but not yet in man.	Psychiatric?
Hypothalamic DI (DI; true DI).	Acquired: (1) unknown; (2) neoplastic; (3) traumatic, e.g., automobile accidents; (4) Neurosurgical procedures; (5) Nonneoplastic, e.g., histiocytosis X, sarcoidosis, syphilis, Sheehan's syndrome, encephalitis, leukemia, and others.	Amelioration or elimination of the primary lesion if possible. Various drugs: ADH or one of its synthetic analogues; chlorpropamide (potentiates cellular effect of ADH and, hence, can be used only in partial hypothalamic DI).
	Hereditary.	Same as for acquired.
Nephrogenic DI (vasopressin-resistant DI).	Acquired: Drugs, hypokalemia, hypercalcemia, sickle cell anemia, and other causes.	Withdrawal of offending agent or correction of the primary disorder.
	Hereditary.	Unsatisfactory in most cases; however, the following are used: (1) adequate fluid intake at all times; (2) thiazide diuretics; and (3) reduction of protein and NaCl intake and, hence, of renal solute output.

Reprinted with permission from Valtin, H. 1979. Renal Dysfunction: Mechanisms Involved in Fluid and Solute Imbalance. Little, Brown & Co., Boston.
ADH, antidiuretic hormone; DI, diabetes insipidus.

WDT serves as a good example of the principles involved in the differentiation of DI (Table 6-14).

The child undergoing the WDT is restricted from drinking any water. The patient's weight, urine output, urine specific gravity, and vital signs are monitored hourly. A maximum weight loss of 3 percent of the original body weight is allowed. This results in an increase in the plasma osmolality of approximately 15 mOsm/kg of water. At this point, there is no need to continue the test since maximal stimulation of the hypothalamo-neurohypophyseal system occurs. Special precautions must be taken in infants and young children since severe dehydration can occur rapidly. In the face of no water intake and continuing renal losses of water, the body normally signals the release of ADH in response to the hypernatremia and hyperosmolality. The result is a decrease in urine volume and an increase in urine osmolality. The patient with primary polydipsic DI will respond to the WDT by exhibiting all of these features, whereas patients with pituitary or nephrogenic DI will not. Patients with primary polydipsic DI have a hypothalamo-neurohypophyseal system that can release ADH appropriately and kidneys that respond properly to this ADH.

The more common test used to differentiate between the three forms of DI is a modified Hickey-Hare test. Following the establishment of a high urine flow rate (accomplished by administration of 5 percent dextrose water at a rate of 0.3 ml/kg/min) in the patient, an intravenous infusion of hypertonic saline (2.5 percent) is administered (at a rate of 0.2 ml/kg/min). Only patients with primary polydipsic DI will show a decrease in urine output and an increase in urine osmolality. Patients with pituitary or nephrogenic DI can be differentiated by the subsequent administration of exogenous vasopressin (1 milliunit of aqueous Pitressin in glucose and water per minute). Patients with pituitary DI will exhibit a decrease in urine output and an increase in urine osmolality, whereas patients with nephrogenic DI remain unresponsive. Patients with primary polydipsic DI will show no further decrease in urine output or increase in urine osmolality with the administration of exogenous ADH.

Pituitary DI

Pituitary DI results from an insufficiency of ADH, either in production or release of ADH from the posterior pituitary gland. The causes of pituitary DI are listed in Table 6-13. In approximately 50 percent of children who develop pituitary DI, the etiology is unknown. In addition, children undergoing neurosurgical procedures that involve structures near the hypothalamo-neurohypophyseal region constitute another group of patients at high risk for the development of DI.

Pathophysiology and clinical manifestations. Pituitary DI is characterized by the absence of ADH. As a result, the production of copious amounts of diluted urine leads to contraction of ECF and plasma volume. Even though the thirst mechanism is intact or operative in patients with pituitary DI, their fluid intake is unable to keep up with the urine output in the face of continuing negative water balance. As the negative water balance of the patient becomes more severe, the kidneys show an increase in the reabsorption of sodium ions. Hypernatremia results, stimulating the thirst mechanism. Even if the patient has free access to water, is alert and old enough to drink a large volume of fluid on his own, dehydration may ensue if renal loss of water progresses more rapidly than fluid intake. If dehydration continues, prerenal azotemia may develop and disguise the diagnosis. Clinical

TABLE 6-14 Differentiation of the Different Types of Diabetes Insipidus Using the Water-Deprivation Test and/or Modified Hickey-Hare Test

Type of DI	Effect of water deprivation on urine volume and osmolality	Effect of exogenous ADH	Normal hypo-thalamo-neurohy-pophyseal function	Normal renal functioning
Primary polydipsic DI	Urine volume decreases; osmolality increases; specific gravity increases.	None	Yes	Yes
Hypothalamic DI	Urine volume does not decrease.	Response is a decrease in urine flow and an increase in urine concentration. Urine osmolality increased beyond value achieved with water deprivation.	No	Yes
Nephrogenic DI	Urine volume does not decrease.	None	Yes	No

ADH, antidiuretic hormone; DI, diabetes insipidus.

features common to patients with this type of DI include a urine osmolality that is less than the plasma osmolality, a negative water balance, a high urine flow rate, hypernatremia, and thirst.

Other clinical conditions associated with a high urine flow rate may initially confuse the diagnosis of pituitary DI. For example, a clinician may suspect pituitary DI in a child excreting large volumes of diluted urine, but if the child has recently received mannitol, his body is responding appropriately to the osmotic load that mannitol produces. In this situation, hypernatremia is usually not present.

Critical care management. Treatment of pituitary DI involves the administration of ADH as replacement therapy. Currently, a variety of preparations are available for use, although Pitressin Tannate in Oil (5 U/ml) is often used because its duration of action is 24 to 48 hours. The usual dose is 5 units intramuscularly. DDAVP, which is an analogue of vasopressin, is occasionally used in children. It is dispensed in 2.5-milliliter bottles (100 μg/ml), with the usual dose being 10 to 20 μg intranasally. The duration of action is approximately 12 to 24 hours.

Transient pituitary DI, which often occurs secondary to neurosurgical procedures, is difficult to manage in children. Rapid, marked shifts in fluid balance may prevent the establishment of good fluid control in these patients.

In caring for patients with pituitary DI, it is necessary that the nurse carefully monitor urine flow rate, the intake and output of fluid, and the plasma electrolyte concentrations. Monitoring the overall fluid balance of the child is an important nursing function. Measuring and recording fluid intake and output on an hourly schedule are necessary for the child receiving fluid and exogenous ADH as replacement therapy. In particular, the nurse should watch for signs and symptoms of excess fluid retention in patients receiving this regimen.

Nephrogenic DI

Nephrogenic DI is a disorder characterized by a defect in the response of the renal tubular epithelium (distal tubule and collecting duct) to ADH. Although ADH is present in ample amounts in the plasma, a defective renal mechanism prevents the normal reabsorption of water from the renal tubules into the renal interstitium. This form of DI can be acquired or inherited. For example, severe nephrogenic DI is acquired secondary to some drugs and conditions such as hypokalemia. Nephrogenic DI is inherited as a sex-linked trait in male infants. This form is quite rare.

Pathophysiology and clinical manifestations. The mechanism to explain the resistance of renal tubules to the action of ADH has not been well identified. The clinical manifestations of nephrogenic DI include those described in the section on pituitary DI. If nephrogenic DI goes undiagnosed and untreated, the chronic dehydration and hypernatremia would be life threatening.

Critical care management. Since the kidney will not respond to the administration of exogenous ADH, treatment involves the administration of feedings that consist of large volumes of fluid and a low renal solute load of sodium, potassium, chloride, and protein. This will decrease the amount of free water excretion and urine output. The majority of calories needed for growth and development are best provided by carbohydrates and fats in these children. Thiazide diuretics may be used in some patients to decrease the urine flow. The exact mechanism of action of these diuretics in patients with nephrogenic DI is unknown.

HYPERTENSION

Hypertension is a frequently encountered condition in children who require intensive care. Hypertension in this patient population often develops secondary to renal disorders and, less commonly, to cardiovascular, endocrinologic, or neurological disorders. In order to define nursing strategies that are effective in caring for the hypertensive child, it is necessary for the pediatric critical care nurse to possess an understanding of the pathophysiology and current treatment modalities of hypertension. The following pages will describe (1) factors that govern the normal regulation of arterial pressure, (2) definitions of primary and secondary hypertension, and (3) critical care management of the child with hypertension.

Physiology

Blood pressure is a function of cardiac output and peripheral resistance. The relationship between arterial blood pressure (BP), cardiac output (CO), and peripheral resistance (PR) is described by the following equation:

$$BP = CO \times PR.$$

Blood pressure or systemic arterial pressure is the force exerted by the blood on the vessel wall. Cardiac output is the amount of blood ejected by the left ventricle into the aorta per unit time and is expressed in milliliters per minute. Cardiac output (CO) is equal to the heart rate (HR) (beats per minute) multiplied by the stroke volume (SV) (milliliters per beat): $CO = HR \times SV$, and is indirectly controlled by venous return, which in part, is influenced by the cellular needs of body tissues.

Peripheral resistance refers to the impediment to blood flow through a vessel. Peripheral resistance is, therefore, influenced by such factors as the size of the vessel lumen, the length of the vessel, and the viscosity of blood. For example, the longer the vessel, the greater the blood viscosity, and the smaller the vessel lumen, the greater the resistance. The major physiological control variable is the size of the vessel lumen. Under normal conditions, the body can alter the size of the vessel lumen and, thus, affect peripheral resistance. This is accomplished through the action of the autonomic nervous system on smooth muscle fibers in the vessel wall, causing either vasoconstriction or vasodilation.

Nervous system control of blood flow. The normal control of blood pressure is accomplished through the action of three related reflex loops in the CNS. One regulates cardiac function (heart rate and stroke volume), one controls arteriolar tone (vasodilation and vasoconstriction), and the third influences blood volume through the renal regulation of sodium and water. Afferent impulses to these centers are inhibitory and serve to reduce the excitatory impulses that arise from higher brain centers.

The effector limb of these systems uses the peripheral autonomic nervous system. There is rich sympathetic innervation to the effector organs required for blood pressure control: the heart, the peripheral vasculature, the kidney, and the adrenal medulla are all involved. When sympathetic neurons are stimulated (fever, stress, or decrease in blood pressure), norepinephrine is released from postganglionic neurons and norepinephrine and epinephrine are released from the adrenal medulla.

Adrenergic receptors are the cellular sites located on effector organs where catecholamines bind. These receptors, when bound to catecholamines, induce changes that result in the characteristic physiological effect of that effector organ. Adrenergic receptors are subdivided into alpha (α) and beta (β) types. These types are further subdivided into α_1, α_2, β_1, and β_2 types. The α_1 and β_1 effects on blood vessels are generally vasoconstrictive in nature, whereas the β_2 receptors cause vasodilation. When stimulated, the α_2 receptors (which are located in the presynaptic sympathetic neurons) cause inhibition of further norepinephrine release. Stimulation of beta-adrenergic nerve endings that innervate cardiac muscle (β_1) causes an increased force of contraction (inotropic effect) and increased heart rate (chronotropic effect).

Maintenance of Normal Blood Pressure

Guyton and others have identified eight important arterial pressure regulating systems.[33] These systems function continually to help maintain blood pressure within normal limits. Although they are all believed to play a role in the maintenance of normal blood pressure, the renal-body fluid mechanism is believed to be the principal determinant of long-term arterial pressure regulation.

1. *Baroreceptor mechanism:* An increase in arterial pressure stimulates baroreceptors located in the walls of large systemic arteries (carotid sinuses and the aortic arch). The receptors then send afferent signals to the vasomotor center in the medulla of the brain. Efferent fibers are routed through fibers of the autonomic nervous system in order to slow heart rate, decrease the strength of ventricular contraction, and dilate peripheral blood vessels by inhibiting the vasoconstrictor center of the medulla. Consequently, arterial pressure is decreased.

2. *Chemoreceptor system:* This system operates when arterial pressure falls below 80 mmHg. The chemoreceptors located in the aortic arch and carotid sinuses are stimulated by the decreased delivery of oxygen and the decreased removal of carbon dioxide that occurs with decreased cardiac output. Signals are sent through the autonomic nervous system to increase arterial pressure toward normal.

3. *Central nervous system ischemic response:* A decrease in arterial pressure to an extremely low level (less than 40 mmHg) will cause ischemia of the vasomotor center of the brain and subsequent stimulation of the sympathetic nervous system. As a result, cardiac activity is enhanced, peripheral vessels are constricted, and blood pressure increases toward normal.

4. *Renin-angiotensin-vasoconstrictor mechanism:* When mean arterial pressure falls below 100 mmHg, the kidneys form increased amounts of renin. This compound increases synthesis of angiotensin II from angiotensin I and exerts three effects: (1) increased sympathetic nervous system activity (increased secretion of norepinephrine), (2) direct vasoconstrictor activity, which increases peripheral resistance, and (3) increased sodium and water retention by the kidneys secondary to stimulation of aldosterone secretion. These effects result in an increased blood volume and an increased blood pressure.

5. *Stress relaxation mechanism:* When arterial pressure increases, blood vessels stretch (stress relaxation). This stretching allows the pressure in these parts of the circulation to fall, decreasing peripheral resistance and arterial pressure.

6. *Capillary fluid shift mechanism:* When arterial pressure increases, capillary pressure also increases. Elevated intracapillary pressure may result in transudation of fluid out of the bloodstream into the interstitium. As blood volume decreases, arterial pressure gradually decreases toward normal.

7. *Renal-body fluid mechanism:* A decrease in arterial pressure below normal has a direct effect on the kidneys to decrease the excretion of salt and water. A progressive retention of salt and water causes an increase in the ECF volume. This returns the arterial pressure toward normal.

8. *Vasodilator mechanism:* Recent evidence points to the fact that the kidney may have a blood pressure lowering effect that is independent of its control of salt and water excretion. There may be a vasodepressor substance normally present in the kidney that has an antihypertensive effect. The renal kallikrein system may play a role in this antihypertensive effect, which may be decreased in patients with hypertension.

These control mechanisms will interact when necessary. Each system has unique characteristics that make it particularly valuable under specific physiological conditions. Some are involved in short-term arterial pressure regulation and respond rapidly, whereas other systems directly affect the long-term regulation of arterial pressure and respond more slowly (Table 6-15).

Short-term regulation of arterial pressure. Short-term regulation is maintained by the effects of the sympathetic nervous system on peripheral resistance and cardiac output, and by hormonal mechanisms. For example, a decrease in blood pressure will stimulate the sympathetic nervous system and cause vasoconstriction and enhance cardiac activity. These combined actions will increase arterial pressure toward normal. The hormones involved in raising arterial pressure include norepinephrine, epinephrine, angiotensin II, aldosterone, and ADH.

Long-term regulation of arterial pressure. The renal and adrenal systems are largely responsible for the long-term maintenance of normal arterial pressure. The renal-body fluid mechanism is responsible for the long-term regulation of arterial pressure. There is a direct relationship between arterial pressure and the excretion of salt and water by the kidneys. The difference between the net intake of salt and water and the renal excretion of salt and water determines the rate of change of ECF volume. The size of the ECF compartment, in turn, controls the level of arterial pressure.

The renal-body fluid mechanism can be influenced in many ways to alter arterial pressure. As can be seen from Figure 6-22, the dependent variables can be increased or decreased as needed to affect a change in the net intake and output of salt and water and, thus, in arterial pressure. The determinants of arterial pressure (Fig. 6-23) can alter arterial pressure independently. A change in any one of these variables will alter the level at which arterial pressure will stabilize, because it can affect the net intake and output of water and salt. For example, a decrease in arterial pressure will increase renin secretion, which in turn, affects the renal output of salt and water through a direct effect on the kidneys. The kidneys will increase the reabsorption of salt and water and restore ECF volume and arterial pressure toward normal.

Hypertension is defined as a systolic and/or diastolic blood pressure that exceeds the 95 percent confidence limits (approximately 2 standard deviations from the mean) of a given population. For adults, this limit is 140/90 mmHg, but the value is progressively less for adolescents and children (Fig. 6-24, p. 366).[34] There are relationships between the degree of hypertension and morbidity and mortality. Therapy is, therefore, directed toward lowering the pressure to normal.

Hypertension can be a primary or secondary process. Secondary hypertension results from renal disease and, less often, from a cardiac, adrenal, endocrine, or neurological disorder. Essential (or primary) hypertension is a condition for which there is no clear identifiable cause.

Hypertension may result when either the arterial vascular bed is overfilled from excess fluid, or when the vascular bed is inappropriately vasoconstricted, relative to the fluid volume. The relationship of these two components is expressed by the following equation:

$$BP = EV \times VC,$$

where BP is blood pressure, EV is effective volume, and VC is vasoconstrictor components. The effective circulating blood volume in relation to the total vascular capacity is determined by ECF volume and, therefore, by sodium balance. The vasoconstrictor components are influenced by angiotensin and nonangiotensin pressor factors. Hypertension may thus be categorized as volume dependent or vasoconstriction dependent, if one mechanism or the other is predominant. The dynamics of these different forms of hypertension are described in the following section.

Pathophysiology

Definitive mechanisms that describe the pathogenesis of hypertension are not well understood. Current speculation suggests that hypertension is a disorder characterized by a multifactorial derangement of regulation.

Volume-dependent hypertension.   Although the exact mechanism is unknown, the development of volume-dependent hypertension is thought to result from the retention of excess salt and water. This retention may result from one of two causes: excess mineralocorticoid activity for the amount of dietary sodium, or an inability to excrete dietary sodium. Retention of salt and water for whichever reason results in an increased total ECF volume and an increased cardiac output. As autoregulatory vasoconstriction acts to increase the total peripheral resistance, cardiac output decreases toward normal and high blood pressure is maintained by vasoconstriction.

Little is known about hemodynamic disturbances in children with hypertension. The generalization that in hypertension a state of high cardiac output and normal peripheral resistance precedes a state of high peripheral resistance and normal cardiac output, holds true for some children, but not for all. Once arterial pressure is elevated, it remains high because peripheral resistance remains high. When ECF volume is expanded, arterioles become more sensitive to circulating pressor substances. This may aggravate the hypertension. This type of hypertension is treated with drugs that regulate the effective plasma volume (e.g., diuretics). A

TABLE 6-15 Blood Pressure Control Mechanisms

Control mechanism	Description	Responds to	Effect on BP	Short-term regulation*	Long-term regulation*	Example
Baroreceptor mechanism	Baroreceptors in aortic arch and carotid sinus stimulated.	↑ BP	↓ BP	Seconds‡		Rapid bleeding or posture changes
Chemoreceptor system	Stimulated by decreased O_2 and increased CO_2 levels.	↓ BP	↑ BP	Seconds‡		
Central nervous system ischemic	Vasomotor center in brain becomes ischemic.	↓ BP (< 40 mmHg)	↑ BP	Seconds‡		
Renin-angiotensin vasoconstrictor	Kidneys secrete renin when BP is decreased below 100 mmHg.	↓ BP (< 100 mmHg)	↑ BP	Minutes to hours		Hemorrhage

Stress-relaxation	Blood vessels stretch.	↑ BP	→ BP	Minutes to hours	Overtransfusion
Capillary fluid shift	Intracapillary pressure increased. Transudation of fluid and decreased blood volume	↑ BP	→ BP	Minutes to hours	Overtransfusion
Renal-body fluid	Decreased excretion of salt and water by kidneys. ECF volume increased.	→ BP	← BP	Hours to indefinite duration	
Vasodilator	May be a depressor substance deficient in hypertension.	← BP	→ BP		

BP, blood pressure; ECF, extracellular fluid.

*The expressions short- and long-term regulation describe the onset and duration of the specific control mechanism.

‡Nervous system feedback mechanism.

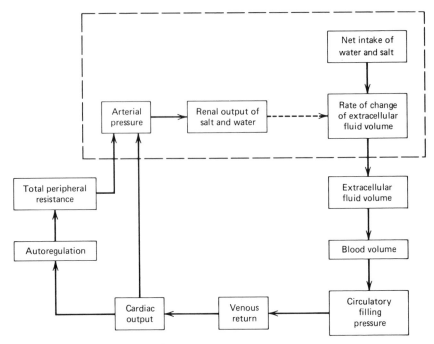

Figure 6-22. The feedback control loop of the renal-body fluid arterial pressure mechanism. The dashed arrow indicates a negative effect. Those portions of the diagram within the dashed enclosure represent the determinants of arterial pressure. Those outside the enclosure represent the dependent variables of the system. *Reprinted with permission from* Guyton, A. C., T. G. Coleman, A. W. Crowley, K. W. Scheel, R. D. Manning, and R. A. Norman. 1974. Arterial pressure regulation: overriding dominance of the kidneys in long-term regulation and in hypertension. In Laragh, J. H., editor. 1974 Hypertension Manual. Dun-Donnelley, New York. 119.

low-salt diet is often used in conjunction with diuretics. Ultrafiltration with hemodialysis is another method that may be used in patients with chronic renal failure to remove the excess salt and water that contributes to the development of hypertension.

Vasoconstriction-dependent hypertension. Arteriolar vasoconstriction is the predominant factor in this type of hypertension. Vasoconstriction results from renin secreted in response to low renal perfusion pressure (causing ischemia) or excess beta-sympathetic stimulation. Renin generation causes increased production of angiotensin II and secretion of aldosterone. The control of renin release is not completely characterized. It involves a number of factors, including intrarenal sodium receptors (macula densa and renal afferent arterioles), renal sympathetic nerves, and a number of humoral agents. The effects of angiotensin II and aldosterone result in vasoconstriction and sodium retention. The renin-angiotensin system is implicated in the pathogenesis of renovascular hypertension, hypertension secondary to renin-secreting tumors, and malignant hypertension. The treatment of vasoconstriction-dependent hypertension involves the use of agents that indi-

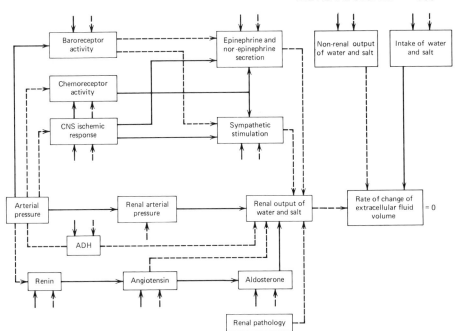

Figure 6-23.   The determinants of long-term arterial pressure regulation. This figure is an expansion of the dashed enclosure of Figure 6-22. *Reprinted with permission from* Guyton, A. C., T. G. Coleman, A. W. Crowley, K. W. Scheel, R. D. Manning, and R. A. Norman. 1974. Arterial pressure regulation overriding dominance of the kidneys in long-term regulation and in hypertension. In Laragh, J. H. editor. 1974 Hypertension Manual. Dun-Donnelley, New York. 122.

rectly neutralize or eliminate excess renin secretion (e.g., beta-adrenergic blocking agents, such as propranolol).

An additional factor that may play a role in hypertension generated by either mechanism discussed above is the composition of the arteriolar wall.[35] The sodium chloride content of the wall increases in hypertension, causing thickening of the wall and narrowing of the vessel lumen. These vessels may then develop ischemia and fibrinoid necrosis. As a result, peripheral resistance and blood pressure increase. It is unknown whether this change in the vascular wall is secondary to hypertension or whether it precedes the hypertensive state.

Secondary forms of hypertension.   Secondary hypertension in children is most often due to renal disease.[36,37] The types of renal disease that can cause hypertension can be divided into three categories: renovascular, glomerular, and tubulointerstitial.

The most common disorder in the first category is renal artery stenosis. In this condition, either one or both renal arteries (or a branch) becomes stenosed. The kidney distal to the stenosis becomes ischemic, which results in the release of renin, increased tubular reabsorption of salt and water, and increased blood pressure. The GFR remains normal in this disease.

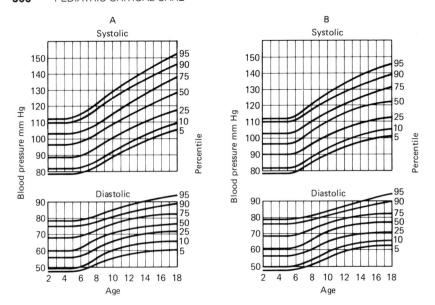

Figure 6-24. Blood pressure distributions for normal children. Percentiles of blood pressure measurement in (A) boys and (B) girls (right arm, seated).

Loss of renal mass may occur in glomerular diseases such as pyelonephritis, acute and chronic glomerulonephritis, polycystic disease, and hydronephrosis. Most of these conditions are associated with mild hypertension, although when renal mass is decreased by 70 percent or more, blood pressure becomes markedly elevated. The decrease in renal mass prevents the kidneys from excreting excess amounts of salt. When a large amount of salt is consumed, hypertension develops. The treatment includes natriuretic agents and, possibly, other antihypertensive drugs.

Lesions of the kidney that cause increased salt and water reabsorption are rare. Renal tumors such as Wilms's or a tumor of the JGA (hemangiopericytoma) can cause excessive secretion of aldosterone. Primary aldosteronism caused by an adrenal adenoma or adrenal hyperplasia is also characterized by excessive aldosterone secretion. The excess aldosterone results in hypokalemia and excess sodium conservation, which expands the ECF volume and increases blood pressure.

Tubulointerstitial nephritis can occur as a result of a variety of diseases, such as medullary cystic disease and polycystic disease, or secondary to drugs (e.g., furosemide) and radiation. Although these conditions are uncommon, damage to the renal tubules and interstitium can severely compromise tubular functions. The fluid and solute imbalances that result from tubular dysfunction contribute to the development of hypertension. Therapy is directed toward correcting the underlying disease process or removing the offending substance.

Chronic renal failure (CRF) develops most often when the GFR is less than 10 ml/min/1.73 m². The child is characteristically seen at some point with hypertension. Hypertension results from sodium and/or renin excess. It has been suggested that the mechanism for this form of hypertension is a renin level that is inappropriate for the level of exchangeable sodium in the body. The mechanism that normally increases arterial pressure to excrete excess sodium is reset at a higher level. Thus, sodium is retained and the arterial pressure will increase to the point where sodium balance is restored. Renal functioning in children with CRF is inadequate to maintain life without dialysis. Treatment consists of a form of dialysis — either hemodialysis or continuous ambulatory peritoneal dialysis.

Adrenal disorders that may cause hypertension include Cushing's syndrome and pheochromocytoma (a catecholamine-producing tumor arising from cells of the sympathetic nervous system).

The cardiac lesion most often associated with hypertension is coarctation of the aorta (*see* p. 138). A narrowing of the aorta results in compromised renal blood flow and increased renin secretion, with consequent increase in salt and water resorption by the kidney. Hypertension is characteristically found in the upper extremities, with normal or low blood pressure in the lower extremities and the presence of delayed or absent femoral pulses.

Neurological disorders associated with hypertension include familial dysautonomia, Guillain-Barré syndrome (*see* p. 282), and expanding lesions of the CNS.

Various medications are known to induce hypertension in some individuals: oral contraceptives, high-dose corticosteroids, and sympathetic stimulants (amphetamine, ephedrine, phenylephrine hydrochloride). Other agents, such as lead and mercury, can also cause hypertension as part of their effect on renal functioning.

Essential hypertension. Essential hypertension is a condition of unknown origin that affects target systemic arterioles and transitional small arteries. The development and maintenance of essential hypertension involves the kidneys, adrenal hormones, and the central and autonomic nervous systems. Predictors of essential hypertension — blood pressure, age, relative weight for height, family history, etc. — suggest that there are genetic determinants of the tendency toward familial aggregation of blood pressure in childhood.[38,39]

The mechanism of essential hypertension is unknown, but it is generally accepted that the kidney plays a key role. Although there is no intrinsic renal pathology, kidney functioning in essential hypertension may not be normal. Early in the course of the development of essential hypertension, a person may be unable to excrete sodium and water in a normal fashion. Instead, to excrete normal amounts of salt and water, the arterial pressure must be considerably higher than normal. A new steady state is reached in which the intake equals the net output, cardiac output is normal, and the kidneys maintain normal GFR at the expense of greatly increased arterial pressure. If arterial pressure decreases, solute retention occurs.

The role of the renin-angiotensin system in the development of essential hypertension is not well understood. Attempts have been made to quantitate the role of this system and define its significance in terms of the prognosis of patients with essential hypertension. Individuals have been classified according to their plasma renin activity (PRA) value. Because renin is not easily measured directly in the plasma, it is measured indirectly. Renin normally reacts with renin substrate to produce angiotensin I, which is then quantitated by radioimmunoassay. The rate of formation of angiotensin I is an index of renin activity. Thus, PRA reflects the capacity of the blood to generate angiotensin I. PRA is affected by many factors, such as posture, sodium balance, excitement, and drugs. Normal values in children are difficult to define, and therefore, appropriate reference standards are needed in order to interpret PRA values.

Hypertensive emergencies. Hypertensive encephalopathy is a syndrome consisting of an abrupt, severe elevation of arterial pressure, which may cause severe headaches, convulsions, and/or a variety of transitory cerebral phenomena.[40] These cerebral manifestations may result from a defect in the autoregulation of cerebral blood flow. This may result in overregulation with ischemic injury to the brain or underregulation with overperfusion of the brain. No decisive mechanism for the pathogenesis of hypertensive encephalopathy exists. Accelerated hypertension, hypertensive encephalopathy, and left ventricular failure are all considered emergencies and demand prompt attention. Symptoms associated with an acute increase in arterial pressure are frontal headache, seizures, blurred vision, decreased visual acuity or other visual disturbances, lower motor neuron facial palsy, dizziness, nausea, vomiting, irritability, hyperactivity, personality changes, anxiety, tachycardia, sweating, weight loss, polyuria, polydipsia, peripheral edema, congestive heart failure, and weakness. Ophthalmologic symptoms are less common in children than in adults, but may include papilledema, retinal hemorrhages, exudates, and transient blindness. A sustained severe increase in arterial pressure may initiate intracranial hemorrhage (either intracerebral or subarachnoid).

The cause of accelerated hypertension is most often renal disease, e.g., poststreptococcal glomerulonephritis, hemolytic-uremic syndrome, end-stage renal disease, unilateral or bilateral renal disease, reflux nephropathy, renovascular hypertension, and renin-secreting tumors.

Critical Care Management

Nursing assessment. Hypertension in children most often develops in association with an acute illness or as an acute manifestation of a chronic illness. The prior experience of the child and his family with high blood pressure and hospitalization may influence their response to the child's hypertensive crisis. The recognition of high blood pressure as a major public health problem in the United States in recent years has led to the development of advertising campaigns to heighten public awareness of the potential morbid sequelae of sustained hypertension and the role of preventive health care. It is important for the nurse to ascertain the extent of the child's and family's understanding of hypertension.

The formulation of nursing interventions that are appropriate to the care of the hypertensive child is decribed in subsequent paragraphs. The description of the process is necessarily general because many factors — including the child's previous health status, the type of hypertension present, the child's age, and the course of hospitalization — determine the child's specific needs.

Base-line data regarding the child's personality should be obtained early in the course of his illness. This data should include information on development up to the present, emotional responses to strange people, situations and environments, reactions to previous illnesses, normal sleep/rest patterns, and normal play activities and interactions with family members and peers. Also of importance is information on family members' responses to and relationships with the child. This would include, for example, identification of the primary caregiver, family support systems, methods of discipline, and family dynamics.

Organization of this information into a framework will enable the nurse to more accurately assess symptoms expressed by the child and to better interpret the meaning of specific behavioral responses. The symptoms of hypertension (headache, anxiety, and dizziness) are often similar to symptoms associated with side effects of antihypertensive medications. These same symptoms may also be an expression of a child's normal reaction to hospitalization, illness, or another situation. Because the etiology of the symptoms may not be apparent initially, all avenues must be investigated. Information that is gathered must be interpreted in light of what are normal behavioral and coping mechanisms for that individual child.

The next step in the process involves the compilation of objective data. The measurement of blood pressure is the most important piece of information. Measurement of parameters that provide information regarding the status of the cardiovascular (*see* p. 98), renal, neurological (*see* p. 210), and respiratory (*see* p. 33) systems is also essential. These systems indirectly influence arterial pressure and, therefore, are involved to varying degrees in hypertension.

Measurement of blood pressure.   Before discussing the measurement of blood pressure, a review of the different types of pressure readings is indicated.

1. *Systolic pressure:* The peak pressure during systole, or the highest pressure generated by ventricular contraction. Cardiac output is a major determinant of systolic pressure.

2. *Diastolic pressure:* The peak pressure during diastole, or the lowest pressure determined by ventricular relaxation and peripheral resistance. The resistance in arterioles is a major determinant of the diastolic pressure.

3. *Pulse pressure:* The difference between the systolic and diastolic pressures, or the amplitude of the pulsations of the arterial pressure. Pulse pressure in large arteries is influenced by the heart rate. For example, if the heart rate slows, the pulse pressure will increase.

4. *Mean pressure:* The average driving force for blood flow to tissues during the entire cardiac cycle. It is approximately equal to one third the pulse pressure plus the diastolic pressure.

Blood pressure can be measured directly or indirectly. Although hemodynamic monitoring is frequently used in pediatric critical care settings (*see* p. 108), the indirect measurement of blood pressure (via blood pressure cuff) continues to be relied upon heavily for assessment of blood pressure in children. In conjunction with monitoring other vital signs, nurses have the responsibility to measure, record, and evaluate blood pressure in patients. Consequently, the nurse should not only know how to obtain an accurate blood pressure in a child, but also be aware of what factors can potentially affect accuracy.[41]

Accuracy in the measurement of blood pressure is important because it often determines whether a child is treated, when treatment begins and ends, and at what drug dosage blood pressure is stabilized. An accurate blood pressure reading is often difficult to obtain because of the child's anxiety over unfamiliar conditions or environment and because of the size of the child. Several factors may serve as sources of error in the measurement of blood pressure (Table 6-16). The reliability of indirect measurement can be increased through the use of standardized conditions.

TABLE 6-16 Potential Sources of Error in Measuring Blood Pressure

Factor	Problem
Equipment	
Sphygmanometer	Mercury level not at 0; leak in tubing.
Cuff	Inflatable bladder incorrect size; tear or crack in bladder.
Stethoscope	Kinked tubing; blocked ear pieces; ear pieces do not fit well.
Environment	
Temperature	Ambient temperature that is excessively warm or cool will cause vasodilation or vasoconstriction.
Noise	Noise in surrounding environment makes it difficult for the clinician to distinguish Korotkoff sounds.
Diurnal variation	May be present.
Subject	
Position	Supine and sitting positions result in different blood pressure readings; support the extremity in which blood pressure is measured, should be at the level of the heart.
Activity	Physical activity will elevate blood pressure; have patient rest before taking blood pressure measurement.
Stress	Pain, anxiety, and/or a distended bladder will elevate the blood pressure; allow sufficient time for recovery or document the presence of these symptoms when recording blood pressure.
Other	Ingestion of alcohol, coffee, tea, certain drugs, smoking, and fever.
Technique	
Examiner	Inadequate knowledge of proper technique; decreased visual or hearing acuity may prevent accurate measurement of blood pressure; poor coordination.
Digit preference	A preference for rounding to certain numbers when recording blood pressure (usually round to measurements ending in 0).
Observer bias	A preconceived notion or prejudice on part of examiner as to what reading should be heard. (Might expect to hear sounds within the hypertensive range in a patient previously noted to be hypertensive and presently not taking all antihypertensive medications.)

Precautions. The nurse should begin by explaining the procedure to the child and family. If the child expresses the desire, he or she should be allowed to manipulate the blood pressure equipment and stethoscope to become familiar with them. Demonstrating how the equipment functions and that it does not hurt may alleviate some fears within the child. It is advisable that the child be in a comfortable position and relatively quiet. If it is difficult to calm the young child or infant, an accurate blood pressure reading can often be obtained if the child falls asleep with the blood pressure cuff in place. The extremity in which the blood pressure is to be measured should be fully exposed to allow the proper placement of the cuff.

The size of the inflatable bladder within the cuff (rather than the cloth covering) is of paramount importance in measuring blood pressure accurately.[34] The bladder should be long enough to completely encircle the arm without overlapping or

TABLE 6-17   Dimensions for Appropriate Size Cuff

Cuff name	Dimension range of bladder*	
	Width	Length
	cm	cm
Newborn	2.5–4.0	5.0–10.0
Infant	6.0–8.0	12.0–13.5
Child	9.0–10.0	17.0–22.5
Adult	12.0–13.0	22.0–23.5
Large adult	15.5	30.0
Adult thigh	18.0	36.0

Reprinted with permission from American Academy of Pediatrics. 1977. Report of the Task Force on Blood Pressure Control in Children. *Pediatrics.* **59**(Suppl.)**:**801.

*Dimensions may vary according to the manufacturer, although the cuff name is the same.

leaving a gap. A bladder that is at least one half the circumference of the arm and that is centered over the brachial artery will also work well. The bladder should be wide enough to cover two-thirds of the upper arm, leaving approximately 1 centimeter in the antecubital space for placement of the stethoscope. The blood pressure cuff sizes that are currently available for use are listed in Table 6-17. If the clinician is unsure of what cuff size to use, it is always best to select the largest cuff that will encircle the child's arm snugly without overlapping. A cuff that is too narrow for the child's arm will give a falsely high reading.

Technique.   A variety of methods to measure blood pressure in children have been developed. The method of choice in children and adolescents is auscultation, and in infants, it is the Doppler method. The technique of blood pressure measurement using auscultation and a mercury manometer is outlined below.

1. Apply the appropriate size cuff snugly to the child's upper arm.
2. Position the extremity so it is at heart level.
3. The mercury column should be at the examiner's eye level.
4. Palpate the radial artery for pulse.
5. Rapidly inflate the cuff to the point just above where the radial pulse disappears (this corresponds to a point approximately 30 mmHg above systolic pressure).
6. Deflate the cuff.
7. Palpate the brachial artery and place the stethoscope directly over the artery.
8. Rapidly reinflate the cuff to the approximate systolic level.
9. Deflate the cuff at a rate not greater than 2 to 3 mmHg/sec.
10. Auscultate over the brachial artery to detect Korotkoff sounds.

Steps 4 to 6 are not necessary to perform, but may be helpful in obtaining an approximation of systolic pressure in a hypertensive child.

The Korotkoff sounds are separated into five phases:

Phase 1: Corresponds to the distention of a previously collapsed vessel wall. Clear but often faint tapping sound.

Phase 2: Turbulent flow through a vessel. Sounds progress to a murmur.

Phase 3: Vessel closes for a brief time. Intensity of sounds increase as vessel reopens.

Phase 4: Sounds become muffled.

Phase 5: All sounds disappear.

Although the definition of systolic pressure is generally agreed upon, there is some controversy regarding whether diastolic pressure best corresponds to phase 4 or 5. The Task Force for Blood Pressure Control in Children has recommended that phase 1 define the systolic pressure and phase 4 the diastolic pressure.[34] Phase 4 and 5 may occur simultaneously in some children. Confusion may arise when there is inconsistency on the part of the nurse in using a specific phase (4 or 5) to identify diastolic pressure. If the nurse can clearly identify both phase 4 and 5 it is best to record both pressures. Other information that needs to be recorded is the position of the patient, the cuff size used, and the extremity used for blood pressure measurement. For example: "R arm, sitting, 9-cm child cuff, 120/82/60 (1/4/5)."

Doppler method. The Doppler method is often used to obtain reliable blood pressure measurements in acutely ill infants. This method is more accurate than auscultation in small infants because Korotkoff sounds are of lower frequency and more difficult to hear in the smaller child.

The Doppler method consists of a small electronic transmitting and receiving transducer, which may be either contained in the cuff or separate. This transducer is placed over the brachial artery. Ultrasound waves are then directed toward the vessel wall and are reflected back. The frequency of the reflected waves is amplified and transmitted through a loudspeaker or headphones. The systolic pressure is identified by the onset of high-frequency sounds. The sounds become muffled at the diastolic pressure. The Doppler method gives accurate and reliable systolic measurements, but may not consistently give accurate measurements of the diastolic pressure. The technique of obtaining blood pressure with a Doppler device is, therefore, quite similar to that previously described. The only difference between the Doppler method and the auscultation method is that a transducer, rather than a stethoscope, is used to hear Korotkoff sounds.

Flush method. This method has largely been replaced by the Doppler method for the measurement of blood pressure in infants. The nurse may encounter situations in which blood pressure cannot be obtained by the methods described above. The flush method may prove useful in these situations. A blood pressure cuff is applied in the normal fashion to the upper arm. The arm is elevated and an elastic bandage is wrapped around the arm distal to the cuff. When the hand becomes pale, the cuff is inflated. The elastic bandage is removed and the cuff is deflated slowly. The pressure is recorded at the point where the hand and forearm become pink. This level is approximately equal to the mean pressure. Normal values for the mean pressure by age using the flush method are available.[42]

Digital palpation. This method is rarely used. The technique is the same as described above except that no auscultation is performed. Instead, as the blood pressure cuff is deflated, the examiner palpates the brachial artery. The first point at which pulsations appear is the systolic pressure. The diastolic pressure is not identifiable with this method. A measurement is recorded, for example, as 120/p.

Interpretation of blood pressure measurements.   Graphs have been prepared by several investigators for blood pressure distributions in children.[34,37,43] The grids developed by the Task Force for Blood Pressure Control in Children depict blood pressure distributions for normal children and are often used as a rough guideline to assess blood pressure levels in individual children (*see* Fig. 6-24). These grids allow the clinician to compare blood pressure values in one child with the pressure range for normal children of the same age and sex. These blood pressure charts are intended for the longitudinal assessment of blood pressure rather than for the assessment of blood pressure at a single point in time. Although blood pressure does not necessarily follow percentile tracks in all chidlren, the annual measurement and recording of blood pressure in a child allows the clinician to observe a pattern over time, which can be quite important in the evaluation of hypertensive children.

The dividing line for separating children with increased blood pressure is somewhat arbitrary. In general, a blood presure reading (systolic or diastolic) that is greater than 2 standard deviations from the mean for the child's sex and age is considered abnormal. Although blood pressure measurements may persistently fall within 2 standard deviations of the mean for age and sex, a child may be considered hypertensive or at risk if other conditions (such as renal disease) coexist.

The critical care nurse clearly plays an important role in the assessment of the hypertensive child. Nurses have a shared responsibility to assess how different organ systems affect blood pressure. The nurse must also obtain accurate blood pressure measurements and observe how the daily blood pressure pattern relates to the child's activity, medication schedule, sleep patterns, interaction with family members, and emotional responses to various treatments and personnel.

Treatment of hypertension.   The goal of treatment in hypertension is to control the blood pressure within a normal range for the child's age. The patient being treated should experience a minimum of side effects. The treatment of hypertension in children is empirical. There is a lack of studies that investigate the effect of combined medication regimens on the treatment of hypertension in children. Information on the long-term effects of antihypertensive medications in the pediatric age group is also not available.

Treatment of hypertensive emergencies.   The goal of treatment in malignant hypertension is to decrease blood pressure to near normal levels and to avoid severe hypotension, which would cause a decrease in cerebral perfusion. The responsibilities of the nurse in the treatment of malignant hypertension include the measurement of blood pressure and the administration of antihypertensive medications. Treatment of hypertensive emergencies in children involves the use of vasodilating medications, namely diazoxide, hydralazine, and nitroprusside. The repeated use of these agents causes retention of sodium and water. A diuretic such as furosemide (Lasix) will often reverse this action, thereby enhancng the effectiveness of vasodilators. Both the vasodilators and diuretics are administered intravenously.

Diazoxide is the drug of choice in the initial treatment of children with severely elevated blood pressure. It should be administered rapidly (in less than 30 seconds) by the intravenous route at a dose of 5 mg/kg/dose.[40,44] The onset of action of diazoxide is rapid, and it should produce a decrease in blood pressure within 5 to 15 minutes. If no response is seen in 15 to 30 minutes, the dose may be increased by 25 to 50 percent and repeated. The effect of diazoxide may last anywhere from 4 to 24 hours. Children rarely experience hypotension when diazoxide is used.

Diazoxide produces a prompt reduction in blood pressure by relaxing smooth muscle in peripheral arterioles. Although children rarely experience hypotension secondary to diazoxide, caution must be exercised when it is given to children in combination with other drugs that act to produce vasodilation, since severe hypotension could result. After diazoxide is administered, the nurse must maintain the patient in a recumbent position and monitor blood pressure every 5 to 15 minutes until it stabilizes. Hourly measurements of blood pressure should then be taken. Since repeated doses of diazoxide may cause hyperglycemia and glycosuria, it is wise to routinely monitor plasma and urine concentrations of glucose.

Hydralazine is another antihypertensive drug that is commonly used in children for the management of hypertensive crises. The onset of action of parenterally administered hydralazine (15 minutes to 1 to 2 hours) is slower than diazoxide. At a dose of 0.2 mg/kg/dose, hydralazine is often effective in controlling moderate elevations of blood pressure in asymptomatic children.[45] The dosage can be increased by 50 to 100 percent and repeated every 3 to 4 hours if necessary.

As with diazoxide, hydralazine acts to decrease blood pressure by causing vasodilation of peripheral arterioles. In addition, hydralazine produces reflex tachycardia. Therefore, it is often administered in combination with a drug that inhibits sympathetic reflex stimuli (e.g., a beta-adrenergic blocker). Possible side effects of hydralazine include headache, palpitations, anorexia, nausea, vomiting, flushing, and postural hypotension. The nurse should warn the child and family that side effects may develop within a few hours after the first dose. Rapid changes in posture should be avoided, and patients should be instructed to lie down if they feel dizzy. Blood pressure is monitored closely every 2 minutes until stable, then hourly.

In addition, the nurse must observe the patient for signs and symptoms of decreased urinary output and edema that may develop secondary to excessive sodium and water retention caused by hydralazine and diazoxide. Accurate measurement of fluid intake and output is important in these patients. Furosemide at a dose of 2 to 10 mg/kg/dose is often given to patients who receive diazoxide and hydralazine, in an attempt to prevent the retention of excess sodium and water.

Children receiving intravenous hydralazine are often changed to the oral form within 24 to 48 hours after therapy is initiated, with titration of the dosage to a level where blood pressure is maintained within a normal range.

Sodium nitroprusside is reserved for the management of severe hypertension that is unsuccessfully controlled by the measures described above. This powerful antihypertensive drug must be dissolved in a 5 percent dextrose and water solution and administered by a carefully regulated continuous intravenous infusion. The duration of action of this drug is very short (seconds to minutes). Although the dose and rate of infusion must be titrated against the arterial blood pressure, a dose of 1 μg/kg/min is generally effective in decreasing and maintaining a normal blood pressure.

Because sodium nitroprusside causes a rapid decrease in arterial and central venous pressure, hemodynamic monitoring must be used in patients who receive this drug. There are several points the nurse must remember when caring for a child receiving nitroprusside. Since nitroprusside may be deactivated by light, the nurse should cover the infusion bottle and tubing with an opaque material. A new solution of nitroprusside should be mixed and hung every 24 hours and the old bottle discarded because of the instability of the drug. Nitroprusside should be administered by a constant infusion pump and via a separate intravenous line since it is incompatible with many drugs. An intravenous line that contains nitroprusside should never be flushed. If hypotension develops, the infusion should be stopped immediately. Plasma thiocyanate levels should be monitored since values greater than or equal to 10 mg/dl indicate toxicity and warrant reevaluation of the child.

Long-term treatment of hypertension in children. The present forms of treatment include diet, medications, and surgery. Attempts to control hypertension by restriction of salt and caloric intake are rarely successful in children when used alone. In many Western cultures (e.g., the United States), the daily dietary consumption of salt far exceeds the amount required for optimum health. The important contribution of sodium chloride to the development and maintenance of hypertension has long been emphasized. Thus, in all forms of hypertension it is wise to restrict the dietary intake of salt. A common medicinal method of treating hypertension in children is the "stepped care" approach. Each step in the treatment is begun with a low dose of a specfic medication. The dosage is increased to therapeutic levels. If after a certain period of time there is minimal or no response to the medication, a different medication is added and the old medication is either withdrawn slowly or continued. The stepped care approach is outlined below.

Step 1: Usually, therapy is initiated with a thiazide diuretic; although a potassium-sparing diuretic may be used.

Step 2: Initiated if diuretics do not give normal blood pressure with no side effects after 6 weeks to 3 months. Methyldopa or propranolol hydrochloride are added.

Step 3: If diuretics and propranolol or methyldopa are unsuccessful, a vasodilator (such as hydralazine hydrochloride) is added.

This approach of adding only one medication at a time allows the clinician to evaluate the effectiveness and side effects of each medication at different dosages.

Nearly all medications that are used for the treatment of hypertension affect the cardiovascular system, the adrenergic nerves, the renin-angiotensin system, and the volume-regulating systems of the body. These medications can be divided into three main categories: diuretics, autonomic nervous system medications, and vasodilators. These will be described briefly below. For additional information, the reader is referred to Table 6-18.

Diuretics. Diuretics are the mainstay of treatment for essential hypertension. They are also used as adjunctive agents in the treatment of children with secondary hypertension. Diuretics deplete the ECF volume by decreasing the reabsorption of salt and water from kidney tubules. Diuretics accomplish this by promoting excretion of sodium. Three groups of diuretics that are often used act at different sites in the kidneys; they are the thiazides, loop diuretics, and potassium-sparing diuretics (*see* Table 6-18). Diuretics may be effective in the control of mild hypertension. They may also be used in conjunction with other antihypertensive medications.

TABLE 6-18 Medications Used to Treat Hypertension

Drug class	Description of action	Indications for use	Precautions
Diuretics			
Thiazides and related diuretics Chlorothiazide Hydrochlorothiazide	Promote diuresis by decreasing rate at which sodium chloride is reabsorbed by the distal renal tubule. Also has antihypertensive effect, mechanism unknown. May potentiate effects of other antihypertensive drugs. Potassium excretion enhanced. Do not affect GFR.	Hypertension, edematous states (e.g., CHF, corticosteroid or estrogen therapy, nephrotic syndrome, acute GN, CRF).	Not effective in severe kidney decompensation when GFR is ≤50 ml/min/1.73 m². May cause hypokalemia. Use with caution in patients receiving other drugs that cause potassium loss. Check serum potassium level frequently.
Chlorthalidone	Diuretic with prolonged action. Differs chemically from thiazides. Increases excretion of sodium chloride by kidneys by acting on cortical-diluting segment of ascending limb of the loop of Henle. Can potentiate effects of adrenergic blocking agents.	Same as above.	Requires adequate renal functioning for initial effect. In large doses, can decrease blood pressure in patients with renal insufficiency.

Action time	Dosage	Side effects	Nursing implications
			General implications for all diuretics listed
Onset, 2 hr; peak, 6 hr; duration, 12 hr.	Oral tablets: 250 and 500 mg. Oral suspension: 250 mg/5 ml. Daily starting dose: 10 mg/kg. Daily maximum dose: 20 mg/kg.	Hypokalemia, hyperglycemia, hyperuricemia, hypercalcemia.	1. Weigh patient daily or bid on same scale, at the same time, and under standard conditions. 2. Maintain accurate intake and output records. 3. Examine patient for edema. This may shift, depending on the child's activity and position (e.g., sacrum, abdomen).
Onset, 2 hr; peak, 6 hr; duration, 12 hr.	Oral tablets: 25 and 50 mg. Daily starting dose: 1 mg/kg. Daily maximum dose: 2 mg/kg.		4. Observe for diuresis. Report absence of diuretic effect. 5. Explain to the child and/or family that diuretics may cause frequent urination of
Onset, 2 hr; duration, 24–72 hr.	Oral tablets: 25, 50, and 100 mg. Daily starting dose: 1 mg/kg. Daily maximum dose: 2 mg/kg.	Hypokalemia, hyponatremia, hypochloremic alkalosis.	large volumes. 6. Assist the child to bathroom as needed. Make sure urinal is within reach. 7. If diuretic given once a day, administer in morning so that main diuretic effect occurs before bedtime. 8. Observe the child for signs and symptoms of fluid and electrolyte imbalances: dehydration, hypokalemia, metabolic acidosis/alkalosis. 9. Observe children receiving other antihypertensive agents for hypotension because some diuretics will potentiate their effect. Caution patients to change body position slowly. 10. If supplemental potassium is needed, encourage dietary sources with high potassium content. 11. Observe children receiving digitalis for signs of digoxin toxicity because potassium disorders may potentiate the effects of digoxin. 12. Use caution in patients losing fluid through gastric suctioning, vomiting, high fever, diarrhea.

TABLE 6-18 (Continued)

Drug class	Description of action	Indications for use	Precautions
Diuretics			
Spironolactone	Diuretic and potassium-sparing agent. A steroid compound that blocks the sodium-retaining effects of aldosterone. Excretion of sodium and water promoted, while excessive loss of potassium prevented. Works in distal tubule of kidney. Diuretic and antihypertensive effect.	Hypertension. Used alone or with other diuretics in the treatment of edematous states.	Not for use in patients with acute renal failure, anuria, or significant renal impairment or hyperkalemia. Avoid concomitant use of potassium supplements. Watch for signs of hyperkalemia.
Metolazone	A potent diuretic and antihypertensive drug that interferes with renal tubular electrolyte reabsorptive mechanisms. Inhibits sodium reabsorption at proximal tubule and cortical-diluting site. Increases distal delivery of sodium and may promote potassium excretion.	Used alone or with other diuretic and antihypertensive drugs. Edematous states. May need to decrease dose of other antihypertensive drugs.	Not for use in patients with anuria or hepatic coma. Observe for fluid and electrolyte imbalances. Use with caution in patients with renal failure.
Loop diuretics Furosemide	Diuretic that inhibits reabsorption of sodium chloride in the loop of Henle. Potassium and bicarbonate excreted in smaller proportions. Antihypertensive effect. Potentiates effects of other antihypertensive drugs.	May be effective for patients resistant to thiazides or those with a decreased GFR. Can use with potassium-sparing diuretics. Edematous states. Can use alone or with other antihypertensive drugs in the treatment of hypertension.	Not for use in anuric children. Use with caution in patients receiving sodium-depleting steroids or digitalis glycosides.
Autonomic nervous system agents			
Propranolol hydrochloride	A nonselective beta-adrenergic blocking agent. The chronotropic, inotropic, and vasodilator responses to beta-adrenergic stimulation are decreased. Results in decreased cardiac output, heart rate, and blood pressure. Causes constriction of bronchioles. Mechanism of antihypertensive effect unknown.	Hypertension. Often used with a thiazide diuretic.	Do not use in children with bronchial asthma, allergic rhinitis, sinus bradycardia or heart block greater than first degree, CHF, cardiogenic shock, and right ventricular failure secondary to pulmonary HTN. May block ability of heart to respond to reflex stimuli. Can prevent premonitory signs of hypoglycemia.

Action time	Dosage	Side effects	Nursing implications
Onset, gradual with maximum diuresis in 3 days.	Oral tablets: 25 mg. Daily starting dose: 2 mg/kg. Daily maximum dose: 4 mg/kg.	Hyperkalemia.	**Specific Implications** No supplemental potassium needed.
Onset, 1 hr; peak 2–3 hr; duration, 12–24 hr.	Oral tablets: 2.5, 5.0, and 10.0 mg. Daily starting dose: 0.1 mg/ kg. Daily maximum dose for children not established.	Hypokalemia, azotemia, hyperuricemia, hypochloremia, hyperglycemia, increased BUN and creatinine.	
PO: onset, 1 hr; peak, 1–2 hr; duration, 4–8 hr. IM or IV: onset, 5 min; peak, 30 min; duration, 2 hr.	Oral tablets: 20, 40, and 80 mg. Daily starting dose: 0.5–1.0 mg/kg. Daily maximum dose not established, but is approximately 8 mg/kg. 2-, 4-, and 10-ml ampules: 1 ml = 10 mg.		1. Monitor blood pressure closely. 2. Observe child with rapid diuresis for dehydration, circulatory collapse, pulmonary embolism. 3. Monitor for signs of ototoxicity, particularly if the patient has renal impairment or is receiving ototoxic drugs.
Onset, 2 hr.	Oral tablets: 10, 20, 40, and 80 mg. Daily starting dose: 1 mg/kg. Daily maximum dose: 4–6 mg/ kg.	None.	Observe the child for untoward effects on the cardiovascular system (bradycardia, symptoms of CHF).

TABLE 6-18 (Continued)

Drug class	Description of action	Indications for use	Precautions
Autonomic nervous system agents			
Methyldopa	Unique antihypertensive drug. Mechanism of action probably metabolism of drug to α-methylnorepinephrine, which lowers blood pressure by stimulation of central inhibitory α-adrenergic receptors. Reduces cardiac output and peripheral resistance. Blood pressure lower in upright than supine position.	Hypertension. Useful in patients with impaired renal functioning, renal hypertension, and resistant forms of hypertension.	None.
Clonidine hydrochloride	A central alpha-adrenergic stimulant. Result of action is inhibition of bulbar sympathetic cardioaccelerator and sympathetic vasoconstrictor centers. Sympathetic outflow from brain decreased. Initially a peripheral vasoconstriction. Heart rate decreases. Cardiac output decreases. Effect enhanced when administered with a diuretic. Tolerance may develop in some patients.	Hypertension.	Reduce dose over 2–4 day to prevent possible increase in blood pressure if drug is withdrawn rapidly (due to release of catecholamines).
Metroprolol tartrate	A selective beta-adrenergic receptor blocking agent. Affects primarily bronchiolar and vascular musculature. Results in decreased heart rate, decreased cardiac output, decreased blood pressure, bronchial dilation, decreased reflex orthostatic tachycardia. Mechanism of antihypertensive effect unknown.	Hypertension.	Not for use in patients with overt heart failure, or severely impaired renal or liver functioning. Use with caution in patients with ischemic heart disease, sinus bradycardia, and heart degree greater than first degree. Can slow AV conduction.

Action time	Dosage	Side effects	Nursing implications
Onset, 2 hr.	Daily starting dose: 10 mg/kg. Daily maximum dose: 40 mg/kg.	GI cramps, constipation.	Observe the child for retention of sodium and water (edema). Caution the child to rise from supine to standing position slowly. May experience dizziness and faintness. Drowsiness may occur. Urine may turn darker color than normal if exposed to open air for any length of time.
Onset, 30–60 min; peak, 2–4 hr; duration, 6–8 hr.	Oral tablets: 0.1, 0.2, and 0.3 mg. Daily maximum dose: 0.1 mg/day.	Sedation can enhance the depressive effects of alcohol and barbiturates. Dry mouth, drowsiness, headache, fatigue, all common.	Monitor blood pressure closely after initial dose because blood pressure decrease occurs within 30–60 min. Observe the child in first week of therapy for retention of salt and water. Note daily blood pressure pattern. Drug should not be withdrawn abruptly because rebound hypertension can occur.
Onset, 1 hr; duration, dose-related.	Oral tablets: 50 and 100 mg. Daily starting dose: 0.50–0.75 mg/kg. Daily maximum dose: not established.	Fatigue, dizziness, shortness of breath, bradycardia, wheezing.	Observe for symptoms of CHF. May become drowsy. In children with diabetes, observe for signs of hypoglycemia, because symptoms can be masked. Observe for signs of disorientation, behavioral changes, and sensory impairment.

TABLE 6-18 (Continued)

Drug class	Description of action	Indications for use	Precautions
Autonomic nervous system agents			
Prazosin hydrochloride	An α_2-stimulator. Causes a decrease in total peripheral vascular resistance. Unlike conventional alpha-blockers, the antihypertensive action of this drug is not accompanied by reflex tachycardia. Blood pressure lowered in supine and standing positions. Used alone or with other antihypertensives. Effect enhanced with a diuretic and a beta-blocker.	Mild to moderate hypertension.	May cause syncope with sudden loss of consciousness; may be preceded by tachycardia. Syncope may occur within 30–90 min of initial dose. Not always associated with postural hypotension. Headache, nausea, and palpitations may occur.
Vasodilators			
Diazoxide	Rapid acting. Produces prompt reduction in blood pressure by direct relaxation of smooth muscle in peripheral arterioles. Cardiac output increased. Coronary and cerebral blood flow maintained. Renal blood flow decreases as well as GFR and urine output. Used with a diuretic for chronic use.	Malignant hypertension. Emergency reduction of blood pressure required.	Use cautiously in patients receiving drugs that act by producing vasodilation. Severe hypotension may occur.
Hydralazine hydrochloride	As above. Produces myocardial stimulation. Reflex tachycardia. Should administer with drugs that inhibit sympathetic reflex symptoms (a beta-blocker).	Hypertensive emergencies. Essential hypertension when diuretics insufficient to control blood pressure.	Not for use in patients with coronary artery disease or rheumatic heart disease. Use with caution when used in combination with other potent antihypertensive drugs.

Action time	Dosage	Side effects	Nursing implications
Peak, 3 hr.	Capsules: 1 and 5 mg. Daily starting dose: 0.5–1.0 mg tid. Maximum pediatric daily dose: not established.	Dizziness, drowsiness.	Sympathomimetic drugs administered concomitantly may interfere with action of drug. Administer initial dose in evening or keep the child in a supine position for approximately 1 hr after initial dose, because syncope may occur without warning. Have the child avoid rapid postural changes until he has been on the drug for 1–2 days.
IV: onset is immediate; peak, 30 sec; duration, 4–12 hr.	20-ml ampules: 20 ml = 300 mg. Dose: 3–5 mg/kg rapidly. Can repeat at 15-min intervals. Maximum single dose: 300 mg.	In chronic use, hyperglycemia can occur. Sodium and water retention. Hyperuricemia.	After drug administration, monitor blood pressure frequently until it stabilizes, then measure every hour. Maintain the patient in recumbent position after the drug is administered. Monitor urine for glucose content while the child is on chronic therapy.
IV: onset, 30–40 min.	Oral tablets: 10, 25, 50, and 100 mg. IV ampules: 1 ml = 20 mg. Daily starting dose: 0.75–1.50 mg/kg PO, and 0.1–0.2 mg/kg IV. Daily maximum dose: 5–6 mg/kg PO.	Headache, palpitations, anorexia, nausea, vomiting, tachycardia, diarrhea, angina pectoris, flushing, nasal congestion, postural hypotension.	Warn the patient and family that side effects may occur after the first dose (headache, nausea, vomiting). Monitor blood pressure within 5 min after injection until stable. Observe for decreased urine output and edema.

TABLE 6-18 (Continued)

Drug class	Description of action	Indications for use	Precautions
Vasodilators			
Minoxidil	Potent antihypertensive agent that decreases total peripheral resistance to cause vasodilation. Reflex sympathetic phenomena include, increased cardiac output, increased heart rate, salt and water retention secondary to increased renin release. Use a diuretic and beta-blocking agent concomitantly.	Severe refractory hypertension that is symptomatic or associated with target organ damage and is not manageable with maximum doses of a diuretic plus two other antihypertensive drugs.	Adverse reactions include hypertrichosis, severe sodium retention, and reflex tachycardia.
Sodium nitroprusside	Powerful antihypertensive agent. Effect almost immediate and ends when infusion stops. Causes a rapid fall in arterial and central venous pressures. Moderate increase in heart rate.	Hypertensive emergencies.	Acute toxicity is secondary to excessive vasodilation and hypotension. Thiocyanate may accumulate in plasma with long-term use (greater than 96 hr). Must continually monitor blood pressure.

Adapted from Physicians' Desk Reference. 1981. Medical Economics Co., Oradell, N. J.; and S. Loebl, G. Spratto, and E. Heckheimer. 1980. The Nurse's Drug Handbook. John Wiley & Sons, Inc., New York. Second edition.

AV, atrioventricular; bid, twice per day; CHF, congestive heart failure; CRF, chronic renal failure; D5W, 5 percent dextrose in water; GFR, glomerular filtration rate; GI, gastrointestinal; GN, glomerulonephritis; tid, three times per day.

Autonomic nervous system agents. This group of medications exerts its antihypertensive effects by acting on the central nervous system or on peripheral adrenergic receptors. In general, the mechanisms of action of these various medications are not well understood. Treatment is often initiated with either propranolol or methyldopa if diuretics fail to produce an acceptable decrease in blood pressure in the hypertensive individual.

Vasodilators. Vasodilators are often used alone in hypertensive emergencies or in conjunction with a diuretic and autonomic nervous system agent to control

Action time	Dosage	Side effects	Nursing implications
Onset, 30 min; peak, 2–3 hr; duration, 72 hr.	Oral tablets: 2.5 and 10.0 mg. Daily starting dose: 0.2–0.5 mg/kg. Daily maximum dose: 1–2 mg/kg.	Sodium and water retention.	Administer under close supervision. All patients develop hypertrichosis, assist the family and child in the resolution of feelings regarding this. This will disappear within 3–6 mo after drug is discontinued. Hair removal products may be useful.
Onset, immediate.	IV vial: 5 ml = 50 mg. Infuse with D5W at rate of 0.5–8.0 µg/kg/min.	None.	Continuous intra-arterial blood pressure monitoring necessary to safely administer this potent vasodilator. Dosage is calculated and regulated in µg/kg/min and must be provided by continuous intravenous infusion via a mechanical pump. Nitroprusside is unstable in combination with most other drugs and must be delivered via a separate IV line. May be deactivated by light, therefore the infusion bottle and tubing should be protected from the light by an opaque covering. In addition, the solution should be discarded and a new solution mixed at least every 24 hr. If hypotension occurs, stop the infusion immediately. An IV line containing nitroprusside should never be flushed.

chronic hypertension. Vasodilators act directly on arteriolar smooth muscle to cause relaxation. This results in a decrease in total peripheral resistance and a decrease in blood pressure.

Guidelines for nursing management of the hypertensive child. A nursing care plan for the hypertensive child in the ICU should contain short- and long-term goals. Although hypertension often resolves if it develops secondary to an acute illness, it can recur as a long-term complication of an illness that is long past the acute phase (e.g., hemolytic uremic syndrome and poststreptococcal glomerulonephritis). The parameters that need to be monitored by the nurse include cardiovascular status (blood pressure, apical pulse, peripheral circulation, left ventricular functioning; renal-fluid status (including intake and output, skin turgor, presence of edema); respiratory status (quality and rate of respirations); and neurological signs of hypertensive encephalopathy, which include headache, convulsions, and blurred vision (*see* p. 368).

In a child with secondary hypertension, different symptoms would be expected to be present, depending on the disease causing the hypertension. The systems affected by the disease will characterize the symptoms displayed by the child.

Other information that is important to document includes the action and side effects of the antihypertensive medications that the child is receiving, dietary intake, activity level, the child's response to illness and hospitalization, the family's response to the child's illness, and the symptoms the child exhibits with an increase in blood pressure.

The care plan should also address the educational needs of the child and family regarding what high blood pressure is, what factors are known to increase blood pressure, medications, diet, and activity. Plans for family participation in the child's care need to be individualized. Family members can contribute in a positive manner to the child's care by providing the child with a sense of security and by creating a calm atmosphere for the child. Parents are often anxious to participate in activities such as feeding, bathing, and playing with the child; rocking them to sleep or reading to them; and explaining procedures and situations to them. The nurse should determine with the family what activities they would like to assist with, and then plan the child's daily schedule to incorporate their requests as much as is realistically possible.

ACUTE RENAL FAILURE

Children and adolescents who require intensive medical and nursing care are at high risk for the development of acute renal failure (ARF). The complex medical and surgical conditions that exist in these children predispose them to a variety of cardiovascular, respiratory, neurological, and infectious complications that can affect kidney functioning. Although there are different forms of ARF, this section of the chapter will deal primarily with one form: acute tubular necrosis (ATN). Other forms of ARF will be described as they relate to the differential diagnosis of ATN. The etiology, pathogenesis, history, and clinical course of ATN will be described. The hemolytic-uremic syndrome, a clinical disorder that is often characterized by ARF, will be reviewed later in this chapter. The role of the nurse in the critical care management of children with ARF and hemolytic-uremic syndrome will be described as it pertains to both the conservative medical management and the use of dialytic therapy.

In infants and children, ARF is a clinical syndrome characterized by a sudden deterioration in renal functioning that results in abnormalities in body homeostasis. The acute change may occur in previously normal kidneys or may be superimposed upon previously damaged kidneys. ARF may be accompanied by a reduced, normal, or high urine flow; although in the majority of cases (90 percent) of children over 1 year of age, there is a decreased urine volume and increased solute retention.

There are a number of terms defined below that are important for the nurse to understand before beginning this section.

1. *Oliguria:* A somewhat arbitrary term wherein a patient excretes less than the minimum volume of maximally concentrated urine that would have to be excreted in a given period of time to maintain osmotic balance. The usual frame of reference is 300 ml/m^2 of body surface area per 24 hr or 0.75 to 1.0 ml/kg/hr.

2. *Anuria:* A urine output of less than 50 to 100 ml/24 hr.

3. *Polyuria:* A urine output of greater than 1,000 to 2,000 ml/24 hr or more than 1,500 ml/m^2.

4. *Nephrotoxin:* A specific toxin that destroys renal cells.

5. *Azotemia:* Refers to an elevated value of BUN. A value of 20 mg/dl is abnormal for older infants, and 50 to 60 mg/dl is abnormal for older children.

6. *Uremia:* Refers to the clinical symptoms associated with ARF and CRF. The syndrome involves multiple body systems. Some clinical symptoms associated with azotemia include nausea, vomiting, GI bleeding, confusion, and disorientation.

Pathophysiology

A basic understanding of the pathophysiology of ARF will provide the nurse with information and a rationale for developing patient management strategies and identifying nursing interventions that are effective in children with acute renal disorders.

Etiology. The causes of ARF in children include the clinical entities listed in Table 6-19. This list includes prerenal (preglomerular), postrenal, and renal (vascular, glomerular, interstitial, and tubular) causes of ARF in pediatric practice. There are three forms of renal failure: prerenal, renal, and postrenal. Prerenal and postrenal failure will be discussed only as they relate to the differential diagnosis of the renal type of ARF. The focus of this section will, therefore, be a detailed description of the renal form of ARF, more commonly referred to as acute tubular necrosis (ATN). In the child who presents with oliguria and/or azotemia, it is of paramount importance to rapidly assess the presence of treatable lesions. Prompt differentiation of ATN from other reversible forms of ARF may allow sufficient time to institute corrective measures in order to prevent the development of ATN and the accompanying potential morbidity and mortality. The pre- and postrenal forms of ARF will be described before the differential diagnosis of ATN is detailed.

The prerenal form of ARF develops as the result of (1) a decrease in the ECF volume, or (2) a decrease in the effective circulating volume. Extrarenal loss of water and electrolytes can be caused by diarrhea, vomiting, nasogastric suctioning, or sweating. A decrease in the effective circulating volume or the intravascular volume can result from loss of water and electrolytes into a third space (as in congestive heart failure) or from hemorrhage. Hypovolemia and circulatory insufficiency then lead to reduced renal perfusion. The body responds by activating the renin-angiotensin-aldosterone system, thereby increasing the reabsorption of sodium and water from kidney tubules. As a result of the decrease in RBF and GFR, there is a decrease in the filtered load and an increase in the fraction of glomerular filtrate (largely sodium, water, urea) reabsorbed in the nephron. The combination of oliguria and solute retention that now develops is referred to as prerenal azotemia. The extent of oliguria depends primarily on the water required for obligatory solute excretion. If renal perfusion is reduced over a period of time,

TABLE 6-19 Causes of Acute Renal Failure in Pediatric Practice

1. *Glomerulonephritis (especially necrotizing, proliferative, membranoproliferative, rapidly progressive):*
   Streptococcus* and other bacteria, viruses, lupus erythematosus, Wegener's granulomatosis, eclampsia
2. *Vascular and thrombotic disease:*
   Malignant hypertension, Wegener's granulomatosis, hypersensitivity angiitis, periarteritis nodosa, thrombotic thrombocytopenic purpura, hemolytic-uremic syndrome,* Shwartzman reaction (cortical necrosis),* collagenosis, scleroderma, acute allograft rejection, fat embolism, renal venous*-vena caval thrombosis, post-traumatic arterial thrombosis or avulsion, aortic coarctation with arterial thrombosis, renal artery dysplasia
3. *Interstitial disease:*
   Allergic, postinfectious, and idiosyncratic interstitial nephritis, fulminating pyelonephritis, papillary necrosis
4. *Functional renal failure ("prerenal" renal failure):*
   Severe volume depletion,* shock,* sepsis,* trauma,* heart failure
5. *Vasomotor nephropathy (acute tubular necrosis, acute renal failure):*
   All causes of functional renal failure (e.g., nephrotic syndrome, hemorrhage, vomiting, diarrhea, hypotension) if not adequately treated;* blunt trauma, burns, surgery, fractures, intravascular hemolysis, heat-stroke, malaria, snake bite, electric shock, dissecting aneurysm (e.g., Marfan's, homocystinuria), septicemia, rhabdomyolysis; poisons,* especially antibiotics, mercury, bismuth, phosphorus, lead, carbon tetrachloride, ethylene, glycol, methanol, mushrooms, Lysol, methoxyflurane, other poisons are rare.
6. *Hepatorenal syndrome*
7. *Urinary obstruction:*
   Ureter, bladder, or urethra, including inflammation stone, blood clot, urate crystallization, tumor, retroperitoneal mass or fibrosis

Reprinted with permission from Oken, D. E. 1978. Clinical aspects of acute renal failure (vasomotor nephropathy). *In* Edelmann, C. M., editor. 1978. *Pediatric Kidney Disease.* Little, Brown & Co., Boston. 1110
* Common cases in children.

constriction of renal vessels may result in a selective reduction in blood flow to the superficial cortex of the kidney and severe ischemia. The prerenal form of ARF may be reversed if the cause of renal ischemia is corrected before renal cell damage occurs. Reversal may be accomplished with restoration of depleted ECF volume and/or the effective circulating blood volume. This should increase renal perfusion and the filtration and reabsorption functions of the kidney to normal.

One method that is often used to aid in the differentiation of the prerenal form of ARF from other types is a fluid challenge. This usually consists of administering a 0.9 percent saline solution intravenously to the patient at 10 to 20 ml/kg body weight over 20 to 60 minutes. The goal is to restore depleted body fluids and to reestablish urine flow. A positive response is considered to be a urine output of 6 to 10 ml/kg/hr within 1 to 2 hours. The fluid challenge may be repeated, depending on the urine output response and the characteristics of the urine. Failure to respond to a fluid challenge may mean that ATN is present. A fluid challenge is contraindicated in patients with congestive heart failure, severe hypertension, edema secondary to sodium retention, or respiratory compromise. The fluid challenge may be followed by the administration of a diuretic (furosemide, 1 to 3 mg/kg intravenously). It is important for the first voided urine specimen (before the

TABLE 6-20   Laboratory Values That Aid in the Differentiation of Prerenal Oliguria and Acute Tubular Necrosis

Value	Prerenal oliguria	Complete renal failure (ATN)
Specific gravity	≥1.015–1.020	1.010
U_{Na}, mEq/liter	<10	>40
U_{osm}, mOsm/kg H_2O	>500	<350
U_{osm}/P_{osm}	>1.5	<1.0
FE_{Na}	<1	>1
U_{urea}/P_{urea}	>20:1	<10:1
U_{cr}/P_{cr}	>40:1	<15:1
$U_{Na}/(U_{cr}/P_{cr})$	<1	>5
BUN/P_{cr}	>20:1	10:1

ATN, acute tubular necrosis; BUN, blood urea nitrogen; FE_{Na}, fractional excretion of sodium; P_{cr}, plasma concentration of creatinine; P_{osm}, plasma osmolality; P_{urea}, plasma concentration of urea; U_{cr}, urine concentration of creatinine; U_{Na}, urine concentration of sodium; U_{osm}, urine osmolality; U_{urea}, urine concentration of urea.

administration of a diuretic) to be saved because, once diuretics are administered, the significance of urine characteristics is greatly reduced.

Urinary laboratory values are important in the differentiation between prerenal ARF and ATN (Table 6-20). The fractional excretion of sodium provides a reliable means of differentiating reversible, prerenal azotemia from ATN. It has been suggested to be the most effective noninvasive test for a differential diagnosis of ARF. The fractional excretion of sodium is calculated in the following manner:

$$FE_{Na} = \frac{U_{Na}/P_{Na}}{U_{cr}/P_{cr}} \times 100,$$

where FE_{Na} is the fractional excretion of sodium — a measure of tubular sodium ion reabsorption, U_{Na} is the urine concentration of sodium (in mEq/liter), P_{Na} is the plasma concentration of sodium (in mg/dl), U_{cr} is the urine concentration of creatinine (in mg/dl), and P_{cr} is the plasma concentration of creatinine (in mg/dl). Since there is no volume component in the formula for the fractional excretion of sodium, the clinician can use either a spot urine sample or an incomplete collection.

Under normal circumstances, the fractional excretion is approximately equal to 1. A fractional excretion of sodium of much greater than 1 is suggestive of ATN, nonoliguric ATN, and urinary tract obstruction in which sodium ions are not reabsorbed by the kidney tubules in the normal fashion. A value of much less than 1 is found, for example, in patients with prerenal azotemia and certain forms of acute glomerulonephritis, in which tubular functions are intact. Calculation of the fractional excretion of sodium is, therefore, a valuable test for early evaluation of ARF and identification of its cause. This enables prompt institution of corrective measures in potentially reversible disorders, such as prerenal azotemia.

A careful history and physical examination often reveal information that aids in the differentiation of prerenal azotemia from ATN. For example, questions like, What is the history of fluid and solute intake over the last few days?, What has been the duration of oliguria?, Has the child ingested or been exposed to a nephrotoxic agent?, and Is there reason to suspect decreased cardiac functioning or adrenal insufficiency?, may provide the clinician with important clues. The physical examination will provide objective data that may help pinpoint the etiology of ARF. Once a diagnosis of prerenal azotemia is established, steps should be taken to correct the systemic cause of renal ischemia, systemic hypotension, and hypovolemia, and to improve cardiac functioning in the hope of increasing urine output and improving renal functioning.

The postrenal form of ARF is a condition that is caused by an obstruction to urine flow distal to the kidney tubules. An obstruction can occur at any point in the urinary tract or bladder, and may, for example, be a congenital obstruction or a calculus. An abrupt decrease or cessation in urine flow occurs with postrenal obstruction. The child with obstruction may have a history of intermittent anuria alternating with widely fluctuating rates of urine output, or difficulty initiating and terminating the urinary stream. Normal renal functioning can be restored if the cause of obstruction is removed. Chronic obstruction in a child can lead to irreversible renal parenchymal damage.

History

ATN is a clinical syndrome that encompasses several different disease entities. The two primary pathogenic events that initiate renal damage are acute ischemic injury and acute nephrotoxic injury. Although ATN has characteristic features and follows a fairly well-defined course, it continues to pose a serious threat to life in the pediatric patient.

Adverse reactions to antibiotics (e.g., gentamicin, neomycin), blood transfusion reactions, and the accidental exposure to or ingestion of toxic substances (e.g., carbon tetrachloride, chlorodane paraquat) are common etiologic events that may cause a pediatric patient to develop acute nephrotoxic renal failure or ATN. Nephrotoxic injury occurs after exposure of renal cells to a variety of substances that include heavy metals, drugs, and organic solvents. The kidneys possess certain characteristics that make them vulnerable to damage from toxic substances. These characteristics include (1) renal parenchyma exposed to a high proportion of toxins because of the large blood flow, (2) the resorption of water along nephrons leaves high concentrations of toxins in the tubules, (3) the countercurrent mechanism results in high concentrations of certan toxins in the interstitium, and (4) the proximal tubules reabsorb high-molecular-weight substances. The renal cells most often affected by toxins are those of the proximal tubules. The lesion that results is referred to as nephrotoxic tubular necrosis. Even though necrosis may occur, regeneration of tubular epithelial cells is possible if the tubular basement membrane remains intact.

Shock, hemolysis, infection, and dehydration are examples of disorders that often lead to the development of acute ischemic renal failure or ATN in the pediatric ICU patient. The disordered fibrinolytic activity (intravascular coagulation) that results from these conditions affects renal cells by causing hypoxia and ischemia. ATN is a consequence of the ischemia when the insult is of mild to moderate severity, but bilateral cortical necrosis may occur if ischemia is prolonged (Fig. 6-25).[46] The pathological lesion that results from intense renal ischemia is referred to as tubulorrhexis — widespread and random necrosis in scattered portions of the renal tubule. If destruction of the basement membrane occurs with ischemic injury to renal cells, epithelial regeneration is patchy.[47] The prognosis for the child with ischemic ATN is, therefore, dependent on the extent of tubulorrhexic necrosis.

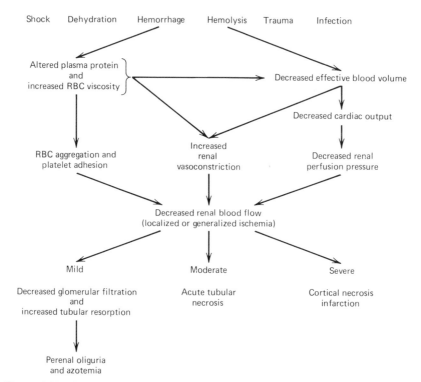

Figure 6-25.   Role of renal ischemia in the pathogenesis of prerenal azotemia and acute renal failure. RBC, red blood cell. *Reprinted with permission from* Franklin, S. S., and M. H. Maxwell. 1980. Acute renal failure. In Maxwell, M. H., and C. R. Kleeman, editors. 1980. Clinical Disorders of Fluid and Electrolyte Metabolism. McGraw-Hill Book Co., New York. Third edition. 748.

The pathogenesis of oliguria in ARF remains an enigma. The fundamental disturbance in ATN is a severe reduction in the amount of plasma being filtered at the glomerulus. The mechanisms that lead to a decrease in the GFR after renal cell injury have yet to be clearly defined. The following theories have been proposed to explain diminished GFR and oliguria:

1. Intratubular obstruction from casts and cellular debris sloughed from damaged tubular epithelial cells. Tubular obstruction results in increased tubular hydrostatic pressure that opposes glomerular filtration pressure and results in a secondary decrease in the GFR.
2. Passive back diffusion of filtrate out of tubular lumen and through damaged tubular epithelium into renal interstitium.
3. Selective reduction in blood flow to the superficial cortex of kidney (mechanism not defined), results in a change in glomerular arteriolar resistances and a

primary decrease in GFR. Renal cortical blood flow of patients with ARF is reduced by 50 to 70 percent.[48]

4. Damage to tubular epithelium reduces the amount of sodium chloride reabsorbed. An increased amount of sodium chloride is then delivered to the distal nephron, causing increased amounts of renin and angiotensin II to be released.

Although tubular obstruction augments renal insufficiency, it is not currently believed to play a major role in the pathogenesis of oliguria. Hemodynamic alterations appear to hold the most promising explanation of the mechanisms involved in the development of oliguric ATN. From the evidence currently available, it is concluded that the oliguria that accompanies ATN probably results from several different mechanisms. The relative contribution of each mechanism varies with the situation and is highly dependent on the severity of the initial insult as well as the course of the disease process.

Clinical Presentation

Children with ATN often present with an abrupt onset of azotemia and oliguria. Although in most cases of ATN there is prior documentation of normal renal functioning, children with chronic renal failure can develop ARF. There are three phases that characterize the clinical course of ATN: oliguria, diuresis, and recovery.

Oliguric phase. The onset of the oliguric phase may immediately follow exposure to a nephrotoxic agent or an ischemic event, or it may develop several days after renal cell damage of unknown etiology occurs. This phase is most often characterized by an abrupt reduction in urine output that continues over 24 to 48 hours. Although severe oliguria may last from 1 day to 8 weeks, the average duration is 7 to 14 days.[49] During the oliguric phase, the BUN rises approximately 10 to 20 mg/100 ml/24 hr, and the serum creatinine increases 0.5 to 1.0 mg/100 ml/24 hr. If the catabolic rate is high, the BUN will increase more rapidly (25 to 35 mg/100 ml/24 hr). The normal BUN:creatinine ratio is 10:1. A much higher ratio suggests either catabolism or prerenal azotemia. Potential complications that the nurse must be aware of during this phase include congestive heart failure and/or pulmonary edema secondary to volume overload; hyperkalemia; a decrease in the hematocrit and hemoglobin values; and metabolic acidosis. The critical care management of hyperkalemia and metabolic acidosis in ARF are discussed later in this chapter.

Diuretic phase. The diuretic phase can be divided into early diuresis and late diuresis. The mechanism of diuresis is presently unknown. The early diuretic phase is characterized by an initial abrupt increase in urine volume. There continues to be a gradual stepwise increase in urine volume over the next several days. During this early phase, which lasts only 4 to 7 days, it is not unusual for the BUN level to continue to rise. The increase is due to depressed glomerular filtration and a urea clearance that does not keep pace with endogenous urea production. The late diuretic phase is marked by the initial decrease in BUN and the eventual disappearance of azotemia. Because glomerular functioning (filtration) is the first mechanism to recover, extremely large volumes of urine that are rich in electrolytes (especially sodium and potassium ions) are often responsible for fluid and electrolyte disturbances during this phase. The nurse must monitor the child for clinical signs and symptoms of dehydration, hypovolemia, and electrolyte imbalances (*see* p. 337). Tubular functioning (reabsorption) returns next and contributes significantly to the overall improvement in renal functioning.

Recovery phase.   The recovery phase usually lasts 2 to 3 months, although for some children, a convalescent period of up to 1 year is necessary before normal renal functioning exists and full activity resumes. The BUN and urine laboratory values return to normal during this phase. For the most part, patients regain full renal functioning, but there are some who are left with relatively benign residual damage, such as a permanent decrease in renal functioning or a urine concentrating defect. The nurse must continue to closely monitor the child with ARF during the recovery phase. The principal causes of death during this period are infection and complications of the primary illness that was present when ARF developed.

Children with ARF have the potential to develop serious physiological complications. The disturbances that frequently occur secondary to AFR include hypervolemia, hyperkalemia, hypocalcemia, hyperphosphatemia, hypermagnesemia, azotemia, anemia, hematologic abnormalities, infection, metabolic acidosis, and neurological and nutritional complications.

Critical Care Management

The goal of treatment for the child with ARF is to reestablish normal urine flow. Until normal urine flow resumes, it is important to maintain a physiologically balanced internal environment. The two broad categories of treatment are conservative medical management and dialytic therapy. Nurses play a crucial role in management of the child with ARF. Because of their close contact with these critically ill children, nurses are in the best position to observe subtle changes in patient status. Signs and symptoms may be observed sufficiently early to permit reversal of prerenal ARF. Nursing observations will provide early detection of the complications of ARF or its treatment and permit rapid intervention when necessary.

Knowledge of the specific clinical settings associated with the development of ATN (e.g., diagnostic radiology, surgical procedures, transfusion reactions) and recognition of children who are at high risk for developing this condition are both important factors in the prevention of ATN. For example, inadequate tissue perfusion resulting from a decreased plasma volume and cardiac insufficiency is a hallmark of ATN. Therefore, the preventative plan should include measures that will ensure an adequate circulating blood volume, cardiac output, RBF, and urinary volume.

Fluid management.   In children with oliguric ATN, iatrogenic and physiological events will result in the retention of a large amount of excess body water. The sources of water intake in an acutely ill person under stress are (1) oral, intravenous, and/or nasogastric fluids, (2) water of oxidation formed from metabolism of fat and protein, and (3) water released from cells during catabolism. Water is lost through the skin, lungs, urine, GI tract, and other routes (e.g., vomiting or nasogastric suctioning). In the presence of excess body water, dilutional hyponatremia and hypochloremia may exist. Hypervolemia is most often treated by restricting fluid intake. The amount of fluid intake allowed each day is determined by estimating intake and output and obtaining serial body weights. The following equation is used to approximate the daily exogenous fluid intake allowance. The amount of fluid intake allowed (IA) is equal to the insensible water loss (IWL) plus the urine output (UO) minus the water of oxidation (WO) plus the preformed water (PW):

$$IA = (IWL + UO) - (WO + PW).$$

Under normal conditions this amount approximates the insensible water loss plus the urine output because the amounts of preformed water and water of oxidation are minimal.

The insensible water loss usually equals 30 to 40 ml/100 calories expended in 24 hours or 30 to 40 percent of maintenance fluids. This is usually equal to 300 to 400 ml/m²/24 hr. In addition to replacing the insensible water loss, urine output is replaced. Urine output is measured, and the previous 8 hours' output is replaced milliliter for milliliter over the subsequent 8 hours. Fluid intake may need to be further reduced if the child is in a high catabolic state. Abnormal fluid loss from excessive sweating, diarrhea, vomiting, nasogastric drainage, or wounds should be quantitatively replaced with the appropriate fluids and electrolytes. Overall fluid balance is reflected in the body weight. A weight loss of 0.5 to 1.0 percent per day during the oliguric phase is to be expected and assures the clinician that treatment has been successful. Fluid balance must be assessed frequently during the first few days of ARF, and decisions regarding fluid intake may need to be revised often. Fluid retention may be so severe as to compromise a child's cardiovascular or respiratory status. The use of diuretics (*see* p. 376) and/or dialytic therapy may be the treatment of choice under these circumstances.

Electrolyte imbalances.   Hyperkalemia is potentially the most life-threatening electrolyte disturbance that may occur in patients with ARF. A number of circumstances contribute to the rapid accumulation of potassium ions in the ECF of patients with ARF: (1) loss of the normal route of potassium ion excretion (the kidneys), (2) cellular catabolism releases intracellular potassium ions into the ECF (occurs with tissue breakdown or trauma and infection), (3) transfusion of hemolyzed (bank) blood, (4) acidosis causes extrusion of potassium ions from cells into ECF space, (5) transfusion reactions, and (6) iatrogenic sources (medications).

The clinical signs that may be present with hyperkalemia include bradycardia, hypoactive tendon reflexes, falling blood pressure, restlessness, and apprehension. Symptoms include numbness and tingling of hands, feet, and around the mouth, and generalized weakness. The electrocardiogram (ECG) provides the nurse with the most accurate information regarding the effects of hyperkalemia on the cardiac muscle. The ECG changes that result from hyperkalemia follow a very predictable and definite pattern. The progressive ECG changes the nurse would observe in a child with potassium intoxication are as follows (Fig. 6-26):

1. Tall, peaked T waves with a narrowed base.
2. A depressed RST segment.
3. Decreased amplitude of R wave and increased depth of S wave.
4. A prolonged P-R interval followed by disappearance of the P waves (at serum potassium levels of approximately 8.5 mEq/liter).
5. Progressive widening of QRS complex with prolongation of the QT interval.
6. Gradual formation of sine wave configuration.

Conservative medical treatment of hyperkalemia (Table 6-21) is often begun when the serum potassium value is 5.5 to 6.0 mEq/liter. Therapy involves severe

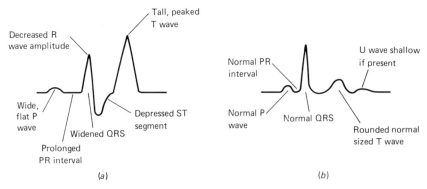

Figure 6-26. The effects of (A) hyperkalemia and (B) normokalemia of the electrocardio-gram. *Adapted from* Holloway, N. M., editor. 1979. Nursing the Critically Ill Adult. Addi-son-Wesley Publishing Co., Menlo Park, Calif. 232.

restriction of potassium intake and the use of ion-exchange resins. Sodium poly-styrene sulfonate (Kayexalate) is an example of such a resin. This particular resin exchanges sodium ions for potassium ions (1 milliequivalent of potassium ions is removed with each gram of resin). Kayexalate can be administered orally or in combination with sorbitol as a high-retention enema. The usual dose is 1 g/kg orally or rectally. It is important to monitor the serum concentration of calcium and magnesium ions because the exchange resin is not specific for potassium ions.

If hyperkalemia is advanced and the ECG depicts cardiac conduction distur-bances, a medical emergency exists and the following treatment is instituted to lower the serum potassium level quickly and stabilize the heart:

1. Infuse a (25 to 50 percent) glucose solution (0.25 to 0.50 g/kg) intravenously plus 1 U of regular insulin per 5 g of dextrose (1 U/kg). Glucose and insulin lower extracellular levels of potassium ions by transferring potassium ions into cells during spurred gluconeogenesis. This may take 30 minutes to work.
2. Infuse 10 percent calcium gluconate (0.5 ml/kg) over 2 to 4 minutes. The effect of calcium as an antagonist to potassium ions is transient.
3. Rapid infusion of 7.5 percent sodium bicarbonate (1 to 3 mEq/kg) over 30 to 60 minutes. This works by correcting acidosis, thereby moving potassium into the intracellular spaces. The effect, however, is transient.

The prevention of hyperkalemia can be aided by taking certain extra measures, including treating infection promptly, debriding necrotic tissue, draining of blood accumulation, restricting potassium intake, and providing nonprotein calories as carbohydrates and fats.

Metabolic acidosis is nearly always present in children with ARF. It results from a failure of the kidneys to excrete hydrogen ions, reabsorb bicarbonate, and produce sufficient amounts of ammonia and titrable acids. The endogenous pro-duction of sulfuric, phosphoric, and organic acids (fixed acids) and acids that are produced as by-products of protein catabolism accumulate in the body. The in-creased amounts of hydrogen ions in the ECF are initially buffered by serum bicarbonate in an effort to maintain serum pH. The plasma bicarbonate concentra-tion decreases by approximately 1 to 3 mEq/day and often drops below 15 mEq/

TABLE 6-21 Treatment of Hyperkalemia

Severity	Agent	Onset	Duration	Mechanism
Mild (serum K^+ = 5.5–6.5 mEq/liter)	Decreased intake	Variable	Variable	Restriction
	K^+ exchange resin	1–2 hr	4–6 hr	Excretion
Moderate (serum K^+ = 6.5–7.5 mEq/liter)	Glucose and insulin	10–30 min	2–4 hr	Redistribution
Severe (serum K^+ > 7.5 mEq/liter)	$NaHCO_3$	≤1 hr	1–2 hr	Redistribution or antagonism
	Calcium gluconate	5 min	30–60 min	Antagonism
	Dialysis	5 min	Variable	Excretion

Reprinted with permission from Franklin, S. S., and M. H. Maxwell, 1980. Acute renal failure. *In* Maxwell, M. H., and C. R. Kleeman, editors. 1980. Clinical Disorders of Fluid and Electrolyte Metabolism. McGraw-Hill Book Co., New York. Third edition. 781.

liter. As a result, the serum bicarbonate concentration is decreased, the amount of carbonic acid is increased, and there is a temporary increase in the $PaCO_2$. The respiratory system attempts to compensate for the acidosis by increasing the rate and depth of breathing. By blowing off excess carbon dioxide, the serum concentration of carbonic acid is lowered. It is important to monitor the child for signs and symptoms of metabolic acidosis that were detailed in the previous section. Severe acidosis may be treated with sodium bicarbonate solutions or dialysis.

Hypocalcemia and hyperphosphatemia may coexist in the patient with ARF. The mechanism for hypocalcemia has not been clearly defined, although hyperphosphatemia causes a decrease in the serum calcium concentration. The metabolic acidosis that may also be present in a child with ARF will increase the amount of calcium that is ionized (physiologically active form) and may forestall the development of hypocalcemia. Hypocalcemic tetany is rare, but it may occur during rapid correction of acidosis. Aluminum hydroxide gels (Amphojel, Basaljel) may be used to bind phosphate in the intestinal tract and correct hyperphosphatemia.

Magnesium accumulates in the ECF during the oliguric phase of ARF. Hypermagnesemia is usually not severe, but because of the possibility of magnesium intoxication, it is necessary to avoid the use of antacids that contain magnesium (Mylanta, Maalox, Gelusil).

Anemia and abnormal bleeding.   Erythropoietin is normally secreted by the kidney in response to hypoxia. This stimulates the production and maturation of RBCs in bone marrow. In severe, prolonged ARF, the release of erythropoietin is diminished and a normochromic normocytic anemia results. A folic acid deficiency and poor utilization of iron slow the maturation of RBCs. A hemoglobin of 7 grams and a hematocrit of 21 percent are not unusual findings. Therapy consists of blood transfusions of packed RBCs (10 ml/kg) and the administration of folic acid and ferrous sulfate. Blood products are infused slowly and the nurse watches for signs of fluid overload. Nursing care is directed toward helping the patient to conserve energy (*see* p. 95). Other hematologic abnormalities may develop as azotemia progresses. Spontaneous ecchymoses and internal bleeding may occur secondary to decreased platelet survival, inadequate production and availability of platelet factor III, inadequate clotting factors and cofactors needed for clotting mechanisms, and decreased platelet adhesiveness. It is important that the nurse monitor the patient for signs and symptoms of abnormal bleeding and limit the number of procedures and treatments that may precipitate bleeding. Therapeutic nursing interventions would include the use of stool softeners to prevent constipation; testing the stools, urine, and all other drainage for blood; careful handling of the patient; limiting the frequency of intramuscular injections; administering antacids as ordered in order to decrease the risk of serious bleeding from stress ulcers (*see* p. 226); and providing meticulous mouth care.

Immunosuppression. Normal immune processes are known to be depressed in patients with acute uremia. The reason for T-cell suppression and altered leukocyte functioning is currently unknown. These disturbances make the child more susceptible to infection and substantiate the fact that the most frequent cause of morbidity and mortality in ARF is infection. Sites that are often infected include the urinary tract, wounds, respiratory tract, and the peritoneum. Signs of infection may not be easily recognized because a lack of temperature elevation is a characteristic feature of ARF. The use of antibiotic therapy needs to be evaluated in relation to how specific medications are excreted. Reduced doses of antibiotics may be needed to avoid the accumulation of dangerously high amounts in the body. Medications that warrant particular attention include gentamicin sulfate, polymixin B sulfate, kanamycin sulfate, penicillin, penicillin derivatives, and erythromycin. Nursing interventions are directed toward preventing infection. Good hand washing is a basic but crucial step in accomplishing this goal. If a urinary catheter must be used, catheter care may be indicated 3 to 4 times each day. Various procedures are currently used for catheter care. Meticulous care should be used when providing mouth and skin care to children. Lemon-glycerine swabs are often used in mouth care in order to prevent stomatitis. Strict aseptic technique should be used when caring for open wounds and when changing dressings that are covering arterial and intravenous lines.

Nutritional support. Nutrition plays a prominent role in the critical care management of children with ARF. A principal strategy is to provide a major portion of the caloric intake from nonprotein sources. Under normal circumstances, when caloric sources are inadequate, protein is metabolized and used for energy. Water, potassium, phosphate, hydrogen, metabolic acids, magnesium, and urea are distributed in the ECF as a result of the metabolism of proteins. Protein catabolism may lead to malnutrition, which further complicates the course of ARF. The nurse should take measures to prevent conditions that result in excess protein breakdown such as tissue necrosis, infection, immobilization, and fever. Protein restriction will slow the rate of rise of the BUN. Treatment involves providing at least 25 to 40 percent of the daily caloric requirements as carbohydrates and fats. The symptoms of anorexia, nausea, vomiting, or diarrhea that often accompany uremia may prohibit adequate oral intake of food and fluids. In these cases, intravenous nutrition is provided. Total parenteral nutrition (TPN) solutions — which contain a combination of dextrose, essential amino acids, and vitamins — will provide the ARF child with the elements needed to meet nutritional requirements. The use of essential amino acids in the nutritional management of patients with ARF has been shown by clinical and experimental means to significantly decrease overall mortality from 66 to 25 percent.[50] Amino acid formulas (Amin-Aid) specially produced for renal patients are currently available for enteral administration (*see* p. 480 and Table 8-4).

Dialytic therapy. Dialysis is the diffusion of dissolved solute particles and water through a selective semipermeable membrane that is placed between two solutions. The principles of dialysis are based on the forces of diffusion, osmosis, and hydrostatic pressure. Diffusion of solute occurs when a concentration gradient exists between two solutions. Although osmosis occurs when there is an osmotic gradient, water and solute can be moved either with or against existing chemical or osmotic gradients if sufficient hydrostatic pressure is present. By controlling osmotic and hydrostatic pressures, dialysis can be effectively used to meet individual patient needs. In peritoneal dialysis, the peritoneum serves as the semipermeable membrane that separates fluid on the visceral side of the peritoneum from the dialysate infused into the peritoneal cavity. Hemodialysis requires the use of an artificial semipermeable membrane. This separates extracorporeal blood from dialysate in the dialyzer. Dialytic therapy is indicated in the following clinical conditions:

Hyperkalemia unresponsive to conservative treatment
Severe metabolic acidosis
Hypervolemia
Severe uremia
ARF
Chronic renal failure
Drug intoxication
Electrolyte disorders (hyperphosphatemia)
BUN value >150 mg/100 ml
Anuria for greater than 24 to 48 hours
CNS disturbances
Congestive heart failure
Bleeding secondary to uremia
Serum creatinine greater than 10 to 15 mg/dl

Peritoneal dialysis. Peritoneal dialysis has been used successfully in children to manage ARF and chronic renal failure. In peritoneal dialysis, the peritoneum functions as a passive dialyzing membrane as water and solutes move between the vascular supply of the peritoneum and the dialysate in the peritoneal cavity. The composition of the dialysate in large part determines the direction of movement of fluid and solutes. The introduction of dialysate into the peritoneal cavity (which contains a high osmolality and a low concentration of nonelectrolyte solutes) enables removal of solutes from the blood in an efficient manner. Commercial dialysate is made in 1.50 and 4.25 percent glucose solutions, both of which are hypertonic to plasma. Dialysate contains approximately the same electrolyte concentrations that are present in the ECF (Table 6-22). Dialysate does not contain any potassium ions because hyperkalemia is a frequent complication of ARF. Potassium (1 to 4 mEq/liter) is often ordered to be added to the dialyzate for individual patients. Dialysate is essentially void of substances that must be removed from the patient, contains high concentrations of those substances that

TABLE 6-22 Peritoneal Dialysis Solution

Factor	Value
Na^+	140 mEq/liter
K^+	0 mEq/liter
Ca^{++}	3.5–4.0 mEq/liter
Mg^{++}	1.5 mEq/liter
Sodium acetate	45 mEq/liter
Cl^-	103 mEq/liter
Dextrose	1,500–4,250 mg/dl
Osmolarity	370–510 mOsm/liter

must be added to the patient, and has the same concentration as plasma for substances that will remain at the same concentration. The goal of dialysis is to remove excess water, potassium ions, urea, creatinine, and uremic toxins (middle molecules), while maintaining plasma concentrations of sodium, chloride, calcium, and magnesium. Warming the dialysate to 37°C (98.6°F) has been shown to increase peritoneal clearance of solutes by 35 percent.[51] If substantial fluid removal is required, dialysate with a higher osmolality (4.25 percent) is used or two different concentrations of dialysate (1.50 and 4.25 percent) are used alternately. Heparin (250 to 500 U/liter) is frequently added to dialysate to prevent fibrin clots from forming inside the lumen of the dialysis catheter.

Initiation of peritoneal dialysis.   After the decision is made to dialyze a patient, a peritoneal catheter is inserted by the physician. The general procedure for catheter insertion is outlined in Table 6-23. Once the catheter is in place, the dialytic process begins. The dialysate is warmed to 37°C (98.6°F) before infusion. Dialysis is divided into three distinct time periods: the inflow time, the dwell or equilibration time, and the outflow or drainage time. A cycle usually lasts 1 hour and begins with the inflow or infusion of 15 to 30 ml/kg of dialysate. This phase is relatively rapid, lasting about 10 minutes. The dwell time lasts approximately 15 to 30 minutes. During this period equilibration occurs between the blood contained in the peritoneal vessels and the dialysate. The outflow period usually lasts 20 minutes. The dialysate may be blood-tinged for the first few cycles, but it should clear. Cloudy or bloody dialysate obtained during the outflow period may be a sign of infection or internal bleeding. Protein loss (1 g/liter of dialysate) occurs routinely with peritoneal dialysis.

Peritoneal dialysis may be performed either manually or by machine. Although the manual method is the simplest, it takes an extraordinary amount of nursing time. It requires the nurse to regulate infusion, monitor the dwell period, regulate the outflow, and drain, measure, and discard the effluent. The two automated peritoneal dialysis machines are the multiple cycler and the reverse osmosis machine. The cycler connects eight 2-liter bottles or bags of dialysate in series, warms the fluid, regulates the infusion and dwell time, and drains and weighs the dialysate effluent. In both the manual method and the multiple cycler, sterility is broken each time a new dialysate bottle is hung and the drainage containers are emptied. The reverse osmosis machine is more complicated to operate, but it has the advantage of providing several different glucose concentrations of dialysate if needed. During the acute early phase of ARF, dialysis is usually continuous. Once the patient becomes stabilized, dialysis is often performed for 24 to 48 hours three times each week.

TABLE 6-23   Procedure for Insertion of a Peritoneal Dialysis Catheter

Locus of responsibility	Procedure
Nurse	Explain procedure to patient/parents and describe common sensations associated with dialysis and sterile technique to be used.
	Measure and record baseline vital signs and weight.
	Have patient empty bladder, or insert urinary catheter to drain urine from bladder.
Physician	The abdomen is surgically prepared.
	1 percent Xylocaine is injected into the skin and subcutaneous tissue.
	An 18-gauge needle or angiocath is inserted at the midline and between the umbilicus and symphysis pubis.
	When the needle has perforated the peritoneum, dialysate (40 ml/kg) is run into the peritoneal cavity. This fluid serves as a cushion to prevent perforation of vital organs during catheter insertion.
	A small incision is made (after the needle is removed), and a catheter and trocar are advanced.
	The trocar is removed and the peritoneal catheter is advanced to a desired location. The catheter is sutured in place at the skin surface.
	The entry site of the catheter is covered with a sterile dressing.

Nursing responsibilities in caring for the child receiving peritoneal dialysis are as follows:

1. Assess the patient before peritoneal dialysis begins. Usually a sedative or analgesic is ordered to be given to the patient before the procedure begins.
2. Monitor vital signs and record every hour. Be particularly aware of changes in the pulse, blood pressure, and the rate and quality of respirations that may be associated with the development of fluid imbalances.
3. Weigh the patient at least daily. Always weigh the patient before and at the completion of dialysis if dialysis is not continuous.
4. Accurately measure the dialyzate intake and output and record on peritoneal dialysis record (Fig. 6-27).
5. Calculate the cumulative balance each hour on the dialysis record.
6. Observe the dialyzate outflow for qualities that may indicate peritonitis (e.g., cloudy or blood tinged). Obtain a culture of peritoneal fluid every 24 hours and send it to the lab for culture and sensitivity.
7. Observe the patient for signs of abdominal distention and respiratory distress secondary to excess peritoneal fluid.
8. Provide food and fluid intake in small amounts in order to avoid increased distention of abdomen. Constipation should be avoided because it will cause abdominal distension and discomfort.
9. Observe the patient for signs and symptoms of electrolyte and acid-base disorders and hyperglycemia.

DIALYSIS CYCLE

Inflow _____   Amount of dialysate each cycle _____ _____

Equilibration _____   Weight prior to dialysis _____ ___ __ __

Drainage _____   Cultures sent _____ _____ __ __ __

Date	Cycle no.	Dialysis fluid		Medication added	Remarks	INFLOW			DRAINAGE			Balance	Cumulative balance
		1.5%	4.25%			Start time	Finish time	Volume in	Start time	Finish time	Volume out		

Figure 6-27. Peritoneal dialysis record. (Courtesy of the Children's Hospital of Philadelphia.) Guidelines for use are listed below:

Cycle number: 1, 2, 3, etc.

Dialysis fluid: Check for concentration of dialysate used each cycle.

Medication added: Note any medications added (heparin, antibiotics).

Remarks: Note if dialysate is blood-tinged, cloudy, etc., or if this cycle is used as a reservoir.

Inflow start and finish: Note the time dialysis fluid begins to run in and when the inflow is completed.

Volume in: Chart the total number of milliliters infused into the peritoneal cavity.

Drainage start and finish: Note the time dialysis fluid begins to drain and the time drainage is completed.

Volume out: Chart the total number of milliliters drained from the peritoneal cavity.

Balance: Chart the difference between volume in and volume out. If the volume in is larger than the volume out, the balance will be positive (+), and if the volume out is larger than the volume in, the balance will be negative (−). If both volumes are the same, the balance will be zero. (0).

Cumulative balance: Chart the balance between each cycle. For example if cycle 1 balance is +100 ml, and cycle 2 balance is −200 ml, the cumulative balance will be −100 ml. The cumulative balance can therefore be + or −

10. Change the dressing around the peritoneal catheter every 24 hours. Use strict sterile technique when changing the catheter dressing daily. Observe the catheter insertion site for signs of infection (redness and/or drainage around the site, or tenderness).
11. Change the dialysate administration tubing every 24 hours.
12. Determine where the dialysis can be carried out (patient in bed, in chair, or ambulating). Provide age-appropriate diversional activities.
13. Instruct the patient on peritoneal dialysis.
14. Evaluate the results of the peritoneal dialysis.

There are several potential complications that may occur in patients receiving peritoneal dialysis. These complications and the nursing interventions directed toward correcting them are listed in Table 6-24. Contraindications to peritoneal dialysis include recent bowel or abdominal surgery, known peritoneal adhesions, extensive burns, and an intraperitoneal hematoma.

The treatment of ARF usually requires continuous dialysis (24 hours a day), in which dialysate fluid is infused through an acute peritoneal dialysis catheter. During this type of dialysis, fluid remains in the peritoneal cavity for a maximum of 30 minutes. If the patient's condition stabilizes and continuous dialysis is not warranted, he or she may be switched to a schedule in which dialysis is performed 12 hours out of each 24 hours, only two to three times per week. This type of dialysis is known as intermittent peritoneal dialysis. Continuous ambulatory peritoneal dialysis (CAPD) is a relatively new method of dialysis used almost exclusively in the treatment of patients with CRF. Although nurses working in an ICU setting are responsible for caring for patients who receive continuous or intermittent peritoneal dialysis, patients who are on a CAPD program at home may be hospitalized in an ICU at some point. There are some articles available that offer a good explanation of the principles of CAPD (*see* Arenz, 1981; Sorrels, 1979 in the Bibliography for this chapter).

Hemodialysis. The goal of hemodialysis is to correct fluid and electrolyte imbalances, acid-base disorders, and remove uremic toxins. In hemodialysis, blood is pumped outside the body (extracorporeally) through a dialyzer and then returned to the vascular system. A hemodialysis unit consists of a dialyzer, dialysate, and a dialysate delivery system. There are three types of dialyzers: hollow fiber, parallel flow plate, and coil. The dialyzer contains a semipermeable membrane made from cellophane or cuprophane. The dialysate is an isotonic electrolyte solution. The dialysate delivery system consists of a proportioning pump that mixes the water and dialysate to a proper concentration and pumps the heated solution through the dialyzer. The flow of blood and dialysate is countercurrent. Fluid and solutes move out of the blood because of hydrostatic and osmotic pressures. Two hydrostatic pressures exist within a dialyzer: (1) In the blood, hydrostatic pressure pushes fluid across membrane; and (2) in the dialysate, a negative hydrostatic pressure pulls fluid from the blood. The combination of these two pressures equals the transmembrane pressure (TMP). The greater the TMP, the greater the ultrafiltration. The movement of solute is determined primarily by the chemical concentration gradient between the two solutions and the movement of water by hydrostatic and osmotic pressures.

Pediatric-sized hemodialyzers (which have a low priming volume and low compliance) are readily available for children who weigh more than 10 kilograms (22 pounds). A dialyzer that requires no more than 10 percent of the patient's blood volume to be extracorporeal at any time is probably the safest type to use for pediatric patients.[52] The rate of ultrafiltration on hemodialysis depends on the characteristics of the dialyzer membrane and the increase in pressure in the blood compartment relative to that in the dialysate compartment (TMP). The clinical condition of the individual patient will determine the type of dialyzer, blood flow rate, and length of dialysis.

Vessel size is often a limiting factor in establishing vascular access for hemodialysis in infants and children. Access to the circulatory system is by creation of an arteriovenous (AV) fistula or shunt. An AV fistula is created surgically by the direct anastomosis of the radial artery to the cephalic vein (Fig. 6-28). Maturation of the fistula takes 2 to 8 weeks after surgery. Maturation results from the thickening and dilation of superficial veins in the forearm in order to accommodate arterial blood flow. The blood in the fistula flows directly from the artery to the vein, bypassing the capillary bed. The nurse can assess the fistula for patency by palpating over the fistula site for a thrill and by auscultating for a bruit. The blood in the fistula is arterial. When the fistula is needed for hemodialysis, two venipunctures are required to gain access to the vascular system. The arterial side is connected to the side going to the dialyzer and the venous side receives blood coming from the dialyzer. Fistulas have several advantages over shunts. They last longer (3 to 4 years), fewer restrictions on activity are required, and there is less danger and fewer complications.

An AV shunt is the cannulation of an artery and a vein, with an external connection between the two (Fig. 6-29). The different shunts that are available are the Schribner and Buselmeier. Activity is limited for 2 to 3 days after the shunt is created, but it can be used for hemodialysis almost immediately. There must always be two shunt clamps attached to the dressing that covers the cannula. Accidental separation of the cannula could result in exsanguination if the clamps are not available. When hemodialysis is required in an emergency, a subclavian or femoral site is used for access using a shaldon catheter.

Potential complications of vascular access include infection, clotting, hemorrhage, aneurysm formation, ischemia, hematoma, and femoral vein thrombosis.

Complications of hemodialysis are (1) hypovolemia resulting from rapid removal of fluid, (2) hypotension secondary to hypovolemia, (3) hypertension from fluid overload, (4) electrolyte imbalances, (5) infection (shunt), (6) excessive bleeding resulting from anticoagulant therapy, (7) air embolism, and (8) disequilibrium syndrome. The disequilibrium syndrome results from a rapid lowering of the serum osmolality. An abrupt decrease in the concentration of serum solutes is not accompanied by as rapid a fall in brain osmolality. Because the brain is hypertonic, cellular swelling occurs. This syndrome is clinically manifested by vomiting, nausea, headache, stupor, and convulsions.

Nursing responsibilities in caring for the child receiving hemodialysis are the same as for peritoneal dialysis, with the following additions: In patients receiving hemodialysis, the blood pressure and blood samples should not be taken in the extremity that contains the shunt or fistula. It is important that the dressing covering the shunt is changed every day with aseptic technique, and that shunt care is provided. The shunt should also be checked for patency, which can be accomplished by observing the tubing for clotting (blood will appear darker) and auscultation for a bruit.

The decision to use peritoneal or hemodialysis in a pediatric patient is based on evaluation of the current clinical status of the patient and consideration of the

TABLE 6-24 Potential Complications of Peritoneal Dialysis

Complication	Nursing intervention
Fluid retention: Results in increased fluid balance that may cause CHF or hypertension.	Determine the maximum allowable positive balance for each individual patient. Consult the physician if the balance exceeds this amount. Assess the patient for signs and symptoms of fluid overload and/or dehydration. Monitor vital signs hourly.
Catheter obstruction: May result from a clogged catheter due to fibrin, omentum, or kinkage. Result is inadequate inflow and disrupted outflow.	Change the patient's position, turn the patient from side to side, elevate the head of the bed, gently massage the abdomen. Send specimen of the peritoneal fluid to the lab for culture and sensitivity.
Peritonitis: Abdominal pain, fever, rebound tenderness, cloudy peritoneal fluid, inflammation at catheter exit site, evidence of redness, swelling, or tracking subcutaneously along site of catheter.	Use strict aseptic technique when changing the catheter dressing daily. Change the dressing if it becomes wet. Send culture of the peritoneal fluid once a day (obtain specimen on first outflow). Send gram stain of fluid if infection is suspected. Administer antibiotics as ordered.
Abdominal pain: May occur secondary to abdominal distention from dialysate or from chemical irritation from the dialysate.	Slow the rate of inflow or outflow of the dialysate. Instill smaller amounts of fluid into the peritoneal cavity each cycle. Serve meals in small portions when the fluid is draining out. Provide diversional activities (family, reading, games, etc.)
Dyspnea and atelectasis: May be the result of restricted diaphragmatic movement secondary to pressure from dialysate volume.	Elevate the head of the bed. Eccourage deep breathing and coughing exercises. Decrease the amount of dialysate instilled. Reposition the patient at frequent intervals to encourage maximal expansion of the lungs.
Bowel or bladder perforation during catheter insertion.	Monitor the patient for sudden increase in urine volume, signs of sepsis, a change in color or consistency of dialysate effluent from the abdominal catheter, and diarrhea.
Hyperglycemia.	Monitor the plasma and urine concentrations. Observe the patient for signs of polyuria or polydipsia.
Leakage around the peritoneal catheter.	Observe the catheter insertion site for drainage. Weigh the dressing material to estimate the fluid loss. Additional sutures may be needed to secure the skin around the catheter in order to prevent leakage. Check the catheter site dressing frequently for abnormal drainage.

TABLE 6-24   (Continued)

Complication	Nursing intervention
Hypotension: Results from excessive removal of fluid. Hypertonic dialysis solution (4.25% dextrose) will remove fluid more rapidly than one with a comparatively lower osmolarity (1.5% dextrose).	Monitor vital signs for an increased pulse rate, decreased blood pressure, and postural hypotension. Weigh the patient more often if hypotension is suspected. The magnitude of weight loss will often correspond to the amount of fluid lost in a short period of time (24 hours).
Hypertension: Results from retention of excess fluid.	Monitor the child for an increase in body weight. Watch for increased blood pressure, signs of respiratory distress, and impending CHF.

CHF, congestive heart failure.

advantages, disadvantages, risks, and benefits of each method (Table 6-25). Peritoneal dialysis is generally preferred over hemodialysis in pediatric patients because of the risk of rapid, severe depletion of ECF volume and hypotension with hemodialysis. The use of peritoneal dialysis may, for example, be preferable under acute life-threatening emergencies (hyperkalemia) because it can be instituted rapidly. Hemodialysis may be better suited for chronic dialysis and in cases where rapid removal of a dialyzable toxin is needed. There is growing evidence that early and frequent dialysis of patients with ARF may have a positive effect on their prognosis.

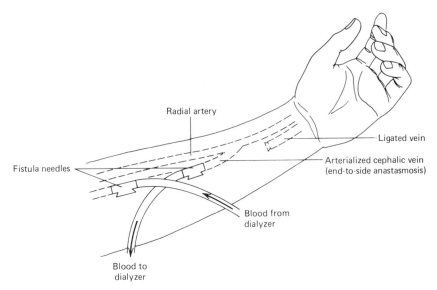

Figure 6-28.   The arteriovenous (AV) fistula. *Adapted from* Holloway, N. M., editor. 1979. Nursing the Critically Ill Adult. Addison-Wesley Publishing Co., Menlo Park, Calif. 269; and Holmes, A. Herrick Memorial Hospital, Berkeley, Calif.

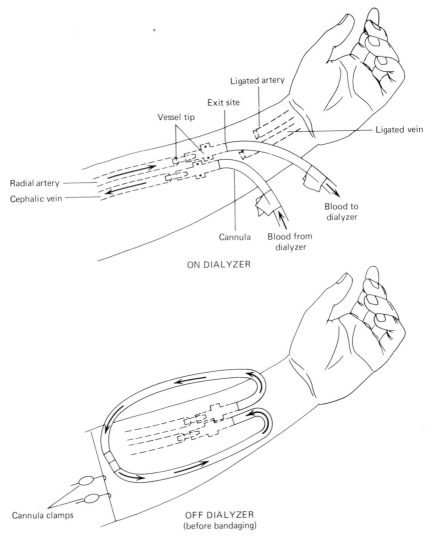

Figure 6-29. The arteriovenous (AV) shunt. *Adapted from* Holloway, N. M., editor. 1979. Nursing the Critically III Adult. Addison-Wesley Publishing Co., Menlo Park, Calif. 267.

The actual techniques of peritoneal dialysis and hemodialysis are relatively simple. It is the nuances of therapy and the management of the complications of dialysis and of the underlying disease that require a great deal of knowledge and expertise on the part of nurses.

Patient outcomes. In the 1940s, the overall mortality rate in patients with ATN was approximately 90 percent. There was a subsequent dramatic decline in the mortality rate to 50 to 60 percent in the 1960s. The decrease in mortality rate is

TABLE 6-25 Comparison of Peritoneal Dialysis and Hemodialysis

Type	Advantages	Disadvantages
Peritoneal dialysis	Simple technique and equipment. Can institute rapidly. No systemic heparinization needed. Less likely than hemodialysis to cause fluid and electrolyte disturbances. Can use in infants and children. Efficient removal of middle-molecular-weight solutes. Peritoneum appears more permeable to these molecules.	Requires abdomen free of recent surgery, adhesions, etc. Large amounts of protein lost. Procedure slower. Takes three to six times longer to achieve the solute removal achieved by hemodialysis. Usually conducted for at least 24–48 hr initially. Peritonitis a risk.
Hemodialysis	Chronic intermittent dialysis possible. Rapid treatment procedure. Efficient.	Equipment is complex. Specially trained registered nurses and physicians necessary. Requires circulatory access; may be difficult in infants and children. Systemic heparinization required. Disequilibrium syndrome can occur. Hemodialysis can cause rapid and dangerous hemodynamic changes in pediatric patients. Air embolus and hemorrhage are potential complications.

related to the introduction of antibiotics, effective treatment of hyperkalemia, and the development of effective dialysis techniques. Despite the progress in management with the availability of modern therapeutics, the mortality rate remains at 50 percent. One study of ARF in infants and children has examined the outcome of 53 patients treated with hemodialysis.[53] Of 23 patients with ATN, 14 developed ATN during the postoperative period after major surgery. Of these 14 children, 10 died. The main cause of death was neurological injury secondary to hypotension or severe cardiac dysfunction. The remaining 9 of the 23 patients had ATN that was associated with major catastrophic illness. All 9 of these children died. The remaining 30 of the 53 patients had ARF due to a primary nephrologic disorder. Of these patients, 90 percent survived. All of the patients who died had hemolytic-uremic syndrome (*see below*). It was not specifically the ARF, but the severity of the underlying disorders, that for the most part determined the outcome of these patients. It is important to note that the patients who died had predialysis BUN levels that were significantly higher than in the children who survived. In addition, nonsurvivors received their first dialysis significantly later after the onset of their illness than did the survivors. In another study of 70 children with ARF, the mortality rate was somewhat lower (20 to 30 percent).[54] Although the majority of cases developed secondary to renal hypoperfusion, hemolytic-uremic syndrome, glomerulonephritis, septicemia, and congenital abnormalities were other causes of ARF. Of the 70 patients, 37 fully recovered, 10 were discharged with chronically impaired renal functioning, 17 died, and 6 entered the dialysis and transplantation program.

The prognosis for children with ATN is largely determined by the initial event that led to its development. Mortality most often stems from complications of the underlying disease. Sepsis is the primary complication and cause of death.

The Hemolytic-Uremic Syndrome

The first communication about the association of hemolytic-uremic syndrome (HUS) and bilateral cortical necrosis was published in 1955. HUS is often the cause of ARF in infants. There has been an increase in the number of cases of HUS reported in the last 10 years. The average age of onset is 2 years, with the range being 2 months to 8 years old. There is no racial predilection, and the sexes are equally affected. HUS has been reported to occur in small sporadic epidemics, and more than one family member may be affected at the same time.[55]

HUS is characterized by the presence of microangiopathic hemolytic anemia, thrombocytopenia, and azotemia. The diagnosis of HUS usually depends on the presence of (1) hemolytic anemia with fragmentation of RBCs on the peripheral blood smear, (2) thrombocytopenia ($<140,000/m^3$), (3) a BUN level of greater than 40 mg/100 ml, (4) elevated serum creatinine, (5) oliguria or anuria, and (6) hypertension.

The etiology of HUS is unknown at present, although viral, bacterial, immunological, and hormonal factors have been suggested by researchers as potentially contributing to the onset. In the pathogenesis of HUS, an unknown agent causes vascular endothelial damage. This leads to fibrin and platelet deposition in the vessels, resulting in microangiopathic hemolytic anemia, thrombocytopenia, and impaired renal functioning. There is thought to be a primary event that causes injury to vascular endothelium and then secondary activation of the coagulation mechanism. As blood flows through vessels that are lined with fibrin deposits, RBCs are fragmented because of the mechanical stress they undergo. The high RBF per unit of the kidney mass explains the severity of the anemia in HUS. Damaged RBCs are then destroyed by the liver and spleen. Fibrin deposition in renal vessels may be followed by proliferative and sclerotic glomerular changes.

Symptoms of HUS usually develop in a previously healthy infant or child and progress in severity over a period of several days. The two phases of HUS are the prodromal and the acute phase. The prodromal phase lasts approximately 1 to 7 days and is associated with the following symptoms: vomiting, diarrhea, abdominal pain, mild fever, pallor, irritability, and restlessness.[56] Other symptoms include upper respiratory infection, pharyngitis, lymphadenopathy, rash, and edema. Although the diarrhea may subside in 24 to 72 hours, the abdominal pain may persist for 3 to 4 days beyond this period.

The onset of the acute phase of HUS is characterized by the presence of oliguria, severe gastroenteritis (often bloody diarrhea), seizures, and hemolytic anemia. The hemolytic anemia is usually severe from the onset, although the number and severity of the episodes tend to decrease over time. The hemoglobin may decrease by 2 g/mm^3/24 hr, whereas the reticulocyte count increases.

ARF is present in approximately 90 percent of the cases of HUS, and oliguria and/or anuria persist for a different number of days in each child. Any or all of the complications described under the section on ARF may be present with HUS. Nearly 50 percent of children with HUS develop major CNS symptoms during the course of the disease. Neurological complications may be mild (irritability) or severe (convulsions).[57] The cause of the seizures is unknown, but it may result from, for example, hypoxia, ischemia, or bleeding. There is no strict correlation between the degree of neurological involvement and either the severity or the intensity of renal impairment.

Most patients with HUS present with GI problems. Therefore, HUS should be recognized as a cause of serious GI disease.[58,59] GI disease is a major cause of morbidity in HUS. Bloody, mucousy stools often result secondary to mucosal irritation and ulcerated areas in the cecum and ascending colon. The vascular process in the colon is similar to that in the kidneys.

Hematologic values that are altered in HUS vary, but may include decreased hemoglobin, increased reticulocyte count, low or absent haptoglobin, negative Coombs's test, increased WBC count with a shift to the left, shortened platelet half-life, and an increased amount of fibrin degradation products. The clotting factors are generally normal but in some cases the prothrombin time and the partial thromboplastin time are prolonged.

Critical care management.   The goals of treatment for HUS are to improve the hematologic indicies, control the renal failure, and manage the neurological manifestations. The treatment of HUS, therefore includes many of the same modalities used for the treatment of ARF. The indications for early dialysis are similar for ARF and HUS.[60] Dipyridamole and aspirin (which inhibit platelet function) have been used in the treatment of HUS.[61] Although the platelet count may increase temporarily following the administration of these drugs, ongoing hemolysis suggests that only secondary phenomena are affected by these drugs without altering the actual course of the disease.[62]

The three factors that appear to have the greatest influence on prognosis are (1) the period of oliguria, (2) the presence of hypertension (late vs. early onset), and (3) the severity of the nervous system symptoms. The early institution of dialysis seems to positively influence the prognosis of patients with HUS.[63] Recovery from HUS is identified by the presence of a normal blood pressure for 1 to 2 years after the disease, no proteinuria or hematuria, and normal renal functioning. The extent of nonrenal involvement becomes an important determinant in the ultimate prognosis of children with HUS.

The majority of children (80 to 90 percent) who develop HUS recover completely. The morbidity (5 percent of cases) is most often due to bilateral cortical necrosis, severe hypertension, and neurological sequelae. Mortality from HUS remains relatively high at 10 to 20 percent of all cases.

SUMMARY

Nurses who work in pediatric ICUs play an important role in the care of children and adolescents with renal disorders. Children who are acutely ill often develop fluid and/or solute disturbances secondary to pathological processes originating in other organ systems. For this reason, it is important that the nurse identify patients at risk for the development of such disorders so that treatment can begin early in the course of the disease. Early and vigorous intervention is often necessary to forestall the progression of disease to a point where the renal damage is irreversible. Not only are nurses important in the identification of patients at risk, but since they are present with the patient 24 hours a day, they have the opportunity and responsibility to assess the onset and progression of signs and symptoms associated with fluid and electrolyte disturbances.

The mechanisms that exist in the body to preserve fluid and solute balance are complicated. Although these renal mechanisms may be difficult to grasp, it is important that the nurse working in an ICU setting have a working knowledge of the concepts, since how the renal system functions has a profound effect on both the cardiovascular and respiratory systems.

REFERENCES

1. Pitts. (1974) 20.
2. Burton-Opitz and Lucas.
3. Spitzer. 36–38.
4. Spitzer. 29–30.
5. Valtin. (1979) 393–395.
6. Thurau.
7. Thurau et al.
8. Deen et al.
9. Burg and Green.
10. Morgan et al.
11. Valtin. (1973) 57–58.
12. Relman and Schwartz.
13. Lindheimer et al.
14. Brenner et al.
15. Dougharty et al.
16. Earley et al.
17. Fitzgibbons et al.
18. Martino and Earley.
19. Davidson et al.
20. Malnic et al.
21. Agus et al.
22. Rocha and Kokko.
23. Bricker et al. 253–256.
24. Albert and Winters.
25. Pitts and Alexander.
26. Pitts et al.
27. Pitts and Lotspeich.
28. Fuller et al.
29. Chantler et al. 515.
30. Schwartz et al.
31. Bartter and Schwartz.
32. Auger et al.
33. Guyton et al.
34. American Academy of Pediatrics.
35. Santos-Buch. 14–29.
36. Loggie. (1977) 645–660.
37. Londe.
38. Biron and Mongeau.
39. Voors et al.
40. Balfe and Rance.
41. Hill.
42. Moss.
43. Loggie. (1975)
44. Siegel and Mulrow. 462.
45. Siegel and Mulrow. 463.
46. Bernstein. 1105–1107.
47. Chapman and Legrain. 383–410.
48. Oken. (Clinical) 1108.
49. Franklin and Maxwell. 770–774.
50. Abel et al.
51. Gross and McDonald.
52. Mauer. 487–502.
53. Hodson et al.
54. Counahan et al.
55. Goldstein et al.
56. Dolislager and Tune.
57. Crisp et al.
58. Whitington et al.
59. Berman.
60. Kaplan et al.
61. Thorsen et al.
62. O'Regan et al.
63. Upadhaya et al.

BIBLIOGRAPHY

Abel, R. M., C. H. Beck, Jr., W. M. Abbott, J. A. Ryan, Jr., G. O. Barnett, and J. E. Fischer. 1973. Improved survival from acute renal failure after treatment with intravenous essential L-amino acids and glucose. Results of a prospective, double-blind study. *New England Journal of Medicine.* **288:**695–699.

Agus, Z. S., L. B. Gardner, L. H. Beck, and M. Goldberg. 1973. Effects of parathyroid hormone on renal tubular absorption of calcium, sodium, and phosphate. *American Journal of Physiology.* **224:**1143–1148.

Albert, M. S., and R. W. Winters. 1966. Acid-base equilibrium of blood in normal infants. *Pediatrics.* **37:**728–732.

American Academy of Pediatrics. 1977. Report of the Task Force on Blood Pressure Control in Children. *Pediatrics.* **59**(Suppl.):797–820.

Arnez, R. 1981. Do-it-yourself dialysis. RN. **44:**57–60.

Auger, R. G., J. E. Zehr, R. G. Siekert, and W. E. Segar. 1970. Position effect on antidiuretic hormone: blood levels in bedfast patients. *Archives of Neurology.* **23:**513–517.

Balfe, J. W., and C. P. Rance. 1978. Recognition and management of hypertensive crises in childhood. *Pediatric Clinics of North America.* **25:**159–174.

Bartter, F. C. and W. B. Schwartz. 1967. The syndrome of inappropriate secretion of antidiuretic hormone. *American Journal of Medicine.* **42:**790–806.

Berman, W. 1972. The hemolytic-uremic syndrome: Initial clinical presentation mimicking ulcerative colitis. *Journal of Pediatrics.* **81:**275–278.

Bernstein, J. 1978. Renal cortical and medullary necrosis. *In* Edelmann, C. M., editor. 1978. *Pediatric Kidney Disease.* Little, Brown & Co., Boston.

Biron, P., and J. G. Mongeau. 1978. Familial aggregation of blood pressure and its components. *Pediatric Clinics of North America.* **25:**29–33.

Brenner, B. M., and F. C. Rector, Jr., editors. 1976. *The Kidney.* Vol. I. W. B. Saunders, Co., Philadelphia.

Brenner, B. M., J. L. Troy, and T. M. Daugharty. 1971. On the mechanism of inhibition of fluid reabsorption by the proximal tubule. *Journal of Clinical Investigation.* **50:**1596–1602.

Bricker, N. S., R. G. Schultze, and A. Light. 1980. Renal function: general concepts. *In* Maxwell, M. H., and C. R. Kleeman, editors. 1980. Clinical Disorders of Fluid and Electrolyte Metabolism. McGraw-Hill Book Co., New York. Third edition.

Brundage, D. J. 1976. Nursing Management of Renal Problems. C.V. Mosby Co., St. Louis.

Burg, M. B., and N. Green. 1973. Function of the thick ascending limb of Henle's loop. *American Journal of Physiology.* **224:**659–668.

Burton-Opitz, R., and D. R. Lucas. 1911. The blood supply of the kidney. Part V. The influence of the vagus nerve upon the vascularity of the left organ. *Journal of Experimental Medicine.* **13:**308–313.

Chantler, C. 1976. Evaluation of laboratory and other methods of measuring renal function. *In* Lieberman, E., editor. 1976. Clinical Pediatric Nephrology. J. B. Lippincott Co., Philadelphia.

Chapman, A., and M. Legrain. 1979. Acute tubular necrosis and interstitial nephritis. *In* Hamburger, J. C., J. Crosnier, and J. P. Grunfeld, editors. 1979. Nephrology. John Wiley & Sons, Inc., New York.

Counahan, R., J. S. Cameron, C. S. Ogg, P. Spurgeon, D. G. Williams, E. Winder, and C. Chantler. 1977. Presentation, management, complications, and outcome of acute renal failure in childhood: five years' experience. *British Medical Journal.* **1:**599–602.

Crisp, D. E., R. L. Siegler, J. F. Bale, and J. A. Thompson. 1981. Hemorrhagic cerebral infarction in the hemolytic uremic syndrome. *Journal of Pediatrics.* **99:**273–276.

Daugharty, T. M., L. J. Bellau, J. A. Martino, and L. E. Earley. 1968. Interrelationship of physical factors affecting sodium reabsorption in dogs. *American Journal of Physiology.* **215:**1442–1447.

Davidson, D. G., N. G. Levinsky, and R. W. Berliner. 1958. Maintenance of potassium excretion despite reduction in glomerular filtration during sodium diuresis. *Journal of Clinical Investigation.* **37:**548–555.

Deen, W. M., C. R. Robertson, and B. M. Brenner. 1974. Glomerular ultrafiltration. *Federal Proceedings.* **33:**14–20.

Dolislager, D. and B. Tune. 1978. The hemolytic uremic syndrome: Spectrum of severity and significance of prodrome. *American Journal of Diseases in Children.* **132:**55–58.

Dossetor, J. B. 1966. Diagnosis and treatment: creatininemia versus uremia — the relative significance of blood urea nitrogen and serum creatinine concentrations in azotemia. *Annals of Internal Medicine.* **65:**1287–1299.

Earley, L. E., J. A. Martino, and R. M. Friedler. 1966. Factors affecting sodium reabsorption by the proximal tubule as determined during blockade of distal sodium reabsorption. *Journal of Clinical Investigation.* **45:**1668–1684.

Fitzgibbons, J. P., F. J. Gennari, H. B. Garfinkel, and S. Cortell. 1974. Dependence of saline-induced natriuresis upon exposure of the kidney to the physical effects of extracellular fluid volume expansion. *Journal of Clinical Investigation.* **54:**1428–1436.

Franklin, S. S., and M. H. Maxwell. 1980. Acute renal failure. *In* Maxwell, M. H. and C. R. Kleeman, editors. 1980. Clinical Disorders of Fluid and Electrolyte Metabolism. McGraw-Hill Book Co., New York. Third edition.

Fuller, G. R., M. B. MacLeod, and R. F. Pitts. 1955. Influence of administration of potassium salts on the renal tubular reabsorption of bicarbonate. *American Journal of Physiology.* **182:**111–118.

Gamble, J. L. 1954. *Chemical Anatomy, Physiology, and Pathology of Extracellular Fluid.* Harvard University Press, Cambridge. Sixth edition.

Goldstein, M. H., J. Churg, L. Strauss, and D. Gribetz. 1979. Hemolytic uremic syndrome. *Nephron.* **23:**263–272.

Gordon, A., and M. H. Maxwell. 1980. Water, electrolyte, and acid-base disorders associated with acute and chronic dialysis. *In* Maxwell, M. H., and C. R. Kleeman, editors. 1980. Clinical Disorders of Fluid and Electrolyte Metabolism. McGraw-Hill Book Co., New York. Third edition.

Gross, M., and H. P. McDonald. 1967. Effect of dialysate temperature and flow rate on peritoneal clearance. *Journal of the American Medical Association (JAMA).* **202:**215–217.

Guyton, A. C., T. G. Coleman, A. W. Cowley, K. W. Scheel, R. D. Manning, and R. A. Norman. 1974. Arterial pressure regulation: overriding dominance of the kidneys in long-term regulation and in hypertension. *In* Laragh, J. H., editor. 1974. Hypertension Manual. Yorke Medical Books, New York.

Hamburger, J. C., J. Crosnier, and J. P. Grunfeld. 1979. Nephrology. John Wiley & Sons, Inc., New York.

Hill, M. N. 1980. Hypertension: what can go wrong when you measure blood pressure. *American Journal of Nursing.* **80:**942–945.

Hodson, E. M., C. M. Kjellstrand, and S. M. Mauer. 1978. Acute renal failure in infants and children: outcome of 53 patients requiring hemodialysis treatment. *Journal of Pediatrics.* **93:**756–761.

Holliday, M. A., and W. E. Segar. 1957. The maintenance need for water in parenteral fluid therapy. *Pediatrics.* **19:**823–832.

Holloway, N. M., editor. 1979. Nursing the Critically Ill Adult. Addison-Wesley Publishing Co., Menlo Park, Calif.

Kaplan, B. S., J. Katz, S. Krawitz, and A. Lurie. 1971. An analysis of the results of therapy in 67 cases of the hemolytic uremic syndrome. *Journal of Pediatrics.* **78:**420–425.

Langley, L. J., I. R. Telford, and J. B. Christensen. 1980. Dynamic Anatomy and Physiology. McGraw-Hill Book Co., New York. Fifth edition.

Laragh, J. H., editor. 1974. Hypertension Manual. Yorke Medical Books, New York.

Lieberman, E. 1972. Hemolytic uremic syndrome. *Journal of Pediatrics.* **80:**1–16.

Lieberman, E. 1976. Workup of a child with azotemia. *In* Lieberman, E., editor. 1976. *Clinical Pediatric Nephrology.* J. B. Lippincott Co., Philadelphia.

Lindheimer, M. D., R. C. Lalone, and N. G. Levinsky. 1976. Evidence that an acute increase in glomerular filtration has little or no effect on sodium excretion in the dog unless extracellular volume is expanded. *Journal of Clinical Investigation.* **46:**256–265.

Loebl, S., G. Spratto, and E. Heckheimer. 1980. The Nurse's Drug Handbook. John Wiley & Sons, Inc., New York. Second edition.

Loggie, J. M. H. 1975. Hypertension in children and adolescents. *Hospital Practice.* **10:**81–92.

Loggie, J. M. H. 1977. Systemic hypertension. *In* Moss, A. J. and G. C. Emmanouilides, editors. 1977. Heart Disease in Infants, Children, and Adolescents. Williams & Wilkins Co., Baltimore. Second edition.

Londe, S. 1978. Causes of hypertension in the young. *Pediatric Clinics of North America.* **25:**55–65.

Londe, S., and D. Goldring. 1980. High blood pressure in children: problems and guidelines for evaluation and treatment. *In* Laragh, J. H., editor. 1980. Topics in Hypertension. Yorke Medical Books, New York.

Malnic, G., M. de Mello-Aires, and G. Giebisch. 1971. Potassium transport across renal distal tubules during acid-base disturbances. *American Journal of Physiology.* **221:**1192–1208.

Martino, J. A., and L. E. Earley. 1967. Demonstration of the role of physical factors as determinants of natriuretic response to volume expansion. *Journal of Clinical Investigation.* **46:**1963–1978.

Mauer, S. M. 1978. Pediatric renal dialysis. *In* Edelmann, C. M., editor. 1978. Pediatric Kidney Disease. Little, Brown & Co., Boston.

Morgan, T., F. Sakai, and R. W. Berliner. 1968. In vitro permeability of medullary collecting ducts to water and urea. *American Journal of Physiology.* **214:**574–581.

Moss, A. J. 1978. Indirect methods of blood pressure measurement. *Pediatric Clinics of North America.* **25:**3–14.

Oken, D. E. 1978. Pathogenetic mechanisms of acute renal failure (vasomotor nephropathy). *In* Edelmann, C. M., editor. 1978. Pediatric Kidney Disease. Little, Brown & Co., Boston.

Oken, D. E. Clinical aspects of acute renal failure (vasomotor nephropathy). *In* Edelmann, C. M., editor. 1978. Pediatric Kidney Disease. Little, Brown & Co., Boston.

O'Regan, S., R. W. Chesney, J. G. Mongeau, and P. Robitaille. 1980. Aspirin and dipyridamole therapy in the hemolytic-uremic syndrome. *Journal of Pediatrics.* **97:**473–476.

Pitts, R. F. 1959. The Physiological Basis of Diuretic Therapy. Charles C. Thomas, Publisher, Springfield, Ill.

Pitts, R. F. 1974. Physiology of the Kidney and Body Fluids. Year Book Medical Publishers, Inc., Chicago. Third edition.

Pitts, R. F., and R. S. Alexander. 1945. The nature of the renal tubular mechanism for acidifying the urine. *American Journal of Physiology.* **144:**239–254.

Pitts, R. F., J. L. Ayer, and W. A. Schiess. 1949. The renal regulation of acid-base balance in man. Part III. The reabsorption and excretion of bicarbonate. Part III. *Journal of Clinical Investigation.* **28:**35–44.

Pitts, R. F., and W. D. Lotspeich. 1946. Bicarbonate and the renal regulation of acid-base balance. *American Journal of Physiology.* **147:**138–154.

Price, S. A., and L. M. Wilson. 1978. Pathophysiology. McGraw-Hill Book Co., New York.

Relman, A. S., and W. B. Schwartz. 1952. The effect of DOCA on electrolyte balance in normal man and its relation to sodium chloride intake. *Yale Journal of Biology and Medicine.* **24:**540–558.

Rocha, A. S., and J. P. Kokko. 1973. Sodium chloride and water transport in the medullary thick ascending limb of Henle: evidence for active chloride transport. *Journal of Clinical Investigation.* **52:**612–623.

Santos-Buch, C. A. 1977. The pathology of high blood pressure. *In* Alderman, M. H., editor. 1977. Hypertension: The Nurses Role in Ambulatory Care. Springer Publishing Co., Inc., New York.

Schwartz, G. J., G. B. Haycock, C. M. Edelmann, and A. Spitzer. 1976. A simple estimate of glomerular filtration rate in children derived from body length and plasma creatinine. *Pediatrics.* **58:**259–263.

Siegel, N. J., and P. J. Mulrow. 1978. The management of hypertension. *In* Edelmann, C. M., editor. 1978. Pediatric Kidney Disease. Little, Brown & Co., Boston.

Smith. H. W. 1935. The Kidney. Oxford University Press, New York.

Sorrels, A. J. 1979. Continuous ambulatory peritoneal dialysis. *American Journal of Nursing.* **79:**1400–1401.

Spitzer, A. 1978. Renal physiology and functional development. *In* Edelmann, C. M., editor. 1978. Pediatric Kidney Disease. Little, Brown & Co., Boston.

Thorsen, C. A., E. C. Rossi, D. Green, and F. A. Carone. 1979. The treatment of the hemolytic-uremic syndrome with inhibitors of platelet function. *American Journal of Medicine.* **66:**711–716.

Thurau, K. 1964. Renal hemodynamics. *American Journal of Medicine.* **36:**698–719.

Thurau, K., W. Nagel, M. Horster, and M. Wahl. 1967. Composition of tubular fluids in the macula densa segment as a factor regulating the function of the juxtaglomerular apparatus. *Circulation Research.* **21**(Suppl. 2):79–90.

Upadhyaya, K. K., Barwick, M. Fishaut, M. Kashgarian, and N. J. Siegel. 1980. The importance of nonrenal involvement in hemolytic-uremic syndrome. *Pediatrics.* **65**:115–120.

Valtin, H. 1973. Renal Function: Mechanisms Preserving Fluid and Solute Balance in Health. Little, Brown & Co., Boston.

Valtin, H. 1979. Renal Dysfunction: Mechanisms Involved in Fluid and Solute Imbalance. Little, Brown & Co., Boston.

Vander, A. J., J. H. Sherman, and D. Luciano. 1975. Human Physiology: The Mechanisms of Body Functions. McGraw-Hill Book Co., New York. Second edition.

Voors, A. W., L. S. Webber, and G. S. Berenson. 1978. Epidemiology of essential hypertension in youth: implications for clinical practice. *Pediatric Clinics of North America.* **25**:15–27.

Whitington, P. F., A. Friedman, and R. W. Chesney. 1979. Gastrointestinal disease in the hemolytic-uremic syndrome. *Gastroenterology.* **76**:728–733.

Winters, R. W. 1973. The Body Fluids in Pediatrics: Medical, Surgical and Neonatal Disorders of Acid-Base Status, Hydration and Oxygenation. Little, Brown & Co., Boston.

CHAPTER 7

MULTISYSTEM DISORDERS: SHOCK AND TRAUMA

Kathleen M. Corse
Linda E. Lambert

Shock, or the acute disruption of coordinated organ functioning associated with severe hypoperfusion and hypoxia, remains one of the most challenging conditions to which the medical and nursing clinician may be exposed. Although the causes of shock may be similar in any age group, there are considerable variations in clinical onset and manifestation of the shock state that depend on the age of the patient. The first major division of this chapter will deal primarily with hypovolemia and sepsis, the most common causes of shock in the pediatric population.

Traumatic injuries, which are responsible for approximately one half of the deaths in children aged 1 to 15 years in the United States, will be discussed in the last part of this chapter.

SHOCK SYNDROME*

Selected Aspects of Hemodynamic Physiology

To comprehend and anticipate the needs of the child in shock, the clinician must first have an understanding of certain physiological principles. These include various aspects of hemodynamic physiology, such as the interrelationships among flow, pressure, and resistance, the determinants of myocardial pump function, capillary dynamics, and controls of mean arterial pressure. Although it is beyond the scope of this text to provide an in-depth discussion of hemodynamic physiology, those concepts and variables that are most significant in understanding the pathophysiology of shock and in managing the care of children in the shock state will be the focus of this section.

Flow, pressure, and resistance. The circulatory system is one continuous circuit with two major subdivisions: the systemic (or peripheral) circulation and the pulmonary circulation. The function of the circulatory system is to provide blood flow to all body tissues, thereby sustaining and promoting cellular growth and

---

*The section on Shock Syndrome was written by Kathleen M. Corse; Traumatic Injuries in Childhood (*see* page 447) was written by Linda E. Lambert.

metabolism. The concepts of flow, pressure, and resistance are central to any understanding of the circulatory system. The study of the interrelationships of these three concepts, as well as of other basic principles of blood circulation, is known as hemodynamics.

Blood flow through a vessel is dependent on a driving pressure gradient. That is, there must be a difference in pressure between one end of the vessel and the other in order for blood flow to occur. This concept applies not only to the individual vessel but to the cardiovascular system as a whole. In the heart various pressures are generated during the cardiac cycle that allow for the filling of the heart chambers and the ejection of blood from those chambers into the peripheral and pulmonary circuits. Blood flow continues through these systems and returns to the heart, by way of capacitance (venous) vessels, as a result of pressure gradients.

Impedance to this flow is known as resistance. Many variables influence or determine resistance: the velocity of flow, the change in pressure or pressure gradient, the viscosity of blood, the length of the vessel, and the cross-sectional area.

The above variables can be expressed as mathematical equations. This first equation expresses the basic interrelationships among flow, pressure, and resistance:

$$Q = \frac{\Delta P}{R},$$

where Q is blood flow, ΔP is the pressure gradient, and R is the resistance. A second equation expresses the relationship between the mean velocity of blood flow and vascular diameter. The mean velocity (an integration of all measured velocities within one given vessel) can be expressed as

$$V = \frac{Pr^2}{8nl},$$

where V is the mean velocity, P is the pressure, r is the radius of the vessel, l is its length, and n is the blood viscosity. The third equation incorporates the concept that flow equals velocity times the cross-sectional area of the blood vessel (Q = $V\pi r^2$), substituting the value for velocity from the equation presented above. This third equation is known as Poiseuille's law:

$$Q = \frac{\pi \Delta P r^4}{8nl}.$$

These fluid dynamic equations have many applications to children in the shock state. For example, in the child with hypovolemia it is apparent that there is a significant decrease of the intravascular volume, which will result in a decreased pressure gradient and decreased flow. Within certain limits, the body can compensate for this and maintain flow by increasing peripheral resistance (i.e., by decreasing the diameter of peripheral vascular resistance vessels). If the body is unable to compensate adequately, it is possible to intervene with medical, surgical, or pharmacological therapy if the relationships presented above are kept in mind.

Cardiac output and venous return. Cardiac output and venous return (preload) are two important parameters of myocardial pump function. Because it is frequently necessary to invasively monitor these values in critically ill children in shock states, clinicians must be aware of their derivation in order to deliver optimally informed patient care.

Cardiac output (CO) is defined as the quantity of blood ejected from the left ventricle in 1 minute and is equal to the heart rate times the stroke volume (the volume of blood ejected from the left ventricle in one heart beat). It can be measued as liters per minute or liters per square meter of body surface area, the latter measurement referred to as the cardiac index (CI). Normal CI values range from 2 to 5 liters/min/m^2. The CI is a more useful measurement than the CO because it incorporates body size and differences in metabolic activity. Thus, measured values are noted to be higher in younger age groups and lower in older age groups.

The Frank-Starling law of the heart relates venous return to CO. This law states that the heart has the intrinsic ability to adapt to changing volumes of inflowing blood by generating a more forceful contraction in direct proportion to the amount of left ventricular and diastolic stretch of the myofibrils (i.e., within physiological limits). The ability of the heart to contract with increasing force as the preload increases is known as the heterometric autoregulation of the heart.

Preload, which in most instances is directly proportional to the left ventricular end-diastolic pressure (LVEDP), represents the rate of venous return to the heart and is the most significant determinant of CO (Fig. 7-1). It is important to note that venous return from the peripheral circulation will control the CO whenever the pumping action of the heart is greater than the rate of venous return. That is, the healthy heart will accept and circulate all inflowing volume within its physiological limits.

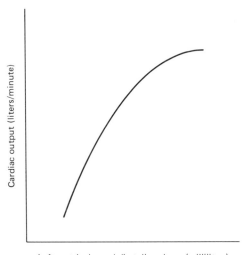

Left ventricular end-diastolic volume (milliliters)

Figure 7-1. Diagram of a Frank-Starling curve, relating ventricular end-diastolic volume to ventricular performance (cardiac output).

Capillary dynamics and transcapillary exchange. Blood flow is directed into the microcirculatory unit by way of a single, muscular arteriole, then through smaller-diameter, less muscular metarterioles. Capillaries arise at the level of the metarteriole, then undergo profuse branching. Capillaries can be divided into two types: (1) the preferential or thoroughfare capillaries, which potentially serve as shunt vessels, and (2) the true capillaries, across which nutrient and gas exchange actually occurs. The profuse branching of the capillaries results in a greatly increased surface area across which exchange can take place. In addition, the branching results in a much slower velocity of blood flow, thereby allowing more time for exchange to occur. Blood flow into the network is largely controlled by precapillary sphincters — muscular bands surrounding the point of origin of the capillaries from the metarterioles. Once blood passes through the capillary bed, it is collected by venules and directed back to the heart by the venous capacitance system.

Precapillary sphincter tone is primarily controlled by tissue oxygen concentration. As tissue oxygen demands increase, the precapillary sphincter relaxes and allows greater blood flow to the subserved capillary bed. Other controls of precapillary sphincter tone include various vasoactive substances (carbon dioxide, electrolytes, histamine, lactic acid, and humoral factors).

The control of precapillary sphincter tone is clinically significant with regard to the different types and stages of shock. In high output shock, the capillary system is overwhelmed with a large volume of blood flow. This results in large amounts of blood being shunted away from the capillary bed, with little net flow available for nutrient and gas exchange. In low output shock states, there is a compensatory peripheral vasoconstriction in an attempt to maintain blood pressure, adversely decreasing blood flow to the capillary network. This results in tissue hypoxia and lactic acidosis.

Transcapillary exchange takes place across the capillary membrane through fenestrations. The net bidirectional flow across the membrane is dependent on two factors: the *hydrostatic* and *osmotic* pressure differences between intravascular and interstitial fluid. Plasma osmotic pressure is determined principally by plasma proteins, particularly albumin.

Any alteration in capillary membrane integrity could result in large fluid shifts between the intravascular and interstitial compartments. This alteration in membrane integrity occurs in shock and predisposes the child to intravascular volume loss (*see* Pathophysiology of Shock, p. 425).

Cellular physiology. The major function of the circulatory system is to provide oxygen to the tissues perfused. Oxygen is necessary for the highly efficient catabolism of glucose (by means of aerobic glycolysis) through which the bulk of the body's energy is produced in the form of adenosine triphosphate (ATP). Without available oxygen, as with the decreased tissue perfusion of shock states, the body resorts to the much less efficient anaerobic form of glycolysis. Anaerobic glycolysis results in the accumulation of toxic products, especially lactic acid. Without sufficient amounts of ATP available, numerous cell functions cannot occur. One of the more important ATP-dependent mechanisms that is adversely affected is the sodium-potassium pump. Without its proper functioning, cells can be lysed by the influx of sodium and water. Once the cell is lysed, toxic substances (e.g., potassium and enzymes) are released into the general circulation, and this can further potentiate the shock state.

Controls of mean arterial blood pressure. Common to all types of shock is a state of hypotension. The body attempts to compensate for this drop in pressure through the use of hormonal and neurological controls. These compensatory responses can be further divided into rapid-acting and long-term pressure control mechanisms.

Rapid-acting neurological responses: The most important rapid-acting neurological mechanism is the baroreceptor reflex. Baroreceptors are highly specialized nerve endings located in the aorta, internal carotids, and carotid sinuses, which sense changes in arterial pressure. When these receptors are stimulated by increased intravascular pressure, they reflexly decrease heart rate and the force of contraction by increasing vagal tone, and they cause vasodilation by inhibiting the vasoconstrictor region of the medulla. Conversely, hypotension causes decreased stimulation of the baroreceptors, decreased vagal tone, and a concomitant increase in the sympathetic tone of the heart, resulting in more rapid and forceful contraction. In addition, there occurs a deinhibition of the vasoconstrictor region of the medulla, permitting an increase in vascular tone.

Another rapid-acting neurological mechanism is the central nervous system (CNS) ischemic response. When there is a significant drop in the mean arterial pressure beyond the autoregulatory control range of the cerebral vascular system, cerebral ischemia occurs. Consequently, carbon dioxide and other toxic metabolites accumulate in the vasomotor center. This is thought to cause overactivation of the vasomotor center in an attempt to maintain an adequate mean arterial pressure and to ensure sufficient cerebral blood flow. The end result, however, is massive peripheral vasoconstriction, which can be so profound that the peripheral vessels become almost completely occluded. The CNS ischemic response is the most powerful sympathetic vasoconstrictor response to hypotension. The chemoreceptor response also plays a significant role in the maintenance of mean arterial blood pressure (*see* p. 359).

Rapid-acting hormonal responses: In addition to causing direct stimulation of vascular tissue, the sympathetic vasoconstrictor response also results in the release of epinephrine and norepinephrine from the adrenal medulla. These catecholamines can be considered an extension of the sympathetic nervous system because they circulate to the heart and cause an increase in heart rate and force of contraction. They also circulate to other areas within the body that have no direct sympathetic nervous innervation (such as the metarterioles), resulting in vasoconstriction.

When kidney perfusion is decreased, the juxtaglomerular cells begin to secrete renin into the bloodstream. Renin converts angiotensinogen (a plasma protein) into the peptide angiotensin I, which, in turn, is converted into the hormone angiotensin II by a specific converting enzyme found predominantly in the lungs. Angiotensin II is the most powerful vasoconstrictor known and has direct vasoconstrictor effects on vascular tissue, especially the arterioles. Constriction of the arteries will result in an overall increase in peripheral vascular resistance, thereby raising the arterial pressure (*see* p. 359).

There is also some vasoconstriction of the venous capacitance vessels by angiotensin II. This improves the overall circulation by increasing venous return to the heart, thereby aiding the heart in pumping effectively against the increased resistance. Other effects of angiotensin II are related to the regulation of fluid via the release of aldosterone and are considered long-term compensatory mechanisms.

The last rapidly acting mechanism for arterial pressure control is vasopressin or antidiuretic hormone (ADH). This hormone is released by the posterior pituitary gland when hypoperfusion exists. The released vasopressin has direct vasoconstrictor effects on the circulatory vessels and increases arterial pressure by increasing total peripheral resistance. Vasopressin also plays an important role in the long-term maintenance of arterial pressure by means of its antidiuretic effect.

Long-term pressure control: The long-term control of arterial pressure is dominated by the renal-body fluid system, which incorporates the aldosterone control system. Aldosterone is a mineralocorticoid secreted by the adrenal cortex that acts on the renal tubules to increase the reabsorption of sodium and water. Thus, aldosterone functions to control arterial pressure through the regulation of intravascular volume.

The renal-body fluid system controls pressure and regulates vascular volume through a series of feedback mechanisms. When the arterial pressure falls, the kidneys attempt to increase vascular volume through the reabsorption of salts and water. This increase in volume results in increased venous return and, therefore, increased CO.

Conversely, if the arterial pressure increases, the kidneys will excrete large quantities of fluid. This fluid will markedly reduce both extracellular and intravascular volume, with a subsequent decrease in venous return and CO (*see* p. 360).

It is vital for the clinician to be able to recognize when compensatory mechanisms are called into action to maintain adequate tissue perfusion during shock states. Furthermore, it is equally necessary for the clinician to have sufficient understanding of the mechanisms to be able to discern when the patient is failing to compensate — a situation that would require early effective intervention to be implemented.

Principles of Care

Shock is a pathophysiological state characterized by profound tissue hypoperfusion and hypoxia, resulting in the disruption of coordinated organ functioning. The primary principle of care for children in shock is to prevent hypoperfusion and hypoxia, and thereby to preserve organ functioning. To achieve this primary goal efficiently, the critical care team must manage their patient according to a carefully planned, systematic approach that is based on more tangible secondary principles.

First, the accurate diagnosis of shock must be established. Second, any remaining organ functioning must be optimized to prevent further decompensation. Finally, coordinated organ functioning must be reestablished in order to return the child to his premorbid state.

The most important information used to make the diagnosis of shock is obtained by meticulous physical examination. The intensive care nurse plays a key role in the diagnosis of shock by continually monitoring the child at the bedside. Thus, the nurse is able to perceive subtle, early indicators of impending shock, thereby allowing early aggressive intervention to occur. With this responsibility comes that of having a firm grasp of normal human physiology. This is particularly important because, in general, abnormal pathophysiological events cannot be fully understood without first comprehending the normal physiological state. With this knowledge, deterioration to a catastrophic state can often be avoided.

The most significant variable for the prevention of further organ damage is the early establishment of the diagnosis of shock, which allows for the early application of specific shock measures. These specific modalities are most notably cardiovascular and respiratory support — frequently in the form of volume replacement, the use of vasoactive amines, and oxygen therapy. The intensive care nurse is responsible for monitoring the effects of the therapy initiated and to be aware of potential untoward effects of the specific therapeutic modalities that are used. Furthermore, the nurse must be aware of the different available treatment options so that the institution of a specific treatment can be facilitated. If these efforts are successful, normal coordinated organ functioning can be restored.

The critical care nurse with refined physical assessment skills is a valuable member of the critical care team and may (1) assist in making the early diagnosis of shock, (2) initiate the specific therapeutic intervention chosen, and (3) coordinate the efforts of the critical care team.

Assessment of the Child in Shock

The effectiveness of care rendered to shock patients depends largely on the skills possessed by the intensive care clinician. Excellent fundamental skills, insightful assessment skills, and a working knowledge of the various technically complex support systems are all necessary. Of these, however, assessment skills are probably the most important because the shock state is one of dynamically changing organ dysfunction.

Because of the multisystem involvement, the following discussion of initial assessment will adopt the review-of-systems approach. This section will deal only with specific assessments associated with shock states. (*See* Chapters 2, 3, 4, and 6 for more detailed information on respiratory, cardiac, neurological, and renal assessments.)

Respiratory system.   The most essential respiratory assessment skill is the ability to evaluate airway patency. This is of special concern in those children presenting with shock associated with multiple trauma. Soft tissue swelling, direct cervical and thoracic trauma, and mechanical obstruction can result in complete airway blockage. Auscultation of the lungs and monitoring of chest excursion will allow the clinician to determine effective airway entry.

The child's respiratory rate must be monitored at all times because the stressed child in shock may exhibit great variance in rate. Depending on age, the physical maturity of the child, and the stage of shock, this variance can range from apnea to hyperventilation. Infants and younger children will most likely present with apnea because of their inability to sustain an effective intrinsic response to the metabolic acidosis associated with shock states. The older child's presentation is much like that of an adult, usually exhibiting an initial period of hyperventilation, which is attributed to the body's attempt to compensate for a state of metabolic acidosis. In the initial stages of shock, one can expect little or no deviation in arterial blood gas values although a slight respiratory alkalosis may exist. This alkalosis is a direct result of a lowered partial pressure of arterial carbon dioxide ($PaCO_2$) during hyperventilation. It is vital to note when the hyperventilating child begins to tire, for if the intrinsic ability to compensate is lost, the child rapidly becomes acidotic and may die unless there is the intervention of mechanical assistance.

Auscultation of the lungs for adventitious or diminished breath sounds is an important aspect of the complete clinical assessment of respiratory functioning. The presence of rhonchi, rales, pleural friction rubs, and diminished breath sounds should provide the impetus for a more extensive evaluation. For example, an infant can rapidly develop sepsis secondary to pneumonia, particularly with a fulminant type such as that caused by beta-hemolytic *Streptococcus*. The pneumonia may have initially presented as a few localized rhonchi. Thoracic trauma can result in a life-threatening hemopneumothorax, which initially may have been manifested by diminished apical and basilar breath sounds.

Additional signs of hypoxic distress include the use of accessory muscles for respiration, nasal flaring, cyanosis, and alterations in consciousness.

Routine chest x-rays and frequent arterial blood gas determinations are a necessity. The responsible clinician should be able to detect deviations from the patient's base-line status and to interpret arterial blood gas values in relation to the patient's clinical status.

Cardiovascular system. Measurement of systolic, diastolic, and mean arterial blood pressures provides the clinician with a rough estimate of the amount of circulating volume within the cardiovascular system. If the arterial pressure is within the normal range, one can, in general, assume that adequate tissue perfusion exists. Any deviation within this system, whether it be volume depletion or structural alteration, will be reflected in the pressure reading.

It may be difficult to auscultate a cuff pressure on an infant or small child, especially if the child is indeed in shock. An alternative is the palpation method, but, if the child's pressure cannot be palpated, ultrasound or invasive monitoring is necessary.

It is of clinical importance to note that low arterial pressure alone does not confirm the diagnosis of shock. Cuff pressures are frequently inaccurate because of peripheral vasoconstriction secondary to the excessive release of catecholamines triggered in the stressed patient. In addition, cuff pressures can differ from true arterial pressure by an average underestimation of 15 mmHg, with an even greater deviation in some patients.[1]

The diagnosis of shock is established by demonstrating either directly or indirectly that a state of tissue hypoperfusion exists. Thus, it is possible to have two patients of the same age with equally low arterial blood pressures, yet one may have no difficulties whereas the other may be in a state of shock. It is apparent, then, that there are other cardiovascular parameters besides arterial pressure that can be monitored in order to assess the patient's clinical status (i.e., the perfusion of specific organs, the character of the peripheral pulse, and capillary refill).

An important feature of tissue perfusion is blood flow. The monitoring of vital organ functioning is essential in determining if flow is adequate. Intact cerebral and renal functioning is the most important indicator of perfusion adequacy because these organs are the most sensitive to disruption of flow: level of consciousness and urine output are the two most important parameters to be monitored in patients in shock.

Also part of a complete cardiovascular evaluation is the palpation and evaluation of central and peripheral pulses, capillary refill, and skin temperature. These three parameters are reliable indicators of total blood flow (CO) and peripheral perfusion. Peripheral pulses should be graded on a standardized scale to ensure consistency and accuracy (Table 7-1). Capillary refill is easily assessed by depressing nail beds until blanching occurs. With the release of pressure, base-line color should return within 3 seconds. If color return exceeds 3 seconds, capillary refill is sluggish and indicates an alteration in peripheral perfusion.[2]

As vital as it is to monitor the respirations of children in shock, it is equally vital to monitor their heart rate. Again, depending on age, the physical maturity of the child, and the stage of shock, there can be a great variance of heart rate. Infants and younger children cannot effectively respond to hypotension and subsequently become bradycardic in response to this stressful state. Older children should

TABLE 7-1 Standardized Scale for Clinical Assessment of Peripheral Pulse Volume

Numerical value	Description
0	The pulse cannot be palpated.
1	The pulse is difficult to locate. It is weak and thready and obliterates easily with light pressure.
2	The pulse is difficult to locate; however, once it is located, it is stronger than 1. The pulse may also be obliterated, so light palpation is necessary.
3	The pulse is easily located. It does not become obliterated as easily with pressure. It is considered to be of normal volume.
4	The pulse is easily located. It is strong, bounding, and hyperactive. It does not obliterate with pressure. In some cases (e.g., aortic regurgitation), it may be considered pathological.

Adapted with permission from Miller, K. M. 1978. Assessing peripheral perfusion. *American Journal of Nursing.* **78:**1674.

exhibit an effective intrinsic response to hypotension through an induced tachycardia. This tachycardia is an important catecholamine-mediated compensatory response to hypovolemia and a baroreceptor-mediated response to various types of shock. It should be noted, however, that a number of other factors may induce tachycardia (e.g., pain, anxiety, fever, and various sympathomimetic and anticholinergic medications).

Renal system.   As mentioned above, urine output is one of the best indicators of adequate CO, because CO is directly related to renal blood flow, and renal blood flow is directly related to urine production. A urinary catheter should be inserted in all children in shock so that hourly urine flow can be monitored. Frequent measurement of specific gravity and screening of urine samples for gross hematuria, proteinuria, glycosuria, ketonuria, and pH should be considered routine. In addition, base-line renal function studies, urine and serum electrolytes, and urine and serum osmolality should be obtained and monitored. In situations in which such laboratory data are not readily available, monitoring the urine for gross hematuria and concentration, as well as monitoring the traumatized child for flank tenderness and guarding, assume a greater degree of importance. Clinical evaluation of hydrational status is also necessary in determining patient management in terms of fluid replacement. Because infants and small children exhibit a greater percentage of water per body weight than adults, they are extremely sensitive to fluid loss. Signs of dehydration include sunken orbits, depressed fontanels, dry mucous membranes, poor skin turgor, and oliguria.

Gastrointestinal system.   There are numerous medical and surgical pediatric gastrointestinal disorders that may precipitate the shock state in children. Among the medical disorders are (1) severe diarrhea and/or persistent vomiting resulting from a number of enterotoxic viruses and bacteria, (2) pseudomembranous enterocolitis associated with antibiotic usage, (3) dietary intolerance (e.g., lactose intolerance), and (4) any acute gastrointestinal insult. The surgical problems include abdominal trauma, bowel obstruction, perforation, volvulus, and intussusception. Necrotizing enterocolitis can also precipitate shock. Any infant or child exhibiting signs of shock associated with the above disorders requires a complete gastrointestinal evaluation consisting of a thorough physical examination, blood chemistry studies, hematologic surveillance studies, blood cultures, appropriate radiographic studies, and nasogastric and peritoneal lavage in the face of abdominal trauma (*see* p. 450).

It is apparent that a wide range of gastrointestinal disorders can be associated with hypovolemic, hemorrhagic, and septic shock states. Strict attention must be paid to the following nursing assessments to allow for early warning of impending gastrointestinal decompensation. All stools should be evaluated for hematochezia, melena, and occult blood. Rectal swabs should be sent for bacterial culture and sensitivity whenever diarrhea becomes apparent. Bowel sounds should be assessed for quality to aid in the recognition of paralytic ileus or mechanical obstruction. If a nasogastric tube is in place, gastric fluid should be monitored for the presence of blood. In addition, the gastric pH should be checked frequently, since a pH of less than 5 is associated with an increased incidence of stress ulcer. Abdominal girths may be measured at regular intervals to check for the accumulation of fluid within the peritoneal cavity.

CNS. Persistent hypoxia and hypotension can alter the level of consciousness. This alteration can range from lethargy to combativeness, disorientation, or coma. Strict attention must be given to the neurological functioning of those in shock. (*See* Chapter 4 for nursing assessment of the CNS.)

Miscellaneous assessments. There are a number of other important manifestations of shock that cannot be easily categorized within one system. Ischemic and/or traumatized tissue can result in a bleeding disorder known as disseminated intravascular coagulopathy (DIC) (*see* p. 431). It is important to monitor children for signs of occult and frank bleeding. This should include testing stools and vomitus for blood, monitoring for prolonged bleeding from venipuncture sites, watching for oozing at indwelling catheter sites, and assessing the skin for bruising, petechiae, and purpuric rashes. The clinician should also monitor the child for signs of cerebral bleeding manifested by a change in level of consciousness, tenseness of the fontanels, evidence of temperature instability, pupillary changes, and seizurelike activity. As an adjunct to clinical assessment of bleeding disorders, coagulation studies including prothrombin time (PT), partial thromboplastin time (PTT), fibrin split products (FSP), platelet count, hemoglobin, and hematocrit should be followed closely.

Stress causes an increase in catecholamine release from the adrenal medulla. This results in a transient hyperglycemic state, followed by a prolonged hypoglycemia. Any increase in glucose metabolism is of special concern when dealing with infants because they become hypoglycemic quite rapidly as a result of liver immaturity and deficient glycogen stores. Hypoglycemia can result in irreversible brain damage and should be monitored clinically by watching for drowsiness or lethargy, for signs of catecholamine excess such as tachycardia and tremulousness, and for seizurelike activity. Blood glucose levels can also be easily followed by Dextrostix determination and by serum glucose as measured by laboratory analysis.

In addition, the presentation of septic neonates is often nonspecific. These infants can present with unexplained apnea and bradycardia, seizures, jaundice, diarrhea, abdominal distention, hepatomegaly, splenomegaly, lethargy, and temperature instability. Hypothermia can be the first sign of stress, such as sepsis, in infants and small children. This drop in body temperature can result from a large surface area to body mass ratio, a relative deficiency of subcutaneous fat, and a decreased ability to produce heat by shivering. In most instances, hypothermia can be reversed through the use of Isolettes, overbed warmers, and warming blankets.

Pathophysiology of Shock

The following discussion will provide an overview of the pathophysiology of shock, especially with regard to septic and hypovolemic shock, since these are most common in the pediatric age group. The greater part of this section will deal with septic shock as a prototype of the shock syndrome.

Epidemiology of septic shock.   All children exposed to certain infectious agents, but particularly those children with impaired host defense mechanisms, are susceptible to infection and, ultimately, to a state of septic shock. The human body has an armamentarium of defenses against bacterial, fungal, viral, and parasitic invasion. These mechanisms include normal skin integrity, nasal cilia and tracheobronchial mucus, secretory immunoglobulin (IgA), gastric acidity, the humoral and cellular immune systems, and bacterial interference by the normal flora with which the host is colonized. When there is a disruption in any of these mechanisms, an avenue for infection is established. Clinical examples of altered host defense mechanisms leading to an increased susceptibility to infection include artificial airways, operative incisions, and second- and third-degree burns. Any child in an intensive care unit with invasive monitoring lines in place is at increased risk for developing localized and systemic infections. Sepsis, in particular gram-negative sepsis, has increased to such an extent that it is now a common complication of the critically ill.[3] Other children who are at particular high risk for infection are those who are immunosuppressed as the result of a primary immunologic disorder or, more commonly, who are iatrogenically immunosuppressed via oncological chemotherapy or for organ transplantation.

Infants are also more susceptible to septicemia because of the immaturity of their immune system, as compared with that of older individuals. This increased susceptibility is thought to be due to deficient serum levels of IgM, impaired phagocytosis resultant from less opsonization, and complement levels 50 to 75 percent less than that of adults.[4]

Inappropriate antibiotic choice or use may be responsible for the development of more virulent and resistant organisms, and this renders a child more prone to developing a septic state as opposed to a simple infection. More importantly, however, the vast proliferation of different antibiotics within the past decade has been responsible for more virulent organisms, especially in nosocomial infections.

Finally, children demonstrating localized infection are more susceptible to seeding and, ultimately, to sepsis.

Epidemiology of hypovolemic shock.   The *sine qua non* of hypovolemic shock is the loss of intravascular volume, which can be caused by fluid shifting, hemorrhage, or general volume depletion. Specific examples of these causes include second- and third-degree burns, acute gastrointestinal decompensation, severe dehydration, intra- and postoperative hemorrhage, traumatic hemorrhage, and postoperative and traumatic fluid shifting.

Clinical presentation.   Common to all types of shock are three classical presenting signs — hypotension with subsequent oliguria and altered sensorium. However, it is clinically important to recognize, for diagnostic purposes as well as for management purposes, that the individual child's presentation will vary according to the specific stage of shock in which the child can be categorized.

TABLE 7-2 Clinical Presentation of Shock: Initial (Compensated) Stage

Clinical presentation	Septic shock	Hypovolemic shock
Vital signs		
Heart rate	Increased*†	Increased*†
Respiratory rate	Increased*†	Increased*†
Blood pressure	Decreased*	Decreased*
Skin temperature	Increased	No Change or decreased
Skin color	Flushed	Pale
Urine output	Decreased	Decreased
Level of consciousness	No change or decreased*	No change or decreased*
Hemodynamic parameters		
Mean arterial pressure	Decreased*	Decreased*
Central venous pressure	Increased	Decreased
Calculated systemic vascular resistance	Decreased	Increased
Cardiac index	No change or increased	Decreased
Arterial blood gas determinants		
pH	No change or slightly increased	No change or slightly increased
PaO₂	No change	No change
PaCO₂	Decreased*	Decreased*
Calculated shunt	Normal: 3–8%	Normal: 3–8%

$PaCO_2$, partial pressure of arterial carbon dioxide; PaO_2, partial pressure of arterial oxygen.
*Degree depends on neural and hormonal compensation.
†Varies depending on the age and physical maturity of the child.

There are three established stages of shock.[5,6] The initial stage can be referred to as the compensated stage, in which there is a significant reduction in arterial pressure that is adequately compensated for by neural and hormonal factors. The second stage of shock can be identified as the progressive (or the noncompensated) stage. With the development of this stage, the body can only partially compensate for the drop in blood pressure, and outside intervention (e.g., fluid resuscitation and pharmacological support) is required. This is a survivable state. The third stage is the end (or irreversible) stage of shock. In this stage, the fall in blood pressure is so profound that the body's intrinsic compensatory mechanisms fail, intervention with fluids and pressor agents have only transient beneficial effects, irreversible tissue damage is present, and the blood pressure will continue to fall until death occurs. (Tables 7-2, 7-3, and 7-4 offer a comparative overview of septic and hypovolemic shock throughout the clinical stages described above.)

Pathogenesis of septic shock. Septic shock can be defined as the shock state associated with overwhelming septicemia. This section will focus primarily on gram-negative bacillary sepsis because it is the most common type of septic shock seen in the hospital setting. Septic shock can occur with septicemia caused by gram-positive organisms and gram-negative cocci, as well as by fungi and viruses.

The shock state in gram-negative sepsis is thought to be caused by endotoxins found in the cell walls of gram-negative bacilli.[4] Endotoxin is a lipopolysaccharide (LPS) that exerts its deleterious effects when it is released from the cell walls of bacteria after they are lysed.

TABLE 7-3   Clinical Presentation of Shock: Progressive Stage

Clinical presentation	Septic shock	Hypovolemic shock
Vital signs		
Heart rate	Increased*†	Increased*†
Respiratory rate	Increased*†	Increased*†
Blood pressure	Decreased*	Decreased*
Skin temperature	Decreased	No change or decreased
Skin color	Pale	Pale
Urine output	Decreased‡	Decreased‡
Level of consciousness	Decreased*	Decreased*
Hemodynamic parameters		
Mean arterial pressure	Decreased*	Decreased*
Central venous pressure	Decreased	Decreased
Calculated systemic vascular resistance	Increased	Increased
Cardiac index	Decreased	Decreased
Arterial blood gas determinants		
pH	Decreased	Decreased
PaO_2	Decreased	Decreased
$PaCO_2$	Increased*	Increased*
Calculated shunt	>10%	>10%

$PaCo_2$, partial pressure of arterial CO_2; PaO_2, partial pressure of arterial oxygen.

*Degree depends on neural and hormonal compensation.

†Varies depending on the age of the child.

‡May be increased during the diuretic phase of renal failure.

TABLE 7-4   Clinical Presentation of Shock: End Stage

Clinical presentation	Septic shock	Hypovolemic shock
Vital signs		
Heart rate	Decreased	Decreased
Respiratory rate	Decreased	Decreased
Blood pressure	Markedly decreased	Markedly decreased
Skin temperature	Decreased	Decreased
Skin color	Pale	Pale
Urine output	Markedly decreased	Markedly decreased
Level of consciousness	Markedly decreased	Markedly decreased
Hemodynamic parameters		
Mean arterial pressure	Markedly decreased	Markedly decreased
Central venous pressure	Markedly decreased	Markedly decreased
Calculated systemic vascular resistance	Increased or decreased	Increased or decreased
Cardiac index	Markedly decreased	Markedly decreased
Arterial blood gas determinants		
pH	Markedly decreased	Markedly decreased
PaO_2	Markedly decreased	Markedly decreased
$PaCO_2$	Markedly increased	Markedly increased
Calculated shunt	>20–40%	>20–40%

$PaCO_2$, partial pressure of arterial carbon dioxide; PaO_2, partial pressure of arterial oxygen.

Biological characteristics of endotoxin: Endotoxin is known to cause fever, although the exact mechanism of this action is not clear. One possible mechanism is a direct action on the thermoregulatory center of the hypothalamus by which it may cause hypothermia or, more commonly, hyperthermia.[4] It is also possible that endotoxin may have an indirect hyperthermic effect by causing the release of endogenous pyrogens from leukocytes, reticuloendothelial cells, and possibly other tissues.

Many host defense mechanisms are affected by their interaction with endotoxin. These interactions can either cause harmful inflammation or interfere with the normal functioning of these defense mechanisms. LPS is known to activate the alternate (and possibly the classical) complement pathway.[4] Activated factors and complexes produced by activation of the complement pathway cause such varied effects as leukostasis and clumping, neutrophil chemotaxis, and direct endothelial damage. It is important to note that endotoxin is a prototype for septic shock and that the same state can be caused by direct injury of host tissue by fungi, viruses, and parasites.

It is thought that endotoxin may interact with factor XII (the Hageman factor) of the clotting cascade and with complement factor 3, thus causing DIC.[4,7] with the onset of DIC, further microvascular damage can occur as the result of microembolization, which can aid in the propropagation of DIC and the original shock state. From the cellular and endothelial tissue damage noted above, a number of substances with potent effects on vascular smooth muscle and endothelial integrity are released (e.g., histamine, serotonin, and kinins).

Cardiovascular effects of septic shock.   The following are the cardiovascular effects of septic shock for each of the three stages.

Initial stage: physiological events: The primary initiating cardiovascular event in the septic shock state is a marked peripheral vasodilatory response to the release of substances such as histamine and bradykinin. With the onset of peripheral vasodilation, the metarterioles and precapillary sphincters relax, allowing the capillary bed to become engorged. Because the capillary bed is unable to physiologically accommodate this increased flow, blood is shunted away from the capillary bed via arteriovenous shunt vessels. This shunting causes decreased oxygen exchange and increased lactic acid production by a reversion to anaerobic metabolism. With the use of kinetically less efficient anaerobic form of metabolism, less energy is available to cells. Specifically, the highly energy-dependent sodium-potassium pump begins to fail, allowing potassium to leak out of cells into the intravascular space. The free potassium and the increased hydrogen ion concentration produced by the acidosis both further potentiate arteriolar vasodilation.

Initial stage: clinical presentation: The marked peripheral vasodilation is evidenced clinically by a state of hypotension — the degree of which will be determined by the amount of neural and hormonal compensation that occurs. The hypotensive state is also manifested by oliguria secondary to decreased renal perfusion, by dulling of the sensorium if the intrinsic cerebral autoregulatory capacity is overcome by a sufficiently marked hypotension, and by the skin appearing warm and flushed because of the vasodilation.

Initial stage: hemodynamic parameters: There is a decrease in the mean arterial pressure (MAP) because of the peripheral vasodilation and a concomitant normal to increased central venous pressure because of the lowered total vascular resistance. This combination of events causes an increase in CO of up to two to three times the normal value.

Progressive stage: physiological events: The marked hypotension in the initial stage of shock persists in the progressive stage, causing further tissue and organ hypoperfusion. The disruption of capillary dynamics is more profound in this second stage of shock. Relative constriction of the postcapillary sphincters results in pooling and sludging of blood in the capillary bed. These effects cause an imbalance in the transcapillary exchange, yielding a net loss of fluid into the interstitium. This, compounded with the fluid loss caused by the endothelial damage and the resultant loss of plasma proteins (and thus of colloid osmotic pressure), further potentiates intravascular volume depletion. The body attempts to maintain an adequate MAP by peripheral vasoconstriction. In the progressive stage of shock, the most significant physiological event is vasoconstriction in response to intravascular volume loss. This vasoconstriction takes place far beyond compensatory parameters because numerous vasoactive substances are now circulating. Consequently, capillary beds are now greatly hypoperfused, even less oxygen exchange takes place, and tissue damage becomes more advanced.

Progressive stage: clinical presentation: The hypotension, altered sensorium, and oliguria of the initial stage of shock are still evident in the progressive stage. In addition, the skin is now cool and clammy because of the relative hypovolemia and peripheral vasoconstriction.

Progressive stage: hemodynamic parameters: Decreased MAP persists in the progressive stage of shock. There is an increase in overall vascular resistance because of an overwhelming vasoconstriction. Furthermore, venous return is diminished because of volume depletion and peripheral vasoconstriction. The net result is a decrease in central venous pressure and, depending on the extent of hypovolemia, the CO may be normal or decreased.

End stage: physiological events: The end stage of septic shock is marked by profound hypotension that cannot be compensated for by the body's intrinsic mechanisms or by medical intervention. There is persistent capillary leakage, leaving the intravascular compartment lethally depleted. At this point, the cells are so hypoperfused that they are totally dependent on anaerobic metabolism, which causes an irreversible state of lactic acidosis. With the depletion of energy stores, the sodium-potassium pump fails completely, resulting in an efflux of potassium from the cells, subjecting the child to lethal hyperkalemia and concomitant cardiac dysrhythmias. A host of toxic metabolites causes cellular lysis and death. DIC also progresses to the point at which multiple organ infarction commonly occurs. These events combine to cause irreversible cardiac depression until death occurs.

End stage: clinical presentation: In the end stage of shock, there is progressive clinical deterioration with multisystem failure marked by renal shutdown, coma, and myocardial depression.

End stage: hemodynamic parameters: There is progressive cardiovascular collapse evidenced by a profoundly decreased MAP, loss of vascular tone, and decreased venous return with a subsequent fall in CO.

Respiratory effects of septic shock.   Adult respiratory distress syndrome (ARDS), or shock lung, is a common, devastating complication of septic shock, as well as of shock states of any etiology. The primary site of insult in ARDS is the terminal respiratory unit of the lung (i.e., the alveolar-capillary unit). ARDS is acute respiratory failure (in the absence of upper airway disease) evidenced by (1) alveolar infiltrates, (2) decreased lung compliance, (3) decreased functional residual capacity (FRC), and (4) hypoxemia due to intrapulmonary shunting.[8,9]

It should be noted that the respiratory effects of septic shock, unlike the cardiovascular effects, do not lend themselves easily to physiological staging that is meaningful in terms of the overall progression of the shock state.

The first event to occur in the onset of ARDS is damage to the alveolar membrane. The exact underlying mechanism for this injury is unknown, but a number of possible explanations have been proposed, including microembolization, complement-mediated damage, and vasoactive substances.[9] All of these factors tend to directly alter membrane integrity. With the loss of membrane integrity, there is leakage of fluid as well as of plasma protein into the interstitium. This accumulation physically widens the space between the alveolar membrane and the capillary membrane, thus making diffusion of gases more difficult and increasing the alveolar-arteriolar oxygen difference (A-aDO$_2$). As the fluid accumulation between the alveolus and the capillary increases, pressure within this space is also increased, causing collapse of the alveolus. This results in worsened gas exchange. In the normal steady state, the lymphatics are able to compensate for minor increases in interstitial fluid. When ARDS first begins, they may initially handle this increased volume of fluid. As ARDS progresses, however, the lymphatics become engorged with fluid, either resulting in further alveolar collapse or in backflow of fluid into the alveoli (by mechanisms that remain unknown). The lungs are now stiff or less compliant, which results in a decrease in the FRC. This, in turn, causes a decrease in the ventilation to perfusion ratio and increases intrapulmonary shunting of oxygen. The end result of these pathophysiological changes is severe hypoxemia.

Initial stage: clinical presentation: In the initial stages of shock (that is not caused by a primary respiratory infection), there is no readily apparent respiratory distress. The patient, however, may clinically present with hyperventilation as an appropriate compensatory response. The lungs are found to be clear on auscultation. The chest x-ray is usually free from infiltrates.

Initial stage: blood gas determinants: The arterial blood gas will show that the patient has adequate oxygenation of blood at the alveolar-capillary site, demonstrated by a normal partial pressure of arterial oxygen (PaO$_2$) value and by an A-aDO$_2$ value of less than 20 mmHg. The PaCO$_2$ is found to be decreased, reflecting the hyperventilation that serves to compensate for the already developing metabolic acidosis. At this point, the pH is within a normal range.

Progressive stage: clinical presentation: There can be a wide range of pulmonary manifestations of shock during the progressive stage, depending on the extent of pulmonary insult. All children, however, evince some degree of respiratory distress, ranging from mild to severe. Clinical evidence of respiratory distress includes cyanosis, retractions, grunting, nasal flaring, and CNS dysfunction (e.g., lethargy or combativeness). Auscultation of breath sounds may reveal scattered rhonchi, basilar rales, and diminished breath sounds. Chest x-rays may demonstrate diffuse infiltrates.

Progressive stage: blood gas determinants: The arterial blood gas will show that the patient now has a disruption in oxygen exchange at the alveolar-capillary level, as evidenced by a falling PaO$_2$ and a rising A-aDO$_2$ of 25 to 40 mmHg despite the administration of supplemental oxygen. There will also be evidence of an increasing intrapulmonary shunt, with a calculated shunt of 10 to 20 percent. The child may still be able to compensate for the metabolic acidosis and exhibit a normal pH, or the pH may reflect a metabolic acidosis.

End stage: clinical presentation: Cyanosis, retractions, grunting, nasal flaring, and adventitious breath sounds are present as in the progressive stage of shock, but are now more pronounced. In addition, there is clinical evidence of severe hypoxemia to the extent that coma may be present. The chest x-ray now shows the confluence of previous infiltrates.

End stage: blood gas determinants: As with the progressive stage, there is poor oxygen exchange demonstrated by a decreasing PaO_2 in the face of escalated support, that is, higher inspired oxygen concentrations and positive end-expiratory pressure (PEEP). The A-aDO_2 continues to rise above 40 mmHg with a concomitant increase of the calculated shunt, which can now be greater than 20 to 40 percent. The patient is now hypercapneic (due to a persistent state of hypoventilation with a lowered tidal volume), and the pH reflects both a respiratory and a metabolic acidosis.

Renal effects of septic shock. Renal insufficiency is not an infrequent development in the progressive stage of shock. Renal compromise results most commonly because of renal hypoperfusion. This may occur either as a result of loss of intravascular volume (e.g., by hemorrhage, vomiting, or diarrhea) or because of redistribution of intravascular fluid, as occurs in septic shock. If this insult is prolonged, acute tubular necrosis may result.

Neurological effects of septic shock. Persistent hypoperfusion beyond the capability of the CNS to autoregulate may cause severe neurological insult. There may be clinical evidence of increased intracranial pressure due to an anoxic encephalopathy, precipitated by the accumulation of toxic metabolites such as potassium, lactate, and hydrogen ions.

Miscellaneous effects of shock. DIC, or consumptive coagulopathy, represents a series of syndromes associated with a very complex pathogenesis, diagnosis, and clinical management. It can be defined as a hypocoagulable state following a hypercoagulopathy. In general, DIC is characterized by the following: hypofibrinogenemia; thrombocytopenia; reduced levels of coagulation factors II, V, and VIII; the presence of fibrinolytic split products in the serum; and clinical evidence of bleeding. Although it is inferred that thrombin acting on fibrinogen is the basis for the disorder, there is no substantial amount of evidence to prove this. Exactly what activates the intravascular clotting is not known, but the conversion of fibrinogen to fibrin is the common denominator of all clinical entities with DIC.

Intravascular coagulation can occur to a variable degree in any child or newborn with infection, hypoxia, hypovolemia, or a metabolic derangement. The most common cause in the pediatric population, however, is bacterial septic shock.[10] The following is a complete listing of other precipitating causes:

Severe respiratory distress syndrome in newborns

Giant hemangiomas

Leukemia (especially promyelocytic leukemia)

Massive trauma

Burns

Snakebite

Rickettsial infections

Heatstroke

Viral illnesses

In order to understand the pathogenesis of DIC, it is necessary to be familiar with normal coagulation and fibrinolysis. At the center of normal coagulation is thrombin, which is produced by the cleavage of prothrombin by either the intrinsic or extrinsic coagulation system. The intrinsic system is activated by endothelial activation of factor XII and is analyzed by the PTT. The extrinsic system

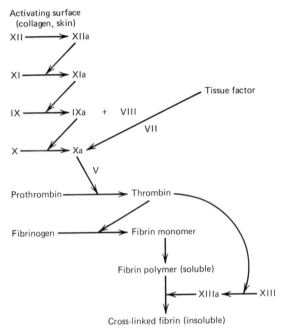

Activating surface
(collagen, skin)

Figure 7-2. Normal clotting pathways. (*See* text for discussion.)

is initiated by the activation of factor VII by tissue thromboplastin substances and is analyzed by the PT (Fig. 7-2). Thrombin has a number of different specific activities. First and foremost, it causes the cleavage of fibrinogen, resulting in the release of fibrin monomer (a substance that is soluble in plasma), fibrinopeptide A, and fibrinopeptide B. The fibrin molecules then polymerize and assume an insoluble configuration when acted on by activated factor XIII.

Factor XIII assumes an activated state by the action of thrombin, which also causes platelet aggregation. During their aggregation, platelets release platelet factor 4 and thromboglobulin. In large amounts, thrombin also causes the degradation of factors V and VIII.

The procoagulant activity of thrombin is normally balanced by the fibrinolytic activity of plasmin, which is formed by the cleavage of plasminogen by extrinsic factors released when cells are damaged. The activity of circulating plasmin is normally blocked by circulating plasmin inhibitors. When a fibrin clot forms, however, small amounts of plasmin are trapped within the clot, separate from the inhibitors, thus allowing plasmin to lyse fibrin. Plasmin can also lyse fibrinogen, fibrin monomer, and the unstabilized fibrin polymer. The products of these reactions are known as fibrinolytic split products (FSP) and possess anticoagulant properties of their own. They both slow the rate of fibrin polymerization and cause a disordered, weakened thrombus to form.

The occurrence of DIC in association with shock states is common, although the exact mechanism of activation remains unknown at present.[4] With specific regard to gram-negative bacterial septic shock, endotoxin has been shown experimentally to cause DIC by two mechanisms.[4,7] First, endotoxin may result in a

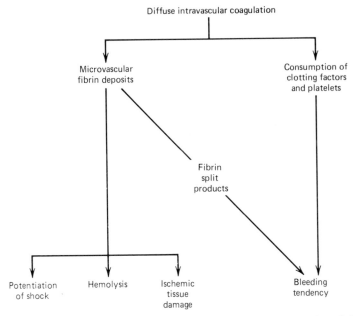

Diffuse intravascular coagulation

Microvascular fibrin deposits

Consumption of clotting factors and platelets

Fibrin split products

Potentiation of shock

Hemolysis

Ischemic tissue damage

Bleeding tendency

Figure 7-3. Disseminated intravascular coagulation: mechanisms producing clinical disease. *Adapted with permission from* Williams, W. J., E. Beutler, A. J. Erslen, and R. W. Rundles. 1972. Hematology. McGraw-Hill Book Co., New York. 1235.

coagulopathy through the direct activation of factor XII. Second, endotoxin may interact with platelets to cause the release of platelet factor 3 which, with calcium and factor V, may act on activated factor X to form thromboplastin complex. This, in turn, cleaves prothrombin to form thrombin. It is apparent, then, that septic shock may activate both the intrinsic and extrinsic pathways.

Once the clotting pathways become activated, diffuse intravascular clotting may occur, leading to deleterious effects by means of a number of different mechanisms. With diffuse clot formation, stores of platelets and clotting factors II, V, and VIII are depleted. This, in turn, causes an increased bleeding tendency. The formed microvascular clots may be partially lysed to yield FSP. These degradation products have anticoagulant properties and may also enhance the bleeding diathesis. Intravascular fibrin deposits within the microcirculation may also cause ischemic tissue damage and microangiopathic hemolytic anemia. The above events combine to potentiate the original shock state (Fig. 7-3).

The most common clinical manifestation of DIC is bleeding, usually from multiple sites. The hemorrhagic diathesis may manifest itself by petechiae of the skin and mucous membranes, oozing from venipuncture sites, and as gastrointestinal or CNS hemorrhage.

Pathogenesis of Hypovolemic Shock

Hypovolemic shock is caused by the loss of intravascular volume, which can result from hemorrhage, trauma, burns, or dehydration. The net effect of these different pathogenic mechanisms is loss of circulating volume and resultant tissue hypoperfusion. In this setting, the body attempts to maintain an adequate MAP by increasing peripheral vascular resistance. This compensatory vasoconstriction leads to a reduction in capillary blood flow and thus to a diminution of tissue nutrient and gas exchange. This relative tissue hypoxia causes a change from predominantly aerobic to anaerobic metabolism, resulting in further lactic acidosis. In addition, vasoactive substances such as kinins, histamine, and potassium are released. From this point, hypovolemic shock follows the same pathogenesis as septic shock, with the exception of the vasodilatory phase and its concomitant hemodynamic variables (*see* Tables 7-2, 7-3, 7-4).

Critical Care Management

When a child presents in a state of shock, the critical care team must make speedy but accurate assessments and then implement appropriate treatment in order to achieve an overall effective resuscitation. It is vital that the critical care team individualize and organize treatment priorities to best meet the demands of the child in shock. Because patient management depends on the patient's presenting clinical situation, it is often useful to separate critical care management into stages that correspond to the progression of the shock states.

Initial stage. Critical care management during this stage comprises two actions: resuscitation and stabilization.

Cardiovascular support: The first priority of cardiovascular support is the establishment of intravenous access via large-bore peripheral or deep femoral catheters to permit rapid fluid resuscitation. Initially, 10 to 20 milliliters of fluid per kilogram of body weight should be administered by rapid intravenous infusion. It is important to note, however, that 10 to 20 ml/kg should be used only as a guideline: enough fluid should be administered to raise the blood pressure to an acceptable level as determined by improved organ functioning.

The fluids used for resuscitation can be classified into three types: crystalloids, colloids, and whole blood products. Generally, fluid losses are replaced with fluid of the same composition. For example, with intra- and postoperative hemorrhage, volume losses are replaced with whole blood or blood products. However, in the emergent situation of acute shock states, any type or combination of fluid replacement is deemed acceptable. It is after the initial resuscitative phase, when the child is being stabilized, that the clinician has the responsibility to use more sophisticated determinants in selecting fluid replacement solutions. The direct or calculated measurement of the colloid osmotic pressure (COP) enables the clinician to determine when colloid solutions such as albumin and dextran are preferable to crystalloid solutions such as saline and lactated Ringer's solutions.[11,12] This is of special concern to clinicians caring for shock victims in the progressive stages with evidence of respiratory decompensation (*see* p. 429).

During the stabilization phase it is helpful to determine the intravascular volume status, which will help determine the rate of fluid replacement. This can be achieved by the utilization of specific clinical assessments, specific laboratory values (hemoglobin and hematocrit, serum/urine osmolality, and electrolytes), the insertion of a urinary catheter, and the placement of a central venous catheter. The central venous pressure (CVP) reading not only provides a rough estimate of intravascular volume but can also be used as a guide for fluid management. In general, vigorous replacement should persist if the CVP reading is 15 mmHg or less. When the CVP is 15 mmHg or greater, each case must be examined individually, frequently with the aid of additional invasive monitoring (i.e., pulmonary artery catheter) in order to determine the optimal CVP and whether vigorous fluid replacement should continue.

Respiratory support: The first priority of respiratory management during the initial shock state is the establishment of airway patency. Once this is ensured, it is necessary to evaluate aeration and ventilation. This is determined by specific physical assessments and diagnostic studies, i.e., arterial blood gas analysis and chest x-ray (*see* p. 33). In general, if the initial shock state presents in the absence of thoracic trauma or direct pulmonary insult, treatment priorities should be directed toward providing optimal cardiovascular support. However, because the shock state is one of metabolic or physiological hyperdynamics, the child's increased metabolic demands are best met with the administration of supplemental oxygen. Even if the arterial blood gas shows no evidence of acute respiratory decompensation, it is beneficial to institute oxygen therapy for the reasons mentioned above.

Renal support: The best way to ensure adequate renal functioning and to prevent significant insult is to ensure adequate perfusion, which is achieved through fluid support. Base-line renal function studies, intake and output, and routine dipstick testing will alert the clinician to early evidence of renal dysfunction.

Neurological support: The CNS is extremely sensitive to disruption in blood flow. In order to protect the child in shock from significant neurological insult, cerebral perfusion must be maintained through fluid intervention. Protection of the airway assumes priority if neurological impairment exists. The testing of airway reflexes is essential. Any evidence of a dulled sensorium with weak or absent airway reflexes necessitates intubation of the trachea for airway protection. In addition to checking for the metabolic causes of obtundation (e.g., hyponatremia, hypocalcemia, hypoxemia, or hypoglycemia), it is necessary to obtain blood and urine specimens for toxicology screening for any child who presents with an altered mental status.

Metabolic support: Shock is a hypermetabolic state that increases the need for available nutrients, especially oxygen. Fever can exacerbate this hyperdynamic state, thereby raising the cellular need for oxygen to an even greater extent. In addition, fever promotes a state of acidosis. Consequently, it is vital to control febrile episodes, which commonly occur in children with septic shock. The antipyretic of choice for the pediatric patient is acetaminophen, administered in doses of 10 mg/kg of body weight. The rectal route is suggested for administration in order to minimize the risk of aspiration if the need for tracheal intubation should arise. Aspirin compounds are contraindicated because of their effect on platelet adhesiveness and because of the child's already increased tendency to bleed (*see* p. 424).

Hyperthermia can also be controlled through the use of an electric cooling blanket. This method should be used with extreme caution in the pediatric patient because it is not without certain risks. Children treated with cooling blankets can experience the "drift phenomenon;" that is, after the blanket is turned off, the child's temperature may drop an additional 1 to 2°C (1.8 to 3.6°F). In addition, hypothermic injuries to the skin from prolonged direct contact with the cooling blanket are not uncommon.

Infants and small children in shock may present with hypothermia (*see* p. 424). It is vital that hypothermia be reversed because it results in a three- to fourfold increase in the minute volume of oxygen required and in impaired tissue perfusion with a reversion to anaerobic metabolism and acidosis. Prolonged hypothermia predisposes the child to lethal hyperkalemia, hypoglycemia, irreversible acidosis and, ultimately, death. Hypothermia can be reversed through the use of overhead warmers, Isolettes, and electric warming blankets.

Hyper- and hypoglycemic states are commonly seen in the child in shock regardless of its etiology. Profound hypoglycemia is particularly prevalent in the infant and small child, and can further exacerbate the already existent shock state. Frequent determinations of serum glucose levels are necessary in the prudent management of shock victims. These values are also used to determine the type of fluid support for the child. All infants should receive a 10 percent dextrose solution as intravenous maintenance, unless otherwise contraindicated. If the child is profoundly hypoglycemic (serum glucose level of less than 25 mg/dl), 4 ml/kg of a 25 percent dextrose solution should be administered over 5 minutes, and 2.5 ml/kg of a 10 percent dextrose solution should be administered over 5 to 10 minutes to neonates.[13] If hyperglycemia arises, management should include restriction of dextrose solutions and administration of insulin as necessary.

Miscellaneous support: The cause of shock must be eradicated in order to treat shock states effectively. For example, a child may hemorrhage postoperatively secondary to intra-abdominal arterial bleeding. The child may be stabilized with volume and inotropic agent support, but the only way to completely arrest the shock process would be to correct the bleeding sites surgically. Similarly, antibiotic therapy is one of the most important medical interventions in septic shock. One may halt septic shock by selecting the appropriate antibiotic(s) to eradicate the etiologic organism(s).

Often, the clinician is confronted with situations in which a patient clinically appears septic, but the source of the sepsis is not readily apparent. In these circumstances, cultures of blood, urine, sputum, stool, and cerebrospinal fluid should be obtained immediately. Once these specimens are collected, broad-spectrum antibiotic coverage — frequently with multiple-drug regimens — should be initiated. Once the organism is isolated and an antimicrobial sensitivity profile is obtained, it is often possible to select fewer (and/or less toxic) antibiotics to which the causative organism is susceptible.

Progressive stage. Critical care management during the progressive stage of shock involves (1) supportive therapy (an extension of the stabilization phase of the initial critical care management) and (2) aggressive anticipatory therapy directed toward halting the progressive clinical deterioration of the patient.

Cardiovascular support: The primary goal of shock management is to ensure adequate tissue perfusion. From the cardiovascular standpoint, this is achieved by maintaining adequate pump functioning in direct relationship to an appropriately compensated vascular system. The net result of the various pathophysiological processes that occur in the shock state can be depression of myocardial pump functioning with total vascular collapse. Certain specific interventions in patient management can potentially terminate or at least slow down the progressive stage of shock. The first of these interventions is intravascular fluid volume support. Beyond the initial fluid resuscitation, the clinician must consider more sophisticated physiological principles in order to deliver optimal cardiovascular support. Specifically, the clinician must fully understand the ramifications of the Frank-Starling law of the heart. This concept deals with the importance of venous return and its effect on CO (*see* p. 417). It is necessary to think beyond the obvious repletion of the volume of the vascular system and to consider the effects of various fluid volumes on myocardial functioning. That is, enhanced venous return ultimately results in increased ventricular filling, increased stretch of the myocardial musculature, and a more forceful contraction, yielding a higher CO. This indirectly results in improved tissue perfusion and improved cellular functioning.

More invasive monitoring techniques are required to obtain measurements of cardiac dynamics. The technique that provides the greatest amount of information is the use of the pulmonary artery catheter (Swan-Ganz catheter). It can be used to measure pulmonary artery occluded pressure, to obtain thermodilution CO measurements, and to determine pulmonary artery blood gas values. The pulmonary artery occluded (wedge) pressure (PAOP) is a measurement of the transmitted pressure of the left atrium and, during diastole, of the left ventricle. Hence, the PAOP is a very good estimate of the left ventricular filling pressure, which reflects venous return or preload status and myocardial contractility (see p. 113). CO can be measured by applying a hemodynamic principle called Fick's law, which, in essence, states that the rate of flow can be established by measuring the rate of dilution of a tracer substance. This is accomplished by injecting a fixed amount of solution at a specified temperature at the proximal lumen and measuring the change in temperature at the distal lumen (see p. 117). Base-line CO is established by this method and is frequently reassessed in order to objectively monitor the adequacy of volume and inotropic agent support.

Mixed venous oxygen tension can only be accurately measured in the pulmonary artery. This is an averaged measurement of the oxygen in venous blood from throughout the body. It is useful because it reflects tissue perfusion as considered with other hemodynamic variables such as CO and the arterial-venous oxygen content difference (CaO_2-CvO_2).[14] Normal mixed venous oxygen pressure ($P\bar{v}O_2$) is 40 mmHg, and therapeutic modalities should be aimed at maintaining the $P\bar{v}O_2$ at this pressure. If the $P\bar{v}O_2$ begins to fall, this indicates that tissues are being hypoperfused and thus are extracting more oxygen per unit of blood. This drop in the $P\bar{v}O_2$ and an increase in CaO_2-CvO_2 are ominous signs of impending cardiovascular decompensation. The $P\bar{v}O_2$ and the CaO_2-CvO_2 will vary, depending on the patient's cardiac reserve or,.in essence, on their ability to increase the CO in response to increased physiological demands (Table 7-5).

In the progressive stage of shock, if the patient has not responded adequately to volume replacement and attempts to correct metabolic abnormalities, vasoactive drugs to correct hypoperfusion are indicated. To fully understand the actions and advantages of the different vasoactive drugs, one must first know the effect of stimulation of the different adrenergic receptors. Alpha-adrenergic (α-adrenergic) receptors are found predominantly in the arterial tree. Stimulation of these receptors results in vasoconstriction. In addition, α-adrenergic receptors are also found in the intestine and the iris, and stimulation at these sites causes intestinal relaxation and mydriasis, respectively. Beta-adrenergic (β-adrenergic) receptors are of two types: β-1 and β-2. The β-1-adrenergic receptors are found solely in the heart. Stimulation of β-1-adrenergic receptors causes increased heart rate, increased rate of contraction, and increased force of contraction. The β-2-adrenergic receptors are found in the bronchi, the arterial tree, and a number of other locations. Stimulation of these receptors causes bronchodilation and vasodilation, respectively.

The most commonly used vasoactive agent to treat shock is dopamine hydrochloride (Intropin).[15,16] This is a unique drug in that it has dramatically different actions, depending on the dosage at which it is administered. At low doses (1 to 2 μg/kg/min), dopamine stimulates specific dopaminergic receptors in the renal and mesenteric vasculature, causing increased renal blood flow and, thus, increased

TABLE 7-5 Predicted Pulmonary Artery Blood Gas Values in Health and Disease

Condition	$P\bar{v}O_2$		% Hb sat		CaO_2-$C\bar{v}O_2$	
	range	average	range	average	range	average
Healthy resting volunteer	37–43	40	70–76	75	4.5–6.0	5.0
Critically ill patient; cardiovascular reserves excellent	35–40	37	68–75	70	2.5–4.5	3.5
Critically ill patient, cardiovascularly stable; limited cardiovascular reserves	30–35	32	56–68	60	4.5–6.0	5.0
Critically ill patient; cardiovascular decompensation	<30	<30	<56	<56	>6.0	>6.0

Reprinted with permission from Shapiro, B. A., R. A. Harrison, and J. R. Walton. 1977. Clinical Application of Blood Gases. Year Book Medical Publishers, Inc., Chicago. Second edition. 232.

CaO_2-$C\bar{v}O_2$, arterial-venous oxygen content difference; % Hb sat., percentage of hemoglobin saturation; $P\bar{v}O_2$, mixed venous oxygen content.

glomerular filtration rate, urine flow, and sodium excretion. In the dose range of 2 to 10 μg/kg/min, the β-1-adrenergic receptors of the heart are stimulated to increase contractility and CO without a significant change in the heart rate or blood pressure, both by direct stimulation and by causing the release of endogenous stores of catecholamines. At 10 to 20 μg/kg/min, there is some α-adrenergic effect in addition to the β-1-adrenergic effects, resulting in increased heart rate and blood pressure. Above 20 μg/kg/min, alpha-stimulatory effects are predominant, causing marked vasoconstriction, increased blood pressure, and, perhaps, a counteracting of the dopaminergic effects on renal perfusion. Dopamine increases ventricular irritability and may occasionally induce dysrhythmias.

Isoproterenol hydrochloride (Isuprel) is an agent that possesses pure β-adrenergic stimulatory effects, affecting both the β-1- and β-2-adrenergic receptors. Hence, it causes vasodilation, a markedly increased heart rate (both directly and reflexly by its vasodilating effects), increased contractility, and increased CO (both by direct stimulation and by decreasing afterload by its vasodilating effect). Because of the vasodilating effects, however, the MAP may actually decrease with this agent, particularly if fluid replacement is not adequate. An additional adverse effect of isoproterenol is that it greatly increases myocardial irritability and susceptibility to potentially lethal dysrhythmias. The recommended dose of isoproterenol is 0.1 to 2.0 μg/kg/min, but it is important to titrate the dose to the desired effect.[17]

Dobutamine hydrochloride (Dobutrex) is the newest of the cardioactive sympathetic amines.[18] Although it is chemically related to isoproterenol, its actions are much more selective. Like dopamine, dobutamine acts directly on β-1-adrenergic receptors in the heart to increase the force and velocity of myocardial contractility, but it does not cause the release of norepinephrine from nerve endings. When administered in doses of less than 20 μg/kg/min, dobutamine has little effect on heart rate, slightly decreases peripheral arterial resistance, and causes a significant increase in CO. At high doses (20 μg/kg/min), dobutamine tends to act more like isoproterenol, causing more tachycardia and more vasodilation than at moderate doses. Although dobutamine may slightly increase the risk of ventricular dysrhythmias, it does not do so to nearly the same extent as either dopamine or isoproterenol.

Epinephrine is a naturally occurring catecholamine that is the prototypical vasoactive substance with which other vasopressors are usually compared. Epinephrine has both α- and β-adrenergic effects. The β-adrenergic effects, however, are predominant. In the doses commonly administered, epinephrine causes increased peripheral resistance and a concomitant increase in CO — both by increased inotropic and chronotropic effects. This combination of events results in an increased MAP. A significant disadvantage of epinephrine as opposed to dopamine, however, is that epinephrine decreases splanchnic perfusion. Another disadvantage includes marked peripheral vasoconstriction, resulting in decreased capillary perfusion and an increased heart rate, eventually leading to a decreased CO. The recommended dose range for epinephrine is 0.1 to 1.0 μg/kg/min.[18]

Sodium nitroprusside (Nipride) is an extremely potent vasodilating agent that acts independently of autonomic innervation of the vasculature. It causes direct dilation of both venous and arterial systems, and thus is useful in the treatment of cardiogenic pulmonary edema and advanced shock lung. Nitroprusside also reduced peripheral vasoconstriction, therefore increasing capillary blood flow. The usual dose range is 0.2 to 10 μg/kg/min, titrated accordingly.[20]

In summary, it is vital for all members of the critical care team to be familiar with the actions of the vasoactive drugs in order to allow for intervention with the appropriate drug and at the optimal time to yield the most beneficial results. In addition, a knowledge of the vasoactive drugs allows the health care team to quickly identify the potentially lethal adverse effects of these agents. A summary of the pharmacological actions of these drugs is provided in Table 7-6.

Respiratory support: Shock lung frequently results from the prolonged ischemia associated with shock states. Thus, a major part of the respiratory management of children in shock is oriented toward preventing or curtailing the primary etiology for the shock state. (*see* p. 429 for the pathophysiology of shock lung.) If the shock process has progressed to the point of causing significant pulmonary insult, the goal of management then becomes a supportive one and is essentially directed to ensuring ventilation-perfusion equality.

During the resuscitative phase of cardiovascular management, large amounts of fluid may be required to restore systemic perfusion. If significant pulmonary capillary damage has already occurred, excessive fluid administration can produce or exacerbate the formation of pulmonary edema. This sequence of events can quickly proceed to acute respiratory failure. It is apparent then that volume replacement must proceed carefully and with appropriate hemodynamic monitoring, particularly when the potential for shock lung exists.

The relative advantages and disadvantages of crystalloid versus colloid fluid replacement in ARDS remain very controversial and, hence, will not be discussed here. The relationship of the plasma COP to left atrial pressure has been used to assess the extent of fluid losses across the pulmonary capillary membrane.[21] In the early stages of ARDS, the pulmonary capillary wedge pressure is generally low or normal while pulmonary edema is present. This points to a defect in the pulmonary capillary membrane (as opposed to an elevated left atrial pressure secondary to decreased left ventricular functioning) as the cause of the noncardiogenic edema in shock lung. It is believed that a rapid equilibration of protein content occurs across the pulmonary capillary membrane during major leaks in the pulmonary capillary membrane. Therefore, it is suggested that crystalloid solution be administered in the early phase of ARDS and that colloid replacement be the fluid of choice in the later stages of shock lung.[21]

If there is clinical and roentgenologic evidence of interstitial pulmonary fluid after cardiovascular stability has been attained, then a potent diuretic such as furosemide should be administered. By decreasing the interstitial fluid with the use of a diuretic, one may improve oxygenation, as reflected by an increased PaO_2. The recommended dose of furosemide is 1 mg/kg of body weight, titrated to its expected response. In addition, an afterload reducing agent such as nitroprusside can be employed to reduce the pulmonary hypertension that may accompany shock lung. This potent vasodilator must be used with extreme caution in shock states. If severe or persistent hypotension develops, nitroprusside must be discontinued until the blood pressure is stabilized. Various sympathetic amines may be used in conjunction with nitroprusside to maintain peripheral perfusion.

Children who develop advanced shock lung will invariably require endotracheal intubation and ventilation. Because of the rapidly progressive nature of the onset of shock lung (from tissue damage to pulmonary edema, loss of lung volume, and hypoxemia), early intubation is a rational approach to respiratory management.

One of the means to determine the ventilation-perfusion equality is the arterial blood gas determination — specifically the PaO_2. Each child's expected PaO_2 should be calculated by taking his age and base-line pulmonary status into consideration. If concentrations of inspired oxygen greater than 50 to 60 percent are

TABLE 7-6 Pharmacological Actions of Various Agents Used to Treat Shock States

Parameter	Epinephrine	Dopamine	Isoproterenol	Dobutamine
Heart rate	Moderately increased	No appreciable change, or slightly increased	Markedly increased	No appreciable change
Cardiac contractility	Increased	Increased	Increased	Increased
Peripheral resistance	Increased	Slightly decreased	Decreased	No appreciable change, or slightly increased
Cardiac output	Increased	Increased	Increased	Increased
Mean blood pressure	Increased	No appreciable change, or slightly increased	Decreased	No appreciable change
Renal blood flow	Decreased	Markedly increased	No appreciable change	Slightly increased
Ventricular irritability	Markedly increased	Increased	Markedly increased	

required to maintain an acceptable PaO_2 or if the PaO_2 continues to drop or becomes unresponsive to such high oxygen concentrations, then endotracheal intubation is necessary — both to improve oxygenation and to prevent oxygen toxicity caused by exposure to high oxygen concentrations (*see* p. 46).

Restoration of the FRC by using PEEP or continuous positive airway pressure (CPAP) results in the reestablishment of small-airway and alveolar patency by producing a constant positive distending pressure.[9] Gas exchange is improved by expanding the alveoli and displacing an equal volume of fluid occupying the alveolar lumen back into the pulmonary interstitium. This fluid displacement results in improved gas diffusion. PEEP also improves the ventilation of gas-exchange units, thereby eliminating previous sites of intrapulmonary shunting. An additional benefit of PEEP is that it allows adequate oxygenation to occur at lower oxygenation concentrations, thus decreasing the risk of oxygen toxicity.

Children with shock lung as evidenced by increased intrapulmonary shunting usually respond well to incremental increases in PEEP with increased FRC and PaO_2. The use of PEEP, however, is not without significant risks. PEEP increases the mean airway pressure, which is transmitted to the pleural space and the great veins in the chest. This increased pressure results in decreased venous return to the heart and decreased CO. The occurrence of decreased CO with the use of PEEP has significant clinical implications. Even though PEEP may increase the PaO_2, the reduction in CO may actually decrease the total amount of oxygen delivered to the tissues. The systemic oxygen transport can be calculated by multiplying the CO by the arterial oxygen content (CaO_2). The effect of PEEP on systemic oxygen transport can be determined by the CO and CaO_2, or by monitoring the $P\bar{v}O_2$ (*see* p. 42). It should be noted, however, that in most instances reductions in CO by PEEP can be compensated for with the use of volume expanders such as albumin and fresh frozen plasma.

Another complication of PEEP is barotrauma, resulting in pneumothorax or pneumomediastinum. This occurs from the overdistention and rupture of less diseased alveoli. The incidence of barotrauma with different levels of PEEP is variable but should be anticipated in any child receiving PEEP. Once the diagnosis of pneumothorax is made, a chest tube must be inserted promptly.

It is vital to achieve a balance between the beneficial effects and the complications of PEEP therapy. At present, there is no agreement as to what level of PEEP is considered optimal and even what criteria should be used to define such suggested PEEP levels.[21] One proposal suggests that the optimal PEEP, or "best PEEP," is the level associated with maximal oxygen transport (Fig. 7-4).

If the child requires mechanical assistance, high tidal volumes (10 to 15 ml/kg of body weight) are preferred. Controlled ventilation (with or without neuromuscular blockage) is often required.

The use of corticosteroids in the treatment of shock lung remains controversial.[9] The possible beneficial effects of steroids are as follows: (1) prevention of complement activation; (2) stabilization of lysosomal membranes; (3) decreased tissue fibrosis; and (4) decreased alveolar hemorrhage and edema.[9] However, there is little clinical data to substantiate these effects at present.

Renal support: The first concern of the critical care clinician in dealing with the renal problems of the child in the progressive stage of shock is to correct the prerenal factors — those that cause renal hypoperfusion. In general, these factors are related to those that cause decreasing intravascular volume (e.g., vomiting, diarrhea, hemorrhage, third-space fluid losses, inadequate fluid intake, and

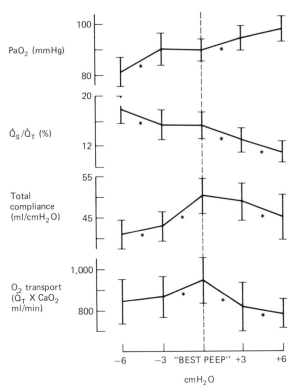

Figure 7-4. Effects of incremental increases in the positive end-expiratory pressure (PEEP) on the arterial oxygen tension (PaO$_2$), intrapulmonary shunt ($\dot{Q}_S/\dot{Q}_T$), total lung compliance, and oxygen (O$_2$) transport ($\dot{Q}_T \times CaO_2$ [arterial O$_2$ content]) in patients with acute respiratory failure requiring mechanical ventilation. "Best PEEP" is the point at which there is maximal respiratory compliance. Any increase in PEEP above the point identified as "best PEEP" will result in an increased PaO$_2$, a decreased $\dot{Q}_S/\dot{Q}_T$, and a decrease in O$_2$ transport. This decrease in O$_2$ transport is a direct result of a decreased cardiac output ($\dot{Q}_T$). The asterisks indicate significant change. $\dot{Q}_S$, shunted blood flow. *Reprinted with permission from Suter, P. M., H. B. Fairley, and M. D. Isenberg. 1975. Optimum end-expiratory airway pressure in patients with acute pulmonary failure. New England Journal of Medicine.* **292:**286.

diuretic therapy). Prerenal factors are directly corrected, if possible, and sufficient fluid volume is administered to return the patient to normovolemia. Another cause of renal failure that is particularly important in children with septic shock is hypotension that is beyond the ability of the kidneys to autoregulate. This problem can be much more difficult to manage, particularly when hypotension persists after volume replacement. In this setting, vasopressors (particularly low-dose dopamine) may help to maintain adequate renal perfusion.

Also important in renal management is the search for potentially toxic agents in the child's therapy, such as aminoglycoside antibiotics (especially in the hypoperfused kidney or with the concomitant use of cephalosporin antibiotics), iodinated contrast dyes, chemotherapeutic agents, and nonsteroidal anti-inflammatory agents. In addition, vasopressors used to maintain an adequate MAP may cause constriction of the renal vasculature.

Occasionally, patients recovering from acute renal failure may enter a diuretic phase (*see* p. 392). In this setting, adequate fluids must be administered to prevent dehydration.

Potent loop diuretics and mannitol are frequently used early in acute renal failure to try to turn an oliguric state into a nonoliguric one. The rationale behind this approach is to minimize morbidity and mortality, because nonoliguric renal failure has a more favorable prognosis than oliguric renal failure. Dialysis is indicated in acute renal failure to treat resistant hyperkalemia, severe acidosis, symptomatic uremia, and volume overload (*see* p. 398).

Metabolic support: The progressive stage of shock is characterized by a metabolic acidosis, which can cause a life-threatening diminution in myocardial contractility, diminished myocardial responsiveness to endogenous and exogenous catecholamines, and cation shifts resulting in potentially lethal hyperkalemia. It is felt that once tissue perfusion is reestablished, there will be a decrease in anaerobic metabolism, a decrease in lactic acid production, and a self-correction of the pH. Severe metabolic acidosis (pH ≤7.10), however, should be corrected with appropriate buffers, generally sodium bicarbonate. Sodium bicarbonate should be administered to correct one third of the base deficit by using the following calculation:[22]

$$\frac{\text{Base deficit} \times \text{weight (kg)} \times 0.3}{2}.$$

(For a newborn, the constant is 0.5; for a small child, 0.4.)

Overcorrection of acidosis must be avoided because severe alkalemia can be more dangerous than the original state of acidosis. When the arterial pH is greater than 7.80, the myocardium is much more prone to developing fatal dysrhythmias, cation shifts can cause severe hypokalemia, cerebral vasoconstriction decreases cerebral blood flow by one third, and the oxyhemoglobin curve is shifted to the right, resulting in less delivery of oxygen to tissues (*see* p. 29).

Hyperkalemia is a common, but life-threatening, electrolyte imbalance frequently associated with shock states. Hyperkalemia can result from failure of the cellular sodium-potassium pump, acidosis, or tissue necrosis, or it may be iatrogenic. Electrocardiographic abnormalities in hyperkalemia depend on the degree of the electrolyte disturbance. Mild hyperkalemia is associated with peaked T waves. Moderate hyperkalemia may result in flattening of the P wave, ST segment elevation or depression, slight widening of the QRS complex, first-degree atrioventricular (AV) block, and hemiblock (bundle branch block). Advanced hyperkalemia can cause various bi- and trifascicular blocks, premature ventricular contractions, ventricular dysrhythmias, and ventricular standstill.[23]

The treatment of hyperkalemia follows a twofold approach. Initially, attempts to temporarily reduce the serum potassium level are instituted. By shifting the extracellular potassium back into the cell and thereby lowering the serum potassium levels, myocardial irritability and the propagation of lethal dysrhythmias can be minimized. This can be accomplished by raising the serum pH with intravenous sodium bicarbonate (1 mEq/kg) and/or controlled hyperventilation, intravenous administration of 10 percent calcium gluconate (0.5 ml/kg) over 3 minutes, and, finally, the intravenous use of a solution which combines 8 milliliters of 50 percent

TABLE 7-7 Normal Pediatric Coagulation Laboratory Values

Factor	Value*
PT†	11–14 sec
PTT†	25–35 sec
Platelet count	150,000–400,000/ml
Fibrinogen	150–450 mg/dl
Fibrin split products	<10 μg/ml

PT, prothrombin time; PTT, partial thromboplastin time.

*May vary depending on the laboratory and the age of the child.

†Normal newborns may have a longer PT and PTT than older children.

dextrose solution in water with 1 unit of regular insulin (1 ml/kg).[24] Once the immediate danger of the initial hyperkalemic state is controlled, more definitive therapy can be employed. This involves decreasing the total body potassium supply through (1) restricting potassium intake, (2) administering potassium-binding ion exchange resins (i.e., sodium polystyrene sulfonate [Kayexalate], 1 g/kg via nasogastric lavage or an enema), and (3) using dialysis in the critical situation[25] (*see* p. 394).

Miscellaneous support: The first concern in the management of DIC is establishing a definitive diagnosis, which is made in the laboratory, although the presence of DIC can be strongly suggested by certain screening tests. Examination of the peripheral blood smear reveals fragmented red blood cells and a reduced platelet count. Other abnormal screening tests include prolonged PT and PTT values and a reduced fibrinogen concentration. The most commonly used specific tests for the diagnosis of DIC are (1) the measurement of factors II, V, and VIII and of the fibrinogen levels, and (2) detection of elevated levels of fibrin monomer and its complexes in the serum. In addition, the presence of fibrinopeptide A, platelet factor 4, or β-thromboglobulin in plasma, the short survival of platelets and fibrinogen *in vivo*, and evidence of fibrin deposition by biopsy all strengthen the diagnosis of DIC.

The differential diagnosis of DIC includes liver disease, vitamin K deficiency, dilutional states caused by massive volume replacement with coagulant and platelet poor materials, and sepsis without shock. Although these entities may have abnormal screening tests that are very similar to those of DIC, they do not have elevated levels of fibrin split products and fibrin monomers.

The management of DIC can be as difficult as making the diagnosis. The most important step in clinically managing DIC is to attempt to remove the initiating cause, which may consist of antibiotics for bacterial sepsis, surgery for trauma, chemotherapy and radiation therapy for malignancies, and general supportive measures. The second step in the management of DIC is to replace the depleted coagulant factors. Replacement therapy is initiated when the child exhibits hemorrhage, thrombosis, and abnormal laboratory values: platelets <20,000/ml, fibrinogen <75 mg/dl, and PT and PTT that are prolonged to twice the normal value. (Normal values are listed in Table 7-7.)

Platelets can be replaced by administering approximately 1 unit of platelet concentrate for each 5 kilograms of body weight. Fibrinogen and factor VIII can be replaced with 3 to 4 bags of cryoprecipitate for each 10 kilograms of body weight, and other coagulant factors are replaced with fresh frozen plasma at 10 to 15 ml/kg. Subsequent replacement is determined by the half-lives of the factors and platelets.[10] Neonates and children with overwhelming DIC who cannot tolerate the large fluid volumes of replacement factors can possibly be corrected with exchange transfusions.

Treatment of DIC with heparin remains controversial, although more recent studies suggest that while heparin therapy may arrest DIC and improve laboratory values, morbidity and mortality are unaffected.[10] Hence, the more current management protocols do not include heparinization. It should be noted, however, that when there is marked thrombosis present, or when there is massive hemorrhage unresponsive to replacement therapy, heparin can be administered with extreme caution. Suggested doses include a loading dose of 50 U/kg and a maintenance dose of 10 to 20 U/kg/hr by continuous infusion. If the child is being heparinized, routine screening studies (i.e., PT and PTT) are rendered useless, and other specific values need to be monitored closely (i.e., platelets, FSP, factor V), along with prudent clinical observation.

The use of corticosteroid in shock states remains controversial. Although most studies suggest that steroids may be useful, there have been no studies proving that they significantly affect mortality. The exact mechanism by which they may be beneficial has not been well defined, but it is thought that corticosteroids stabilize cellular and capillary membranes to maintain their integrity and prevent the release of cellular lysozymes and the loss of proteinaceous fluid to the interstitium. It is also felt that they may shift the oxyhemoglobin dissociation curve to release more oxygen to tissues. When they are administered, it is generally considered that high-dose methylprednisolone sodium succinate (Solu-Medrol) is the drug of choice. It is usually administered in four divided doses over 24 hours, using 30 mg/kg for each dose. If no clinical response is obtained in that time, they are discontinued to prevent any possible deleterious effects from their long-term use.[11,12,26]

Irreversible stage. During the irreversible stage of shock, critical care management assumes a supportive role.

Cardiovascular support: In this terminal stage of shock, complete cardiovascular collapse is both hemodynamically and clinically evident. The MAP and CI values are lethally decreased. Failing left ventricular functioning is apparent by a rising PAOP.

Progressive cellular dysfunction is reflected in a narrowed CaO_2-CvO_2, caused by the inability of tissue to extract oxygen from blood. Arterial vascular resistance is maximally increased, causing decreased perfusion of subserved capillary beds. Clinical evidence of cardiovascular collapse includes: sluggish capillary refill, diminished pulse volume, cool extremities, coma or severe neurological impairment secondary to prolonged cerebral hypoperfusion, and cardiogenic pulmonary edema further compounding ARDS, as evidenced by rales, an S_3 gallop, and enlarged cardiac silhouette and engorged pulmonary vasculature on chest x-ray. These clinical and hemodynamic markers of cardiovascular collapse are not responsive to management protocols.

Respiratory support: This stage of shock is marked by severe respiratory failure, largely as the result of cardiogenic and noncardiogenic pulmonary edema. The PaO_2 is decreased, and the $PaCO_2$ is increased despite maximal ventilatory support (fraction of inspired oxygen [FIO_2] = 1.0, and maximally tolerated PEEP). The serum pH now reflects both a respiratory and a metabolic acidosis.

The primary goal of respiratory support in this stage of shock is continuance of ventilation. Attempts to wean the child from respiratory support are halted because the toxic effects of the support are not a concern at this time. In conjunction with providing the child with maximum ventilatory support, narcotic sedatives are commonly used to provide optimal comfort without concern for depressing the respiratory drive.

Renal support: With the onset of complete cardiovascular collapse, acute renal failure is prevalent. Because of the irreversibility of the cardiovascular failure, further aggressive renal management may be halted.

Neurological support: Clinical evidence of increased intracranial pressure or severe neurological insult may be present. In this case, neurological support (as outlined in Chapter 4) is continued until death occurs.

Metabolic support: The serum pH reflects both a severe metabolic and a respiratory acidosis that is unresponsive to hyperventilation and buffers.

Family support: Once all efforts to make the child as comfortable as possible have been provided, preparing the family for the child's death assumes priority and should include various disciplines such as medicine, nursing, social work, and clergy (*see* p. 8).

Summary: In conclusion, shock syndrome — regardless of etiology — is a rapidly progressive devastating state that requires prompt critical care intervention from a variety of disciplines. The critical care nurse assumes the central role in the minute-to-minute care and management of the child in shock and, to be optimally effective in this role, numerous diverse nursing skills must be mastered in concordance with the mastery of basic physiological principles. In addition, it is the critical care clinician's responsibility to update continually his or her knowledge of critical care management as altered by new information regarding newer pharmacological agents and monitoring techniques. Ongoing research with synthetic sympathetic amines and with the relationships among oxygen-transport-related variables, perfusion indices, and volume-and-flow-related variables may improve the critical care management of the child in shock in the future.

TRAUMATIC INJURIES IN CHILDHOOD

Traumatic injuries account for approximately one half of the deaths in children aged 1 to 15 years in the United States. Trauma is the third cause of death in the general population (after cardiovascular disease and cancer) but the *primary* cause of death in childhood. About 15,000 children under the age of 15 years die from accidental injuries each year. In addition, the morbidity and long-term sequelae of injuries in childhood have profound medical and social significance. More than 100,000 children are permanently crippled each year in this country, and more than 19 million are temporarily incapacitated by their injuries. There has been, and will continue to be, an enormous social investment in the rehabilitation and long-term care of traumatically injured children, many of whom may never be fully capable of returning this investment by becoming productive members of society.

The principal agents responsible for accidental death in childhood are motor vehicles, poison, fires, and falls; more than one half of these injuries are related to automobiles and fires. The principal causes of death are shock, respiratory obstruction, and brainstem damage.

The injuries that will be discussed in this chapter are those that result from trauma to the abdomen, chest, and skeleton. The etiology, pathophysiology, and management of these injuries will be addressed at length.

Selected Aspects of Pediatric Physiology

Blunt-impact accidents are responsible for 80 to 90 percent of the serious multiple injuries in childhood.[27,28] These injuries often result from motor vehicle accidents: (1) as passengers, children are light in weight and are easily tossed around the interior of a car; (2) as pedestrians, they are small in size, difficult to see, and quick to move into the path of a vehicle; (3) the protective reflexes and coordination of children are poorly developed and thus prevent them from moving out of danger quickly; and (4) as bicycle riders, they are prone to relatively high-speed collisions and falls.

There are several unique anatomic, physiological, and developmental features of the bodies and minds of children that enhance their vulnerability to serious injury. Abdominal distention, regardless of etiology, may severely compromise ventilatory functioning, due to the child's limited chest volume and large dependence on diaphragmatic breathing. In addition, respiratory reserve is limited because of small lung volumes and the small caliber of the airways, which are especially prone to obstruction with blood and mucus.

The child's smaller blood volume makes blood loss more dangerous. Concurrently, the highly vascular liver and spleen are large compared with the rest of the abdominal organs, predisposing them to laceration or rupture and resulting in massive hemorrhage. Children have an immature neuroendocrine response to the shock state. This inhibits their ability to efficiently and effectively maintain selective perfusion to major organ systems in the presence of a depleted blood volume.

A child has a larger surface area relative to body mass and is, therefore, jeopardized to a greater extent than the adult by exposure and excessive heat loss, especially when exposure is prolonged during emergency management and transport. The administration of cold intravenous fluids or blood during emergency resuscitation may compound the serious and rapid loss of body heat.

Because the child's head is large relative to the rest of the body and the neck and shoulder muscles are relatively weak, there is a predisposition to serious head injury. The high association of head injury with multiple trauma in children produces a situation that increases the difficulty of evaluating associated injuries because of the child's depressed responses during the examination of the rest of the body.

In addition, the child's age and relative inability to communicate may serve as obstacles in the initial assessment and invervention: "The inability of a young child to express his pain and to localize his symptoms places multiple trauma in childhood almost in the category of veterinary medicine."[29]

Finally, there may be preexisting congenital defects (e.g., cardiac defects) that impair the child's response to trauma. Any serious injury to an immature organism may have deleterious effects on the final physical, intellectual, emotional, and social well-being of the mature human being that the injured child will become.

Principles of Nursing Care

The priorities of emergency care of the severely and/or multiply injured patient are summarized in Table 7-8. The initial period of assessment of the trauma victim

TABLE 7-8 Initial Priorities in the Resuscitation of the Traumatically Injured Child

Priority	Intervention
Cardiopulmonary resuscitation if respiratory and/or circulatory failure has occurred	1. Establish an airway; clear debris (e.g., blood, mucus, vomitus) from mouth and pharynx; open airway by positioning the head in a neutral or slightly extended position (note: hyperextension of the neck must be avoided, especially if cervical injury is suspected); assist with intubation if indicated. 2. Ensure that ventilation is adequate (assess by observation and auscultation of the child's ventilatory efforts). If the ventilation is inadequate, insert an oral airway and initiate bag and mask ventilation. If endotracheal intubation has been performed, continue to oxygenate and ventilate with a resuscitation bag. 3. Support the circulation: assess the child's circulatory status; treat shock; initiate external cardiac compression, if indicated.
Rapid assessment of the child's obvious injuries	1. Assess the child's neurological status. 2. Examine the obvious injuries and control hemorrhage, if the source is controllable. 3. Examine for sources of hidden hemorrhage.
Treatment of the most critical injuries	The following injuries require urgent operative intervention: 1. Intra-abdominal visceral injuries causing massive hemorrhage. 2. Intracranial injury with expanding hemorrhage. 3. Thoracic injury resulting in uncontrolled hemorrhage or massive air leak (e.g., ruptured trachea or bronchus). 4. Major vascular injury.

449

TABLE 7-9 Secondary Resuscitation Priorities for the Traumatically Injured Child

1. One or more large-bore central IV infusions should be started. Often, a cutdown must be performed in a small child to accomplish this. Rapid volume replacement with warmed blood, colloids and/or crystalloid can then be accomplished.
2. Blood samples must be sent to the laboratory for the determination of the following: hematocrit; acid-base status, oxygenation, and ventilation (i.e., arterial blood gas analysis); type and cross-match for emergency transfusion; and electrolyte determination.
3. Insertion of an NG or orogastric tube should be accomplished to decompress and evacuate the stomach. This maneuver may improve ventilation and prevent vomiting with subsequent aspiration.
4. Fractured extremities should be splinted.
5. Relevant diagnostic studies should be performed (e.g., peritoneal lavage, x-rays, arteriogram, IVP, and cystogram).
6. A Foley catheter should be inserted if urethral injury is not suspected.
7. Superficial injuries should be repaired, if appropriate.
8. The child's family should be contacted and brought in to see the child before the child is brought to the OR or ICU.

ICU, intensive care unit; IV, intravenous; IVP, intravenous pyelogram; NG, nasogastric; OR, operating room.

serves to establish priorities for subsequent intervention. The appropriateness of this initial decision-making will have the greatest single influence on the effectiveness and, ultimately, the success of the intervention.

The resuscitation should then proceed to include the interventions listed in Table 7-9. The sequence of these activities depends largely on the nature of the child's injury.

There are three major principles of nursing care of the traumatically injured child. The first is that hemodynamic stability must be preserved to provide for tissue viability. This is accomplished by careful attention to the maintenance of circulating blood volume, cardiac performance, and vascular tone.

The second principle of care is that adequate tissue oxygenation is essential to tissue viability. As a consequence, ventilation and transport of oxygen to the tissues must be sufficient. This is accomplished by ventilatory support, maintenance of the capacity of the blood to carry oxygen, delivery of oxygen to the tissues, and preservation of a favorable acid-base environment to promote oxygen release to the tissues.

The third principle is that care must be comprehensive and coordinated. A child with complex, multisystem injuries requires the involvement of many disciplines in an integrated and complementary approach in order to achieve the best outcome.

Abdominal Trauma

Abdominal injuries are the most common sequelae of trauma and account for approximately 5 percent of all childhood accidents. Approximately 75 percent of these injuries occur in male children during times of the year when outdoor play is common. There are two major types of abdominal trauma: blunt and penetrating injuries.

Blunt trauma is the most common form of abdominal trauma. Nonpenetrating abdominal trauma more often injures solid rather than hollow organs. This is due to a solid organ's density, which results in a greater absorption of disruptive kinetic energy. The following are the three major types of blunt abdominal trauma, along with the injuries that most frequently result from them:

1. Crushing injuries in which a crushing force usually squashes solid organs such as the spleen, liver, and pancreas against adjacent bony structures.
2. Decelerating injuries, which result in the shearing of various organs, as well as of mesentery and ligamentous supports for the bowel.
3. Compressing forces, such as a blow to the abdomen, which squeeze mostly hollow viscera into abnormal shapes and locations. The most common organs affected are the stomach and colon; sudden distention will often result in rupture.[30]

Splenic injuries. The spleen is the organ most often injured in closed (blunt) abdominal trauma. Splenic laceration or rupture is the most common source of intraperitoneal bleeding in children.

Parameters for the assessment of a child with suspected splenic injury will include an examination of the child for evidence of superficial injury to the left abdominal or chest wall. The child may complain of left upper abdominal pain. Older children may report pain in the left neck and shoulder (due to diaphragmatic irritation). Other significant, although nonspecific, signs of splenic damage may be those of the "acute abdomen," i.e., distention, firmness, and tenderness of the abdomen. In addition, the child may exhibit indications of hemorrhage, i.e., falling hematocrit, hypotension, and shock.

If the child's symptoms suggest splenic injury, a peritoneal lavage is performed. If the results of this procedure are "positive" (i.e., a bloody fluid return) and indicate evidence of significant and continuous bleeding occurring within the peritoneal cavity, the child will be taken to the operating room (OR) for an exploratory laparotomy.

There are two major surgical procedures that can be used in the event of splenic damage: splenectomy or splenorrhaphy. A splenectomy is performed only if the general condition of the child deteriorates and splenorrhaphy would take too much time, or if the spleen is too badly damaged to salvage. If a splenectomy is necessary, the young child may be placed on long-term antibiotic prophylaxis.

Splenorrhaphy is the procedure of choice because of the importance of the spleen to the young child's immunologic defense. Current research suggests a higher incidence of septicemia (particularly those associated with encapsulated bacteria such as *Pneumococcus* and *Hemophilus*) in splenectomized children.[31] The child must be carefully observed during the postoperative period for signs of recurrent hemorrhage after a splenorrhaphy.

Conservative (nonoperative) management may be the treatment of choice if the child's condition remains stable and if peritoneal lavage indicates no severe or continuing blood loss. A spleen scan is performed to evaluate perfusion to the organ. The danger of a delayed rupture of a subcapsular splenic hematoma necessitates careful observation of the child. In the event of delayed rupture, sudden hemorrhage will require emergency volume replacement and operative intervention for a splenorrhaphy or splenectomy.

Hepatic injuries. The liver is vulnerable to injury because of its large size relative to the child's other visceral organs. In addition, the child's resilient and compressible rib cage offers the liver less protection. Massive hemorrhage is encountered more frequently as a result of hepatic injury than as a result of injury to the spleen.

Assessment parameters will include the evaluation of the child for shock, accompanied by right upper quadrant tenderness and rigidity, and right shoulder and neck pain. With major liver lacerations, the hematocrit will fall rapidly, and peritoneal lavage will be grossly positive.

As with splenic injuries, minor liver trauma may be managed without surgery. Major liver injury requires immediate volume replacement, operative exploration, and repair to control bleeding. If necessary, devitalized tissue will be debrided and the injured area drained.

Gastric injuries.   Most stomach wounds are penetrating in origin. Gastric rupture is a rare problem most often seen with child abuse. Initial assessment will include an examination of the child for evidence of a penetrating injury. The child may complain of left upper quadrant pain, and the abdomen may be tender, rigid, and distended. In the absence of evidence of penetrating injury, there may be a history of an abdominal blow after a meal.

Peritoneal lavage may be productive of gastric contents or may simply be positive. Placement and aspiration of a nasogastric (NG) tube will usually reveal blood in the gastric drainage. If gastric laceration or rupture is diagnosed, operative exploration and closure of the gastric tear should be accomplished immediately.

Duodenal injuries.   The development of an intramural hematoma is a rare but possible consequence of blunt trauma. Trauma to this portion of the small bowel may result in bleeding that occurs primarily in the intramuscular or submucosal layers of the bowel. This injury may result from seemingly minor degrees of trauma. Children are especially vulnerable to this type of injury because of their greater duodenal vascular supply, which results in bleeding rather than necrosis when tissue injury occurs. In addition, the anatomic structure of the child's costal arch is higher and wider; consequently, the duodenum is more exposed and more easily injured.

The history will indicate a gradual onset of symptoms, usually over a period of days. There may be a significant delay between the traumatic event and the development of abdominal pain or vomiting. The child will exhibit symptoms suggestive of intestinal obstruction. The abdomen will be tender and distended, bowel sounds will be absent or hyperactive, and vomiting will frequently occur.

X-ray or fluoroscopy after a barium swallow will demonstrate a typical "coiled spring" appearance of the duodenum or complete obstruction of the intestinal lumen. Conservative management will consist of (1) NG tube insertion and gastrointestinal decompression until the hematoma resolves, and (2) careful observation. Operative intervention is necessary only if symptoms of intestinal obstruction persist, if the serum amylase rises (suggestive of pancreatic involvement), or if there is a suspicion of duodenal rupture.

Penetrating injuries of the duodenum should be managed by operative intervention. The laceration will be repaired, or more extensive surgery will be performed, if necessary.

Small bowel injuries.   Penetrating injuries of the small bowel will manifest themselves in much the same way as other abdominal injuries. The abdomen will be distended and tender. Abdominal x-rays will demonstrate pneumoperitoneum. Peritoneal lavage will be productive of intestinal contents or blood. Operative repair of the lacerated portions of bowel is the treatment of choice. Rupture or mesenteric disruptions may require resection and reanastomosis of the bowel or external diversion as an ostomy.

Colon injuries. Injuries of the colon require special attention because of the danger of fecal peritoneal contamination, resulting in peritonitis. It is also more difficult to achieve satisfactory healing of this portion of the bowel.

The child will demonstrate symptoms of an acute abdomen. Abdominal x-rays will indicate a pneumoperitoneum. Peritoneal lavage will be productive of fecal material and/or blood.

Intervention is always operative in circumstances of fecal contamination of the peritoneum or with evidence of mesenteric damage. Usually, a colostomy will be performed to exteriorize the injured portion of the colon. There may also be a need for surgical repair of rectal, anal, or other perineal injuries, if the cause of the trauma was perineal impalement.

Critical Care Management of the Child with Acute Abdominal Injury

The following are common problems of children with acute abdominal injury. Each plan of care should be individualized, based on an understanding of the principles involved and the specific injuries encountered.

Hemodynamic instability. One of the major objectives in the postresuscitation period is the restoration of hemodynamic homeostasis and adequate organ perfusion. Vital signs should be monitored every 15 minutes in the acute stage and progress to hourly determinations as the patient stabilizes. Vital signs should include blood pressure (by auscultation or intra-arterial catheter and pressure transducer), pulse, and respirations. Other intravascular pressures, such as CVP and pulmonary artery pressure (systolic, diastolic, mean, and wedge), will provide accurate information regarding intravascular volume status and cardiac performance. Left ventricular filling pressures should be maintained by volume replacement to provide adequate organ perfusion.

The child should be observed carefully for clinical signs of hypovolemic shock (*see* p. 433). Intravascular volume should be maintained with blood products and colloid or crystalloid solutions as ordered by the physician. Rapidly administered solutions should be warmed to body temperature. Intravascular pressures, urine output, and clinical status should be carefully monitored as the child receives volume replacement. If the shock state persists despite restoration of blood volume, vasopressor therapy may be indicated (*see* p. 437).

Infection. The child should be carefully observed for any indications of developing sepsis, particularly peritonitis. Signs and symptoms of peritonitis include: (1) fever; (2) tachycardia; (3) extreme lethargy; (4) ileus — signaled by the sudden or continued absence of bowel sounds; (5) peritoneal irritation — abdominal distention, tenderness, and rigidity; (6) intravascular volume depletion resulting from "third space" fluid losses; and (7) purulent drainage from intraperitoneal drains.

The wound should be inspected for evidence of infection. A wound infection should be suspected if the incisions appear reddened, swollen, warm, or if purulent material drains from them.

If the child demonstrates signs of a generalized septicemia, wounds, drainage sites, intravenous sites, sputum, blood, and urine should be cultured. Broad-spectrum antibiotics are administered until specific organisms can be identified.

Postoperative ileus. Because of surgical manipulation of the bowel and the body's response to trauma, ileus often occurs postoperatively in the pediatric patient. The NG tube should be irrigated with saline solution every 2 hours to ensure proper patency, placement, and drainage until normal bowel sounds return. A double-lumen sump tube is preferred to a single-lumen tube in order to avoid traumatizing the gastric mucosa by direct suction. The NG tube should be irrigated with an approximate volume of 0.5 to 1.0 ml/kg of normal saline. The NG drainage should be measured and tested for the presence of occult blood every 4 hours, and that volume should be replaced milliliter for milliliter with balanced salt solution as ordered. The pH of the gastric drainage should be tested every 2 hours, and antacids should be administered to maintain the gastric pH above 6 or 7 to prevent the development of stress ulcers. Abdominal girth should be measured carefully, and serum electrolytes should be maintained in the normal range.

Respiratory compromise. Respiratory toilet should be provided for the intubated child to promote adequate ventilation and prevent pulmonary complications. The extubated child should be turned and encouraged to take deep breaths and cough every 2 hours. If the child is cooperative, this may be accomplished by incentive spirometry and coughing. If the child is unable or unwilling to cough, light pharyngeal suctioning may be effective in producing a cough.

Chest physical therapy may be indicated if the child's condition permits. If there has been any respiratory insufficiency, serial arterial blood gas determinations may be necessary to assess the adequacy of the child's ventilation, oxygenation, and acid-base status.

Ostomy care. If an ostomy has been performed, a referral to an ostomy specialist should be obtained. An ostomy specialist will help to develop a consistent and effective plan of care for the ostomy, the external drainage appliance, and the skin around the stoma.

The parent and child should be included in the plan of care and encouraged to participate to the extent they are able.

All ostomy drainage should be measured and recorded. The character of the drainage should be noted, as well as the appearance of the ostomy site.

Fluid and electrolyte imbalance. Intake and output must be measured accurately and recorded. All of the following should be measured and regarded as output: (1) drainage on dressings (dressings should be weighed if drainage is large in amount), (2) NG drainage, (3) urine output, (4) emesis, (5) diarrhea, and (6) ostomy drainage. The child should be weighed daily to assess third-space losses. Laboratory determination of serum electrolytes should be performed at least daily and more often if indicated.

Inadequate nutritional intake. Adequate nutrients and calories must be provided if wound healing is to occur. If an extended period of nothing by mouth (NPO) is anticipated, calories and nutrients should be provided intravenously through total parenteral nutrition (TPN) (*see* p. 494). When TPN is in progress, the child should be observed carefully for hyperglycemia, hyperlipemia, and acidosis. If the child will only be NPO for a short time, a graduated diet should begin as bowel sounds return to normal, distention resolves, and the NG tube is removed.

Child and/or parent anxiety. The nurse must help the parent and child develop appropriate coping mechanisms in response to the child's sudden illness and to their mutual anxiety in the intensive care unit (ICU) environment.

The following activities can help reduce stress:

1. Offer explanations according to the parent's and child's ability to understand the nature of the child's injuries and the treatments required.
2. Provide consistent nursing caregivers with whom the parent and child can become familiar.
3. Promote trust by being honest about realities, and avoid speculation about the unknown.
4. Allow as much appropriate participation in the child's care as the child and parent want.
5. Provide opportunities for physical closeness between parent and child and for play periods as the child improves.

Special considerations. The following considerations apply to liver trauma, duodenal trauma, and splenorrhaphy:

1. When liver trauma has occurred, the direct and indirect bilirubin, blood ammonia, and liver enzymes should be monitored daily.
2. After duodenal trauma has occurred, the serum amylase should be measured to monitor pancreatic functioning.
3. After a splenorrhaphy has been performed, the child should be carefully observed for delayed splenic rupture.

Genitourinary Trauma

As with abdominal trauma, the two major types of genitourinary (GU) injuries result from either blunt or penetrating trauma. The essence of managing GU injuries, as with other forms of trauma, consists in rapid evaluation of the type and extent of the injury, combined with early and effective treatment.

Renal trauma. The main focus of therapeutic intervention is to preserve the greatest amount of functioning renal parenchyma with a minimal amount of morbidity for the child. Traumatic renal damage may be complicated by preexisting, undiagnosed renal pathology. Pelvic fractures often coexist with renal or other GU injuries.

Renal contusion is associated with a history of trauma to the renal area and is accompanied by hematuria. Intravenous pyelogram (IVP) demonstrates no evidence of depressed renal functioning, pelvicalyceal damage, or extravasation of dye. A urine specimen should be obtained routinely when trauma involves the chest, back, or abdomen. The urine will be positive for the presence of microscopic or gross blood when renal contusion has occurred. The majority of these children are managed conservatively until the hematuria resolves.

Renal cortical laceration is a more severe type of renal injury. The child will have hematuria, often associated with a renal mass, which is usually an extrarenal hematoma that has formed at the site of the tear. The IVP will demonstrate an intact collecting system in the kidney, with extravasation of dye through the torn capsule. The child may require renal angiography and a renal scan to rule out vascular injury. Most of these children are also managed conservatively and require careful observation and monitoring for continued bleeding or deterioration of renal functioning.

Renal calyceal laceration can be a serious injury. There will be marked hematuria with clinical evidence of flank injury. The IVP will demonstrate an intact capsule, with disruption of the pelvicalyceal system and intrarenal extravasation of dye. Initial management is conservative if the angiography and renal scan show no vascular injury and demonstrate intact renal parenchyma. Surgical intervention may be required at a later time if scarring and obstruction occur.

The most lethal form of renal trauma results in complete renal tear or fracture and renal pedical injury. The child will present with shocklike symptoms. The IVP will demonstrate complete separation of renal parenchyma from the pelvicalyceal system and the capsule, with intra- and extrarenal extravasation of dye.

The child will require volume replacement to treat shock while an emergency IVP and renal angiography are being scheduled. Operative intervention is always indicated to avoid total nephrectomy or exsanguination. If possible, the kidney will be resected rather than removed, and the vascular supply will be repaired.

Urinary bladder and urethral trauma. Bladder and urethral trauma is most often associated with pelvic fractures and may be accompanied by massive retroperitoneal hematoma or hemorrhage. Urethral rupture, most common in males, should be suspected when bright red blood is found to be issuing from the urethral meatus. If urethral rupture is suspected, no urinary catheter should be inserted (to avoid further trauma) until a urethrogram is obtained.

If bladder injury is suspected, a cystogram and urethrogram are performed. Operative intervention is indicated in the event of a bladder tear. A temporary suprapubic (SP) drainage tube will be inserted to diminish bladder wall tension and to allow proper bladder wall healing.

Critical Care Management of the Child with Acute GU Trauma

The care of the child with GU injuries will be discussed in the following sections. Problems associated with this form of trauma are in some instances similar to those presented in the previous section.

Hemodynamic instability. (*See* p. 453 for a general description of care.) The child should be carefully observed for shock due to recurrent hemorrhage from renal vascular repair or amputation.

Infection. The child with indwelling splints or drains (e.g., SP or Foley catheters, urethral splints, or nephrostomy tubes) is at risk for the development of urinary retrograde infections. The color, odor, and character of the urine should be noted. A sterilely collected urine specimen should be sent to the laboratory for culture if it appears cloudy or develops a foul odor. All drainage tube irrigations should be performed using sterile technique, and all urinary collection systems should remain closed and sterile. The drainage tubes themselves must be secured properly to avoid trauma to the entrance wound, kidney, or bladder. Antibiotic coverage should be administered as ordered.

Obstruction of urinary drainage tubes. Drainage tubes should be observed carefully and urinary output measured every hour. Diminished urine output may indicate obstruction of the tubes. If there are clots or exudate in the urine, the drainage tubes may become obstructed, causing stasis, pressure on healing structures, and pain. The urinary drainage tubes or splints should be irrigated, as ordered, using sterile technique. The recurrence of fresh bleeding from any drainage tube may precede hemorrhage and must be reported to the physician.

Bladder spasms.   Bladder spasms may be due to irritation by or obstruction of an SP drainage tube or to edema of the operative site. The drainage system should be checked, and urine output measured every hour. The SP tube should be irrigated as ordered if blockage is suspected. The SP tube should be secured to avoid tension on the entrance wound or on the bladder, because movement of the tube will precipitate painful spasms. The child and parents should be assured that the pain of bladder spasms usually passes quickly. Analgesics should be administered as necessary.

Renal insufficiency.   Renal insufficiency is an uncommon complication of unilateral renal damage; however, it is a serious one that deserves careful consideration. The child's fluid and electrolyte balance must be maintained within normal limits. The urine output should remain in the range of 0.5 to 1.0 ml/kg/hr. The urine specific gravity is best maintained in the range of 1.005 to 1.015. (Note: urine specific gravity may be falsely elevated by the hyperosmolar dyes that are used in some diagnostic tests and are excreted in the urine.) The urine should be tested for the presence of protein, blood, or glucose. The color and odor of the urine should be noted, as well as the persistence or recurrence of gross hematuria. In addition, the laboratory results that reflect renal functioning should be monitored (e.g., blood urea nitrogen, creatinine clearance, serum and urine electrolytes and creatinine). *See* p. 386 for the care of the child with acute renal failure, if this condition should develop. Additional information regarding patient/parent anxiety, and respiratory, ostomy, and nutritional status is as discussed in the abdominal injury section (*see* p. 454).

Thoracic Trauma

Chest trauma requires the concomitant examination of the child for external evidence of trauma and a careful assessment of respiratory status. The thorax (including the clavicles, ribs, and scapulae) should be inspected and palpated carefully. In addition, assessment should be made of the stability of the chest wall itself. Auscultation is helpful to judge the adequacy of the child's ventilatory effort and the presence of breath sounds bilaterally; however, detailed auscultation of the chest is generally not beneficial. The chest x-ray will provide more information and is an essential part of the initial diagnostic work-up in the emergency room (*see* p. 39).

Flail chest.   Flail chest is a consequence of blunt or crushing chest trauma that causes segmental, sequential rib fractures and results in paradoxical chest wall motion upon respiration. The flail may worsen after admission as the lung loses compliance; this will result in worsening respiratory distress. It is important, therefore, to observe any child suspected of chest injury for the development of a flail. Isolated flail chest has an excellent prognosis; however, it is frequently found with other severe and often life-threatening pulmonary and cardiac injuries.

Assessment of the child's respiratory pattern will demonstrate paradoxical chest wall motion (i.e., the chest wall will move in on inspiration and out on expiration, the reverse of normal). The degree of chest wall movement will depend on intrathoracic pressures and the child's ventilatory effort.

Intervention is conservative. The child with a severe flail will be managed with intubation and mechanical ventilation until the chest wall is stable enough to allow for effective spontaneous ventilation. A thoracostomy (chest) tube may be inserted if pneumothorax is also present.

Hemopneumothorax. Hemopneumothorax may result from penetrating or blunt chest injuries. The diagnosis is confirmed by chest x-ray. Severe lung contusion and laceration can result from a blow to the chest wall, trauma from a fractured rib, or any of a number of penetrating injuries. Hemorrhage into the pleural space (from vascular damage) will further compress the lung. Hemopneumothorax is particularly lethal if hemorrhagic shock is accompanied by mediastinal shift and severe hypoxemia.

The child will appear to be in shock and in severe respiratory distress. The trachea will be deviated to the side opposite the collapsed lung, and breath sounds will be severely diminished or absent on the affected side. Chest x-ray will confirm the physical findings.

A chest tube should be inserted immediately after chest x-ray confirmation of hemopneumothorax. The child will be managed conservatively if bleeding is not life-threatening and the lung reexpands without evidence of a major air leak. Operative exploratory thoracotomy is necessary if the air leak is due to the rupture of the trachea or bronchus, or if bleeding persists and produces shock. Adequate evacuation of blood from the chest is important to prevent the development of an organized clot, which can cause empyema or pleuritis.

Myocardial contusion. Every chest trauma victim should be observed for evidence of myocardial contusion or cardiac tamponade. An electrocardiogram (ECG) should be obtained on admission and, if it is indicative of myocardial damage, there should be close ECG monitoring of the child for cardiac arrhythmias. If there is reason to suspect cardiac tamponade (*see* p. 188), a pericardiocentesis may be life-saving.

Intervention for simple myocardial contusion is conservative in nature. The child should be observed carefully for arrhythmias, congestive heart failure, or ECG evidence of extending myocardial damage. Pericarditis may occur several days after the trauma.

Operative management is required if cardiac tamponade or major vessel disruption produces refractory hemorrhage or shock. The child will require the same postoperative care as for closed cardiac surgery (*see* p. 184).

Penetrating chest trauma. Penetrating chest injuries result from stabbings, bullet wounds, or impalement. They are seen most frequently in older children and adolescents. Chest tube drainage and volume resuscitation are adequate for the majority of penetrating injuries and should be initiated immediately in the emergency room.

Immediate thoracotomy and/or cardiorrhaphy are indicated when (1) the location of the entrance wound is mediastinal, (2) the child is in shock and unresponsive to volume replacement, (3) there is a large initial and continuing blood loss (greater than 5 to 10 ml/kg), or (4) there is evidence of cardiac tamponade.

Sucking chest wounds. Open sucking chest injuries represent a life-threatening crisis. The lung collapses and the mediastinum shifts toward the uninvolved lung, compromising its functioning. These wounds require occlusion of the defect in the chest wall with petroleum-jelly-impregnated gauze, plastic wrap, and/or a tight dressing. The immediate treatment is to insert a chest tube to reexpand the lung and evacuate the thoracic cavity of air and blood. Major defects in the thoracic wall require reparative surgery, especially if the underlying lung is damaged, causing a major air leak or hemorrhage.

Critical Care Management of the
Child with Acute Thoracic Trauma

Respiratory insufficiency. Trauma to the chest may directly or indirectly jeopardize the child's ability to maintain effective ventilation and adequate tissue oxygenation. In the event that respiratory failure results from thoracic injury, respiratory support will be needed until the child can resume these activities. (The care of the child with respiratory failure is explained in detail in chapter 2, p. 45.)

Severe flail chest injuries will require a period of mechanical ventilation to provide for adequate internal stabilization of the chest wall. The child may have to be temporarily paralyzed with neuromuscular blocking agents (e.g., curare, pancuronium bromide) in order to minimize movement of the fractured sternum and ribs and to aid ventilation. Sedative medications should always accompany such paralyzing agents in order to minimize the child's pain and fear. Staff and parents should be encouraged to talk to the child despite the child's inability to respond (*see* p. 48).

The child should be carefully observed after chest trauma for the sudden occurrence of pneumothorax. This life-threatening complication should be suspected if the child develops (1) subcutaneous emphysema; (2) diminished or absent breath sounds, with a shift of the trachea away from the affected side; and (3) a mediastinal shift away from the affected side, accompanied by diminished cardiac sounds, change in location of the cardiac point of maximum impulse (PMI), hypoxemia, and shock.

Hemodynamic instability. (*See* p. 453 for a general description of care.) A chest tube will invariably be inserted into the pleural space if blood or air has accumulated there. The tube will be connected to water-seal drainage and suction. The volume and character of the drainage should be measured and recorded every 15 minutes during active bleeding, and should progress to every hour after the bleeding has diminished. Volume replacement with blood products or colloids should be initiated if the bleeding is of a sufficient quantity to cause hypovolemia. The chest tube and the collection tubing should be "milked" frequently to prevent clot formation, resulting in tube obstruction, and the tubing should be positioned above the collection chamber to allow for adequate drainage. The chest tube should be secured to the child to prevent tension on the chest wall or accidental displacement.

The child's breath sounds should be evaluated every hour; diminished breath sounds may indicate an accumulation of blood in the pleural space, resulting in lung compression. The collection chamber should be observed for evidence of pulmonary air leak (i.e., bubbling of air in the collection chamber). Additional information regarding infection, patient/parent anxiety, nutritional status, and fluid and electrolyte imbalance is as discussed in the abdominal injury section (*see* p. 454).

Skeletal Trauma

Children with orthopedic injuries usually present with pain, loss of functioning, or obvious bone or joint deformity resulting from trauma. Orthopedic injuries should be considered not only in terms of the bones and joints, but also in a more general sense with relation to the anatomy, particularly of the extremities. In addition to fractures, there must be a consideration of the blood vessels, skin, nerves, tendons, and muscles of the affected limb. Pelvic and facial fractures are frequently associated with major abdominal or neurological damage.

There are two main principles of fracture treatment: (1) fracture healing is dependent on the nature of local soft tissue injury, circulation, apposition, and immobilization; (2) healing may be rapid in the child, but complications may inhibit bone growth, with resulting limb deformities. The goal of fracture treatment is to obtain an optimally functioning extremity (i.e., a functional hand in the upper extremity, and a well-aligned, weight-bearing leg in the lower extremity). The priorities of fracture treatment are to reduce the fracture to an anatomic setting, to immobilize the fracture in such a manner that the healing process occurs at an optimal rate, and to rehabilitate the child during the process of healing. Reduction of fractures in children is usually accomplished by simple traction and manipulation. Open reduction is rarely indicated in closed injuries.

The earlier a fracture is reduced, the easier it will be to attain alignment; often, this must be accomplished under general anesthesia to eliminate pain and achieve adequate muscle relaxation. The following are the methods of fracture reduction: (1) closed reduction with immediate casting or splinting; (2) continuous traction using Buck's, Dunlop, or skeletal traction to reduce pain, restore and maintain limb length, and decrease muscle spasm; (3) external skeletal fixation with Steinmann pins and a cast or Hoffman device; and (4) open reduction and internal fixation.

Most orthopedic and soft tissue injuries seen in children require care that must be integrated with that of injuries to the head, thorax, and abdomen. Because the setting of priorities is difficult, compromise is often essential. Skeletal injuries that do not involve loss of a limb may be the least serious of a child's injuries but may ultimately disable him.

Upper extremity fractures.   The most common site of upper extremity fracture is the radius. Fractures of the humerus or radius and ulna are potentially dangerous because of the proximity of the brachial artery. If the brachial artery has been transected, the arm or hand will be pale and cold, and pulses will be absent. There is usually a large, expanding hematoma over the site of arterial laceration. This condition requires immediate recognition, arteriography, and surgical intervention to restore blood flow to the arm.

Lower extremity fractures.   The most common lower extremity fractures are those of the femoral shaft, which carry a good prognosis. Skeletal traction is applied by means of an overhead traction frame, with weights applied to a pin through the distal femur to obtain reduction. At a later time, a cast is applied.

Femoral neck fractures are rare and more complicated. Surgery may be required to reduce pressure caused by hematoma formation within the femoral capsule in order to prevent avascular necrosis of the femoral head. Despite this approach, various deformities may develop: (1) limb shortening due to damage and premature closure of the epiphyseal plate, (2) coxa vera or loss of proper angle of the femoral head, and (3) malunion. Dislocations and evulsions of the femoral head carry the additional danger of femoral artery transection.

Pelvic fractures.   Pelvic fractures are more frequently associated with mortality in traumatized children than other skeletal injuries. There is a well-documented relationship to urologic trauma, life-threatening retroperitoneal hemorrhage, abdominal visceral injury, neurological lesions, and fat emboli.[32] The high incidence of serious associated soft tissue injuries often poses a more serious problem than the pelvic fracture itself. When pelvic fractures are diagnosed there must be further aggressive investigation to rule out urologic injury. There is a 13 percent known association between urethral or urinary bladder rupture and fractures of the pelvis.[32]

There are four major types of pelvic fractures. These are, in order of increasing severity: (1) iliac wing fractures, (2) acetabular fractures, (3) stable pelvic ring fractures involving breaks in the anterior ring (usually separation of the symphysis pubis), and (4) unstable pelvic ring fractures involving breaks in the anterior and posterior rings. The first three types of fractures require little other than bed rest and/or sling traction. The fourth type is often treated with a combination of skeletal and sling traction, with ultimate spica casting.

Facial fractures. Facial fractures in children are generally regarded as uncommon, perhaps because of the resilient nature of a child's facial bones and small facial size in relation to the head. The most common types of facial fractures in children are those of the nose and mandible. Bicycle trauma in children under 15 years, and automobile trauma in those over 15 years, are the primary causes of these injuries.

The significance of nasal fractures lies primarily in their association with profuse bleeding, which may compromise the airway. The treatment involves nasal splinting and packing. However, if a mandibular fracture requires jaw wiring, the nose may have to accommodate a nasal endotracheal tube or an NG tube, despite a fracture.

Fractures of the mandible are diagnosed by malocclusion, swelling, tenderness, and pain at the fracture site. They are treated by closed reduction and intermaxillary fixation or jaw wiring. Open reduction is rarely necessary.

Critical Care Management of the Child with Skeletal Trauma

Circulatory compromise. Perfusion to injured extremities must be assessed every hour for (1) color, (2) warmth, (3) the presence of distal and proximal pulses, (4) capillary refill, (5) sensory loss, and (6) edema. Any acute change in perfusion to an extremity should be reported immediately to the physician. Casted extremities should be elevated to the level of the heart to promote venous return. The physician should be notified of excessive edema below a cast or site of injury.

Skin breakdown due to immobility with traction. The child's skin should be lubricated and massaged, particularly over bony prominences, every 2 hours. A sheepskin, eggcrate mattress, or alternating-pressure mattress should be placed under the trunk. Position changes must maintain proper body alignment and maximal effectiveness of the traction.

Airway compromise with mandibular fractures and jaw wiring. Inadvertent premature extubation in a nasally intubated ventilator-dependent child is a potentially life-threatening crisis. Wire scissors must be kept at the bedside to cut the jaw wires in the event of accidental extubation. If the child is spontaneously ventilating, a tonsil-tip suction should be available to suction the large amount of oral secretions that will be present. The NG tube must be kept patent to prevent vomiting and aspiration.

Mouth care must be frequent and meticulous. There are often suture lines in and about the mouth that should be gently swabbed or irrigated with one half strength hydrogen peroxide and saline solution.

Pulmonary complications resulting from a fat embolus.   The child should be carefully observed for symptoms suggestive of the occurrence of a fat embolus. These symptoms are (1) tachycardia, (2) chest pain, (3) sudden evidence of respiratory distress and hypoxemia — tachypnea, cyanosis, air hunger, lethargy, or irritability (initially, severe retractions or abnormal breath sounds will not be seen), and (4) laboratory evidence of hypoxemia (arterial blood gases will indicate hypoxemia and, possibly, acidosis, but rarely hypercapnia). The treatment of respiratory failure is described on page 45. Additional information regarding hemodynamic instability, respiratory insufficiency, nutritional status, and infection is as discussed in the abdominal injury section (*see* p. 453).

Summary

Because of the multiplicity of problems compounding the clinical picture associated with severe trauma, there is a need for coordination of disciplines to minimize the physiological and psychological stress of the injury to the child and family. There is a critical need for consistent nursing caregivers and for a common plan of care coordinated with physicians and allied personnel. Consequently, the pediatric intensive care nurse must be able to evaluate and integrate the variety of data gathered about the different organ systems, as well as information on the psychological, emotional, and developmental status of the child.

REFERENCES

1. Thompson. (*The Patient in Shock*) 6.
2. Miller.
3. Rose and Babcock.
4. Elin and Wolff.
5. Tharp.
6. Rice. Parts I and II.
7. Ulevitch and Cochrane.
8. Hopewell.
9. Lind et al.
10. Corrigan.
11. Thompson. (The Organ in Shock). 50–62.
12. Thompson. (The Cell in Shock). 14–17.
13. Formulary of the Children's Hospital of Philadelphia. 15.
14. Shapiro et al. 231–232.
15. Goldberg.
16. Driscoll et al.
17. Formulary of the Children's Hospital of Philadelphia. 28.
18. Sonnenblick et al.
19. Formulary of the Children's Hospital of Philadelphia. 20.
20. Formulary of the Children's Hospital of Philadelphia. 36.
21. Pontoppidan et al.
22. Yabek.
23. Chung. 590–594.
24. Formulary of the Children's Hospital of Philadelphia. XX.
25. Formulary of the Children's Hospital of Philadelphia. 28.
26. Thompson. (The Patient in Shock) 27–31, 36–38.
27. Haller and Talbert.
28. Gratz.
29. Haller (1970).
30. Haller (1966).
31. Weinstein et al.
32. Bryan and Tullos.

BIBLIOGRAPHY

Allen, B. L., A. P. Kant, and F. E. Emery. 1977. Displaced fractures of the femoral diaphysis in children. *The Journal of Trauma.* 17:8–19.
Asch, M. J., A. G. Goran, and P. W. Johnston. 1975. Gastric perforation secondary to blunt trauma in children. *The Journal of Trauma.* 15:187–189.
Barrows, J. J. 1982. Shock demands drugs. *Nursing 82.* 1:34–41.

Bellonti, J. A. 1979. Immunology: Basic Processes. W. B. Saunders Co., Philadelphia.

Bookman, L. B., and J. K. Simoneau. 1977. The early assessment of hypovolemia: postural vital signs. *(JEN) Journal of Emergency Nursing*. **15**:43–45.

Braham, R. L., M. W. Roberts, and M. E. Morris. 1977. Management of dental trauma in children and adolescents. *The Journal of Trauma*. **17**:857–865.

Brantigan, J. W., E. C. Ziegler, K. M. Hynes, T. Y. Miyayawa, and A. M. Smith. 1974. Tissue gases during hypovolemic shock. *Journal of Applied Physiology*. **37**:117–122.

Bryan, W. J., and H. S. Tullos. 1979. Pediatric pelvic fractures: review of 52 patients. *The Journal of Trauma*. **19**:799–805.

Bussey, H. J., R. N. McGehee, and K. R. Tyson. 1975. Isolated gastric rupture due to blunt trauma. *The Journal of Trauma*. **15**:190–191.

Charters, A. C., and N. Stewart. 1981. The management of trauma. *In* Kinney, M. R., C. M. Dear, D. R. Packa, and D. M. Voorman, editors. 1981. American Association of Critical Care Nurse's Clinical Reference for Critical Care Nursing. McGraw-Hill Book Co., New York.

The Children's Hospital of Philadelphia Formulary. 1980–1981. Prepared under the direction of the Therapeutic Standards Committee by the authority of the Executive Committee of the Medical Staff.

Chung, E. K. 1980. Electrocardiography. Harper & Row, Publishers, Inc., New York. Second edition.

Cline, B. A., and M. L. Fisher. 1982. Adult respiratory distress syndrome. *Nursing 82*. **1**:63–67.

Coleman, D. 1979. Disseminated intravascular coagulation: a problem in critical care medicine. *Heart & Lung*. **3**:787–796.

Corrigan, J. J. 1979. Disseminated intravascular coagulation. *Pediatrics in Review*. **1**:37–45.

Driscoll, D. J., P. C. Gillette, and D. G. McNamara. 1978. The use of dopamine in children. *Journal of Pediatrics*. **92**:309–314.

Elin, R. J., and S. M. Wolff. 1976. Biology of endotoxin. *Annual Reviews in Medicine*. **27**:127–141.

Emanuel, B., H. Weiss, and P. Gollin. 1977. Renal trauma in children. *The Journal of Trauma*. **17**:275–278.

Erickson, W. D., E. O. Burgert, and H. B. Lynn. 1968. The hazard of infection following splenectomy in children. *American Journal of Diseases of Children*. **116**:1–12.

Feigenberg, Z., M. Pauker, M. Levy, M. Seelenfreund, and A. Freid. 1977. Fractures of the femoral neck in childhood. *The Journal of Trauma*. **17**:937–942.

Flint, L. M. 1978. Intraperitoneal injuries. *Heart & Lung*. **7**:273–277.

Formulary of the Children's Hospital of Philadelphia. 1982.

Gay, P., J. Thede, G. Suehiro, and J. J. McNamara. 1979. Filtration of debris from banked blood. *The Journal of Trauma*. **19**:806–811.

Goldberg, L. I. 1974. Shock: the overall mechanisms. *American Journal of Nursing*. **74**:2208–2213.

Goodman, L. S., and A. Gilman. 1975. Pharmacological Basics of Therapeutics. Macmillan Publishing Co., Inc., New York. Fifth edition.

Gratz, E. R. 1976. Accidental injury in childhood: a literature review on pediatric trauma. *The Journal of Trauma*. **19**:551–555.

Guyton, A. C. 1981. Textbook of Medical Physiology. W. B. Saunders Co., Philadelphia. Sixth edition.

Haller, J. A. 1966. Injuries of the gastrointestinal tract in children. *Clinical Pediatrics*. **5**:476–480.

Haller, J. A. 1970. Problems in children's trauma. *The Journal of Trauma*. **10**:269–271.

Haller, J. A., and J. L. Talbert. 1976. Trauma workshop report: trauma in children. *The Journal of Trauma*. **16**:1052–1054.

Hopewell, P. C. 1979. Adult respiratory distress syndrome. *Basics in Respiratory Disease*. **7**:1–16.

Jacob, H. S. 1978. Granulocyte-complement interaction. *Archives of Internal Medicine*. **139**:461–463.

Jona, J. Z., and J. R. Goldstein. 1977. Compression hepatic necrosis in a child. *The Journal of Trauma*. **17**:402–404.

Lamy, M., R. J. Fallat, E. Koeniger, H. P. Dietrich, J. L. Ratliff, R. C. Eberhart, H. J. Tucker, and J. D. Hill. 1976. Pathologic features and mechanisms of hypoxemia in adult respiratory distress syndrome. *American Review of Respiratory Diseases.* **114**:267–281.

Lehman, J. A., and N. D. Saddawi. 1976. Fractures of the mandible in children. *The Journal of Trauma.* **16**:773–777.

Lind, T. L., J. A. McDonald, and L. V. Avioli. 1981. Adult respiratory distress syndrome. *Archives of Internal Medicine.* **141**:1749–1753.

Lonzkowski, P. A. 1979. Hematologic emergencies. *Pediatric Clinics of North America.* **26**:918.

Miller, K. M. 1978. Assessing peripheral perfusion. *American Journal of Nursing.* **78**:1673–1674.

O'Brian, B. S., and S. Woods. 1978. The paradox of disseminated intravascular coagulation. *American Journal of Nursing.* **78**:1876–1880.

Pontoppidan, H., R. S. Wilson, M. A. Rie, and R. C. Schneider. 1977. Respiratory intensive care. *Anesthesiology.* **47**:96–116.

Reed, M. H. 1977. Fractures and dislocations of the extremities in children. *The Journal of Trauma.* **17**:351–354.

Rice, V. 1981. Shock, a clinical syndrome. Part I. *Critical Care Nurse.* **1**:44–48.

Rice, V. 1981. Shock, a clinical syndrome. Part II. *Critical Care Nurse.* **1**:4–13.

Rodgers, B. M. 1977. Trauma and the child. *Heart & Lung.* **6**:1052–1056.

Rose, H. D., and J. B. Babcock. 1975. Colonization of intensive care unit patients with gram-negative bacilli. *American Journal of Epidemiology.* **101**:495–501.

Selkurt, E. E. 1976. Physiology. Little Brown & Co., Boston. Fourth edition.

Shaker, I. J., J. J. White, R. D. Signer, E. S. Golladay, and J. A. Haller. 1976. Special problems of vascular injuries in children. *The Journal of Trauma.* **16**:863–867.

Shapiro, B. A., R. A. Harrison, and J. R. Walton. 1977. Clinical Application of Blood Gases. Year Book Medical Publishers, Inc., Chicago. Second edition.

Shoemaker, W. C. 1971. Cardiorespiratory patterns of complicated and uncomplicated septic shock. *Annals of Surgery.* **174**:119–125.

Shoemaker, W. C. 1971. Sequential hemodynamic patterns in various causes of shock. *Surgery, Gynecology and Obstetrics.* **132**:411–423.

Shoemaker, W. C., E. S. Montgomery, E. Kaplan, and D. H. Elwyn. 1973. Physiologic patterns in surviving and nonsurviving shock patients. *Archives of Surgery.* **106**:630–636.

Shoemaker, W. C., P. Chang, L. Czer, R. Blond, M. M. Shabat, and D. Stat. 1979. Cardiorespiratory monitoring in postoperative patients. *Critical Care Medicine.* **7**:237–249.

Shoemaker, W. C., and L. Czer. 1979. Evaluation of the biologic importance of various hemodynamic and oxygen transport variables. *Critical Care Medicine.* **7**:424–430.

Siemens, R., H. C. Polk, L. A. Gray, and R. L. Fulton. 1977. Indications for thoracotomy following penetrating thoracic injury. *The Journal of Trauma.* **17**:493–550.

Sonnenblick, E. H., W. H. Freshmar, T. H. Le Jemtel. 1979. Dobutamine: a new synthetic cardioactive sympathetic amine. *New England Journal of Medicine.* **300**:17–22.

Spinella, J. L. 1979. Clinical assessment of the shock patient. *(JEN) Journal of Emergency Nursing.* **3**:34–37.

Tharp, G. D. 1974. Shock: the overall mechanisms. *American Journal of Nursing.* **74**:2208–2211.

Thompson, W. L. 1975. The Cell in Shock. The Upjohn Co., Kalamazoo, Mich.

Thompson, W. L. 1976. The Organ in Shock. The Upjohn Co., Kalamazoo, Mich.

Thompson, W. L. 1976. The Patient in Shock. The Upjohn Co., Kalamazoo, Mich.

Tunell, W. P., J. Knost, and F. C. Nance. 1975. Penetrating abdominal injuries in children and adolescents. *The Journal of Trauma.* **15**:720–725.

Ulevitch, R. J., and C. G. Cochrane. 1978. Role of complement in lethal bacterial lipopolysaccharide-induced hypotension and coagulative changes. *Infection and Immunity.* **19**:204–211.

Van Stiegmann, G., E. E. Moore, and G. E. Moore. 1979. Failure of spleen repair. *The Journal of Trauma.* **19**:698–700.

Vassy, L. E., R. L. Klecker, E. Koch, and T. S. Morse. 1975. Traumatic gastric perforation in children from blunt trauma. *The Journal of Trauma.* **15**:184–186.

Vogelpahl, R. A. 1981. Disseminated intravascular coagulation. *Critical Care Nurse*. **1**:38–43.

Weinstein, M. E., G. G. Govin, C. L. Rice, and R. W. Virgilio. 1979. Splenorrhaphy for splenic trauma. *The Journal of Trauma*. **19**:692–697.

West, J. B. 1977. Ventilation-perfusion relationships. *American Review of Respiratory Diseases*. **116**:919–943.

Wilson, K. F. 1976. The diagnosis and management of severe sepsis and septic shock. *Heart & Lung*. **5**:422–429.

Yabek, S. M. 1980. Management of septic shock. *Pediatrics in Review*. **2**:83–87.

Yajko, R. D., F. Seydel, and C. Trimble. 1975. Rupture of the stomach from blunt abdominal trauma. *The Journal of Trauma*. **15**:177–183.

CHAPTER 8

NUTRITIONAL SUPPORT OF THE CRITICALLY ILL CHILD

Diane S. Jakobowski

During an acute physiological crisis, the nutritional status of the critically ill child is all too easily overlooked. The critical care team's concerns may be directed toward immediate life-threatening situations such as cardiopulmonary resuscitation, a major system failure, and fluid and electrolyte abnormalities. In many cases, feedings consist of only 5 percent dextrose in water. Eventually, nutritional reserves are depleted, body protein and fats are broken down and used for energy, and lean body mass is lost. Studies have demonstrated that the effects of such starvation increase the child's susceptibility to infections, increase the length of recovery, and increase the rates of both morbidity and mortality.[1,2] Because of their rapid growth rate, children are much more susceptible to the consequences of malnutrition than are adults. Therefore, in the pediatric intensive care setting, it is essential that each child receive a nutritional evaluation and that nutritional support be considered in the initial plan of care — before the signs and symptoms of acute malnutrition are manifested.

PROTEIN-CALORIE MALNUTRITION

Primary protein-calorie malnutrition (PCM) is rarely seen in the hospitals of the United States, but it is prevalent in the developing countries of the world. Poverty, ignorance, a limited availability of food, and a poor environment all lead to diets lacking many of the essential nutrients. PCM has a very high rate of infant mortality, and children who do survive infancy may become "nutritional dwarfs."

The concern in this chapter is not malnutrition resulting from poverty and nutritional ignorance, but rather, semistarvation of the hospitalized child secondary to malabsorption, infection, anorexia, iatrogenic problems, or certain disease processes which may prevent adequate intake of all of the essential nutrients. Recent studies have shown that, in the *general* adult and pediatric hospital population, approximately 50 percent of the patients suffer from some degree of PCM,[3-6] while as many as 90 percent of the *intensive care* patients may be affected.[6] These figures are frightening, considering that PCM is associated with a high morbidity and mortality rate.

Children are admitted to the pediatric intensive care unit with a wide variety of diagnoses such as major gastrointestinal (GI) insufficiencies, severe cardiopulmonary difficulties, cancer, liver disease, renal disease, multiple trauma, and thermal injury. In all of these conditions, nutritional support may be difficult to provide and/or is often ignored. When a child requires intensive care, oral intake is often prohibited. A nasogastric tube may be inserted in order to drain gastric contents and to prevent possible vomiting and aspiration. Ventilatory support is provided as necessary, fluid and electrolyte balance is carefully assessed, invasive monitoring lines may be inserted, and many diagnostic tests are performed. A patient may remain NPO for 1 week or longer until "stable enough to risk" nutritional intervention. Critical illness, therefore, may be complicated by PCM.

Consequences of PCM

PCM occurs in varying degrees from mild to moderate to severe. Even in the mild form, some amount of growth failure and decrease in energy levels will occur. If malnutrition continues, more severe problems can arise: wounds heal poorly, decubitus ulcers develop, and there is generalized muscle atrophy, increased risk of infection, and impaired immune competence.

It has been postulated that chronic PCM early in a child's life is associated with retarded brain growth. The brains of malnourished children who died in the first year of life have shown a reduced number of brain cells and total lipid, cholesterol, and phospholipid content. Animal studies have demonstrated that inadequate nutrition early in life has a permanent effect on the brain size and cell number. These findings have been more difficult to document in human subjects, but reduced brain cell number, as reflected by decreased head circumference, seems to correlate with reduced intelligence scores.[7]

Prevention of PCM

Secondary PCM can have the same devastating effects as the primary PCM that is seen in underdeveloped nations; however, it can be prevented. Major strides in the field of nutritional research have been made over the past 15 years. Nutritional support services have been formed in most medical centers throughout the United States, and, with their expertise, sufficient alimentation (i.e., nutrition) can be provided in a safe and effective manner. It is the responsibility of the health care team to identify the nutritionally "at risk" patient, and the nurse plays a central role in this process. A simple nutritional screening (*see below*) performed by the nurse is the first step in the process. If warranted, a full nutritional assessment should be obtained, followed by appropriate nutritional support.

NUTRITIONAL ASSESSMENT

A nutritional assessment can be quite simple or very detailed, depending on the nutritional status of the patient. An initial screening is performed to determine if there is a nutritional deficit. Depending on the results, this may be all that is needed; however, if a deficit is found, the next step is a comprehensive nutritional assessment.

Initial Screening

Accurate measurements of the patient's height, weight, and head circumference are the first part of the initial screening. Also included are a brief dietary history and serum albumin level.

The admission screening should also include a brief nutritional history. Any recent weight loss of greater than 5 percent should be noted, as well as general dietary patterns, food fetishes, and any cultural differences in eating patterns. A blood sample (to measure serum albumin) should also be obtained to assess protein deprivation.

Any patient with a (1) decreased weight for height, (2) diagnosis associated with PCM (such as burns or catastrophic GI abnormalities), or (3) serum albumin level of less than 3.5 g/100 ml should receive a comprehensive nutritional assessment (Table 8-1).

Height.   Ideally, height is measured in an upright position for children over 2 years of age. The child must stand as straight as possible. The head should be adjusted so that the child is looking straight ahead. The feet should be bare and the heels placed together. Clearly, this will be impossible for many critically ill children. A second procedure for determining height in an older child is the measurement of recumbent length — which is also the preferred method for the small child or infant. This is most accurately performed on a measuring board or a table surface that has a fixed headboard and a movable footboard to which a metric tape is attached. If a measuring surface is not available or if the child's condition prevents placement on such a surface, the position of the child as described above should be duplicated as closely as possible. Height should be measured to the nearest 0.5 centimeter.

Weight.   For accuracy, weight should be obtained with the child in the nude. If privacy cannot be obtained, a light sheet or clothing may be used to cover the child. Any covering, however, should be weighed prior to placement on the child, and then subtracted from the final weight. A beam balance scale should be used. Whenever possible, the child's weight should be obtained before the insertion of ventilatory and monitoring devices, and again after all equipment is attached. The exact equipment should be accurately charted for continual reference. The weight is recorded to the nearest 10 grams in children.

Head circumference.   A metal or flexible plastic tape should be used to measure head circumference. The maximum circumference of the occipital frontal plane is the desired measurement. The tape must be in the same plane on both sides of the head, and it should pass just above the child's eyebrows. Excessive amounts of hair should be excluded. Head circumference should be measured to the nearest

---

TABLE 8-1   Indications for Comprehensive Nutritional Assessment

>5% body weight loss in past month (excluding dehydration).
Weight for height <5th percentile.
Diagnosis associated with development of PCM.
Serum albumin <3.5 g/100 ml

Reprinted with permission from Suskind, R. M., editor. 1981. Textbook of Pediatric Nutrition. Raven Press, New York. 302.

PCM, protein-calorie malnutrition.

0.5 centimeter. This measurement will not be accurate and need not be performed in children with a distorted head size secondary to head trauma or to cranial or craniofacial surgery.

For these measurements to be of maximum value, they must be plotted on a standard growth chart. The National Center for Health Statistics has published charts that are based on accurate physical measurements made on a large, representative group of children from the United States (Figs. 8-1 to 8-8.) There are two sex- and age-dependent charts: birth to 36 months, and 2 to 18 years. Weight, height, and head circumference for age can be plotted as well as weight for height in prepubescent children. A decrease in head circumference for age may be indicative of malnutrition during infancy — the period of greatest head growth velocity.[8] A deficit in height for age may indicate a state of chronic malnutrition.[9] A decreased weight for age can be misleading because the height of two children of the same age can vary significantly. Weight for height and weight for height for age provide a more accurate assessment of nutritional status. It has been found that a child with a decreased weight for height is more likely to have a prolonged hospital course than a better nourished child. Although these findings may reflect the severity of the primary disease process, a similar correlation was not found with height for age.[5]

Comprehensive Nutritional Assessment

A comprehensive nutritional assessment (Table 8-2) should only be performed by a member of a nutritional support service who is specifically skilled in determining nutritional deficits. The comprehensive assessment is presented here to provide the nurse with the information required to interpret the results.

History. This full assessment begins with a history of weight variance. The child's ideal weight, admission weight, current weight, and any recent weight change should be recorded. The primary diagnosis must be considered in conjunction with any coexisting metabolic problems. A thorough dietary history should then be obtained. Pertinent questions would be related to the parent's evaluation of the child's usual appetite, any changes in eating patterns, likes and dislikes, and vitamin supplementation. It may also be useful to record the child's typical intake for 1 day, including the times of meals and snacks, what is eaten, how it is prepared, and the amount consumed.

Evaluation of protein status. Adequate protein reserves are essential for recovery from critical illness to occur. A number of tests can be performed to evaluate the various aspects of protein status.

Serum albumin, transferrin, prealbumin, and retinal-binding protein studies have all been used to evaluate visceral protein status. The latter two studies are probably the most sensitive indicators of protein malnutrition, but many laboratories are not equipped to perform them. Transferrin, with a half-life of 9 days, can be obtained from the total iron-binding capacity (TIBC) by using the following calculation:

$$(0.8 \times \text{TIBC}) - 43.$$

Albumin has a half-life of approximately 20 days and, therefore, probably will not reflect acute protein deprivation or respond quickly to nutritional intervention.

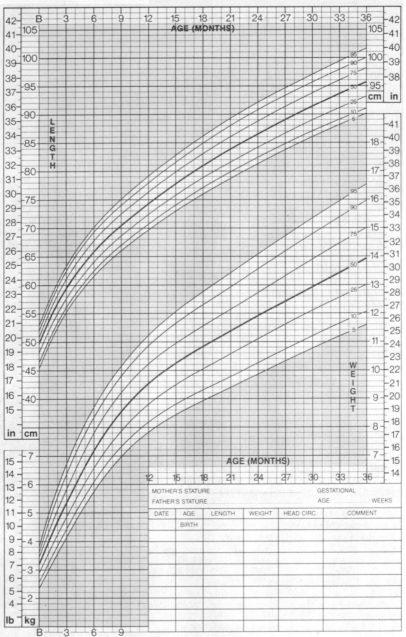

Figure 8-1. Girls: Birth to 36 Months. Physical Growth NCHS Percentiles. Adapted from Hamill, P. V. V., T. A. Drizd, C. L. Johnson, R. B. Reed, A. F. Roche, and W. M. Moore. 1979. Physical growth: National Center for Health Statistics percentiles. *American Journal of Clinical Nutrition* **32:**607–629. Data from the Fels Research Institute, Wright State University School of Medicine, Yellow Springs, Ohio. *Reprinted with permission from* Ross Laboratories, Columbus, Ohio, © 1982.

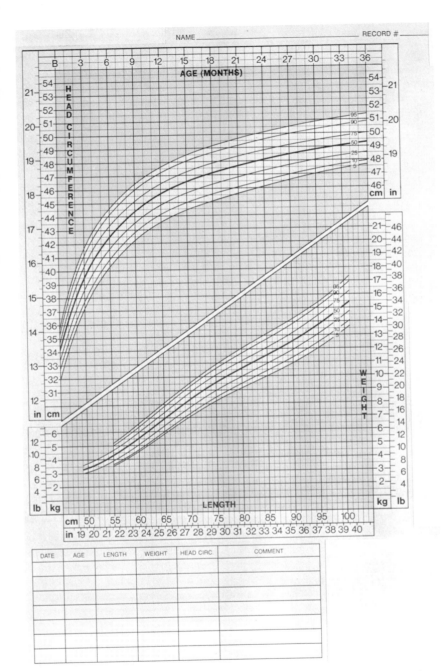

Figure 8-2. Girls: Birth to 36 Months. Physical Growth NCHS Percentiles. Adapted from Hamill, P. V. V., T. A. Drizd, C. L. Johnson, R. B. Reed, A. F. Roche, and W. M. Moore. 1979. Physical growth: National Center for Health Statistics percentiles. *American Journal of Clinical Nutrition* **32:**607–629. Data from the Fels Research Institute, Wright State University School of Medicine, Yellow Springs, Ohio. *Reprinted with permission from* Ross Laboratories, Columbus, Ohio, © 1982.

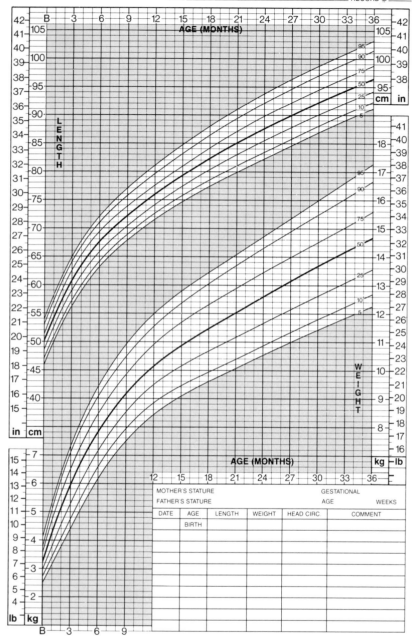

Figure 8-3. Boys: Birth to 36 Months. Physical Growth NCHS Percentiles. Adapted from Hamill, P. V. V., T. A. Drizd, C. L. Johnson, R. B. Reed, A. F. Roche, and W. M. Moore. 1979. Physical growth: National Center for Health Statistics percentiles. *American Journal of Clinical Nutrition* 32:607–629. Data from the Fels Research Institute, Wright State University School of Medicine, Yellow Springs, Ohio. *Reprinted with permission from* Ross Laboratories, Columbus, Ohio, © 1982.

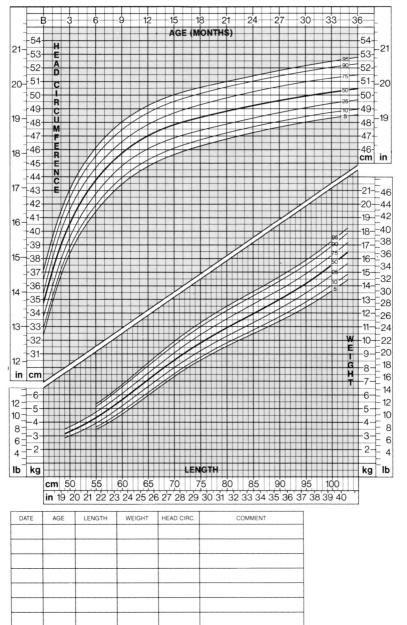

DATE	AGE	LENGTH	WEIGHT	HEAD CIRC.	COMMENT

Figure 8-4. Boys: Birth to 36 Months. Physical Growth NCHS Percentiles. Adapted from Hamill, P. V. V., T. A. Drizd, C. L. Johnson, R. B. Reed, A. F. Roche, and W. M. Moore. 1979. Physical growth: National Center for Health Statistics percentiles. *American Journal of Clinical Nutrition* **32:**607–629. Data from the Fels Research Institute, Wright State University School of Medicine, Yellow Springs, Ohio. *Reprinted with permission from* Ross Laboratories, Columbus, Ohio, © 1982.

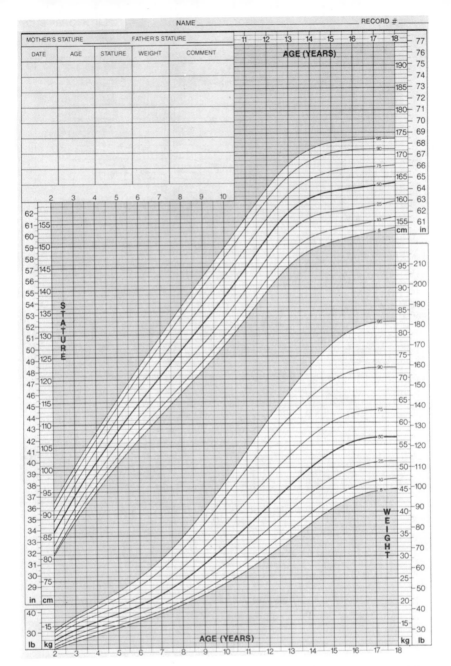

Figure 8-5. Girls: 2 to 18 Years. Physical Growth NCHS Percentiles. Adapted from Hamill, P. V. V., T. A. Drizd, C. L. Johnson, R. B. Reed, A. F. Roche, and W. M. Moore. 1979. Physical growth: National Center for Health Statistics percentiles. *American Journal of Clinical Nutrition* **32**:607–629. Data from the National Center for Health Statistics (NCHS), Hyattsville, Maryland. *Reprinted with permission from* Ross Laboratories, Columbus, Ohio, © 1982.

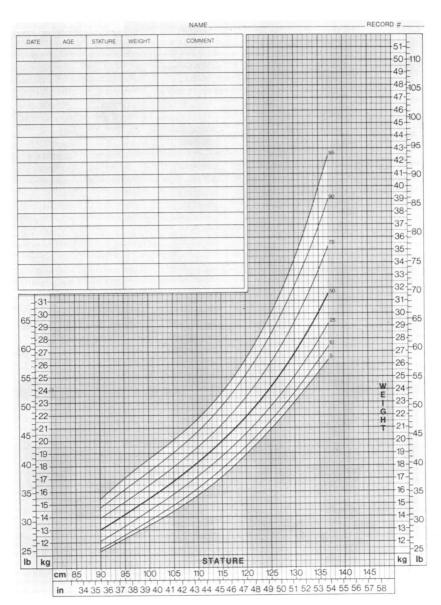

Figure 8-6. Girls: Prepubescent. Physical Growth NCHS Percentiles. Adapted from Hamill, P. V. V., T. A. Drizd, C. L. Johnson, R. B. Reed, A. F. Roche, and W. M. Moore. 1979. Physical growth: National Center for Health Statistics percentiles. *American Journal of Clinical Nutrition* **32:**607–629. Data from the National Center for Health Statistics (NCHS), Hyattsville, Maryland. *Reprinted with permission from* Ross Laboratories, Columbus, Ohio, © 1982.

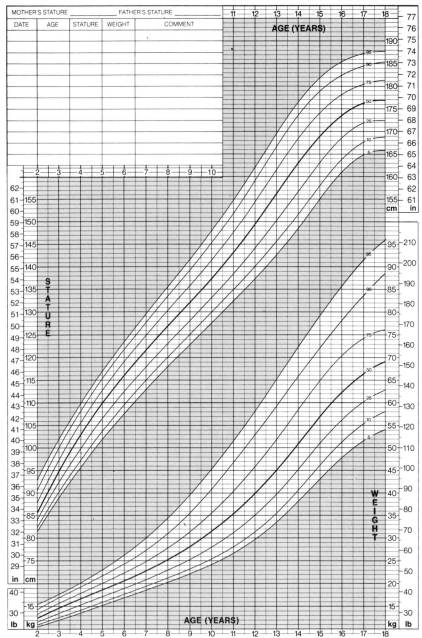

Figure 8-7. Boys: 2 to 18 Years. Physical Growth NCHS Percentiles. Adapted from Hamill, P. V. V., T. A. Drizd, C. L. Johnson, R. B. Reed, A. F. Roche, and W. M. Moore. 1979. Physical growth: National Center for Health Statistics percentiles. *American Journal of Clinical Nutrition* **32:**607–629. Data from the National Center for Health Statistics (NCHS), Hyattsville, Maryland. *Reprinted with permission from* Ross Laboratories, Columbus, Ohio, © 1982.

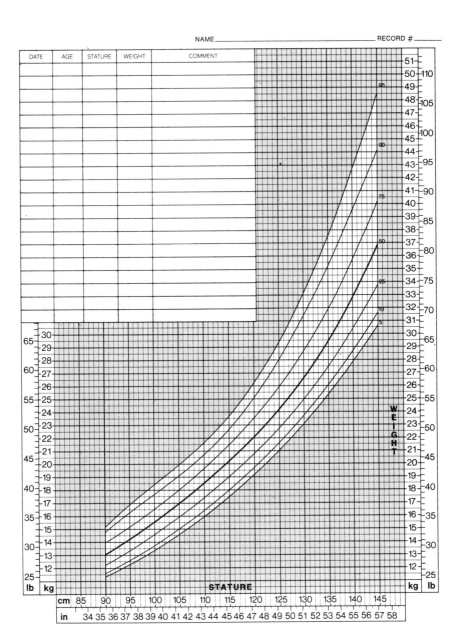

Figure 8-8. Boys: Prepubescent. Physical Growth NCHS Percentiles. Adapted from Hamill, P. V. V., T. A. Drizd, C. L. Johnson, R. B. Reed, A. F. Roche, and W. M. Moore. 1979. Physical growth: National Center for Health Statistics percentiles. *American Journal of Clinical Nutrition* **32:**607–629. Data from the National Center for Health Statistics (NCHS), Hyattsville, Maryland. *Reprinted with permission from* Ross Laboratories, Columbus, Ohio, © 1982.

TABLE 8-2 Comprehensive Nutritional Assessment

Parameter	Assessment
History	Weight (on admission, current, recent change, and ideal)
	Diagnosis (primary; other metabolic problems)
	Dietary history
Anthropometrics	Height for age
	Weight for age
	Height for weight
	Head circumference
	Mid-upperarm circumference
	Triceps skinfold
	Mid-upperarm muscle area
Biochemical analysis	Prealbumin
	Retinal-binding protein
	Transferrin
	TIBC
	Albumin
Protein status	CHI
	Nitrogen-balance study
Immune status	Total lymphocyte count
	Intradermal skin testing

CHI, creatinine height index; TIBC, total iron-binding capacity.

The size of muscle mass is an indirect indication of protein reserve,[10] and therefore, assessment of muscle size should be performed. For a person with a reduced body weight, a decrease in muscle protein would be more dangerous than a loss of fat stores. Height and weight alone may not distinguish between these two body compartments, but anthropometric measurements of the mid-upperarm may. Using the technique described by Grant,[10] the examiner can obtain the circumference of the mid-upperarm and the triceps skinfold thickness. From these measurements, arm muscle circumference and arm muscle area can be calculated and compared with the standard values produced by Frisancho.[11,12]

It has been postulated that daily creatinine excretion is proportional to body muscle size and, therefore, reflects protein status.[13] To evaluate this, the child's 24-hour urinary creatinine excretion is compared with body height (again to exclude the variable of body fat). The actual urinary creatinine excretion level divided by the normal creatinine excretion level for individuals of the same height, multiplied by 100 will provide the creatinine height index (CHI).

$$\text{CHI} = \frac{\text{Mg Urine Creatinine}}{\text{Mg Normal Urine Creatinine}} \times 100$$

This value can then be compared with standard values.[14] This assessment is not always used for the pediatric population for two reasons: (1) the standard values were obtained from a limited, non-American population, and (2) three consecutive 24-hour urine collections are needed for accurate calculation, and can be very difficult to obtain in children.

An evaluation of lean body mass can be performed with a nitrogen-balance study. The intake of nitrogen is compared with nitrogen that is lost through the urine, feces, and skin. Enteral and parenteral intake of protein is then calculated

(6.25 gram of protein is equal to 1.00 gram of nitrogen). Total urine urea nitrogen excretion is determined from a 24-hour urine collection. A constant of 4 is used to estimate the amount of nitrogen lost through the skin, feces, and urinary non-urea nitrogen in the adult population.[15] This constant can also be used for adolescents. For infants and small children, the amount of non-urea nitrogen that is lost is probably negligible, and therefore, no constant is used in this population. In general, it can be assumed that any patient who is starved or infected is in negative nitrogen balance. This tool is especially useful in evaluating the progress of therapy once nutritional support has been initiated. A slow, steady increase from negative to positive nitrogen balance should be seen. As with the CHI, this study may be difficult to complete because of the need for an accurate 24-hour urine collection. Thus, a sustained weight gain and a balanced intake and output is (1) probably equally reliable as an indicator of protein intake and clinical status and (2) easier to measure.

Immune status. It has been documented that malnutrition increases a person's susceptibility to infection because of depressed immunologic defense mechanisms. To complete the nutritional assessment, an evaluation of the child's immune system is needed. This evaluation may be quite difficult in the critically ill child. Whereas a total lymphocyte count of less than $1,500/mm^3$ normally indicates acute malnutrition in the adult population, it has been found to be less reliable in the pediatric population.[6] Another equally sensitive indicator of malnutrition in the adult population is intradermal skin testing with antigens. If the immune system is intact, an inflammatory response will occur after the application of certain antigens. However, successful intradermal skin testing in the child requires prior sensitization to the antigen used. The most reliable antigens are those to which the child is known to have been exposed (e.g., tetanus toxoid or mumps, since virtually all children have been immunized against these diseases). After the age of 1 year, *Candida albicans* antigens may elicit a response, but again, this is dependent on prior exposure.

For a nutritional assessment to be of value to the patient it must be repeated weekly throughout the intensive care course of hospitalization. This continual surveillance will determine changes that need to be made in the patient's dietary formulation, will indicate further monitoring that may be necessary, and will evaluate the adequacies of the nutritional program.

NUTRITIONAL SUPPORT OF THE CRITICALLY ILL CHILD

Once the nutritionally "at risk" patient has been identified, an appropriate diet and the desired route of administration must be selected. Man was created with an alimentary tract for the purpose of ingestion and absorption of nutrients; therefore, usually, "if the gut works, use it." If it cannot be used, the alternative is intravenous-alimentation.

Nutrient Requirements

Protein, energy, water, minerals, trace elements, and vitamins must be supplied to the child. The required amount of each of these elements for the critically ill child is unknown; however, the amounts would certainly depend on the extent of the injury or illness. For example, the protein and energy requirement of a burned child may be the same as that child's normal requirements or may be increased as much as 100 percent, depending on the extent of the injury and the physical activity of the child. In general, the protein requirement for an infant is 2.0 to 2.5 g/kg/day. Lesser amounts (1.0 to 1.5 g/kg/day) are needed for an older child.

Energy requirements change with the metabolic rate. Trauma will increase the metabolic rate, whereas bed rest will decrease the rate. Thermal status also changes energy requirements; for each degree centigrade rise or fall in body temperature, daily energy requirements should correspondingly rise or fall by 12 percent.[16] The following calculation has been used to estimate energy requirements for infants recovering from malnutrition. The kilocalories per kilogram would be less for a well-nourished infant or older child:[17]

$$\text{kcal/kg required} = \frac{120 \text{ kcal/kg(or desired kcal/kg)} \times \text{ideal weight for actual height}}{\text{actual height}}.$$

Water requirements should maintain a state of adequate hydration as indicated by heart rate, urine output and specific gravity, skin turgor, and mucous membrane status. Minerals, vitamins, and trace elements must meet the Daily Recommended Allowances.[18]

ENTERAL ALIMENTATION

A decade ago, most nutritional research was directed at parenteral alimentation, and many patients who could have been fed through their GI tract were not. More recently, this practice was questioned, and the whole field of enteral nutritional support has been revitalized. Solutions have been reformulated, techniques improved, and equipment redesigned with patient comfort and safety in mind.

Critical Care Mangement

Nutritional support must be viewed by the critical care team as a therapeutic modality no less lifesaving than, for example, ventilatory support. This section will review the aspects of the management of the child receiving enteral alimentation, including indications for its use, enteral product classification, methods of administration, general monitoring, measures to ensure patient comfort, and the advantages and complications of this therapy.

Indications

With appropriate management, the GI tract can be used for nutritional intervention for children with a wide variety of disease processes. Table 8-3 reviews circumstances in which enteral feeding can almost always be used, should be delivered with caution, or should not be used at all. Regardless of the situation, close observation of the patient is essential in order to identify potential problems before they become major complications.

TABLE 8-3   Indications/Contraindications of Enteral Therapy

General indications	Use with caution	Contraindications
Intact GI tract Head or neck injury or illness	**Questionable GI** **functioning** Short-bowel syndrome Intractable diarrhea Inflammatory bowel disease Enterocutaneous fistula Pancreatic insufficiency	**Nonfunctioning GI** **tract** Intractable vomiting Intestinal obstruction Upper GI bleeding

GI, gastrointestinal.

Enteral Product Classification

Enteral formulas have been classified in a variety of ways, usually according to their protein, carbohydrate, and fat content. It may be more effective, however, to consider the specific needs of the child. Is a complete diet, a high-calorie supplement, or a single nutrient required? In addition, the nutritional implications of the child's diagnosis must be considered. Does the patient need a low-sodium diet? Must protein be limited? How much fluid can be tolerated?

Complete diets.   Complete diets can be categorized in three basic groups: blenderized (meal replacement), partially hydrolyzed (partially predigested), and chemically defined (elemental). These diets, when administered in volumes needed to meet caloric requirements, contain the Recommended Dietary Allowances for minerals and vitamins.

Blenderized formulas consist of intact nutrients. Digestion and absorption are required, and there is a moderate amount of residue. This type of alimentation was named from the practice of blenderizing a regular house diet in order to provide a tube-fed patient with a liquid preparation that had a proportional amount of nutrients from each of the food groups.

Partially hydrolyzed formulas may contain glucose oligosaccharides rather than the intact carbohydrates found in fruits and vegetables. For the majority of seriously ill children with major GI insult, these formulas are ideal for several reasons. First, they do not contain lactose: After a period of no GI intake, the gut will not produce lactase, the digestive enzyme that is essential for the breakdown of lactose. The administration of lactose to a lactase-deficient child may cause severe diarrhea. Second, many of these formulas are isotonic, which means that the diet can be administered at full volume and concentration within 3 to 4 days without serious GI side effects. Third, the formulas are low in residue: i.e., most of the nutrients are absorbed rather than eliminated. The child's stooling pattern, therefore, may be decreased.

Chemically defined formulas contain nutrients that require little or no digestion before absorption. These diets are primarily used to nourish the child with a shortened bowel surface. The diets have a high osmolality, and therefore, administration must be at a slow, constant rate with close monitoring. In addition, the use of an infusion pump is essential.

High-calorie supplements. High-calorie supplements are usually used for patients who are in the recovery phase of an illness. They are meant to supplement a normal diet, and they contain a fairly large number of calories in a small volume. In general, these supplements taste fairly good and are well accepted by the patient.

Single nutrients. Single nutrients are used to compose a modular type of diet for the child who has severe bowel dysfunction and who has not tolerated conventional formulas. With this modality, a single nutrient such as glucose is administered to the patient. If there are no adverse effects after a specific amount of time, a second, and then a third, nutrient is added. At each step, any feeding intolerance can be clearly identified and appropriate measures can be taken. This type of feeding regimen must be closely supervised by a qualified nutritionist. Single nutrients may also be added to regular enteral products. It must be remembered, however, that this will alter the normal distribution of calories and increase osmolality, therefore, this practice is not recommended for infants.

Special therapeutic formulas. Special formulas are currently available for children with renal and hepatic disease. The renal solution contains a limited amount of protein, and the hepatic formula uses branched-chain aromatic amino acids. For other disease processes, regular formulas may be adapted to meet the metabolic needs of the patient. For example, a formula that is available in the powdered form may be mixed in a more concentrated form for a critically ill child whose fluid intake must be restricted.

Summary. When selecting an enteral product, several factors must be considered. A product that meets one child's needs may not be appropriate for another. The clinician should first consider the child's clinical course; then the route and method of administration; the osmolality and caloric density of the formula; the protein, carbohydrate, and fat source; the electrolyte and vitamin content; the cost; and, finally, the palatability. Table 8-4 (*see* p. 484) lists two or three examples of formulas from each of the classifications.

Methods of Administration

There are three basic methods of administering nutrients to a patient: orally, via nasoenteric feeding tubes, or via tube enterostomies. In the intensive care setting, nasoenteric feedings are probably the most common, and therefore, the majority of this discussion will be concerned with this type.

Oral. If the child's condition permits provision of adequate amounts of nutrients by the oral route, this should be attempted first. Supplements should be added to the diet to increase the calories and/or the protein when necessary. Eating normally is important for conscious, well-oriented children because it is one activity that is related to wellness rather than illness. For the infant, the sucking reflex can be lost without constant reinforcement. Retraining a child to eat normally after a long period without oral stimulation may be a very difficult task. Thus, the oral route of administration of nutrients should be considered to be the most desirable throughout the course of illness.

When children in an intensive care setting are able to eat normally, time should be taken to assist them or to provide company for them. The environment should be as pleasant as possible so that children can look forward to meal times. In addition to providing important social support for seriously ill and recovering children, these simple steps assist them in establishing trust with their nurse, which might otherwise be impossible if their only contact with the nursing staff was during painful or invasive treatments and procedures.

Nasoenteric. If and when oral feedings are unsuccessful and/or dangerous to the infant or child, nasoenteric feedings can be used. When this regimen is indicated, children are best approached in a firm, but positive manner. Far too often, nurses may say to children or parents, "We have to start tube feedings, but it won't be so bad. . . ." This type of situation would not occur if the child were dehydrated and needed intravenous (IV) fluid therapy. Alternatives would not be suggested because there would be none. Likewise, there are rarely better alternatives when a child needs nutritional support, cannot be fed orally, but has a functioning GI tract.

Some children will go to extremes to avoid nasoenteric feedings. Some may make themselves vomit or may continually remove the feeding tube. Neither of these situations should be tolerated. Vomiting, however, may result in a potentially dangerous situation (i.e., aspiration), and the etiology should be investigated: The tube position and function should be checked to be sure that it is not in the esophagus. Was the feeding advanced too rapidly, causing bloating, which may precipitate vomiting? What are the child's medications? Do any of them cause this problem? If this investigation proves negative, the feeding should be continued, but with very careful monitoring. A child who repeatedly removes the feeding tube should know that this action will lead to prompt reinsertion of the tube. Under no circumstances should any alternatives be mentioned, as either a threat or a promise.

Nasoenteric intubation is a far less invasive procedure than other alimentary techniques, such as gastrostomy and parenteral nutrition. At times, IV alimentation may appear to be "easier" than fighting with an uncooperative child over a feeding tube. However, for the patient with a functioning GI tract, this is rarely an acceptable alternative.

It is important for the nursing staff to emphasize the positive aspects of enteral alimentation and to assist children to feel comfortable with it. Many children enjoy fantasizing about the content of their feeding. For example, telling children that peanut butter and jelly, hot dogs, candy, and cookies may all be mixed together in their feeding bags, may increase their acceptance of enteral feedings.

At regular meal times, it may be helpful to distract the children who are receiving enteral alimentation with games and toys so that they are not preoccupied with watching other children eat. In general, any form of positive reinforcement will make this feeding experience more successful.

Insertion techniques: Depending on the needs of the child, nasoenteric feeding tubes may be placed in the stomach, duodenum, or jejunum. Feeding tubes should be composed of polyurethane or silicone (Silastic). A large variety of these tubes are now available in various sizes. The tubes are comfortable, are not usually associated with the erosive complications of polyvinyl chloride, and may remain in place for several weeks without being changed. For patient comfort, the smallest tube that will allow passage of the formula should be selected. Unless a blenderized formula is used, most children will not require a tube larger than size 8 French. The catheter should be radiopaque in order to permit confirmation of tube placement by x-ray.

TABLE 8-4 Enteral Product Classification

Product and manufacturer*	kcal/ml	CHO†	Protein†	Fat†	Osmolality mOsm/kg	Cost dollars/ serving	Comments
Complete diet (blenderized)							
Compleat-B (Doyle)	1	48% Malto-dextrin, lactose, sucrose.	16% Beef, skim milk.	36% Corn oil, beef fat.	390	.04	Can be taken PO. Requires digestion and absorption. Gastrostomy feedings with anticipation for home feedings. Moderate residuals.
Compleat Modified Formula B (Doyle)	1	53% Hydrolyzed cereal, solids, fruit, vegetables, and orange juice.	16% Beef puree.	31% Corn oil, mono- and diglycerides.	300	.12	See comments for Compleat-B.
Vitaneed (Organon)	1	51% Corn syrups, maltodextrin. Pureed green beans, peaches, carrots.	14% Beef, calcium, caseinate.	35% Soybean oil, mono- and diglycerides.	400	.14	Low Na.

Partially hydrolysed

Isocal (Mead Johnson)	1	50% Glucose, oligosaccharides.	13% 80% calcium and sodium caseinate. 20% soybean protein isolate.	37% 80% soybean oil. 20% MCT oil.	300	.06	Low residuals. Low Na. Unflavored.
Osmolite (Ross)	1	55% Corn syrup solids.	14% 88% sodium and calcium Caseinate. 12% Soybean protein isolate.	31% 50% MCT 49% corn oil. 1% soybean oil.	300	.05	Low residuals. Intended for tube feeding. Low Na. Unflavored.
Ensure Plus (Ross)	1	53% 74% corn syrup solid. 26% sucrose.	15% 88% sodium and calcium caseinate. 12% soybean proten isolate.	32% Corn oil.	600	.06	Low residuals. Multiflavored. Hypertonic: not recommended for transpyloric feeding.

TABLE 8-4 (Continued)

Product and manufacturer*	kcal/ml	CHO†	Protein†	Fat†	Osmolality mOsm/kg	Cost dollars/ serving	Comments
Chemically defined							
Vipep (Cutter)	1	68% Corn syrup. Sucrose. Cornstarch.	10% Hydro- lyzed fish protein.	22% MCT oil, corn oil.	520	.12	For children with malabsorption. Absorbed in upper gut.
Vivonex (Eaton)	1	90.5% Glucose oligo- saccharides.	8.2% L-amino acids.	1.3% Safflower.	550	.12	For children with malabsorption. Absorbed in upper gut.
Supplements							
Sustacal Pud- ding (Mead Johnson)	1.7	53% Sucrose, modified food starch, lactose.	11% Nonfat milk.	36% Partially hydro- genated soy- bean oil.	Not applicable.	.09	Contains lactose. Palatable. Multiflavored.
Citrotein (Doyle)	0.66	74% Sucrose, maltodextrin.	24% Egg-white solids.	2% mono- and diglycerides. Partially hydro- lyzed soy- bean oil.	500	.07	Some added vita- mins and minerals. Palatable. Grape and orange flavor.

Single nutrient

Polycose (Ross)	100% glucose polymers.	2	None	None	850	12	For protein- and electrolyte-restricted diets.
MCT Oil (Mead Johnson)	None	7.7	None	100% Fractionated coconut oil, primarily C_8 and C_{10} saturated fatty acid.	Not applicable	04	For use in patients who cannot effectively digest and absorb conventional long chain fatty acids.

Special therapeutic formula

Amin-Aid (McGaw)	75% Maltodextrins, sucrose.	2	40% Crystalline amino acids.	21% Partially hydrogenated soybean oil, lecithin, mono- and diglycerides.	900	.55	For use in renal disease. Low electrolytes. Low amino acids. Contains no vitamins.
Hepatic-Aid (McGaw)	70% Maltodextrins, sucrose.	1.6	10% Branch chain and aromatic amino acids.	20% Soybean oil, lecithin, mono- and diglycerides.	900	1.05	For use in liver disease. High level of branch chain amino acids. Contains no minerals or vitamins.

CHO, carbohydrate; MCT, medium chain triglycerides; Na, sodium; PO, by mouth.

*These formulas are only a few of the many feedings available. Most aspects of formula change frequently. Check company representative for changes in composition and cost.

†The percentages in each column indicate what portion of the total calories provided are in the form of CHO, protein, and fat. Beneath them are the food sources of these percentages.

With a conscious or semiconscious patient, the insertion procedure should be explained to the child and/or family. The nurse should allow children to handle the tube whenever possible and make certain that they and the parents are aware of the reason for the feeding regimen. Both the child and the other family members should be allowed to express their fears and concerns. If possible, older children should not be restrained, but rather, encouraged, to help with the procedure. A cooperative patient will make this task much easier.

Insertion of the soft, pliable tubes may be difficult. There is no all-encompassing set of rules for the insertion of feeding tubes. The clinician should always read the package insert before beginning the procedure because each tube may require different techniques and equipment. For example, some are inserted with removable or dissolvable stylets, whereas others require the installation of water. Freezing of silicone or polyurethane tubes will have little or no effect on decreasing flexibility for easier insertion. Although freezing will affect polyvinyl chloride tubes, it is not recommended because stiffness can cause trauma to the child's mucous membranes. A suggested technique for tube insertion is listed below:

1. Assemble the necessary equipment.
2. Elevate the patient bed to a 45-degree angle or place the child in an infant seat.
3. Select the more patent nostril.
4. For gastric feedings, measure the distance from the patient's ear to his nose and then to the xiphoid process. Add 10 to 15 centimeters of length for transpyloric feedings.
5. Once the appropriate length has been selected, mark the tube with a small piece of tape.
6. Lubricate the tip of the feeding tube.
7. Insert the tube toward the back of the throat. Ask the patient to swallow or have an infant suck on a pacifier to facilitate passage. If the patient experiences any shortness of breath, cyanosis, or inability to speak, the tube should be removed immediately.
8. Continue passing the tube until the desired length is inserted as indicated by the marker tape.
9. Check the position of the tube by aspiration of gut content. Many of the small-bore feeding tubes will collapse when negative pressure is exerted. Therefore, if gastric content can not be aspirated, an abdominal x-ray is indicated to verify proper catheter tip placement.
10. Apply tincture of benzoin to the area of the cheek where the tube is to be taped.
11. Tape the tube securely to the patient's cheek, avoiding pressure on the nares.
12. Document the procedure and the patient's response to it.

After tube insertion, if transpyloric feedings are needed, the patient should be positioned with his right side down for several hours to facilitate passage of the tube into the duodenum. An infusion of water at 1 ml/hr may also assist in the passage. Although content that is aspirated from the tube with pH of 7 indicates likely passage through the pylorus, radiographic confirmation is suggested.

When a tube feeding regimen is discontinued, the tube should be flushed with a small amount of water. The tube should be pinched (to prevent any fluid in the tube from being aspirated into the trachea) and gently but quickly removed.

Enterostomy. When long-term enteric feedings are anticipated, a tube enterostomy may be the best means of providing nutritional support. The feeding tube can be surgically placed directly into the stomach or the intestine. Alternatively, with a small incision in the neck, the tube can be inserted into the pharynx or esophagus and then threaded to the desired location. The major advantage of this type of alimentation is patient comfort and appearance because the nasal area is bypassed.

Feeding Administration

For a critically ill child with altered GI functioning, the preferred method of administration of any nasoenteric feeding is a slow, continual infusion of formula over 24 hours. This usually prevents bloating, vomiting, and gastric retention, all of which are frequently associated with large bolus feedings. Once a continual feeding regimen has been well established for several days and there are no side effects, the regimen can be switched to bolus if desired. In general, the critically ill child will require continual feedings, because this technique facilitates the assessment of fluid and electrolyte balance and glucose tolerance. In addition, a much greater nutrient intake can usually be administered with this method.

Feedings should be delivered into the stomach rather than the small intestines whenever possible. This allows the normal digestive processes to occur and permits selection of a physiologically complete formula with intact protein, complex carbohydrates, and long-chain fatty acids. If the patient does not have a gag reflex or requires mechanical ventilation and aspiration is a major concern, a transpyloric feeding regimen may be selected. A formula with partially hydrolyzed protein but intact carbohydrate and fat is often suitable for duodenal feedings because the majority of the digestive processes take place there. For jejunal feedings, however, nutrients must often be predigested.

Jejunal feedings can be difficult to manage and are not often recommended. Nutrients should be in their simplest form before delivery in order to avoid complications. The osmolality of these predigested formulas is high, and therefore, they must be administered at a very slow and constant rate of infusion in order to be tolerated at all. Meticulous monitoring is essential. Even when an appropriate formula is selected, if the feeding is delivered as a bolus or as a rapid infusion, cramping or diarrhea will probably result.

Feeding regimen. Initiation of enteral feedings, whether into the stomach or the intestine, should begin slowly. Formulas should be diluted to a one-quarter strength concentration and administered at a rate of approximately one-quarter maintenance to start. The remainder of maintenance fluid is administered via the IV route. If no adverse symptoms occur after 12 to 24 hours, the feeding may be advanced in one of the following ways: With delivery into the stomach, it is probably advantageous to initially increase the concentration rather than the volume so that the child's caloric intake is increased as quickly as possible. If energy intake is not at issue, volume can be advanced first. However, whichever method is selected, it is important that only one step in the advancement schedule be taken at a time. For transpyloric feedings, which necessitates the selection of a partially or completely predigested formula with high osmolality, the volume is always advanced first. This measure avoids the problem of a high osmotic load, which would result in water loss in the stools. Table 8-5 is an example of a feeding schedule that a child might readily tolerate.

TABLE 8-5 Sample Enteral Feeding Schedule

Patient information	Weight: 11.2 kg. GI tract: intact. Gag reflex: intact. NPO for past 10 days. Diet: Isocal Liquid Diet. Delivery site: stomach. Fluids: Will calculate maintenance fluids, but initially will deliver only ¼ of that as the formula, the remainder of fluids to be administered intravenously. As the volume of formula is increased the IV fluid volume is correspondingly decreased. Maintenance fluids: 1,060 ml/day (100 ml/kg for first 10 kg, then 50 ml/kg for second 10 kg).

Schedule	Day 1 (8 a.m.): ¼-strength Isocal at 11 ml/hr.
	    (8 p.m.): ½-strength Isocal at 11 ml/hr.
	
	Day 2 (8 a.m.): ¾-strength Isocal at 11 ml/hr.
	    (8 p.m.): full-strength Isocal at 11 ml/hr.
	
	Day 3 (8 a.m.): full-strength Isocal at 22 ml/hr.
	    (8 p.m.): full-strength Isocal at 33 ml/hr.
	
	Day 4 (8 a.m.): full-strength Isocal at 44 ml/hr.
	    (8 p.m.): increase volume as indicated by clinical status and caloric need.

GI, gastrointestinal; NPO, nothing by mouth.

A precise feeding schedule should be established for each child. The patient who falls into the moderately or severely malnourished range in the nutritional assessment will require a longer period for advancement to a full diet than a child who is well nourished before admission and who has only been without adequate nutrition for a short period of time. Many children will tolerate a full feeding regimen in 3 to 4 days, but others will require well over a week to reach an appropriate caloric intake.

One error that is often made in the provision of enteral alimentation is changing the formula at the first sign of intolerance. Many products that are available have very similar formulations, and switching from one to another will probably have little or no beneficial effects. In fact, switching formulas may result in the child receiving an inadequate protein and energy intake for a longer period of time, because changing formulas will probably require returning to the initial step in the feeding regimen. If the child develops diarrhea, nausea, or gastric retention, a decrease in volume or concentration of the formula is recommended before any change in formula itself. An antidiarrheal preparation, if not contraindicated, may be prescribed for persistent diarrhea. If excessive vomiting occurs, however, the feeding must be stopped.

Feeding delivery. Proper tube placement must be confirmed before each feeding, or once per shift for continual feedings. Aspiration of gut content is the best method. Auscultation over the left upper quadrant of the abdomen for air injected into the tube is also acceptable for gastric feedings. The distal end of the feeding tube should not be placed into water, because gas in the stomach may be misinterpreted as air in the lung. In addition, and of greater consequence, if the feeding tube is by any chance in the trachea, the water may be drawn into the lungs during inspiration.

Feeding residuals must be checked at regular intervals. With continual feedings, if more than 50 percent of the previous hour's feeding is aspirated, the volume should be reduced. This should be checked every hour at the initiation of a feeding regimen and then every 4 hours. For bolus feedings, residuals should be checked before each feeding. In general, there should be no residual, but again, if there is greater than 50 percent of the previous feeding, the amount aspirated should be subtracted from the total amount to be administered in the next feeding. Aspirated gut content should always be slowly reinserted to prevent excessive electrolyte loss.

Enteral alimentation solutions should be warmed to room temperature before administration. For continual feedings, they should hang for no longer than 4 hours. At the end of that time, the administration set should be disconnected from the feeding tube and flushed with water. The new formula should then be primed through the administration set and reconnected to the feeding tube. The entire administration set should be changed once every 24 hours. If, at any time, the feeding must be stopped or discontinued, the delivery system should be flushed with an appropriate amount of water (usually 2 to 5 milliliters). All of these measures are intended to decrease the chance of bacterial proliferation.

Oral medications can be administered through most feeding tubes. Solid preparations must be finely crushed before administration. After the administration of either solid or liquid preparations, the tube should be flushed with water to ensure that the entire dose reaches the gut at the appropriate time. If the child is receiving bolus feedings, the tube should be clamped for 20 minutes after the administration of medications.

Enteric feedings may be delivered by gravity drip or an infusion pump. To ensure that the desired volume is delivered at a constant rate, a volumetric or peristaltic pump should be used. Both of these pumps operate with forward pressure that will deliver even viscous solutions through small-bore tubes. Controllers, on the other hand, do not provide forward pressure, but rather, control gravity flow. If the feeding tube becomes clogged with a concentrated solution, the controller will fail to operate. Pumps and controllers were originally designed for total parenteral nutrition, but have now been adapted for use with enteral alimentation. There are also specifically designed enteral pumps that have many of the features of parenteral pumps, such as occlusion and low battery alarms and set flow rates. In general, these are less expensive than the parenteral pumps, and they are ideal for home use.

Battery life is one of the most important aspects in the selection of a pump. This may not seem important in an electronically oriented intensive care unit (ICU), but in an ambulatory care unit, patients who are receiving continual pump feedings do not want to be confined to one place. For this reason, if an institution is selecting only one type of pump for all patient areas, the battery life must be considered. The battery life will also facilitate transport of ICU patients.

Feeding bags should have a large top or side opening for easy filling (Fig. 8-9), and the tubing must be adaptable to an IV system if a parenteral pump is used. The nurse should make sure that the extension set is of adequate length to prevent inadvertent displacement of the tube during procedures and treatments.

With the increased use of IV equipment for the administration of enteral products, the nurse should be absolutely certain that all feeding equipment is clearly marked "Not for IV use," in order to avoid delivery of the enteral product into a

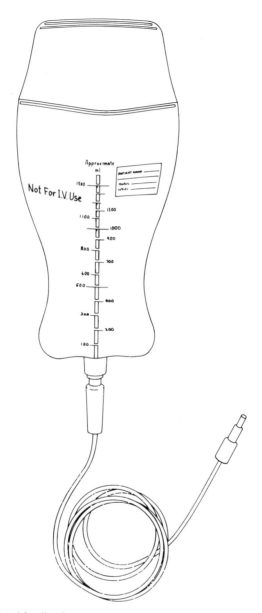

Figure 8-9. Enteral feeding bag.

vein. This is especially important in an ICU setting, where there may be a fairly large number of clinicians caring for one child and as many as three or four of the exact same infusion pump at one bedside. Many centers add 1 milliliter of food coloring to the feeding within the bag so it is more easily distinguished from IV fluids. Regardless of whether food coloring is used, visible labels and diligent nursing care are essential to avoid this potentially fatal complication.

Monitoring of Feeding

Accurate daily monitoring of the patient's tolerance of the feeding regimen is essential to a successful program. This monitoring must include precise recording of intake and output in milliliter increments and measurement of body weight at least three times per week. The patient's urine must be checked routinely for specific gravity and glucose content in order to assess patient tolerance. Further biochemical monitoring is essential when delivering a chemically defined formula. This monitoring schedule would be the same as for a total parenteral nutrition patient (*see* Table 8-14, p. 509). All aspects of the patient's enteral nutrition program should be recorded in a clear and concise manner.

Patient Comfort

The patient's comfort throughout this procedure is of the utmost importance because degree of physical comfort obviously directly effects the individual's behavior and the final outcome of this technique. Measures which may enhance the child's tolerance of the feeding regimen include:

1. Use the smallest bore tube available that will deliver the selected feeding at the prescribed rate.
2. Always warm the feeding to room temperature.
3. Change the patient's position frequently.
4. Wash excessive adhesive marks from the patient's face. Change the external tape as necessary. Never place any pressure on the nares.
5. Provide excellent oral and nasal hygiene.
6. Provide the patient with some type of lip gloss or moisturizing agent.

Advantages

There are many advantages to enteral feeding. First, it is as close to a physiologically normal feeding regimen as possible for many critically ill children. Animal studies have demonstrated that early continual feeding maintains the structural and functional integrity of the small bowels.[19-24] After a period of no GI intake, gut weight, villus height, and mucosal protein are reduced. There is also a depression of digestive enzymes in the brushborder, thereby making the reintroduction of enteral intake a very slow process.

When compared with total parenteral nutrition, enteral nutritional support is a safer mode of therapy. There is little risk of sepsis or anatomic injury. With the use of small-bore silicone tubes, there is very little irritation to the nasopharyngeal or GI areas. Appropriate catheter tip placement can be confirmed by radiography. Once this is accomplished, the tube does not have to be replaced for several weeks, thus eliminating the fairly constant manipulation of the larger polyvinyl chloride tubes.

An enteral feeding regimen is relatively inexpensive when compared with other means of nutritional support. An IV alimentation solution can cost over $100/liter, whereas a simply prepared enteral product may cost as little as $2.00 for the same volume. With the cost of preparation and personnel, even a house diet may be more expensive than enteral alimentation.

Considering all of these factors, as well as the fact that the GI tract is designed for the delivery and absorption of nutrients, enteral alimentation should be considered first for the nutritional support of most critically ill children.

Complications

In general, the complications related to enteral nutrition are divided into three categories: GI, mechanical, and metabolic. Metabolic complications occur rarely, and generally only with the use of chemically defined formulas. (These potential complications are the same as for total parenteral nutrition and are listed in Table 8-17, p. 514.) Table 8-6 (p. 496) outlines the clinical indications (signs and symptoms), probable causes, treatments, and prevention of enteral complications.

Summary

Throughout an ICU course, patients can tolerate and benefit from some form of enteral alimentation. The clinician should select the appropriate formula, begin the feeding slowly, and allow for an adequate period of adjustment. Sufficient nutrients should be provided to sustain weight and nitrogen balance. The clinician must assess the child closely for feeding intolerance. When appropriate enteral alimentation is provided in conjunction with treatment of the primary disease, patient recovery from illness should be hastened.

TOTAL PARENTERAL NUTRITION

Total parenteral nutrition (TPN) is now a well-established, technically acceptable mode of therapy for the critically ill child whose primary or secondary diagnosis has precluded the use of GI feedings. This, however, was not always the case. Before the mid 1960s, isotonic dextrose in water was the accepted method of IV "feeding," but it did not provide an adequate caloric intake or a nutritionally sound diet. With this therapy, the body's protein and energy stores became depleted, PCM developed, and, if this course were not reversed, the patient would succumb to starvation. Experimental IV products of protein and fat were developed, but, without the use of high concentrations of dextrose, anabolism could not be achieved, and hypertonic dextrose could not be administered into a peripheral vein. In 1966, Dr. Stanley Dudrick established a relatively safe technique for the administration of hypertonic dextrose and casein hydrolysates infused directly into the superior vena cava. Using this technique, Dr. Dudrick demonstrated significant growth and development in beagle puppies and then in an infant.[25] After this monumental discovery, an upsurge of interest in nutritional support occurred throughout the medical communities of the world.

Critical Care Management

In many medical centers throughout the country, the delivery of TPN is considered "routine." This delivery, however, can be dangerous if all aspects of nutritional management are not constantly reevaluated and improved. Mature, clinical judgment must be used to determine whether the benefits of TPN outweigh the risks — especially the risk of sepsis. Once a program of aggressive nutritional support in the ICU has been established, close monitoring and meticulous nursing care are essential.

This section will review the aspects of the management of the child receiving TPN, including indications for its use, solution composition, methods of administration, solution delivery, administration of fat emulsion, general monitoring, and a review of the complications of this therapy.

Indications

The indications and uses of TPN for the pediatric population have changed somewhat over the past decade. Initially, this therapy was reserved only for those children with catastrophic GI dysfunctions, such as major small bowel resections secondary to gastroschisis, volvulus, or necrotizing enterocolitis. In these instances, IV alimentation was the only alternative for nutritional support. With the advent of TPN teams, medical centers throughout the country developed such expertise in delivery techniques and monitoring that TPN became the "easier or simpler" way to provide calories and protein in those children with esophageal or gastric dysfunction; pulmonary, cardiac, hepatic, or renal disease; and in conjunction with chemotherapy and radiation. Many of the children with such problems, however, would do very well with a closely monitored program of enteral support, because at least part of their GI tracts are functional. At present, rather than a quick decision to start central vein TPN, a child's entire nutritional situation is considered, and, unless there is almost total bowel dysfunction, nutritional support via the enteral route is attempted first.

The decision to use TPN in the critically ill child is made when enteral nutrition has been considered and determined to be inadequate or inappropriate. Delay in the provision of nutritional support may increase the risk of mortality and morbidity. Therefore, prophylactic use of TPN may be indicated to prevent acute starvation during the initial period of diagnosis, assessment, and treatment of the disease or injury. Once the patient has been stabilized, respiratory functioning is sufficient, and digestion and absorption via the GI tract has been established, slowly advancing enteral feedings can begin in conjunction with tapering TPN. Table 8-7 (p. 498) outlines the general indications for TPN.

Solution Composition

TPN solutions have become quite sophisticated in recent years, and they closely mimic an oral diet. At present, the deficiency states that were seen in the early days of TPN therapy rarely occur with the use of IV fat emulsions and trace element preparations. The main infusion bottle contains a proportionate amount of protein, glucose, and water as well as electrolytes, trace elements, and vitamins. IV fat is prepared and delivered via a separate system. The following section will discuss each of these areas.

TABLE 8-6 Complications of Enteral Alimentation

Complication	Clinical indications	Probable cause	Treatment	Prevention
GI				
Diarrhea	Frequent water loss stools.	Inadequate adaptation of GI tract to enteral feeding.		Begin feeding at a slow rate with a diluted formula.
		Possible causes:		Advance feeding one step at a time.
		1. Rapid advancement of feeding regimen.	Reduce flow rate (may need to add peripheral TPN).	Use an infusion pump for delivery of feeding at a slow, steady speed.
		2. Delivery of hypertonic solution.	Decrease formula concentration.	Do not administer lactose or MCT to a child who has been NPO for a long period of time.
		3. Administration of a milk-base formula to a lactase-deficient child.	Switch to a formula that contains no lactose.	
		4. Use of large amounts of MCT in a fat-intolerant patient.	Decrease or stop administration of MCT.	
			Administer antidiarrheal medications.	
Vomiting		Delivery of large volumes of concentrated formula.	Stop feeding infusion.	Use same preventive measures as for diarrhea.
		Displacement of the feeding tube into the esophagus or pharynx.	Check position of feeding tube.	Check residuals frequency during initial feeding; keep patient in a quiet, comfortable position. Elevate the child's head and trunk. Position on right side.
			Rule out GI obstruction and decreased gastric emptying.	
			If all of the above are negative, restart feeding at a slow continual rate with a diluted formula.	

Mechanical

Complication	Signs and symptoms	Causes	Treatment	Prevention
Pulmonary aspiration	Respiratory distress: Increased respiratory rate Retractions Nasal flaring Cyanosis	Vomited formula. Displacement of the feeding tube into the pharynx or trachea.	Stop feeding immediately. Quickly aspirate all contents from the feeding tube. Suction mouth and pharynx. Check feeding tube position and remove if displaced. May require chest physiotherapy and/or tracheal intubation.	Always check tube position before beginning feeding. Keep head and upper trunk elevated. Use transpyloric feeding for comatose patients without intact gag and swallow reflexes.
Tracheo-esophageal fistulae	Blood in the gastric residual. Formula obtained from tracheal suctioning. Increased respiratory distress.	Use of large-bore polyvinyl chloride feeding tube. Tube remaining in place for long period of time.	Remove feeding tube. May require surgical intervention.	Use of small-bore silicon rubber tubes. Insert tube very gently.
Clogged tube lumen	Inability of the feeding to infuse.	Use of viscous formula.	Remove feeding tube and insert a new one.	For bolus feeding, flush the tube with water after each feeding. Administer feeding via an infusion pump.

GI, gastrointestinal; MCT, medium chain triglyceride; NPO, nothing by mouth; TPN, total parenteral nutrition.

TABLE 8-7 Indications for Total Parenteral Nutrition

Central venous delivery	Peripheral venous delivery
Long-term therapy (>2 wk)	**Short-term therapy (<2 wk)**
Nonfunctioning GI tract	Partial use of GI tract
Abdominal wall deficits	maintained
Congenital or acquired	Transitional feeding from cen-
GI atresias	tral TPN to enteral
Ileus	alimentation
Fistulae	
Severe malabsorption	

GI, gastrointestinal; TPN, total parenteral nutrition.

Protein. The protein source in TPN is either a protein hydrolysate—which contains those essential and nonessential amino acids, as well as di- and tripeptides—or crystalline amino acids, which are composed of free essential and nonessential amino acids. Protein should be provided in adequate quantities to provide at least 1 gram of nitrogen for each 150 non-protein calories (1.00 gram of nitrogen is equal to 6.25 gram of protein). Higher ratios are acceptable when caloric intake must be increased, but lower ratios should not be used because the extra nitrogen cannot be used efficiently. Protein should not be considered caloric intake.

Carbohydrates. Glucose is the major source of carbohydrates in most IV alimentation regimens, and it should make up at least 50 percent of the caloric intake. Each gram of glucose provides 3.4 calories. Concentrations of glucose vary between 5 and 25 percent. Concentrations of 5 percent may be needed for small infants who have an intolerance for glucose because of an immature pancreas. Concentrations of greater than 10 percent should only be infused through a central venous catheter.

Fat. There are three commercially available fat emulsions: Intralipid 10%, Liposyn 10%, and Intralipid 20%. These fat emulsions consist of either soybean oil or safflower oil, an emulsifying agent, glycerin, and water. They contain a mixture of triglycerides of predominantly unsaturated fatty acids. A gram of a 10 percent fat solution provides 11 calories (1.1 cal/ml). A gram of a 20 percent solution provides 20 calories (2.0 cal/ml). An IV fat solution should be administered to any patient requiring TPN for longer than 1 week. These solutions may be administered through a central or peripheral vein.

Special care must be taken when using a 20 percent solution because it is twice as concentrated as the more familiar 10 percent solution. The 20 percent solution is especially useful for patients who are fluid restricted.

Water. Water is the major component of the human body and is maintained in the intercellular, extracellular, and transcellular compartments. To maintain a steady state, the amount of water intake plus water oxidated from carbohydrate, fat, and protein must equal the amount of water loss through the kidneys, lungs, skin, and GI tract. (For calculations of water requirements *see* p. 335.)

Electrolytes. Electrolytes may be needed in a TPN solution in varying amounts. The recommendations in Table 8-8 will meet maintenance requirements. If there are excessive losses from, for example, the GI tract, the sodium content will need to be increased. Care must be taken when adding extra electrolytes to the solution, because the added amounts may disturb the stability of the solution and

TABLE 8-8   Daily IV Electrolyte Requirements

Electrolyte	Requirements
Sodium	3–4 mEq/kg/day
Potassium	2–4 mEq/kg/day
Calcium (elemental)	20–40 mg/kg/day
Phosphate	1–2 mmol/kg/day
Magnesium	1–2 mEq/kg/day

Adapted from Coran, A. G., S. E. Denson, A. B. Fletcher, and B. Bernard, editors. 1980. The Compromised Neonate. Cutter Medical, Berkeley, Calif.

cause a precipitate. Many of the amino acid sources currently available contain a certain concentration of electrolytes, and this must be taken into account when formulating a solution.

Trace elements.   Trace elements are known to be essential to the nutritional status of patients. Initially, trace elements were not added to TPN solutions because they make up a very small percent of total body weight, but without them, many patients developed deficiency states. At present, trace elements are a standard additive to all TPN solutions. Table 8-9 outlines the known trace element requirements.

Vitamins.   The vitamin content of TPN solutions should meet the daily recommended allowances (Table 8-10). At present, there is no commercially available multivitamin preparation completely appropriate for pediatric usage. Multivitamin infusion (MVI) has been adapted for pediatric usage, but it does not contain vitamin K. Vitamin K may be inactivated in the solution and may cause an anaphylactic reaction when administered IV. Therefore, it should be administered intramuscularly once a month to the child who requires long-term TPN.

Methods of Administration

Once a decision has been made to provide IV nutritional support, a route of administration must be selected. Either central vein or peripheral venous nutri-

TABLE 8-9   Daily IV Trace Element Requirements

Trace element	Requirements
	µg/kg/day
Zinc	100–300
Copper	20
Chromium	0.14–0.20
Manganese	2–10

Adapted from American Medical Association, Department of Food and Nutrition. 1979. Guidelines for essential trace element preparations for parenteral use. A statement by an expert panel. *(JAMA) Journal of the American Medical Association.* **241**:2051–2054.

TABLE 8-10 Daily IV Vitamin Requirements

	Requirements	
Vitamin	<11 yr*	>11 yr
A (retinol), IU	2,300.0	3.300.0
D, IU	400.0	200.0
E (tocopherol), IU	7.0	10.0
K$_1$ (phylloquinone), mg	0.2	ND
C (ascorbic acid), mg	80.0	100.0
Folacin, μg	140.0	400.0
Niacin, mg	17.0	40.0
Riboflavin, mg	1.4	3.6
Thiamine, mg	1.2	3.0
B$_6$ (pyridoxine), mg	1.0	4.0
B$_{12}$ (cyanocobalamin), μg	1.0	5.0
Pantothenic acid, mg	5.0	15.0
Biotin, μg	20.0	60.0

Adapted with permission from American Medical Association, Department of Food and Nutrition. 1979. Guidelines for multivitamin preparation for parenteral use. A statement by the Nutrition Advisory Group. Journal of Parenteral and Enteral Nutrition. **3:**258–262.

ND, no standard determined.

*The vitamin requirements for infants should be met by administering 10 percent of the formulation per kilogram of body weight; the total formulation should be administered to children weighing 10 kilograms or more.

tional therapy is possible. In many instances, this choice is not made easily. Four basic criteria must be considered before the selection of a venous route: caloric requirement, anticipated duration of need, venous accessibility, and the benefits of each type of therapy versus the risks. Table 8-11 depicts different situations and indications when these four criteria may need to be evaluated in order to determine the most beneficial route of administration for an individual child.

Central catheter administration.   Because of the high blood flow in the superior vena cava, this vessel is the best site for the infusion of the TPN solution. For a long time, catheter entry was achieved via a cutdown in the internal or external jugular vein or the common facial vein. In order to prevent septicemia from a skin contaminant, the lines were then subcutaneously tunneled to the scalp or anterior chest so the catheter would exit the skin at a separate, distant site from where the catheter entered the venous system. This technique still is a very sound and successful approach. A subcutaneous tunnel (even a short one) is recommended for all nutrition catheters. For long-term nutritional therapy, the cutdown site may be the cephalic vein rather than one of the sites mentioned above. In some centers, the subclavian approach has been found to be very successful, even in very small premature infants.[26,27]

Catheter insertion: Before insertion of a central nutrition catheter (CNC), all aspects of the procedure must be carefully explained to the child and/or family, including positioning, drapes, pre-insertion scrub, and local anesthesia. The equipment used for the catheter insertion and solution administration should be shown to the child. Every effort must be made to relieve any severe apprehension.

TABLE 8-11 Considerations for Selection of Route of Administration

Consideration	Peripheral therapy	Central therapy
Caloric need (100 kcal/kg/day) vs. fluid volume tolerated	Requirement 150 to 250 ml/kg/day plus 3 g/kg/day of fat emulsion	Requirement 80 to 150 ml/kg/day Fat emulsion may or may not be necessary
Anticipated duration of need	<2 wk	>2 wk
Venous access	Multiple venous sticks (rotation q 72 hr) May require maintenance of 2 IV infusions	One catheter insertion may remain indefinitely
Benefits	Avoidance of risks of central line insertion Delivery of minimal amounts of energy and protein	Maintenance or greater than maintenance caloric intake One catheter insertion
Risks	Subcutaneous tissue necrosis and skin sloughing	Complications associated with central line placement Sepsis

IV, intravenous.

Many children will respond positively to the nurse staying with them and just holding their hand; others may require mild sedation. A relaxed, cooperative child is of the utmost importance because any movement during the procedure could cause a major complication.

Elective placement of the CNC is best performed in the operating room, but, in certain cases for acutely ill children, the procedure may be performed at the bedside. The CNC must be inserted using aseptic technique: hood, mask, gown, and gloves are to be worn by those personnel performing the procedure. The cutdown or the percutaneous catheter insertion site must be prepped. Superficial hair should be shaved (if excessive), and the area should be cleaned with an acetone-alcohol solution to de-fat the skin. The area should then be washed for 5 minutes with a providine-iodine solution. This antifungal, antibacterial solution is most effective if allowed to dry on the skin. However, some patients' skin may be irritated by this solution, and it can be removed with 70 percent alcohol.

Proper positioning of the patient is very important for correct catheter placement. For a percutaneous insertion, the patient should be placed in Trendelenburg's position, which will distend the veins in the upper trunk. For a cutdown insertion, a flat position is acceptable.

If the CNC is to be inserted in the ICU, a certain amount of preparation is necessary. All equipment should be assembled on a sterile drape or barrier: the appropriate size catheter, acetone, providine-iodine scrub solution, alcohol, material to perform a cutdown, a sterile dressing, flush solution, and an administration setup. The physician should be assisted with the gown, gloves, and hood.

Once the catheter has been properly placed, it should flush easily and a rapid blood return should be evident. Isotonic solution should be infused at a keep-open rate until an x-ray can be performed to confirm proper catheter tip placement. Many catheters are not radiopaque and will, therefore, require infusion of a small amount of contrast material to be visualized. Ideally, the catheter tip should be in the superior vena cava or the right atrium. During this immediate postcatheter insertion period, the child should be observed for signs of dyspnea, cyanosis, and chest pain (signs of pneumothorax, *see* p. 512).

Once proper catheter placement has been confirmed, the ordered TPN solution may be administered.

Catheter care: After the insertion of a CNC, a sterile dressing must be placed over the catheter exit site. Then, every other day, the old dressing is removed and the area is inspected for drainage, erythema, or any other evidence of infection. In cases where an open, draining wound (e.g., a tracheostomy) is near the catheter exit site, daily dressing changes are indicated. It is not recommended that a site culture be taken routinely. Cultures should only be taken when there is drainage, edema, or erythema at the site. It is essential to culture a suspicious site because many instances of septicemia can be traced to an infected catheter site. If the catheter placement is maintained by sutures, their intactness should be assessed and the site should be cleaned. The following equipment is needed for a dressing change: a surgical mask (optional), sterile gloves, acetone-alcohol swabs, providine-iodine solution, providine-iodine ointment, sterile 2" × 2" gauze pad, tape, and a trash bag. The dressing change procedure is listed below:

1. Assemble necessary equipment.
2. Put on sterile mask.
3. Wash hands.
4. Remove old dressing *carefully,* and place in trash bag.
5. Wash hands.
6. Put on sterile gloves.
7. Clean the skin around the catheter site with acetone-alcohol swabs until the swab comes clean.
8. Clean the site, catheter, and the surrounding skin with providine-iodine solution. This should be a 5-minute scrub. Begin the scrub at the insertion site and work outward in a circular motion, covering a 2-inch area.
9. Remove excess solution from the skin with sterile water.
10. Apply a small amount of providine-iodine ointment to the catheter insertion site (and suture sites, if present).
11. Cover the insertion site (and sutures) with a sterile 2" × 2" gauze pad.
12. Cover the gauze with tape, incorporating the extension tubing into the dressing.
13. Date the dressing.
14. Document the dressing change and the appearance of the site in the patient's chart.

The central line dressing, surrounding area, and tunnel line should be checked every few hours for evidence of problems. No drainage should be present on the dressing, no edema noted at the initial insertion site or exit site, and no erythema or other signs of infection at the tunnel area.

Catheter withdrawal: The child should be properly prepared for the time the catheter is to be removed. Although this is a very simple procedure, a relaxed, cooperate child is important. The dressing over the catheter is removed, and the skin is prepped with providine-iodine solution (as in the routine dressing change procedure). If sutures are present, they are removed. The cathether is then carefully but quickly withdrawn. If the child is able to cooperate, he or she is asked to hold their breath during catheter withdrawal. Pressure should immediately be applied to the exit site and maintained for 5 minutes to prevent air from entering the venous system before closure of the catheter tract. An occlusive dressing is applied to the site.

Peripheral catheter administration. Even though access to the peripheral system is generally quite easy, delivery of TPN solution via a peripheral vein requires as much care and expertise as central vein administration. The veins must be cannulated properly, the delivery system monitored closely, and the same metabolic parameters monitored as in central vein TPN.

Catheter insertion: Proper cannulation of peripheral veins for TPN is essential. Many institutions employ an IV team, but if this service is not available, the most qualified staff member should insert the line. With experienced personnel, one stick is usually all that is necessary, and in terms of vein conservation and alleviation of the child's anxiety, this is very important.

IV catheters are more appropriate for peripheral nutrition support than scalp needles. Catheter insertion may be difficult initially, but once the catheter is in place it generally remains intact for 72 hours. (Three days is the recommended maximum amount of time for one IV catheter to remain in place.) A 24-gauge, 3/4″ catheter that has proven invaluable for children of all ages. Insertion and maintenance of this catheter for the older child is fairly comfortable, and for the premature infant it allows catheter cannulation of even very small veins. Despite the small gauge of this catheter, flow rates of up to 200 ml/hr can be achieved.

The IV should be placed in one of child's upper extremities whenever possible. The vein selection should start with the hand and then slowly work upward toward the antecubital area. Each new cannulation should be performed on the opposite arm. This same basic principle should be employed if the lower extremities are used. There should be a 5-day rest period before reinsertion of a catheter into the same vein.

Catheter care: Once the vein is cannulated, a small amount of providine-iodine ointment should be placed at the insertion site, which is then covered with a small piece of gauze or a bandage. The catheter should be taped securely — but in no way should the tape obstruct visualization of the site, thereby preventing early detection of an infiltration. Arm boards are recommended for small children in order to prevent movement at the insertion site. However, gross movement of the extremity is not a problem. Because the IV remains in place for no longer than 72 hours, dressing changes are not required. Meticulous monitoring of the catheter site is essential for peripheral nutritional support.

If the solution is being delivered via an infusion pump, it is essential that the insertion site be checked for signs of infiltration every 30 minutes. It has been well documented that a hypertonic (10 percent dextrose) parenteral nutritional solution that is pumped into the subcutaneous area can cause severe skin sloughing and tissue necrosis. The need for prevention of this peripheral complication cannot be overemphasized.

Special note: In general, cutdowns of peripheral veins are not recommended for several reasons. The vein may not be reusable, the catheter life is probably no greater than for a well-inserted percutaneous line, and there is a greater risk of infection as with any long-term catheter. Because of these potential problems, when peripheral veins can no longer be cannulated percutaneously, a central line for nutritional support is generally considered.

Solution Delivery

TPN solution must be prepared using aseptic technique under a laminar flow hood by qualified personnel in the pharmacy. Solution is delivered daily to the patient units and refrigerated until needed. The solutions are warmed to room temperature for approximately 1 hour before administration.

The label of the bottle and solution composition must correspond with the physician's order and contain proper patient identification. The solution must be inspected for cloudiness, precipitation, and foreign substances. No changes in the solution should be made on the nursing unit. If a substance such as an electrolyte must be added to the solution, the bottle should be returned to the pharmacy for this service. Nothing should be added to the bottle once it is in use.

TPN is initiated with a solution containing no greater than 10 percent glucose at a maintenance fluid rate (*see* p. 336). The patient is closely monitored for hyperglycemia and glucosuria. If neither of these conditions is present after 24 hours, the glucose concentration is increased at 24-hour intervals to a maximum concentration of 25 percent for central therapy. The concentration should always be at 10 percent for peripheral infusions. After reaching a maximum glucose concentration, the fluid volume can then be increased as tolerated to the volumes necessary for appropriate caloric intake. The protein concentration is regulated by the non-protein calorie: nitrogen ratio, nitrogen balance studies, and the child's clinical condition. In general, the initial protein concentration is 1.0 g/kg/day and is advanced to 2.5 g/kg/day.

The volume and concentration of the TPN solution must be accurately calculated to ensure proper protein and caloric intake. Table 8-12 provides an estimation of needed caloric intake for various weight groups, and Table 8-13 illustrates an example of the calculation that is used to determine caloric and protein intake. (Note that, in this example, the caloric intake may be inadequate, but the non-protein calorie:nitrogen ratio is acceptable.)

Administration Guidelines

The infusion bottle, administration tubing, and filter (if used) should be changed once every 24 hours. If, within that period of time, there is a solution change, or if all of the solution has been delivered, a new infusion bottle may be hung without changing the entire delivery system. Before opening any connection in the nutrition line, the external area should be scrubbed with alcohol. A providine-iodine solution may be substituted for alcohol, but it must dry thoroughly to be totally effective. The catheter or permanent catheter extension tubing must be clamped

TABLE 8-12 Recommended Energy Intake

	Age	Average weight	Energy needs (with range)
	yr	kg	kcal
Infants	0.0–0.5	6	kg × 115 (95–145)
	0.5–1.0	9	kg × 105 (80–135)
Children	1–3	13	1,300 (900–1,800)
	4–6	20	1,700 (1,300–2,300)
	7–10	28	2,400 (1,650–3,300)
Males	11–14	48	2,700 (2,000–3,700)
	15–18	66	2,800 (2,100–3,900)
Females	11–14	46	2,200 (1,500–3,000)
	15–18	55	2,100 (1,800–3,000)

Reprinted from National Academy of Sciences. 1979. Recommended Daily Allowances. National Academy of Sciences — National Research Council, Food and Nutritional Board, Washington, D. C. Ninth edition. 23.

before a routine tubing change or any other disconnection of the nutrition line. This will avoid the very serious complication of an air embolism, which can occur whenever there is communication between the atmosphere and the venous system. Once the new administration set has been attached, all connection points should be securely taped. The tape should be placed in such a way that at least part of the actual connection is visible.

In general, no other solution, medication, or blood product should be delivered through the same catheter. When caring for the critically ill child, however, this is not always feasible. If another solution must be administered through the catheter, a permanent connection should be made with a "y" connector or a multi-flow connector. If blood products are administered through a CNC, the line should be discontinued after the infusion of the blood product because minute amounts of blood fibrin may remain in the catheter and increase the risk of sepsis.

If the TPN solution is abruptly discontinued due to inadvertent displacement of the catheter, occlusion of the line, or infiltration, a peripheral IV should be started immediately with a peripheral TPN solution or a regular 10 percent glucose solution with maintenance electrolytes.

Infusion pumps.   With high concentrations of glucose, it is essential to deliver the solution at a constant, steady rate. Therefore, an infusion pump is recommended. These pumps will accurately control the rate of delivery and eliminate the very serious consequences of a "runaway IV." If an adequate number of pumps are not available, the solution may be dripped through a peripheral IV in an older child (the glucose concentration is no greater than 10 percent).

There is a great variety of infusion pumps available today. A volumetric or peristaltic pump is preferred for TPN because either of these pumps exerts a forward pressure, which is required to maintain a constant rate of infusion. Many of the pumps have an air-detector device and an occlusion alarm. A pump with a long battery life may be very valuable for patients who are being moved frequently for diagnostic studies, procedures, etc.

If two solutions are to be simultaneously delivered into the same vein (e.g., TPN solution and fat emulsion, *see* p. 507), both systems should include infusion

TABLE 8-13 Calculations for Total Parenteral Nutrition

IV caloric values
Protein = 4 kcal/g
CHO = 3.4 kcal/g
Fat = 11 kcal/g

Sample regimen desired for 9 kg child
1. 110 ml/kg/day (excluding fat)
2. 2 g/kg/day of protein (AA)
3. 15% glucose (CHO)
4. 1.5 g/kg/day of fat

Method for determining percentage of AA
1. TPN fluids/day = _____ml/kg/day × _____kg = _____ml
2. AA/day = _____g/kg/day × _____kg = _____g

3. $\dfrac{\text{AA/day (_____ g)}}{\text{fluids/day (_____ ml)}} \times 100 =$ _____% AA

Step 1:
calculate percentage of AA
1. 110 ml/kg/day × 9 kg = 990 ml
2. 2 g/kg/day × 9 kg = 18 g

3. $\dfrac{18\ g}{990\ ml} \times 100 = 1.8\%$ (rounded off to 2% AA)

Step 2:
calculate calories
1. 2% AA = 2 g/100 ml = 19.8 g/990 ml
2. 15% glucose = 15 g/100 ml = 148.5 g/990 ml
3. 10% fat* = 10 g/100 ml (1.5 g × 9 kg = 13.5 g/day)
4. Glucose: 148.5 g/day × 3.4 kcal/g = 504.9 kcal/day

5. Fat: 13.5 g/day × 11 kcal/g = $\dfrac{148.5\ \text{kcal/day}}{653.4\ \text{kcal/day}}$

              or
        72.6 kcal/kg/day

Step 3:
calculate non-protein
calorie:N_2 ratio
(6.25 g of protein = 1 g of N_2)

1. $\dfrac{1\ g\ N_2}{6.25\ g\ \text{protein}} = \dfrac{x\ g\ N_2}{19.8\ g\ \text{protein}}$ $x = 3.17\ g\ N_2$

2. $\dfrac{653.4\ \text{(non-protein calories)}}{3.17\ g\ N_2} = \dfrac{x\ \text{(non-protein calories)}}{1\ g\ N_2}$

$x = 206$ Non-protein calorie: N_2 ratio = 206:1

AA, amino acid; CHO, carbohydrate; IV, intravenous; N_2, nitrogen; TPN, total parenteral nutrition.
*Remember that the fat emulsion is a separate infusion.

pumps to ensure accurate flow rates. When equipment is limited and only one pump is available, the force of gravity must equal the pump pressure.

Filters. Over the past several years there has been much controversy over the use of in-line filters. The 0.22-micron hydrophobic and hydrophilic filters, which will trap both bacteria and fungus, were originally constructed in such a way that they would not withstand the forward pressure of infusion pumps. The filter membrane would rupture during the initial priming of the tubing or after only a few hours of usage. At present, most in-line 0.22-micron filters will withstand pressures as high as 45 pounds per square inch and, therefore, can be used safely and in combination with infusion pumps. Most of the currently available filters also eliminate air. They are strongly recommended for neonates and the immunosuppressed or critically ill child.

Administration sets. Ideally, the administration tubing should be a complete, closed system from the infusion bottle to the patient's permanent catheter connection. The fewer the connections on the line, the less likely the chance of an accidental disconnection. The tubing must also be of adequate length so that the child can move and turn freely.

Intermittent Administration

Although cycling of parenteral nutritional therapy may be beneficial to certain critically ill children, this procedure is usually reserved for the more stable child. A full day's nutritional intake is delivered over 12 to 14 hours. The full concentration of solution is delivered at a maintenance rate for the first hour, then increased sometimes to as much as twice maintenance until the last hour, when it is again decreased. This type of procedure challenges the patient's fluid status and his metabolic response to acute changes in insulin and glucose levels. If venous access is at a critical state and the patient requires a long infusion (8 to 12 hours) of an antibiotic, antifungal agent, or chemotherapy, this type of infusion may be attempted, but only with constant monitoring of glucose levels.

Discontinuing Therapy

Weaning the patient from TPN must occur with the same meticulous care that is used during the initiation of therapy. If another means of nutritional support has not been provided, weaning may take 12 to 24 hours in order to avoid reactive hypoglycemia. In general, however, weaning should occur only when enteral alimentation has been well established. The caloric intake should be maintained at a steady state level while the TPN is decreased and the enteral feedings are increased.

Administration of Fat Emulsions

If a fat emulsion is to be administered, it must not be mixed with any other IV solution in order to avoid disturbing the stability of the emulsion. It can be delivered into the same peripheral or central vein as the amino acid-glucose solution by means of a "y" connector located immediately distal to the catheter exit site. When this is done, the lipid will occasionally flow up into the amino acid-glucose tubing because the specific gravity of the fat emulsion is lower than the other solution. To prevent this problem, the lipid tubing should always be elevated. The initial rate of infusion should be 0.10 ml/min of the 10 percent solution and 0.05 ml/min of the 20 percent solution for the first 10 to 15 minutes. If there are no immediate adverse reactions (*see* Table 8-17, p. 516) the rate can be increased to permit an infusion of 1 g/kg/day. After the first 24-hour period, the child's serum is assessed for hyperlipidemia. If hyperlipidemia is not present, the infusion may be increased to a maximum of 3 to 4 g/kg/day. Once again, the serum should be assessed for lipidemia at each increase in volume and approximately three times a week thereafter. If there is evidence of excessive fat in the blood, the lipid infusion should be slowed or stopped until the serum clears.

IV fat must not constitute more than 60 percent of the total caloric intake. If the fat emulsion is administered as a means of preventing essential fatty acid deficiency, at least four percent of the total caloric intake must be provided as linoleic acid (which is contained in all fat emulsions).[28]

It is recommended that the fat emulsion be administered by means of a continual, slow infusion because the major pediatric complications of this therapy have occurred when large volumes have been administered over a short period of time. The patient receiving IV fat must be closely monitored for immediate and delayed adverse reactions (*see* Table 8-17, p. 516).

General Monitoring During TPN

Vital signs should be assessed routinely every 4 hours. If there is any major complication of therapy, and the patient becomes unstable, the vital signs should be monitored every hour. Precise determination of intake and output must be accurately recorded in order to determine fluid balance, caloric intake, and nitrogen balance. Ideally, the child's weight should be obtained daily but this may be unrealistic for some critically ill children. In such cases, twice-weekly weighings will suffice. The child's urine should be checked routinely for glucose content and specific gravity. In general, when solutions are advanced at a slow rate and the patient is not septic, there is no glucose in the urine. The general range of blood glucose can be determined through a Dextrostix, which may be very useful in an acute situation in which the blood glucose level is shifting rapidly. The exact serum glucose level should be obtained at the same time as the other routine blood studies (Table 8-14).

Patient Comfort

As with enteral feedings, the patient's acceptance of TPN can be greatly facilitated if the patient is made as comfortable as possible. The following is a list of some patient comfort measures:

1. Thoroughly prepare the patient for catheter placement and provide appropriate comfort measures.
2. If necessary, provide pain medications following catheter insertion.
3. Place tape over the dressing site securely, but in such a way that it does not restrict the child's movement or tug at the skin.
4. Provide an adequate length of tubing so that the child can turn easily.
5. If the child is NPO, provide oral and nasal hygiene and lip gloss or a moisturizing agent. Ice chips or gum may be provided, if the child's level of consciousness permits.

Advantages

The discovery of TPN is one of the major medical advances of the 20th century. It has provided a means of survival for persons with temporary or permanent nonfunctioning GI tracts who would otherwise have died of PCM.

Complications

The complications of TPN are divided into three categories: infectious, administrative (mechanical), and metabolic. In general, with an attentive monitoring program, most problems can be identified quickly and treated appropriately. However, infection remains the leading cause of morbidity and mortality related to

TABLE 8-14   Suggested Monitoring

Area	Study	Frequency
General	Vital signs	q 4 hr
	Weight	Daily
	Intake and output	Daily
	Caloric intake	Daily
Blood	Glucose	Daily until stable, then twice a week
	Electrolytes	Daily until stable, then twice a week
	BUN	Weekly
	Ca, P, Mg	Weekly
	Alkaline phosphatase, SGOT, SGPT	Weekly
	Bilirubin (total/direct)	Weekly
	Creatinine	Weekly
	CBC with differential	Weekly
	Zinc, copper	Monthly
	Other trace elements	As indicated
	Serum lipemia	Daily until stable, then 3 times a week
	Triglycerides	As indicated
	Cholesterol	As indicated
Urine	Glucose	q 4 hr until stable, then q 8 hr
	Protein	q 4 hr until stable, then q 8 hr
	Ketone	q 4 hr until stable, then q 8 hr
	Specific gravity	q 4 hr until stable, then q 8 hr

BUN, blood urea nitrogen; Ca, calcium; CBC, complete blood count; Mg, magnesium; P, phosphorus; SGOT, serum glutamic oxaloacetic transaminase; SGPT, serum glutamic pyruvic transaminase.

TPN. Its prevention and/or early detection and treatment merit special attention and will be discussed in the following section.

Infectious complications.   The incidence of infections during TPN therapy varies from one institution to another. However, most researchers have found a positive correlation between catheter-related sepsis and duration of therapy; i.e., the longer the catheter remains in place, the more likely the child is to become septic. In addition, there is strong evidence that violation of catheter care and solution delivery protocols is associated with a higher incidence of sepsis. Therefore, it is imperative that a protocol be established and adhered to strictly during the administration of TPN.

When a critically ill child displays the signs and symptoms of infection, a full sepsis work-up is indicated (Table 8-15). The infusing amino acid-glucose and fat emulsion solutions should be discontinued and sent for culture to rule out the possibility of solution contamination (a rare cause of septicemia). New bottles of nutrition solution should be hung immediately or, if that is not possible, a regular IV solution with a comparable amount of glucose and maintenance electrolytes is an adequate substitute as a temporary measure. The dressing over the central

TABLE 8-15 Infectious Complications of Total Parenteral Nutrition*

Complication	Clinical indications	Probable cause	Treatment	Prevention
Bacterial or fungal infection	Thermal instability, chills, lethargy, restlessness. Sudden glycosuria. Decreased platelet count. Elevated WBC.	Break in aseptic technique during catheter insertion, catheter maintenance (i.e., dressing changes), or preparation of solution.	Septic work-up to ascertain source of infection. This should include the following: 1. Physical examination. 2. Peripheral blood culture. 3. Culture TPN solutions: amino acid-glucose and fat emulsion. 4. Culture central catheter insertion site. 5. Culture any draining wounds, sputum, and urine. 6. Chest x-ray. 7. Lumbar puncture (possible). 8. Central blood culture.	Constant maintenance of strict protocol: 1. Preparation of solution in laminar air-flow area of the pharmacy. 2. Before solution is hung, it should be stored in a refrigerator at 4°C (39.2°F). 3. Nothing should be added to the TPN solution once it has left the pharmacy. 4. Strict adherence to aseptic technique during catheter insertion and maintenance. 5. Catheter exit site dressing changed q 48 hr.

If the infection is catheter related, the catheter should be removed and/or antibiotics initiated.

6. Solution and entire delivery system changed q 24 hr.
7. Maintenance of a continual closed delivery system.
8. Use of an in-line 0.22-micron filter, placed distal to the fat emulsion infusion.
9. Delivery system connections swabbed with alcohol before they are opened.
10. No routine blood sampling through the nutrition catheter.
11. No stopcocks on the nutrition line.
12. Peripheral catheters changed q 72 hr.

TPN, total parenteral nutrition; WBC, white blood count.
*Broad-spectrum antibiotics, radiation, steroids, and immunosuppressants predispose patients to fungal infection.

TABLE 8-16 Mechanical Complications of Total Parenteral Nutrition

Complication	Clinical indications	Probable cause	Treatment	Prevention
Central				
Pneumothorax Tension pneumothorax Hemothorax Hydrothorax	Sharp chest pain, decreased blood pressure, weak and rapid pulse, cessation of normal respirations on the affected side of the chest.	Inadvertent puncturing of the pleura during catheter insertion.	Needle aspiration or insertion of a chest tube.	Central catheter insertion by, or with the supervision of, an experienced physician.
Air embolism	Dyspnea, tachycardia, cyanosis, chest pain, disorientation, cardiac arrest.	Air entering the venous system during catheter insertion or maintenance.	If there is an obvious opening in the delivery system, the catheter should immediately be clamped. Place the child in Trendelenburg's position (left lateral decubitus position) in order to point the right heart up so that the air will exit the heart via the pulmonary artery.	*Always* clamp the catheter when the delivery system is opened. If this is not possible, place the patient in Trendelenburg's position and have the patient perform the Valsalva maneuver (bearing down, holding breath). A padded hemostat must be with the child at all times in case of an emergency, i.e., inadvertent disconnection.

Complication	Clinical signs and symptoms	Probable cause	Treatment	Prevention
Thrombosis of the vena cava	May be undetectable. Edema of the arms, neck, and face.	Fibrin sheath forms around catheter. Occurs most frequently with: Sepsis, Extended therapy, High concentrations of dextrose, Polyvinyl catheters.	Removal of the catheter. Anticoagulation therapy may be ordered.	Avoid the four items listed under "Probable cause."
Dislodgment of the catheter	Leakage of solution on the dressing. Chest pain, edema, or erythema of the catheter area.	Securing sutures that are not intact. Improper taping of the exit-site dressing. Improper movement of the child (tension placed on the catheter). Spontaneous movement.	To ascertain patency of the catheter: Lower the infusion setup to check for backflow of blood. Obtain chest x-ray and/or venogram. Remove the catheter if dislodgment is confirmed	Replace nonintact securing sutures immediately. Incorporate part of the administration set tubing into the dressing. Pay strict attention to the catheter when changing the child's position. Secure (pin) the administration set tubing to the bed linen or the child's clothing.
Peripheral Skin slough Tissue necrosis	Edema of the site and surrounding skin area; may be very extensive. Blister or blanched area at site.	Continual infusion of solution after the catheter has been displaced from the vein. Occurs most frequently with the use of infusion pumps.	Elevate extremity. Do no soak. Treat as a burn if extensive. May require skin graft.	Check catheter site q 1/2 hr for signs of infiltration.

A-V. (Arteriovenous) fistula, cardiac tamponade, thoracic duct injury, and brachial plexus injury are rare mechanical complications of central TPN.

TABLE 8-17 Metabolic Complications of Total Parenteral Nutrition

Complication	Clinical indications	Probable cause	Treatment	Prevention
Hyperglycemia/glucosuria	Pallor, weakness, dizziness, change in disposition, diaphoresis, thremors, sudden hunger, blurred vision, dilated pupils.	Rapid infusion of glucose. Note: Sudden hyperglycemia/glucosuria may be an indication of sepsis.	Reduce the rate and/or concentration of the glucose infusion. Consider administration of insulin. Note: If left untreated may lead to hypernatremia, hyperosmolarity, and osmotic diuresis (nonketotic hyperosmolar coma).	Monitor blood glucose level: Dextrostix q 8 hr Serum level q day Note: Stop dextrostix and decrease monitoring of serum levels to twice a week when maintenance therapy is reached. Monitor urinary glucose level q 4 hr until maintenance therapy is reached, then q 8 hr. Initiation of TPN with a glucose concentration of no greater than 10%. Advance regimen in a slow, step-by-step method. For example, for a 10 kg child: Day 1: D10% at 75 ml/kg/day. Day 2: D10% at 100 ml/kg/day. Day 3: D15% at 100 ml/kg/day. Day 4: D20% at 100 ml/kg/day. Day 5: D20% at 130 ml/kg/day. Deliver solution via an infusion pump.

Complication	Signs/Symptoms	Cause	Treatment	Prevention/Monitoring
Hypoglycemia	Lethargy, nausea, vomiting, dehydration.	Sudden cessation of glucose infusion. Excessive administration of insulin.	Increase rate or concentration of glucose.	Maintain a constant rate of infusion; never "catch up." Monitor blood glucose level. Gradually decrease TPN as enteral alimentation is advanced.
Electrolyte imbalance Hyper- or hyponatremia Hyper- or hypokalemia Hyper- or hypocalcemia Hyperphosphatemia Hypermagnesemia		Inappropriate administration of electrolytes.	Administer appropriate electrolyte.	Close monitoring of electrolyte status (see Table 8-14).
Hypophosphatemia	Anemia, muscular weakness, lethargy, coma.	Inadequate intake. Increased needs with high glucose administration	Increase amount of phosphate.	Monitor phosphate level carefully. Administer adequate amounts of phosphate.
Hypomagnesemia	Twitching, hypertonicity, CNS changes.	Inadequate intake, increased GI losses, anabolism.	Increase amount of magnesium.	Monitor magnesium level carefully. Administer adequate amounts of magnesium.
Hyperchloremic metabolic acidosis	Decreased blood pH. Decreased base excess.	Excessive hydrogen ion load. Excessive delivery of chloride ion. Excessive renal loss of base.	Administration of sodium bicarbonate. Delivery of some acetate salts rather than all chloride.	Monitor acid-base status.
Cholestatic jaundice Note: usually occurs in premature infants.	Direct bilirubin >2 mg/dl.	Unknown; probably related to amino acid imbalance. Usually occurs after intensive IV alimentation without oral intake.	Stop TPN as soon as possible.	Check total and direct bilirubin weekly, as well as other liver function tests. Maintain minimal intake through the GI tract whenever possible.

TABLE 8-17 (Continued)

Complication	Clinical indications	Probable cause	Treatment	Prevention
Essential fatty acid deficiency	Eczematous skin. Poor wound healing. Elevated triene:terraene ratio.	Delivery of fat-free IV alimentation.	Administration of IV fat emulsion or an enteral product containing appropriate amounts of fat.	Administration of IV fat emulsion if child will be NPO for 1 wk.
Excessiver delivery of fat	Immediate: Nausea, vomiting, headache, flushing, increased temperature, chills, chest and back pain, tachypnea, cyanosis, histamine-like reaction, irritation at the site. Delayed: Hepatomegaly, splenomegaly, thrombocytopenia, leukopenia, elevated liver function studies, hyperlipemia.	Excessive rate of administration. Excessive dose. Inadequate metabolism of excessive fat.	Stop fat emulsion infusion. When all symptoms clear, restart infusion as a very slow infusion. Provide fat enterally.	Close monitoring Clinical examination Liver function studies Lipemia checks three times a week.

Zinc deficiency	Dermatitis. Anorexia, growth retardation. Poor wound healing.	Inadequate delivery of zinc with long-term therapy. Excessive renal and GI losses. Seen frequently with chronic diarrhea and excessive ileostomy fluid losses.	Provide adequate zinc to reverse deficiency state.	Administer maintenance zinc therapy.
Copper deficiency	Anemia, leukopenia, neutropenia, bone abnormalities.	Inadequate delivery of copper with long-term therapy.	Provide adequate copper to reverse deficiency state.	Administer maintenance copper therapy.
Chromium deficiency	Glucose intolerance.	Inadequate delivery of chromium with very long-term therapy.	Provide adequate chromium to reverse deficiency state.	Administer maintenance chromium therapy.

CNS, central nervous system; D, dextrose; GI, gastrointestinal; IV, intravenous; NPO, nothing by mouth; TPN, total parenteral nutrition.
Hyperammonia azotemia, other trace-element deficiencies, and vitamin deficiencies are rare metabolic complications of TPN.

catheter site should be changed, and if purulent drainage is present, the drainage should be cultured and (in most cases) the catheter removed because many septicemias have been traced to infected insertion sites. If all of the above findings are negative and the patient continues to manifest symptoms of sepsis, blood should be drawn through the central catheter for culture.

There is much controversy at present regarding when to remove a CNC in the presence of sepsis. Catheters are often removed quickly when there is no positive evidence of catheter-related sepsis. In general, if there is a distant site of infection, the catheter need not be removed, but the blood cultures require very close monitoring because the catheter may act as a focus for bacterial growth. Positive blood cultures or an infected catheter insertion site require treatment. The usual therapy includes catheter removal and/or the administration of organism-specific antibiotics. Once the central line has been removed secondary to sepsis, a 48-hour waiting period between a negative blood culture and reinsertion of another line is recommended.

Mechanical complications.　There are reported administrative (mechanical) complications of both central and peripheral venous delivery. Table 8-16 details the major complications that can occur during catheter insertion and during the following therapy. This table also lists the mechanical complications that are less likely to occur. The use of silicone catheters and radiographic comfirmation of catheter tip placement before delivery of hypertonic solution will eliminate most complications.

Metabolic complications.　Most metabolic complications are related to an excess or deficit in the nutritional formulation of the TPN solution. These problems can be reduced or eliminated by proper estimation of the child's nutritional and metabolic requirements and by continual biochemical monitoring. The major metabolic complications in the pediatric population are detailed in Table 8-17, which also lists the minor (or easily corrected) complications.

Summary

Since its establishment, TPN has become an acceptable mode of nutritional therapy for the child who is unable to tolerate enteral alimentation. The solutions utilized are now more refined, the techniques more widely known, and the equipment more sophisticated. The delivery of TPN can become routine, but the basic guidelines must not be forgotten. First, there must be a need for TPN. The solution selected must meet the nutritional and metabolic needs of the child. Second, all aspects of the child's response to therapy must be closely monitored, and the health care team must be prepared at all times for any of the potential complications that may occur.

CONCLUSION

Critically ill children who suffer from PCM have an increased risk of morbidity and mortality. It is essential that this life-threatening complication be avoided early in the child's course of intensive care hospitalization. Awareness of the existence of PCM in the hospital setting is crucial. There must be an understanding that the general complications of critical illness are intensified in a malnourished child and, therefore, that the signs and symptoms of this must be recognized early. On admission to the ICU, critically ill children must receive a nutritional screening. Those who fall into the area of even mild malnutrition should receive vigorous support with appropriate alimentation.

Nutritional support as a separate entity is a fairly new concept to the medical community. It is clear, however, that the patient benefits from this therapy and that, as research continues, the benefits will become even greater.

REFERENCES

1. Scrimshaw et al.
2. Meakins et al.
3. Hill et al.
4. Bistrian et al.
5. Suskind. 289.
6. Cooper et al.
7. McLaren and Burman. 136.
8. Suskind. 191.
9. Waterlow.
10. Grant. 10–13.
11. Frisancho. 1974.
12. Frisancho. 1981.
13. Suskind. 293.
14. Viteri and Alverado.
15. Blackburn et al.
16. McLaren and Burman. 224.
17. MacLean et al.
18. National Academy of Sciences. 178.
19. Koga et al.
20. Feldman et al.
21. Gray.
22. Levine et al.
23. Heymsfield et al.
24. Johnson et al.
25. Dudrick et al.
26. Filston and Grant.
27. Eichelberger et al.
28. Ghadimi. 35.

BIBLIOGRAPHY

Allardyce, D. B., and A. C. Groves. 1974. A comparison of nutritional gains resulting from intravenous and enteral feedings. *Surgery, Gynecology and Obstetrics.* **139**:179–184.

American Medical Association, Department of Food and Nutrition. 1979. Guidelines for multivitamin preparation for parenteral use. A statement by the Nutrition Advisory Group. *Journal of Parenteral and Enteral Nutrition.* **3**:258–262.

American Medical Association, Department of Food and Nutrition. 1979. Guidelines for essential trace element preparations for parenteral use. A statement by an expert panel. *(JAMA) Journal of the American Medical Association.* **241**:2051–2054.

Andrassy, R. J., R. W. Feldtman, J. A. Ryan, and I. A. Ratner. 1977. Continual catheter administration of an elemental diet in infants and children. *Surgery (St. Louis).* **82**:205–210.

Andrassy, R. J., G. H. Mahour, M. R. Harrison, S. K. Muenchow, H. G. Mishalany, and M. M. Woolley. 1979. The role and safety of early postoperative feeding in the pediatric surgical patient. *Journal of Pediatric Surgery.* **14**:381–385.

Ashworth, A. 1978. Energy balance and growth: experience in treating children with malnutrition. *Kidney International.* **14**:301–305.

Bistrian, B. R., G. L. Blackburn, H. Hollwell, and R. Heddle. 1974. Protein status of the general surgical patient. *(JAMA) Journal of the American Medical Association.* **230**:858–860.

Blackburn, G. L., B. R. Bistrian, B. S. Maini, P. Benotti, A. Bothe, G. Gibbons, and M. F. Smith. 1977. Nutritional and metabolic assessment of the hospitalized patient. *Journal of Parenteral and Enteral Nutrition.* **1**:11–22.

Bode, H. H., and J. B. Warshaw, editors. 1972. Parenteral Nutrition in Infancy and Childhood. Plenum Publishing Corp., New York.

Brown, A. S., D. J. Hoelzer, and S. A. Piercy. 1979. Skin necrosis from extravasation of intravenous fluids in children. *Plastic and Reconstructive Surgery.* **64**:145–150.

Butterworth, C. E., Jr. 1974. The skeleton in the hospital closet. *Nutrition Today.* **9**:4–8.

Chernoff, R. 1980. Enteral feeding. *American Journal of Hospital Pharmacy.* **37**:65–74.

Cooper, A., D. Jakobowski, J. Spiker, T. Floyd, M. M. Ziegler, and C. E. Koop. 1981. Nutritional assessment: an integral part of the preoperative pediatric surgical evaluation. *Journal of Pediatric Surgery.* **16**(Suppl. 1):1052–1058.

Coran, A. G., R. Drongowski, T. M. Sarahan, and J. R. Westley. 1981. Comparison of a new

10% and 20% safflower oil fat emulsion in pediatric parenteral nutrition. *Journal of Parenteral and Enteral Nutrition.* **5:**236–239.

Dobbie, R. P., and O. D. Butterick. 1977. Continuous pump/tube enteric hyperalimentation — use in esophageal disease. *Journal of Parenteral and Enteral Nutrition.* **1:**100–104.

Dobbie, R. P., and J. A. Hoffmeister. 1976. Continuous pump-tube enteric hyperalimentation. *Surgery, Gynecology and Obstetrics.* **143:**273–276.

Dudrick, S. J., D. W. Wilmore, H. M. Vars, and J. E. Rhoads. 1968. Long term total parenteral nutrition with growth, development and positive nitrogen balance. *Surgery (St. Louis).* **64:**134–142.

Eichelberger, M. R., P. G. Rous, D. J. Hoelzer, V. F. Garcia, and C. E. Koop. 1981. Percutaneous subclavian venous catheters in neonates and children. *Journal of Pediatric Surgery.* **16**(Suppl. 1)**:**547–553.

Feldman. E. J., T. J. Peters, J. McNaughton, and R. H. Dowling. 1974. Adaption after small bowel resection: comparison of oral versus intravenous nutrition. *Gastroenterology.* **66:**691.

Feldtman, R. W., and R. J. Andrassy. 1978. Meeting exceptional nutritional needs— elemental enteral alimentation. *Postgraduate Medicine.* **64:**65–73.

Filler, R. M., and A. G. Coran. 1976. Total parenteral nutrition in infants and children: central and peripheral approaches. *Surgery Clinics of North America.* **56:**396–404.

Filston, H. C., and J. P. Grant. 1979. A safer system for percutaneous subclavian venous catheterization in newborn infants. *Journal of Pediatric Surgery.* **14:**564–570.

Fischer, J. E. 1976. Total Parenteral Nutrition. Little, Brown & Co., Boston.

Fletcher, A. B. 1980. Implementation of the neonatal TPN system. *In* Coran, A. G., S. E. Denson, A. B. Fletcher, and B. Bernard, editors. 1980. The Compromise Neonate. Cutter Medical, Berkeley, Calif.

Frisancho, A. R. 1974. Triceps skin fold and upper arm muscle size norms for assessment of nutritional status. *American Journal of Clinical Nutrition.* **27:**1052–1058.

Frisancho, A. R. 1981. New norms of upper limb fat and muscle areas for assessment of nutritional status. *American Journal of Clinical Nutrition* **34:**2540–2545.

Ghadimi, H. 1975. Total Parenteral Nutrition. John Wiley & Sons, Inc., New York.

Grant, A. 1979. Nutritional Assessment Guidelines. Box 25057 Northgate Station, Seattle, Wash. Second edition.

Gray, C. M. 1975. Carbohydrate digestion and absorption: role of small intestine. *New England Journal of Medicine.* **292:**1225–1230.

Greep, J. M., P. B. Soeters, R. I. C. Wesdorp, C. W. R. Phaf, and J. E. Fischer. 1977. Current Concepts in Parenteral Nutrition. Martinus Niuhoff Medical Division, The Hague, The Netherlands.

Hamill, P. V. V. 1977. National Center for Health Statistics Growth Curves for Children. Vital and Health Statistics. (Series 11.) Department of Health, Education and Welfare, Hyattsville, Md.

Hartline, J. V. 1977. Continuous intragastric infusion of elemental diet. *Clinical Pediatrics.* **16:**1105–1109.

Heymsfield, S. B., R. A. Bethel, J. D. Ansley, D. W. Nixon, and D. Rudman. 1979. Enteral hyperalimentation: an alternative to central venous hyperalimentation. *Annals of Internal Medicine.* **90:**63–71.

Hill, G. L., R. L. Blackett, I. Pickford, L. Burkinshaw, G. A. Young, C. J. Scholah, and D. B. Morgan. 1977. Malnutrition in surgical patients: and unrecognized problem. *Lancet.* **I:**689–692.

Jeejeebhoy, K. N., G. H. Anderson, I. Sanderson, and M. H. Byran. 1974. Total parenteral nutrition: nutrient needs and technical tips. *Modern Medicine of Canada.* **29:**1–10.

Johnson, L. R., E. M. Copeland, S. J. Dudrick, L. M. Lichtenberger, and G. A. Casteo. 1975. Structural and hormonal alteration in the gastrointestinal tract of parenterally fed rats. *Gastroenterology.* **69:**1177–1183.

Koga, Y., K. Ikeda, K. Inokuchi, H. Watenabe, and N. Hashimoto. 1975. The digestive tract in total parenteral nutrition. *Archives of Surgery* **110:**742–745.

Koretz, R. L., and J. H. Meyer. 1979. Elemental diets — facts and fantasies. *Gastroenterology.* **76:**394–407.

Levine, G. M., J. J. Deren, E. Steiger, and R. Zinno. 1974. Role of oral intake in maintenance of gut mass and disaccharidase activity. *Gastroenterology.* **67**:975–982.

MacLean, W. C., G. L. deRomano, E. Massa, and G. G. Graham. 1980. Nutritional management of chronic diarrhea and malnutrition: primary reliance on oral feeding. *Journal of Pediatrics.* **97**:316–323.

McLaren, D. S., and D. Burman. 1976. Textbook of Pediatric Nutrition. Churchill Livingstone, Inc., New York.

McLaren, D. S., and W. W. Read. 1975. Weight/length classification of nutritional status. *Lancet.* **I**:219–221.

Meakins, J. L., J. B. Pietsch, O. Bubenick, R. Kelly, H. Rode, J. Gordon, and L. D. MacLean. 1977. Delayed hypersensitivity: indicator of acquired failure of host defenses in sepsis and trauma. *Annals of Surgery.* **186**:241–249.

Merritt, R. J., and R. M. Suskind. 1979. Nutritional survey of hospitalized pediatric patients. *American Journal of Clinical Nutrition.* **32**:1320–1325.

Metz, G., J. Dilawari, and T. D. Kellock. 1978. Simple technique for naso-enteric feedings. *Lancet.* **II**:454.

Mitty, W. F., T. F. Nealon, and C. Grossi. 1976. Use of elemental diets in surgical cases. *American Journal of Gastroenterology.* **65**:297–304.

National Academy of Sciences. 1979. Recommended Daily Allowances. National Academy of Sciences — National Research Council, Food and Nutrition Board, Washington, D. C. Ninth edition.

O'Neill, J. A., M. D. Caldwell, and H. C. Meng. 1977. Essential fatty acid deficiency in surgical patients. *Annals of Surgery.* **185**:535–541.

Page, C. P., J. A. Ryan, and R. C. Haff. 1976. Continual catheter administration of an enteral diet. *Surgery, Gynecology and Obstetrics.* **142**:184–188.

Periera, G. R., J. DeGiacomo, M. Ziegler, K. Roth, and D. Jakobowski. 1981. Hyperalimentation — induced cholestasis. *American Journal of Diseases of Children.* **135**:824–830.

Roche, A. F. 1978. Growth assessment in abnormal children. *Kidney International.* **14**:369–377.

Ryan, J. A., R. M. Abel, W. M. Abbott, C. C. Hopkins, T. M. Chesney, R. Codley, K. Phillips, and J. E. Fischer. 1974. Catheter complications in total parenteral nutrition. *New England Journal of Medicine.* **290**:757–761.

Scrimshaw, N. S., C. E. Taylor, and J. E. Gordon. 1968. Interaction of Nutrition and Infection. Monograph Series No. 57. World Health Organization, Geneva.

Srouji, M. N., W. F. Balesteri, M. H. Caleb, M. A. South, and S. Starr. 1978. Conjugated hyperbilirubinemia in infancy associated with parenteral nutrition: skin manifestations and immune incompetence in a premature infant. *Journal of Pediatric Surgery.* **13**:570–575.

Suskind, R. M., editor. 1981. Textbook of Pediatric Nutrition. Raven Press, New York.

Torosian, M. H., and J. L. Rombeau. 1980. Feeding by tube enterostomy. *Surgery, Gynecology and Obstetrics.* **150**:918–927.

Vaughan, V. C., and R. J. McKay editors. 1979. Nelson's Textbook of Pediatrics. W. B. Saunders Co., Philadelphia. Eleventh edition.

Viteri, F. E., and J. Alverado. 1970. The creatinine height index: its uses in the estimation of the degree of protein depletion and repletion in protein calorie malnutrition. *Pediatrics* **46**:696–706.

Waterlow, J. 1974. Some aspects of childhood malnutrition as a public health problem. *British Medical Journal.* **4**:88–90.

Wilmore, D. W., and S. J. Dudrick. 1968. Growth and development of an infant receiving all nutrients exclusively by vein. *(JAMA) Journal of the American Medical Association.* **203**:860–864.

Winick, M. 1976. Malnutrition and Brain Development. Oxford University Press, New York.

Ziegler, M., D. Jakobowski, D. Hoelzer, M. Eichelberger, and C. E. Koop. 1980. Route of pediatric parenteral nutrition: proposed criteria revision. *Journal of Pediatric Surgery.* **15**:472–476.

CHAPTER **9**

TAKING CARE OF
THE CRITICAL CARE
GIVER

Janis Bloedel Smith

A number of factors in the pediatric intensive care unit (ICU) make its milieu stressful for the individuals who work there: the physical, social, and psychological environment of the ICU; the demands of the physical and emotional care required by children and parents; and other factors related to the level of expertise and knowledge required of the personnel who care for those who are critically ill.

Hans Selye, the noted stress researcher, has pointed out that stress is not necessarily a response to a negative experience. He calls stress "the spice of life" and notes that joy and other positive emotions can also trigger stress.[1] However, the continued, relentless stress of working in a critical care environment often results in a compromising of the clinician's ability to cope positively. Difficulty in coping further compromises the reactions of ICU personnel to their stressors. The result can be alarming not only for the individual concerned, but also for those professionals who are concerned both with the quality of intensive care provided and with the individuals who are the providers.

The purpose of this final chapter is to identify the characteristics that critical care clinicians often share, the stressors inherent in the pediatric ICU, and the common reactions of individuals to those stressors. In addition, based on the data identified, techniques will be presented that will enable the ICU clinician to cope successfully with the stressors inherent in providing intensive care.

CHARACTERISTICS OF THE
ICU CLINICIAN

The ideal ICU nurse has been humorously sketched by an unknown artist (Fig. 9-1). In large part, the humor in this sketch lies in its aptness: individuals who work in critical care settings are often expected to behave like robots with computerized innards. However, the real characteristics shared by many ICU clinicians are undoubtedly responsible for at least some of the stress experienced by these individuals.

Expectations of Self

Not only is the ICU clinician expected to perform perfectly by others, but perfection is often the ego ideal of the individual as well. Though perhaps not a con-

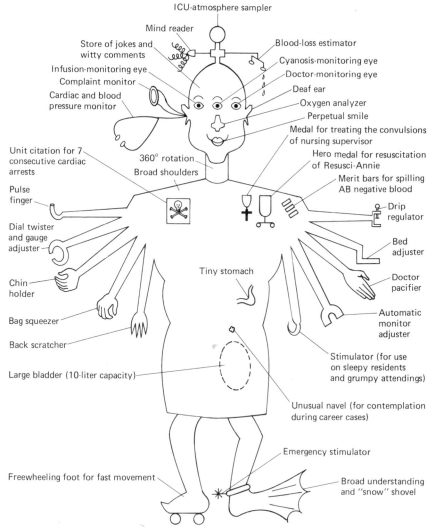

Figure 9-1. The "ideal" ICU nurse (artist unknown).

scious ideal, the concept of perfection may create difficulty for the ICU staff member. People who choose to work in a critical care setting are generally very careful about their work and pay great attention to detail in order to be certain that they are doing their job as well as possible. This characteristic is of obvious benefit to patients because the safe margin for error in the care of the critically ill infant or child is uniquely narrow. On the other hand, as important and valuable as this characteristic is, it can be the source of unreasonable expectations — both by others and by the individual clinicians themselves.

Unreasonable expectations of perfection place the ICU clinician at risk for severe insults to self-esteem in the critical care setting. Errors are made by all human beings, and, in addition, the clinical course of any critically ill child can deteriorate and end in the child's death even when no errors have been made. The clinician who holds an unconscious ideal of perfection can be extremely stressed by deaths in the ICU, feeling an unreasonable and unrealistic responsibility.

Omnipotence

Feelings of responsibility for events that are beyond the control of any human being are likely to be related to feelings of omnipotence. A feeling of omnipotence has been identified as a characteristic of many health care professionals, but it is heightened in the ICU, which is often regarded as the "epitome of modern medical technology".[2] In the pediatric ICU, feelings of omnipotence may be further exaggerated because the patients are "helpless," dependent children and the caregiver can function in the role of "super parent."[3] The greater the clinician's feelings of omnipotence (or unconscious wishes for it), the more vulnerable that individual will be to feelings of personal failure when confronted with the inevitable imperfection of all human beings.

Despite the negative concerns related to omnipotence, it too serves a positive purpose in the critical care setting. Feelings of omnipotence may prevent the ICU staff from becoming overwhelmed by some particularly disastrous accident or other patient situation. Such feelings may also help ICU clinicians to persist in the care of patients for whom the outlook is extremely negative. They have a conscious or unconscious belief in their ability to "work a miracle," returning a child to health despite the gravest prognosis.[2]

Rescue Fantasy

In addition to their unconscious feelings of omnipotence, ICU clinicians, like health professionals in other areas of practice, have the need to "save" lives.[2,4,5] This feeling can be particularly problematic in the critical care setting because the technical means to sustain life are advanced, and physiological functioning can be maintained despite absence of cerebral activity.

Technological Concerns

Because of the high level of technical intervention and the sometimes limited capacity for personal communication with the critically ill patient, ICU clinicians are often oriented toward technological concerns and measurements.[6] In some instances, clinicians may concentrate on various determinations of a child's physiological status (i.e., blood gases, pulmonary artery pressures, cardiac output calculations, etc.) in order to defend against or deny the child's, family's, and their own personal experience of serious illness, pain, and death. Because such behavior permits the individual clinician to maintain functioning despite the stresses inherent in the ICU environment, some purpose may be served by this characteristic. On the other hand, all the individuals involved are deprived of the opportunity for open, honest discourse with regard to their feelings in such circumstances, and the probable result is a disservice to all.

STRESSORS IN THE ICU

The critical care milieu contains a number of factors that contribute to the stress experienced by ICU clinicians. These factors include the physical, social, and psychological aspects of working in an ICU.

Physical Environment

ICUs are generally open, compact units in which many patient beds are visible from a single, central location. Often, each bed can be screened off by curtains, but privacy is often precluded by the urgency of the care being provided. Electronic monitoring equipment abounds, as do intravenous infusion pumps, ventilators, and other pieces of complex equipment. Although an effort is made to dim the lights during the night hours, the ICU is certainly never dark; and the noise from the equipment and the equipment alarm systems persists for 24 hours a day.

There is a continuous traffic of people through the ICU. Physicians and nurses tend to the ongoing needs of their patients, while respiratory therapists, physical therapists, social workers, x-ray technicians, laboratory technicians, intravenous therapists, consultants, housekeepers, and others move in and out of the area. The activity is constant, slowing down slightly at times for some patients who are not as ill as others, but continuing day and night at a fast pace for those whose condition is critical or unstable. The families of seriously ill children add to the number of bodies and to the noise level in the environment.

The physical environment of the ICU often seems highly unsuitable for logical thought or functioning. Fortunately, ICU clinicians are accustomed to the frantic pace and do function; however, two aspects of the effect of the ICU environment on those who work within it are as yet unclear. First, would functioning be improved in an environment that is less distracting? Second, at what price do ICU clinicians maintain functioning despite the chaotic activity surrounding them? ICU patients may experience sensory overload (also referred to as environmental overdose), as well as emotional-touch deprivation in response to the physical environment that surrounds them. Confusion, withdrawal, and hostility may result. To date, studies that clarify the human response to environment have not been extended to include the personnel who work in the same ICU environment. Despite the lack of research in this area, ICU clinicians must become aware of how their environment impacts on them as individuals. It is obvious that removing oneself from the environment to a quiet area for a break or a meal needs to be considered a priority in maintaining quality patient care.

Social Environment

The social organization within an ICU resembles that of a family system — the medical director as "father," head nurse as "mother," and nursing and house staff as "children."[7–9] Although the social environment can provide valuable support for the ICU clinician in the form of work relationships that extend out of the hospital to social events and living arrangements, no social interaction is ever completely satisfactory and free of conflict. The head nurse and staff nurses may come into conflict over areas of control, with the head nurse being so overcontrolling as to prevent staff nurses from developing the ability to function autonomously. Or the head nurse may exercise so little authority that work performance suffers for lack of concerned leadership. Conflict may occur between staff nurses because of competition for advancement within the unit or because of differing philosophies of care.

Differences between the extremely idealistic beginning nurse and the seasoned, experienced nurse may also result in conflict. Often, the experienced nurse is too discouraged or too disillusioned to support the idealism of the younger professional, and what could be an extremely positive force for all concerned becomes instead a negative force that contributes significantly to conflict between nurses.

Conflict between nurses and physicians is often more obvious and more pronounced than that between nurses. Some studies have indicated that conflict with physicians is among the chief sources of stress for ICU nurses.[10,11] Conflict may occur over issues related to the care and treatment of patients or because of the difference between medical and nursing goals. Doctor-nurse conflicts generally involve one of two situations: (1) doctors encroaching on what nurses perceive as their jurisdiction, and/or the reverse, or (2) physicians shifting their responsibility onto nurses.[12] Often, nurses feel as if they have not been provided with complete information about the plan of care for a patient, yet are expected to carry out the physician's orders. Nurses are too often not included in the decision-making process with regard to patient care and/or ICU policy and procedure. This can be especially problematic for the experienced nurse with years of background in critical care. Experienced nurses may also come into conflict with house staff who have less specifically relevant ICU background.

An area of many nurse-physician conflicts that is, as yet, unresolved is based on the larger female-male conflicts in our society. It is a well documented fact that in American society in general, it is men who have power—politically and economically. Within the hospital setting, 91 percent of all physicians (and 56 percent of all hospital administrators) are males and more than 98 percent of all nurses are female.[13] Although the majority of professionals in the health care industry are female and nurses, the work that nurses do is not valued as much as that of physicians. Nurses are not considered equal partners of the doctors and administrators who are managing the health care institutions.

Conflict between female physicians or female administrators and nurses can sometimes be characterized by the Queen Bee Syndrome.[13] These individuals have achieved a great deal of status and prefer to identify up, often to men; rather than with other women, especially with other nurses. Conflict of this nature has an element of destructive and devisive competition, rather than respect for others.

Conflict with the families of children being cared for in the ICU is less common than nurse-nurse or nurse-physician conflict, but it too does occur and can be a source of stress for ICU clinicians. Even when clinicians acknowledge the extreme importance of parents to the seriously ill child and claim to understand the tremendous anxiety experienced by these individuals, defensiveness can arise in conversations when parents ask for repeated explanations or when they appear to be criticizing the care that their child is receiving. Nurses may be audience to, or the object of, more family criticism than are physicians because nurses spend the greatest amount of time with the critically ill child and the child's family and because they include in their role a great deal of family teaching. As a result, parents are often more comfortable with their child's nurse than with the physician, and they may be able to express their concerns and/or negative feelings more openly to the nurse than to the physician. (They have also observed and understood more of the nurse's practice than the physician's). Despite these possible reasons for it, criticism from or conflict with a family member can result in severe stress if the ICU clinician experiences anger, guilt, and feelings of inferiority.[14]

Conflict with parents may cause stress for ICU clinicians when parents must be told that a poor outcome for their child is likely and they react with disbelief or animosity. Parents may seem not to understand or even to be totally unrealistic when told that their child's chances for recovery are very poor.[15] Parents may view nurses and physicians with suspicion, as if they could effect a cure if they really wanted to, but are not doing all that could be done. Even when ICU clinicians recognize that denial on the part of parents may be an extremely important coping mechanism, they may react with guilt and anger to these obviously stressful interactions with parents.

Because of the stressors in the physical environment and the sources of conflict within the social environment of the ICU, critical care clinicians often feel a lack of support from those they work with. They either lack the opportunity to talk about problems on the unit and to share experiences and feelings,[10] or they may perceive the ICU environment as one that prohibits the expression of feelings.[6] In either case, stress is increased.

Work Load

The pace in the ICU varies from frantic and chaotic to so slow and boring that it may result in the temporary assignment of the ICU clinician to another unit. "Floating" to another unit is a frequently identified source of stress for nurses. So, too, are the problems of inadequate staffing, which result in insufficient time to complete all tasks and to provide emotional support to children and families. Nurses especially resent feeling uncertain about the safety of patients in the unit when staffing is short and being nevertheless required to perform nonnursing tasks, such as clerical work, at such a time.

In addition, because of the 24-hour-a-day, 7-day-a-week nature of critical care, the ICU clinician is required to work on weekends, holidays, and during the evening and night hours. Shift rotation can be disruptive of normal biorhythms, whereas weekend and holiday work can disrupt family and social life.

Fear and Anxiety

ICU clinicians are expected to perform at a high level of competency in a variety of complex situations. Less experienced clinicians often report a great deal of stress related to anxiety about their knowledge and/or skills. They may be uncertain about the operation and function of specialized equipment, or they may fear making an error during patient care. During a medical emergency, less experienced clinicians are understandably anxious if a senior staff person is not present. They may feel that they lack the knowledge, experience, or judgment needed to make the astute observations or draw the necessary conclusions with regard to the status of the critically ill child. Finally, they may be uncomfortable about providing children or their families with information and/or emotional support.

Anxiety may also be the result of the inevitable conflicts that occur within the social environment of the ICU. The educational programs that prepare nurses and doctors do little to socialize students of either profession in the skills necessary to deal constructively with conflict. These skills are not inherent; they require formal and specific teaching if they are to be learned and consistent reinforcement if they are to be maintained.

Continued experience in the ICU may assist the clinician in conquering some of the fear and anxiety reported by less experienced individuals. Successfully caring for a variety of critically ill children reassures the clinician that the necessary knowledge and skills are obtainable. This can also be demonstrated by experienced clinicians who are persuaded to continue to practice "bedside nursing," if these individuals are able to demonstrate their skills respectfully and assist the less experienced nurse in obtaining them. In addition, these well-prepared individuals possess the knowledge and skills needed by ICU patients and their families. Finally, experienced ICU clinicians are likely to have methods for dealing constructively with interpersonal conflict.

Patient Care

Caring for critically ill children and their parents is stressful in itself, even without the variety of other stressors in the critical care setting. Being witness to the pain and suffering of a small child or to the sadness of parents who realize that the aspirations they have held for their child will never materialize can fill the clinician with unhappiness. This can be especially difficult when the clinician must continue to carry out invasive or painful procedures. Unreasonable guilt can result, and individuals may also feel angry in a vague, rather undirected way at whatever or whoever is responsible for illness and suffering in children. At times, this anger may be directed specifically at a person who, for one reason or another, is deemed responsible.

ICU clinicians also witness a greater number of deaths than health professionals in other settings. Death in infancy or childhood is difficult for many to justify or accept and is often considered "unfair." The inability to protect children from the harsh realities of death may result in extreme feelings of helplessness and worthlessness in the ICU clinician. The simultaneous responsibility of providing support to the family adds to the stress of these difficult situations. Clinicians may feel inadequately prepared to deal with the emotional needs of dying children and their families. Special skills are required because death can cause the family to experience extreme stress as the result of feelings of failure, guilt, frustration, and depression.

These issues of providing critical care to seriously ill children and their families are complicated by factors in the social and physical environment of the ICU that limit or prohibit opportunities for staff members to share their feelings about the events in which they participate. The ability to provide life-saving technical care is often not accompanied by discourse dealing with the emotional and ethical considerations that result from technological advances.

REACTIONS TO STRESS

The ICU clinician responds in a number of ways to the daily situational stress that characterizes the pediatric critical care setting. The following discussion of "typical" reactions does not necessarily apply in its entirety, to each individual because individual reactions are determined by the interaction between certain characteristics of the stressor and aspects of each ICU clinician's personality.

Inappropriate Attachment

ICU clinicians who care for infants and children have been described as assuming the role of their patients' "surrogate mothers and fathers."[3] When children are removed from their natural family setting by serious illness or accident, they move into the ICU "family" constellation. The physician may unconsciously assume a paternal role, while the nurse assumes a maternal one. Nurses can often be observed playing their assumed role of mother when they speak of "my baby" and defend their patient against all others. Physicians may not appear to be as attached to the children they care for and may, in fact, deny the individuality of the child,[3,6] but their paternal attachment nonetheless exists.

The motives for this inappropriate attachment are complex and varied. They are generally thought to relate to the ICU clinicians' expectations of themselves for perfection and to their unconscious feelings of omnipotence. Nurses and physicians thus assume the responsibility and the power of the child's natural parents.

The establishment of attachments between caregivers and their patients is not pathological in itself; the attachments become pathological or inappropriate when the child's natural parents are excluded from the interaction or when the caregiver becomes so attached to a particular child as to lose competency and objectivity.

Technological Orientation

Some ICU clinicians respond to the stress inherent in the critical care environment by increasing their attention to the technical details of patient care and by excluding any thought of the child or family for whom the care is provided. Such behavior may persist even in the face of an undeniably grave prognosis: diagnostic studies, procedures, and attempts at treatment continue until the time of the child's death. Conflict can result between ICU clinicians because some individuals view this behavior as a responsible attempt to try whatever might be successful, whereas others feel that the dignity of the child and the family is denied by such actions.

The motivation for extreme emphasis on technical data and details is likely to be denial. By concentrating all efforts on technical skills, knowledge, and data, the ICU clinician is able to deny the humanity of the child on whom the procedures are performed. The behavior of the child or family is rarely mentioned, except when either interferes with the solving of technical problems. In a similar way, ICU clinicians deny their own humanity by means of this technological orientation. Intellectualization is a second defense mechanism that is likely to be operational in this type of behavior.

A healthy use of defense mechanisms such as denial and intellectualization is undoubtedly necessary: ICU clinicians must get their work done in an area in which attention to detail may make the difference between recovery and tragedy. Nevertheless, an extreme technological orientation leads to depersonalization of the critically ill child, the family, and the caregivers, which can only result in greater stress for all concerned.

Humor

The use of humor is another way in which individuals may react to the stresses of providing critical care. The movie and television series $M*A*S*H$ illustrates how humor is employed in order to defend against the unacceptable tragedy of war. In the ICU, this kind of humor is used as a way of managing overwhelming situations. It is often employed when ICU clinicians must make a decision regarding the termination of life support.[6] It is also frequently apparent when the pace of work in the critical care unit becomes particularly chaotic or more demanding than what can be managed by the number of clinicians who are present.

The use of humor provides emotional relief and is motivated by the ego's sense of being overwhelmed. It is a form of denial of the reality of a situation — a necessary one in situations in which continued functioning at a high level is demanded. What can be laughed at is less overwhelming and, consequently, more manageable.

In other situations, humor can be risky. The persistent denial of human feelings related to death or frustration does not serve a purpose, but perpetuates the stress associated with providing critical care. In addition, there is always the risk that the "funny" remark or incident related by one ICU clinician to another will be overheard by someone, such as a parent, who cannot possibly see or appreciate the "humor" in the situation, but is instead seriously offended. Such an occurrence could seriously interfere with the process of providing critical care.

Guilt

ICU clinicians often respond to the deterioration in a child's condition or to a child's death with feelings other than sadness. Guilt is the most common reaction. The ICU staff may hold itself responsible for a patient's death, much as the child's parents may blame themselves. Guilty feelings are, of course, accentuated if some technical error or an error in judgment is in any way associated with a patient's death or increased morbidity. Obviously, errors must be corrected and held to a minimum. But it is pertinent to ask whether the critical care staff expects itself to function without errors and whether this level of functioning is humanly possible. When no error is involved, ICU clinicians may still feel guilty when patients do not recover. Guilt is often intensified when clinicians have been called on to perform repeated painful or invasive procedures that they cannot justify when the child dies.

Guilty feelings are undoubtedly related to the expectations of perfection that are held by many ICU clinicians. In cases in which there has been no human error, the guilt may be motivated by a violation of the clinician's unconscious feelings of omnipotence. The members of the ICU staff may feel that they have failed the child, the family, and themselves.

Depression

Depression is a common reaction because of the frequency with which ICU clinicians deal with pain, suffering, and death. Depression is characterized by low spirits, decreased self-esteem, self-depreciation, somatic complaints such as fatigue and appetite disturbances, feelings of guilt and inadequacy, and difficulty in maintaining concentration. The depressed individual also usually withdraws from contact with others. The ICU clinician who is depressed may withdraw from other staff members and may experience difficulties in relationships with family or friends. Gradually, pervasive feelings of apathy and hopelessness can be detected in the entire staff of a closely knit ICU.

Depression, along with the withdrawal and apathy that characterize it, is most often a response to a series of deaths or serious complications in the ICU. In essence, the ICU clinicians have experienced a series of attachments and losses that causes them to defend against the repeated pain by withdrawing from emotional contact with others.[2]

Depression is obviously unpleasant for the individual involved, but can also affect the provision of critical care in a number of ways. Because depression makes concentration difficult, the depressed ICU clinician may be subject to making a greater number of errors by either omission or commission. In addition, the pessimistic outlook of depressed individuals may cause the ICU staff to regard some patients as "beyond hope." Such predictions of failure are related to the clinicians' feelings of worthlessness, but can become self-fulfilling prophecies. Finally, as the depressed individual withdraws from emotional contact with the children and families who are being cared for, the vital "human-to-human" aspect of critical care is lost, and patient care deteriorates immeasurably.

COPING

It is impossible to remove all the stressors inherent in critical care practice or to alter completely the typical reactions that ICU clinicians demonstrate in response to these stressors. (Indeed, because these reactions are defense mechanisms, total change may not be desirable.) Nevertheless, stressors and reactions can be mediated so as to improve staff performance and personal satisfaction. This process involves the active seeking of techniques that promote positive coping with the stressors instead of mere reaction to them. Positive coping can result in improved care of children and their families and in decreased stress for the provider of critical care.

Administrative Techniques

A variety of administrative techniques may lessen the stress of providing critical care. For example, staff members who work 10- or 12-hour shifts rather than the traditional 8 hours can have long weekends away from the stress of the ICU. Rotating the assignment of especially difficult children among staff members may prevent unmanageable stress from building up in one or two individuals. The rotation of shifts should be limited as much as possible. Adequate staffing to permit coffee breaks and dinner away from the ICU is a necessity. This temporary withdrawal to a different environment permits the ICU clinician to conserve and/or restore emotional energy. Adequate staffing is also necessary in order to avoid feelings of inadequacy in meeting the needs of patient care. In addition, avoiding the practice of "floating" the ICU clinician to other units when there is a decreased work load in the critical care setting demonstrates concern for the clinician as an individual.

Undoubtedly, in order for any administrative technique to be successful at reducing the stress experienced by ICU clinicians, good communication between nursing staff and nursing administration is a prerequisite. Staff must clearly articulate its concerns to administration, share the responsibility to investigate areas of practice that are stressful, and develop techniques to reduce stress. For example, nurses in an ICU often identify "floating" as a crucial issue in job satisfaction. Staff might decide to identify for administration the advantages of not removing nurses from the ICU during slow periods by developing unit projects that are worked on when the demands of patient care are reduced. Preparing information for the parents of infants and children who require critical care in the form of pamphlets is an example of one such project. In addition to demonstrating concern for patient care to administration in a concrete manner, unit projects also serve to increase staff satisfaction with their roles.

An administrative technique that can clearly reduce stress and promote coping among ICU clinicians is the provision of a comprehensive orientation program for nurses beginning work in the ICU. An ongoing preceptorship with an experienced ICU nurse is a critical aspect of a thorough orientation program. Identification of a preceptor provides the new ICU nurse with an individual who can be relied on for support and assistance and may ease the transition period experienced by newcomers. In addition, the recognition awarded the preceptors may be an incentive that serves to keep these more experienced nurses at the bedside.

Self-Awareness

The first step in coping positively with the stress of providing critical care is an internal one. ICU clinicians need to reflect on their reasons for having selected the critical care setting for their practice. Often, individuals who choose to work in an ICU enjoy a fast-paced existence and thrive on tension and excitement. A quieter pace might cause greater stress in these people than does the typically rapid tempo of the ICU. Nevertheless, ICU clinicians also need to become aware of those expectations of self (e.g., perfection and omnipotence) that are motivators of many individuals who provide critical care.

Because of individual reactions to stress, ICU clinicians need to become aware of (1) their personal manifestations of stress and (2) what kinds of situations activate their stress responses. Stress produces physiological and psychological responses that can be identified by individuals who learn to attend to their bodies and examine their feelings. An awareness of individual stress responses permits the ICU clinician to gauge how others react to the same or different stressors. It is also a prerequisite to discovering techniques that alleviate stress.

Self-awareness limits the extent to which individuals can use denial as a defense against stress. Although it is often helpful in short-term situations, denial can become persistent, thereby interfering with personal and professional development and with the care of critically ill children and their families.

Stress results in the production of excessive amounts of physical and psychic energy that must be reduced in order for the symptoms of stress to be relieved. Relaxation techniques are routines that provide an approach to drain tension. Some of these techniques, such as autogenic training or simply deep breathing or neck and shoulder rotation, can be used to relieve stress during work in the ICU. Other techniques, including transcendental meditation and progressive relaxation, require greater concentration, a quiet environment, and regular practice. Certain individuals prefer an active alternative (e.g., jogging or swimming) to the internal tension associated with stress. Once again, self-awareness assists each individual in identifying a routine that permits decompression from the stresses of providing critical care.

Positive Outlook

Stress is usually regarded as a negative experience, as is the social or psychological conflict that is often the source of stress in the ICU. However, the ICU clinician should realize that there is nothing inherently "bad" about either stress or conflict. Conflict, which can actually be useful, is inevitable wherever people work together. Stress can be anticipated as a challenge rather than regarded as a threat. From this perspective, it is possible for the ICU clinician to consider a variety of options in dealing positively with either stress or conflict.

Increasing Group Cohesiveness

The opportunity for all members of the ICU staff to meet together regularly provides a forum for the exchange of feelings and ideas and enhances group cohesiveness. Often, at the start of such meetings, staff members are hesitant about sharing their feelings. One possible way of overcoming this initial barrier is to have group meetings led by a psychiatric nurse or a psychiatrist who is familiar with ICU routines, personnel, and patients and who is skilled at eliciting feelings, reflecting them, and providing emotional support. Individual ICU clinicians can thus examine their expectations of themselves, testing the appropriateness of these expectations by comparing them with those of others who have a similar background. Expectations of perfection and omnipotence are often more obvious in a group than in an individual. These expectations can be dealt with by a realistic evaluation of the goals of critical care (in the abstract or for a specific child). Thus, the unrealistic goals of perfection and omnipotence are prevented from damaging the professional self-esteem of the group or the individual.

Other feelings such as guilt, frustration, anger, and sadness can be explored by ICU clinicians through group process. Guilty feelings can often be identified as inappropriate manifestations of omnipotent fantasies by staff members who have not been closely involved in a particular situation. The pain and sadness of repeated attachments and losses can be shared and supported. Inappropriate attachment can be identified. Feelings of anxiety or anger can be examined and may change as their source is understood. The ethical dilemmas that have resulted from our ever-increasing technological ability can be discussed and analyzed with the view of discovering more satisfying solutions to these problems.

In short, group meetings led by an individual who is able to accurately identify important psychological issues among ICU staff members can provide an atmosphere in which both thinking and feeling states can be considered and modified. Self-awareness is likely to increase as the result of such meetings because ICU clinicians are thereby afforded an opportunity for freely expressing troublesome feelings and for gaining greater insight into the source and nature of such feelings. All individuals should be able to receive any extra support that may be needed in order to continue functioning effectively both in the critical care setting and in personal life away from the hospital.

Dealing with Conflict

Conflict between ICU clinicians is a prevalent source of stress that must be dealt with effectively in order to achieve positive coping. As noted above, the first step toward dealing with conflict is to regard it from a positive outlook and to realize that it can be productive: conflict can encourage problem solving, reduce tension, and prevent suppression of feelings and subsequent withdrawal from others.

Effective confrontation is the key to successful resolution of interpersonal conflict.[16] Because conflict cannot be suppressed, differences of opinion, interests, or values must be dealt with openly. Conflict can then be resolved by using problem-solving strategies and communication skills.

Problem-solving strategies define conflict as a mutual problem and encourage individuals who are in conflict to pursue common goals or to find a solution that is mutually acceptable. Differences in individual power are minimized by emphasizing (1) mutual interdependence and (2) an understanding of the other person's feelings or position as being equally plausible. It is also helpful to clarify the issues and all the possible positions around them. Threats are avoided, but hostility is expressed in order to eliminate feelings that might interfere with cooperation, not in order to overwhelm or attack the other person.

Effective problem solving demands open, honest, and accurate communication that leads to effective confrontation. Assertiveness skills can assist the individual to express feelings clearly and directly in a nondefensive yet nonthreatening way. It is important for individuals to use personal statements (e.g., "I think" and "I feel") to reflect what they think or feel, so that misunderstanding can be avoided. Similarly, it is important to clarify the perception that one individual has of the other's feelings, thoughts, or motives. Because behavior is always subject to more than one interpretation, perceptions of the behavior of others must be verified. Communication skills also include listening actively to what another person says and responding in a way that demonstrates understanding.

Problem-solving strategies that are based on open, honest, and accurate communication can promote resolution of conflicts, greater understanding, and closer relationships. Mutual dislike and rejection are not the necessary outcomes of conflict, but can be avoided by effective confrontation and problem solving. Furthermore, the provision of quality critical care is dependent on being able to deal with conflict in a positive way.

Preparation for Providing Critical Care

Preparation for work in a critical care setting may be effective psychoprophylaxis for several reasons. First, educational and practical preparation in the knowledge and skills required of the ICU clinician will eliminate some of the anxiety and stress that may be associated with feeling inadequately equipped to deal with the complex needs of critically ill children. Obviously, no one can learn all that is needed in every situation without actually having experience in the critical care setting. However, it is absolutely necessary that sufficient support be made available for each ICU clinician in order to ensure that no one experiences the anxiety of not being able to adequately care for a child.

In addition to practical preparation in ICU knowledge and skills, the ICU clinician requires preparation in a number of other areas. For example, the bureaucratic procedures that must be followed after the death of a child can be overwhelmingly stressful if they are inadequately understood. Providing support to a child and family through the process of critical illness and assisting the family to grieve, should their child die, require great sensitivity as well as knowledge and skills in psychological processes. These skills can be taught so that the necessary sensitivity can develop in continued helping relationships.

Finally, ICU clinicians should be prepared for the stresses, reactions, and feelings that they are likely to experience as providers of critical care. During the selection and orientation of ICU personnel, staff might be asked to identify factors that they realize are stressful to them and identify the mechanisms that they use to cope with stress. Continued open communication about the stresses encountered in providing intensive care, including feelings of failure or overwhelming sadness, facilitates coping positively with such stressors. As a result, ICU clinicians are helped to provide better care to critically ill children and their families.

REFERENCES

1. Selye. 5.
2. Eisendrath and Dunkel.
3. Kachoris.
4. Cassem.
5. Michaels.
6. Frader.
7. Eisendrath and Dunkel.
8. Kachoris.

9. Gardner et al.
10. Gray-Toft and Anderson.
11. Huckabay and Jagla.
12. Jacobsen.
13. Spengler.
14. Goodell.
15. Waller et al.
16. Nichols.

BIBLIOGRAPHY

Cassem, N. H., and T. P. Hackett. 1975. Stress in the nurse and therapist in the intensive care unit and the coronary care unit. *Heart & Lung.* **4:**252–257.

Eisendrath, S. J., and J. Dunkel. 1979. Psychological issues in intensive care unit staff. *Heart & Lung.* **8:**751–758.

Frader, J. E. 1979. Difficulties in providing intensive care. *Pediatrics.* **64:**10–16.

Gardner, D., Z. D. Parzen, and N. Stewart. 1980. The nurse's dilemma: mediating stress in critical care units. *Heart & Lung.* **9:**103–106.

Goodell, A. S. 1980. Responses of nurses to the stresses of caring for pediatric oncology patients. *Issues in Comprehensive Pediatric Nursing.* **4:**1–6.

Gray-Toft, P., and J. G. Anderson. 1981. The nursing stress scale: development of an instrument. *Journal of Behavioral Assessment.* **3:**11–23.

Huckabay, L. M. D., and B. Jagla. 1979. Nurses' stress factors in the intensive care unit. *Journal of Nursing Administration.* **9:**21–26.

Jacobsen, S. P. 1978. Stressful situations for neonatal intensive care nurses. (MCN) *American Journal of Maternal Child Nursing.* **3:**144–152.

Kachoris, P. J. 1977. Psychodynamic considerations in the neonatal ICU. *Critical Care Medicine.* **5:**62–65.

Michaels, D. R. 1971. Too much in need of support to give any? *American Journal of Nursing.* **71:**1932–1933.

Nichols, B. 1979. Dealing with conflict. *The Journal of Continuing Education in Nursing.* **10:**24–27.

Oskins, S. L. 1979. Identification of situational stressors and coping methods by intensive care nurses. *Heart & Lung.* **8:**953–960.

Scully, R. 1980. Stress in the nurse. *American Journal of Nursing.* **80:**912–915.

Selye, H. 1975. Stress Without Distress. New American Library, Inc. (a Signet Book), New York.

Spengler, C. D. 1978. The challenge of caring. Paper presented at the Third National Pediatric Nursing Conference. University of Pennsylvania School of Nursing, Philadelphia. April 12–14, 1978.

Surveyor, J. A. 1976. The emotional toll on nurses who care for comatose children. *(MCN) American Journal of Maternal Child Nursing.* **1:**243–248.

Waller, D. A., D. Todres, N. H. Cassem, and A. Anderlen. 1979. Coping with poor prognosis in the pediatric intensive care unit. *American Journal of Diseases of Children.* **133:**1121–1125.

INDEX

537